Management of Abdominal Hernias

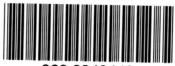

369 0246443

This book is due for return on or before the last date shown below.

Andrew N. Kingsnorth • Karl A. LeBlanc

Editors

Management of Abdominal Hernias

Fourth Edition

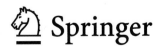 Springer

Editors
Andrew N. Kingsnorth
Department of Surgery
Peninsula College of Medicine & Dentistry
Plymouth, Devon, UK

Karl A. LeBlanc
Surgeons Group of Baton Rouge/
Our Lady of the Lake Physician Group
Baton Rouge, LA, USA

ISBN 978-1-84882-876-6   ISBN 978-1-84882-877-3 (eBook)
DOI 10.1007/978-1-84882-877-3
Springer London Heidelberg New York Dordrecht

Library of Congress Control Number: 2012953269

Preface

The literature in hernia surgery is vast, and keeping abreast of developments is a never-ending task that one or two individuals may find difficult to fit into their daily routine. With this in mind, for the fourth edition of this book, we have recruited selected experts to write each chapter, so that a ray of discerning knowledge is beamed into each crevice of the hernia story to create a comprehensive and authoritative text.

A detailed description of the anatomy of the abdominal wall is of utmost importance and a primary concern for planning all hernia operations. Recent technical developments will influence our decision making now and in the future. More training is needed to increase awareness of the large number of prosthetic meshes, innovative plastic procedures, and the appropriate use of biologic meshes. Each requires a thorough knowledge of the literature and outcomes research rather than the mere use of a technique or product because it is new and "seems like a good idea."

The long-term outcomes of our patients are now an area of important consideration and can no longer be overlooked in the discussion of consent prior to surgery. This discussion includes the issue of postoperative pain, quality of life, recurrence rates, and cosmesis.

Hernia science is a relatively new specialty, and its future will be defined by the introduction of "physiologic" repairs and the prosthetic meshes used. Biologic products may be used for tissue replacement, for tissue reinforcement, or simply as a "bridge" to synthetic materials that will perform as good as or better than the biologic materials.

This text strives to introduce these concepts and to educate readers about the current state of the art in hernia surgery and to prepare them for future considerations of which we should all be aware at this point.

Plymouth, UK   AN. Kingsnorth
LA, USA   K. LeBlanc

Preface to the Third Edition

The first edition of this book was a monograph written by the late H. Brendan Devlin and was a landmark in the scientific analysis of surgery of the abdominal wall, which discarded many of the older out-of-date concepts. We are heavily indebted to Brendan not only for providing the basis for this text but also for the inspiration to follow along a line of inquiry for evidence-based material to present to our readers. At the same time we have not neglected the important historical and economic aspects of hernia surgery and some of our own personal views. Andrew Kingsnorth assisted Brendan in writing the second edition of this book, and Karl Le Blanc now adds an entirely new perspective from North America with particular emphasis on the use of prosthetic materials and laparoscopic techniques.

We have thoroughly revised and added to all the chapters resulting in an increase in material of approximately 50% and the addition of hundreds more up-to-date references. We have also provided the reader with clear line drawings of operative techniques, photographs, and several short video clips on CD-ROM. This extra effort should allow the reader the ability to adopt and apply much of the information and operative techniques that are presented. The technological revolution that began a decade ago and still continues to evolve has therefore been fully recognized in this text which we believe will appeal to surgeons in training and those already experienced in managing abdominal wall hernias. It is hoped that this work will be an effective reference to all those that possess this book.

Contents

Contributors

Brent W. Allain Jr. Surgeons Group of Baton Rouge/Our Lady of the Lake Physician Group, Baton Rouge, LA, USA

Morten Bay-Nielsen Department of Gastroenterology, Surgical Section, Hvidovre University Hospital, Hvidovre, Denmark

Igor Belyansky Surgical Specialist at Anne Arundel Anne Arundel Medical Center Health Sciences Pavilion, Suite 600

David H. Bennett Department of Surgery, Royal Bournemouth Hospital, Dorset, UK

Dieter Berger Department of General Surgery, Stadtklinik, Baden-Baden, Germany

Valentina Bertocchi Surgical Department - Università Insibria, Ospedale di Circolo di Varese, Varese, Italy

L. Michael Brunt Department of Surgery, Washington University School of Medicine, St. Louis, MO, USA

Giampiero Campanelli Surgical Department - Università Insubria, Istituto Clinico Sant'Ambrogio, Milano, Italy

Patrice R. Carter Department of Surgery, Adventist LaGrange Hospital, LaGrange, IL, USA

Marta Cavalli Surgical Department - Università Insubria, Istituto Clinico Sant'Ambrogio, Milano, Italy

Simon Clarke Department of Pediatric Surgery, Chelsea and Westminster Hospital, London, UK

Joachim Conze Department of General and Visceral and Transplantation Surgery, University Hospital RWTH Aachen, Aachen, Germany

Joe Curry Department of Neonatal and Paediatric Surgery, Great Ormond Street Children's Hospital Foundation Trust, London, UK

Andrew C. de Beaux Department of General Surgery, Royal Infirmary of Edinburgh, Edinburgh, UK

Sheila Grant University of Missouri, Columbia, MO, USA

B. Todd Heniford Department of Surgery, Carolinas Laparoscopic and Advanced Surgery Program, Carolinas Medical Center, Charlotte, NC, USA

Leif A. Israelsson Department of Surgery, Sundsvall Hospital, Sundsvall, Sweden

Michael S. Kavic Department of Surgery, St. Elizabeth Health Center, Youngstown, OH, USA

Stephen M. Kavic Department of Surgery, University of Maryland School of Medicine, Baltimore, MD, USA

Suzanne M. Kavic Division Reproductive Endocrinology and Infertility Associate Professor of OB/GYN and Medicine Loyola University Medical Center Maywood, IL 60153

Anjili Khakar Department of Pediatric Surgery, Chelsea and Westminster Hospital, London, UK

Andrew N. Kingsnorth Department of Surgery, Peninsula College of Medicine & Dentistry, Plymouth, Devon, UK

Martin Kurzer Department of Surgery, British Hernia Centre, London, UK

Karl A. LeBlanc Surgeons Group of Baton Rouge/Our Lady of the Lake Physician Group, Baton Rouge, Louisiana, USA

Vishy Mahadevan Department of Education, The Royal College of Surgeons of England, London, UK

Pär Nordin Department of Surgery, Östersund Hospital, Östersund, Sweden

Patrick J. O'Dwyer Department of Surgery, Western Infirmary, Glasgow, Scotland, UK

Dilip Patel Department of Radiology, Royal Infirmary of Edinburgh, Edinburgh, UK

Benjamin S. Powell Department of Surgery, University of Tennessee Health Science Center–Memphis, Memphis, TN, USA

Bruce Ramshaw Department of General Surgery, Transformative Care Institute, Daytona Beach, FL, USA

Aly Shalaby Department of Neonatal and Paediatric Surgery, Great Ormond Street Children's Hospital Foundation Trust, London, UK

Maciej Śmietański Department of General and Vascular Surgery, Ceynowa Hospital in Wejherowo, Wejherowo, Poland

Cristina Sfeclan Surgical Department, University of Pharmacy and Medicine of Craiova, Istituto Clinico Sant'Ambrogio, Milano, Italy

Brian M. Stephenson Department of General Surgery, Royal Gwent Hospital, Newport, Wales, UK

William C. Streetman Surgeons Group of Baton Rouge/Our Lady of the Lake Physician Group, Baton Rouge, LA, USA

V. B. Tsirline Assistant Professor Department of Surgery Northwestern Memorial Hospital Northwestern University USA

Luke Vale Institute of Health and Society, Newcastle University, Newcastle upon Tyne, UK

Guy R. Voeller Department of Surgery, University of Tennessee Health Science Center–Memphis, Memphis, TN, USA

Andrew N. Kingsnorth

Ancient and Renaissance Hernia Surgery

The high prevalence of hernia, for which the lifetime risk is 27% for men and 3% for women [1], has resulted in this condition inheriting one of the longest traditions of surgical management. The Egyptians (1500 BC), the Phoenicians (900 BC), and the Ancient Greeks (Hippocrates, 400 BC) diagnosed hernia. During this period a number of devices and operative techniques have been recorded. Attempted repair was usually accompanied by castration, and strangulation was usually a death sentence. The word "hernia" is derived from the Greek (hernios), meaning a bud or shoot. The Hippocratic school differentiated between hernia and hydrocele—the former was reducible and the latter transilluminable [2]. The Egyptian tomb of Ankhmahor at Saqqara dated to around 2500 BC includes an illustrated sculpture of an operator apparently performing a circumcision and possibly a reduction of an inguinal hernia (Fig. 1.1) [3]. Egyptian pharaohs had a retinue of physicians whose duty was to preserve the health of the ruler. These doctors had a detailed knowledge of the anatomy of the body and had developed some advanced surgical techniques for other conditions and also for the cure of hernia. The mummy of the pharaoh Merneptah (1215 BC) showed a complete absence of the scrotum, and the mummified body of Rameses 5th (1157 BC) suggested that he had had an inguinal hernia during life with an associated fecal fistula in the scrotum and signs of attempts at surgical relief.

Greek and Phoenician terracottas (Figs. 1.2 and 1.3) illustrate general awareness of hernias at this time (900–600 BC), but the condition appeared to be a social stigma, and other than bandaging, treatments are not recorded. The Greek physician Galen (129–201 AD) was a prolific writer, and one of his treatises was a detailed description of the musculature of the lower abdominal wall in which he also describes the deficiency of inguinal hernia. He described the peritoneal sac and the concept of reducible contents of the sac.

Celsus (AD 40) was a prolific writer and although he had no medical training, he documented in encyclopedic detail Roman surgical practice: Taxis was employed for strangulation, trusses and bandages could control reducible hernia, and operation was only advised for pain and for small hernias in the young. The sac could be dissected through a scrotal incision, the wound then being allowed to granulate. Scar tissue was perceived as the optimum replacement for the stretched abdominal wall. A common method of treating hernia at this time was to reduce the contents of the sac and then attempt to obliterate it by a process of inflammation and gangrene by applying pressure to the walls of the sac through clamping the hemiscrotum between two blocks of wood. The last of the Greco-Roman medical encyclopedists, Paul of Aegina (625–900 AD), distinguished complete scrotal from incomplete inguinal herniation or bubonocele. For scrotal hernia, he recommended ligation of the sac and the cord with sacrifice of the testicle. Paul was the last of the great surgeons who wrote several books, which gave detailed descriptions of operative procedures including inguinal hernia.

During the dark time of the Middle Ages, there was a decline of medicine in the civilized world and the use of the knife was largely abandoned, and few contributions were made to the art of surgery, which was now practiced by itinerants and quacks. With the rise of the universities such as the appearance of the school of Salerno in the thirteenth century, there was some revival of surgical practice [3]. At this time three important advances in herniology were made: Guy de Chauliac, in 1363, distinguished femoral from inguinal hernia. He developed taxis for incarceration, recommending the head down, Trendelenburg position [4]. Guy was French and studied in Toulouse and Montpelier and later learned anatomy in Bologna from Nicole Bertuccio. Guy wrote extensively about hernia in his book Chirurgia (Fig. 1.4), principally about diagnosis and methods of treatment. He described four surgical interventions: one of which

A.N. Kingsnorth (✉)
Department of Surgery, Peninsula College of Medicine & Dentistry, Plymouth, Devon, UK
e-mail: Andrew.kingsnorth@nhs.net

A.N. Kingsnorth and K.A. LeBlanc (eds.), *Management of Abdominal Hernias*,
DOI 10.1007/978-1-84882-877-3_1, © Springer Science+Business Media London 2013

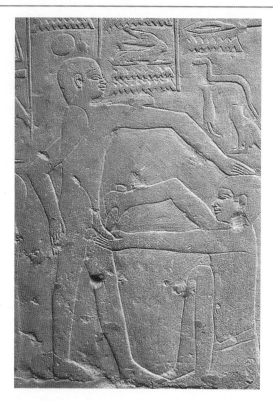

Fig. 1.1 Egyptian Tomb of Ankhmahor (Saqqara). The operator (*bottom right*) rubs in something with an instrument and seems to perform a reduction of an inguinal hernia

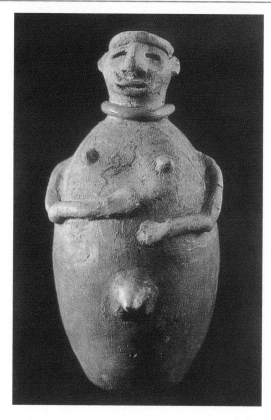

Fig. 1.3 Phoenician terracotta figure (female) shows umbilical hernia (fifth–fourth century BC) (from Museo Arquelogico, Barcelona, Spain)

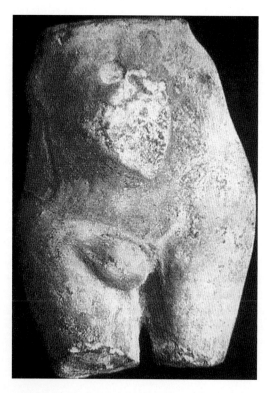

Fig. 1.2 Terracotta ex voto shows femoral hernia (from Geschichte der Medizin, 1922)

was a herniotomy without castration, another consisting of cauterization of the hernia down to the os pubis, and third consisting of transfixion of the sac to a piece of wood by a strong ligature. His fourth method however was conservative treatment with bandaging and several weeks of bed rest accompanied by enemas, bloodletting, and special diet. At the time he was the authoritative expert on hernia.

Franco's book Traites des Hernies [5] standardized the practice of hernia surgery at the time and diminished the influence of the itineran practitioners (Fig. 1.5). Franco popularized the punctum aurium and using this instrument made a small incision in the upper scrotum, isolated the hernia sac from the spermatic cord, and then encircled it with a gold thread, thus sparing the testis. He chose gold thread because this was considered to be the best nonreactive material. In spite of the known hazards and high mortality of operating on a strangulated hernia, Franco advised early intervention and rejected the conservative measures employed such as bloodletting and tobacco enemas. As a result he saved numerous patients with lifesaving operations. He wrote many up as case reports illustrating his management and surgical techniques. He recommended reducing the contents and closing the defect with linen suture (Fig. 1.6). His beautifully written manuscript was rediscovered and published again in 1925 by Walter van

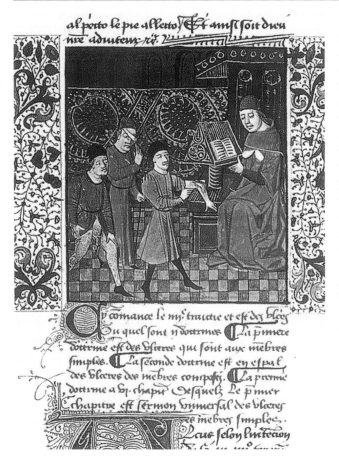

Fig. 1.4 The visit of surgical patients in Chirurgia. Guy de Chauliac, fifteenth-century manuscript (from the Bibliothèque Nationale, Paris, France)

Brunn. As shown in the illustration the unusual feature of the book was the patients posing in everyday attire as if they were going about their everyday life.

In 1559 Stromayr, a German surgeon from Lindau, published a remarkable contribution to surgery. His book Practica Copiosa describes sixteenth-century hernia surgery in great detail and is comprehensively illustrated. Stromayr differentiated direct and indirect inguinal hernia and advised excision of the sac and of the cord and testicle in indirect hernia [6]. Having differentiated and classified the two types of inguinal hernia, Stromayr recommended a testis-sparing procedure for the direct type. His operation for high ligation of an indirect sac at the internal ring is illustrated in Fig. 1.7. Stromayr also advanced the technology of trusses, which he designed to be adapted to the rigors of everyday life. The Renaissance brought burgeoning anatomic knowledge, now based on careful cadaver dissection. William Cheselden successfully operated on a strangulated right inguinal hernia on the Tuesday morning after Easter 1721. The intestines were easily reduced, and adherent omentum was ligated and divided. The patient survived and went back to work [7] (Fig. 1.8).

Without adequate interventional surgery, some patients survived hernia strangulation when spontaneous, preternatural fistula occasionally followed infarction and sloughing of a strangulated hernia. Cheselden's Margaret White survived for many years "voiding the excrements through the intestine at the navel" after simple local surgery for a strangulated umbilical hernia [7]. The closure of such a fistula in the absence of distal bowel pathology was described by Le Dran, who had noted that it was quite common for poor people with incarcerated hernias to mistake the tender painful groin lump for an abscess and incise it themselves. He found that these painful wounds with fecal fistulas required no more than cleaning and dressing. Often the wound would heal, nature preferring to send the feces along the natural route to the anus [8] (Fig. 1.9).

The Anatomical Era

The great contribution of the surgical anatomists was between the years 1750 and 1865 and was called the age of dissection [3]. The main contributors were Antonio Scarpa and Sir Astley Cooper, and few major advances in our knowledge of the anatomy of the groin have been made since this time. The names of these great anatomists are Pieter, Camper, Antonio Scarpa, Percival Pott, Sir Astley Cooper, John Hunter, Thomas Morton, Germaine Cloquet, Franz Hesselbach, Friedrich Henle, and Don Antonio Gimbernat.

The Dutchman Camper was a polymath who described a fascia, which is sandwiched in between the skin and deep fascia and can only be separated from this fascia below the inguinal ligament where the space between them accommodates lymph glands and cutaneous vessels of the groin. Below the external ring, Camper's fascia becomes the dartos muscle of the scrotum, which like the platysma is a muscle of the superficial fascia. Camper was the author of the definitive surgical text on hernia at the time. Antonio Scarpa was educated at the University of Padua (Fig. 1.10), and he occupied the chairs of anatomy at the University of Modena and later Pavia. He was said to be arrogant and tyrannical and as a result despised by his colleagues. Sir Percival Pott described the pathophysiology of strangulation in 1757 and recommended surgical management (Fig. 1.11): "I am perfectly satisfied that the cause of strangulated hernia is most frequently . . . a piece of intestine (in other respects sound and free of disease) being so bound by the said tendon, as to have its peristaltic motion and the circulation through it impeded or stopped" [9]. Pott was trained at St Bartholomew's Hospital and wrote the manuscript a Treatise on Rupture. This publication brought him into conflict with the Hunters who accused him of plagiarism for his description of congenital hernia, which they claimed to have described 2 years previously. He emphasized that the hernia sac was peritoneum

Fig. 1.5 Frontispiece and surgery instruments in Traités des Hernies (by Pierre Franco, Vincent, Lyon, 1561)

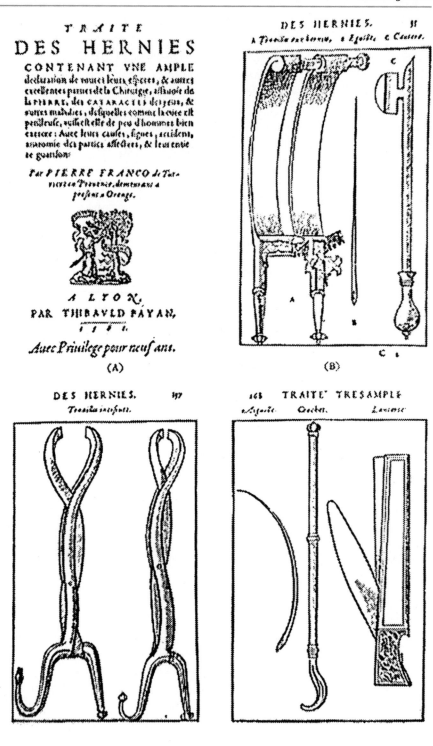

continuous with the general peritoneal cavity and had not been in any way ruptured or broken, which until that time was the popular theory of causation of hernia.

Fifty years later Astley Cooper (Fig. 1.12) implicated venous obstruction as the first cascade in the circulatory failure of strangulation: "By a stop being put to the return of blood through the veins which produces a great accumulation of this fluid and a change of its colour from the arterial to the venous hue." Nevertheless ligature, the insertion of setons, and castration remained the mainstays of treatment prior to the publication of Astley Cooper's monograph in 1804 [10] (Fig. 1.13). Sir Astley Cooper (1768–1841) trained at St Thomas's Hospital, London and became a surgeon at Guy's Hospital and from 1813 to 1815 was professor of comparative anatomy of the Royal College of Surgeons. Cooper published six magnificent books, two of

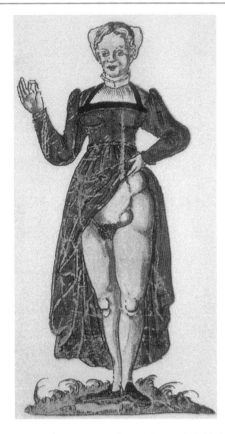

Fig. 1.6   Woman with femoral hernia. In Die Handschrift des Schmitt- und Augenartztes. Caspar Stromayr (by Walter von Brunn, 1925)

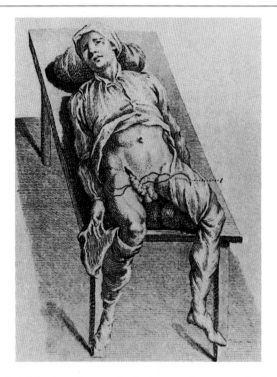

Fig. 1.8   Ligation of strangulated omentum in a strangulated right scrotal hernia. The wound then granulated. The patient survived and the hernia did not recur (operation by Cheselden in 1721 [7])

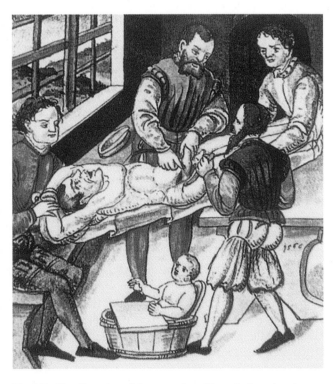

Fig. 1.7   The dissection of the sac and cord in an indirect hernia, carried to the level of the internal ring (in von Brunn, 1925)

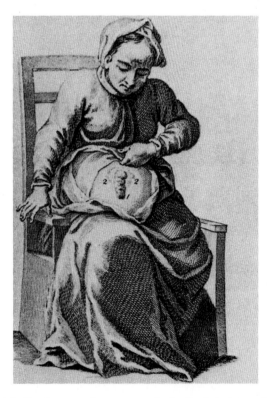

Fig. 1.9   Development of a preternatural colon fistula (colostomy) after strangulation of an umbilical hernia. The wound was trimmed. The patient survived many years "voiding" the excrements at the umbilicus (operation by Cheselden about 1721 [7])

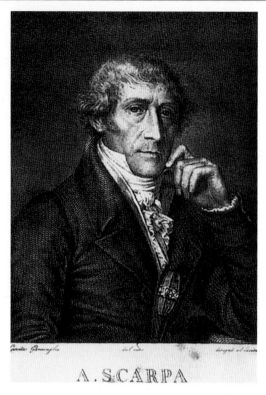

Fig. 1.10 Antonio Scarpa (1752–1832) professor of surgery and anatomy in Pavia, Italy

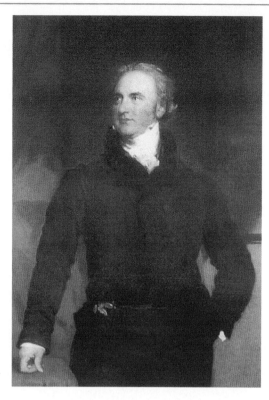

Fig. 1.12 Sir Astley Paston Cooper (1768–1841). Surgical anatomist, London, England

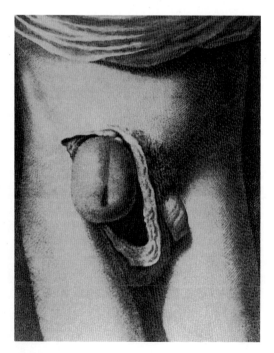

Fig. 1.11 Intestine strangulated by the "tendon" so that the venous circulation through it is stopped, leading to gangrene (described by Pott in 1757 [9])

which covered the subject of hernia, which were liberally illustrated by his own hand from dissections he had performed personally. Cooper was a charismatic lecturer and socialite and had an extensive surgical practice, which included being sergeant surgeon to King George IV. Cooper's recognition of the transversalis fascia positions him as one of the most important contributors to present-day surgery which emphasizes this layer as being the first layer to be breached in groin hernias.

John Hunter (1728–1793) was born in Glasgow but became a pupil at St Bartholomew's Hospital to Percival Pott and later served as a surgeon at St George's Hospital where he established his well-known anatomy lessons and later the Hunterian museum which is now housed in the Royal College of Surgeons of England. Hunter's contribution was to define the role of the gubernaculum testis that directed the descent of that organ with the spermatic vessels into the scrotum around the time of birth. Thomas Wharton (1813–1849), also a London surgeon working at the North London Hospital, in his short life, wrote three anatomical texts, two of which were the subject of inguinal hernia and the groin. He first gave an accurate description of the conjoined tendon of the internal oblique and transversus muscles and their termination and attachment to the outer portion of the rectus sheath.

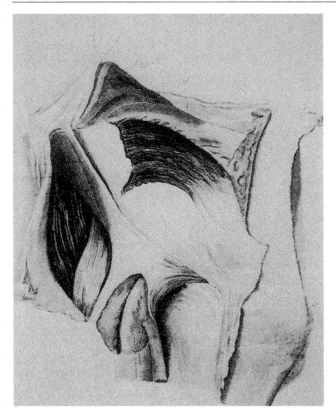

Fig. 1.13 Anatomy of the fascia transversalis. Astley Cooper (1804) demonstrated the fascia extending behind the inguinal ligament into the thigh to be the femoral sheath. He first recognized the fascia transversalis and its importance in groin herniation [10]

The first accurate description of the iliopubic tract, an important structure utilized in many sutured repairs for inguinal hernia, was made by Jules Cloquet (1790–1883). Cloquet was professor of anatomy and surgery in Paris and surgeon to the emperor. Cloquet researched the pathological anatomy of the groin in numerous autopsy dissections and their reconstruction in wax models. He was the first to observe the frequency of patency of the processus vaginalis after birth and its role in the production of a hernia sac later in life. Franz Hesselbach was an anatomist at the University of Wurzburg who described the triangle now so important in laparoscopic surgery which originally defined the pathway of direct and external and supravesical hernias (Fig. 1.14). The triangle as defined today is somewhat smaller. Friedrich Henle (1809–1885) was another German latterly working in the University of Gottingen. Henle described an important ligament running from the lateral edge of the rectus sheath and fusing with the pectineal ligament. This structure when present could be utilized to anchor sutures in herniorrhaphy. Finally Don Antonio Gimbernat (1742–1790) was a Spanish surgeon working in Barcelona and also surgeon to King Charles III and president of the College of Surgeons of Spain. Gimbernat not only defined the lacunar ligament as a distinct anatomical structure but also showed how its division in strangulated

femoral hernia was usually the point of obstruction and allowed reduction of the contents of the sac.

The Era of Antisepsis and Asepsis

Before bacteria were recognized and with it the need for meticulous cleanliness in the environment of the operating theater, postoperative sepsis was virtually routine and mortality rates were extremely high. Oliver Wendell Holmes in 1842 and Semmelweiss in 1849 emphasized the importance of hand washing before operating. However, identifying and understanding the problem of infection and the causal bacteria had to await the discoveries of Louis Pasteur which were later put into practice by Joseph Lister (1827–1912). The application of Lister's principles of providing clean linen and special coats, special receptacles for antiseptic dressings, cleansing sponges soaked in carbolic acid and thymol, and the segregation of postmortem examinations and operating theaters profoundly influenced British and European surgeons and decimated postoperative infection rates. Modern Surgery Commenced with Lister's Discoveries [11].

Other important innovations were acquired before operative surgery presented a minimal danger to the patient. Ernst von Bergman invented the steam sterilizer in 1891 and introduced the word "aseptic." Halsted with the nurse Caroline Hampton introduced rubber gloves in 1896, and together with the introduction of a face mask by von Miculicz, the conversion from antiseptic to aseptic technique was finally set for the techniques of modern hernia surgery to develop [12].

The Dawn of Anesthesia

The removal of pain during surgical operations not only eliminated the terror of the surgical operation from the patient but also enabled more careful anatomical dissection and reconstruction and the evolution of planned surgical procedures [3]. An American dentist Horace Wells pioneered the use of nitrous oxide as an anesthetic, but his first public attempt at demonstrating a painless dental extraction was a failure. It was left to his associate William Thomas Green Morton to demonstrate the first successful anesthetic using sulfuric ether in the theater of the Massachusetts General Hospital in Boston. The operation on Edward Gilbert Abbott was for removal of a tumor angioma in the neck. Following this demonstration on 16 October 1846, the practice spread widely into Europe and Listen in London used it for a thigh amputation on Frederick Churchill on 21 December 1846. With patients no longer fearing pain, the scene was set for the great technological advances of the second half of the nineteenth century.

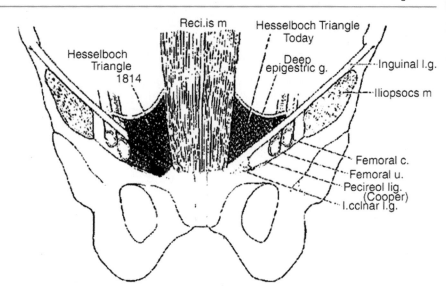

Fig. 1.14 The triangle of Hesselbach described in 1814, and as understood today. In Hernias (by JE Skandalakis, SW Gray, and JS Rowe Jr, 1983)

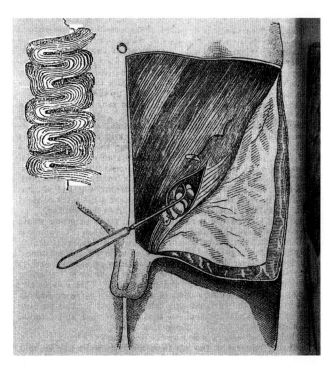

Fig. 1.15 The operation of McEwan 1886. The dissected indirect sac is bundled up and then used as an internal stopper or pad to prevent further herniation along the valved canal [15]

The Technological Era

Initial surgical attempts at hernioplasty were based on static concepts of anatomic repair using natural or modified natural materials for reconstruction. Wood (1863) described subcutaneous division and suture of the sac and fascial separation of the groin from the scrotum [13]. Czerny (1876), in Prague, pulled the sac of an inguinal hernia through the external ring, ligated it, amputated the redundant sac, and allowed the neck

to spring back to the deep ring [14]. MacEwen (1886), of Glasgow, bundled the sac up on itself and stuffed it back along the canal so that it would act as a cork or tampon and stop up the internal ring [15] (Fig. 1.15). Kocher (1907), surgery's first Nobel Prize winner, invaginated the sac on itself and fixed it laterally through the external oblique [16] (Fig. 1.16). Suffice to say, none of these operations have stood the test of time.

As so often in surgery a new concept was needed before further progress could be made in herniology. Two (Figs. 1.17 and 1.18) pioneers—the American Marcy [17] and the Italian Bassini (1884)—vie for priority for the critical breakthrough [18–20]. Both appreciated the physiology of the inguinal canal and both correctly understood how each anatomic plane, transversalis fascia, transverse and oblique muscles, and the external oblique aponeurosis contributed to the canal's stability. Read, having carefully surveyed all the evidence, agrees with Halsted that Bassini got there first [21].

Although both contributed to herniology, Bassini made another seminal advance when he subjected his technique to the scrutiny of the prospective follow-up. Bassini's 1890 paper is truly a quantum leap in surgery [20]; indeed, if it is read alongside the contribution of Haidenthaller, from Billroth's clinic—reporting a 30% early recurrence rate—which appears in the same volume of Langenbeck's Archiv fur Klinische Chirurgie, Bassini's stature is further enhanced [22].

Marcy directed his attention to the deep ring in the fascia transversalis; his operation for indirect inguinal hernia entailed closure of the deep ring with fascia transversalis only, the object being the recreation of a stable and competent deep ring. In 1871, he reported two patients operated on during the previous year "in which I closed the (deep) ring

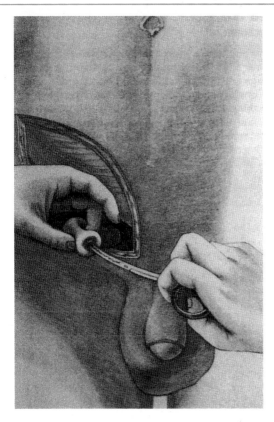

Fig. 1.16 Invagination of the sac which is fixed laterally by suturing its stump to the external oblique. No formal dissection or repair of the deep ring was made (operation by Kocher in 1907 [16])

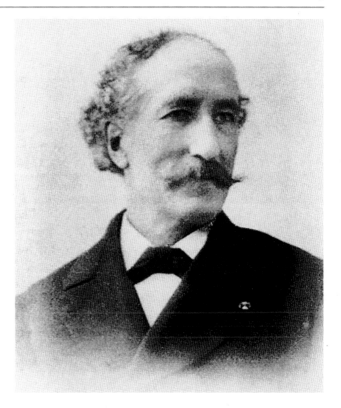

Fig. 1.17 Henry Orville Marcy (1837–1924), Boston surgeon, anatomist, and philanthropist. The first American student of Lister (courtesy of the New York Academy of Medicine Library)

with the interrupted sutures of carbolized catgut followed by permanent cure" [23].

Bassini had become interested in the management of inguinal hernia in about 1883, and from 1883 to 1889 he operated on 274 hernias. After trying the operations of Czerny and Wood, he modified his approach and attempted a radical cure, so that the patient would not require a truss after surgery. He decided to open the inguinal canal and approach the posterior wall of the canal; gradually he was focusing onto the deep ring and fascia transversalis. Seven times he opened the canal, resected the sac, and closed the peritoneum at the internal ring. He then constructed a tampon of the excess sac at the internal ring and sutured this sac stump, or tampon, to the deep surface of the external oblique. One of his seven patients died 3 months after the operation from an unrelated cause. Postmortem examination showed the sutured portion of the neck, the "stopper" or tampon, to be completely reabsorbed. Bassini deduced that although the risk of recurrent herniation was diminished by this technique it did not afford adequate tissue repair, and some external support—a truss—would still be needed to prevent recurrence. He now proceeded to complete anatomical reconstruction of the inguinal canal.

> . . this might be achieved through reconstruction of the inguinal canal into the physiological condition, a canal with two openings one abdominal the other subcutaneous and with two walls, one anterior and one posterior through the middle of which the spermatic cord would pass. Through a study of the groin, and with the help of an anatomical knowledge of the inguinal canal and inguinal hernia, it was easy for me to find an operative method, which answered the above described requirements, and made possible a radical cure without subsequent wearing of a truss. Using the method exclusively I have, during the year 1884, operated on 262 hernias of which 251 were either reducible or irreducible and 11 strangulated.

His series included 206 men and 10 women; the non-strangulated cases were 115 right, 66 left, and 35 bilateral inguinal hernias. The age range was 13 months to 69 years. The operations were performed under general narcosis, and there were no operative deaths; however, three patients who each had strangulated hernias died postoperatively—one of sepsis, one of shock, and one of a chest infection. Bassini's patients were carefully followed up, some to 4¾ years, and seven recurrences were recorded. There were, in fact, eight recurrences; Bassini failed to tabulate case 65, a 54-year-old university professor in Padua with a strangulated right direct inguinal hernia, with a recurrence at 8 months. The wound infection rate was 11 in 206 operations, and the time to healing averaged 14 days [20]. These statistics compare favorably with reports made up to the 1950s.

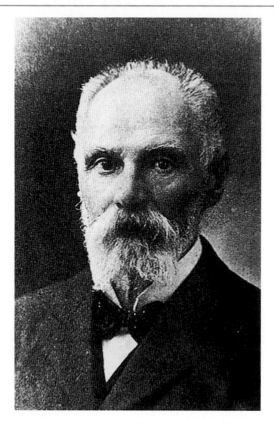

Fig. 1.18 Edoardo Bassini (1844–1924) invented the first successful inguinal hernioplasty

Bassini dissected the indirect sac and closed it off flush with the parietal peritoneum. He then isolated and lifted up the spermatic cord and dissected the posterior wall of the canal, dividing the fascia transversalis down to the pubic tubercle. He then sutured the dissected conjoint tendon consisting of the internal oblique, the transversus muscle, and the "vertical fascia of Cooper," the fascia transversalis, to the posterior rim of Poupart's ligament, including the lower lateral divided margin of the fascia transversalis. Bassini stresses that this suture line must be approximated without difficulty; hence the early dissection separating the external oblique from the internal oblique must be adequate and allow good development and mobilization of the conjoint tendon (Fig. 1.19).

The Bassini legacy was popularized by Attilio Catterina, Bassini's assistant in Padua in 1887 who later became professor in Genoa in 1904. Catterina was entrusted by Bassini to teach the exact surgical technique. To do this he wrote an atlas of "The Operation of Bassini!" This adds 16 life-sized color plates by the artist Orazio Gaicher of Cortina. This book was published in London, Berlin, Paris, and Madrid in the 1930s and described in detail the uncorrupted Bassini technique, especially the division of the transversalis fascia, resection of the cremaster muscle, and complete anatomical survey of all the relevant anatomy nowadays considered so essential [24, 25]—a foretaste of the Shouldice operation [26]. The illustrations show quite clearly that Bassini resected the cremaster muscle (Fig. 1.20) and completed division of

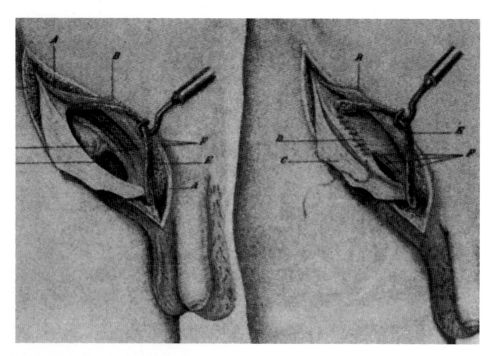

Fig. 1.19 Suturing the "triple layer" (F) (fascia transversalis, transversus tendon, and internal oblique) to the upturned edge of the inguinal ligament. An anatomical and physiological repair of the posterior wall of the inguinal canal preserving its obliquity and function (operation by Bassini in 1890 [20])

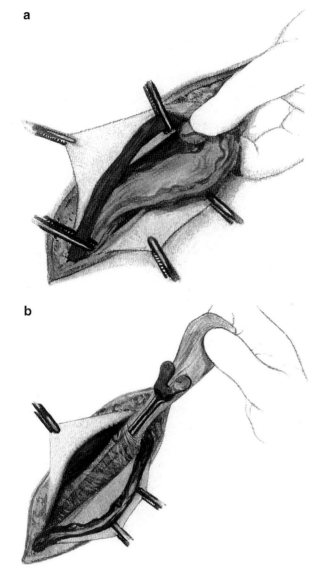

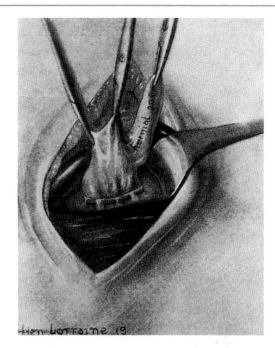

Fig. 1.21 Transabdominal approach to the groin through a muscle-splitting incision above the inguinal canal with subsequent closure of the peritoneal sac away from the canal [39]

Fig. 1.20 (**a**) Bassini completely isolated and excised the cremaster muscle and its fascia from the cord. He thus ensured complete exposure of the deep ring and all the posterior wall of the inguinal canal, an essential prerequisite to evaluate all the potential hernial sites. (**b**) Bassini stressed the complete exposure and incision of the fascia transversalis of the posterior wall of the inguinal canal. To complete the repair he sutured the divided fascia transversalis, together with the transversus muscle, and the internal oblique muscle, "the threefold layer" to the upturned inner free margin of the inguinal ligament [24]

the posterior wall of the inguinal canal (Fig. 1.21). The Shouldice and Bassini hernioplasties are therefore essentially the same.

By contrast, Haidenthaller, from Billroth's Clinic in Vienna, reported 195 operations for inguinal hernia, with 11 operative deaths and a short-term recurrence rate of 30.8% [22]. Although Halsted made important contributions to herniology, his general technical contributions of precise hemostasis, absolute asepsis, and the crucial importance of avoiding tissue trauma are easily overlooked. Halsted was always concerned to achieve optimum wound healing, and he not only practiced surgery but he experimented and theorized. His observation on closing skin wounds is best repeated verbatim: "The skin is united by interrupted stitches of very fine silk. These stitches do not penetrate the skin, and when tied they become buried. They are taken from the underside of the skin and made to include only its deeper layers—the layers which are not occupied by sebaceous follicles" [27, 28]. In today's world, hematoma, sepsis, and damaged tissue leading to delayed healing mean not only a poor surgical outcome but weigh heavily on the debit side of any economic evaluation. These Halstedian principles should be rigidly applied by any surgeon who undertakes hernia surgery.

Halsted must also be given priority for recognizing the value of an anterior relaxing incision, first described by Wolfler in 1892 [29] and subsequently popularized in the USA by Rienhoff [30] and in England by Tanner (1942) [31]. Apart from Halsted, countless other authors have corrupted or simplified the original Marcy–Bassini concept of a review of the posterior wall of the canal and the correction of any deficits in it, the reconstruction of the patulous deep ring for indirect herniation, and the repair of the stretched fascia transversalis in cases of direct herniation. Bull and Coley independently sutured the internal oblique and the aponeurosis over the cord [32, 33], whereas Ferguson (1899) advised against any mobilization of the cord and, therefore, any review of the posterior wall of the canal [34].

Imbrication, or overlapping, of layers was introduced by Wyllys Andrews in 1895 in Chicago [35]. Andrews confessed

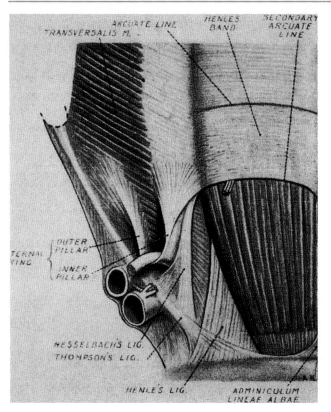

Fig. 1.22 The "shutter mechanism" of canal and the internal anatomy of the deep ring, demonstrating the sling of fascia transversalis which pulls the deep ring up and laterally when the patient strains [50]

that his technique was an outgrowth of experience with MacEwan, Bassini, Halsted and similar operations. Andrews laid great stress on careful aseptic technique: "Finally, I unite the skin itself with a buried suture which does not puncture any of its glands or ducts." Andrews used cotyledon only as a dressing. Again the importance of careful surgical technique is emphasized. Andrews stressed the importance of the posterior wall of the canal: "The posterior wall of the canal . . . is narrowed by suturing the conjoined tendon and transversalis fascia firmly to Poupart's ligament." Andrews recommended the kangaroo tendon introduced by Marcy. Andrews then reinforced the posterior wall with the upper (medial) margin of the external oblique aponeurosis, which he drew down behind the cord and sutured to Poupart's ligament. Andrews' intention was to interlock or imbricate the layers. The lower (lateral) flap of the external oblique aponeurosis was then brought up anterior to the cord. Andrews concluded his article: "Any successful method of radical cure must be a true plastic operation upon the musculo-aponeurotic layers of the abdominal wall. Cicatricial tissue and peritoneal exudate are of no permanent value." Andrews had visited Bassini in Padua on several occasions to acquaint himself with the revolutionary operation. However, in his future descriptions of the operation, Andrews failed to mention that Bassini had divided the posterior wall of the inguinal canal, and these

erroneous observations were passed on to a generation of European and American surgeons because Catterina's atlas was not published in Europe until the 1930s. Andrews' description of Bassini's operation was therefore the only definitive description, and the classical Bassini operation became corrupted until it was reintroduced as the Shouldice operation in the 1950s.

Perhaps we should pause at about 1905 and summarize what empiricism had achieved thus far. First, all authors agree that division of the neck of the sac and flush closure of the peritoneum is imperative to success. Second, dissection of the deep ring with exploration of the extraperitoneal space to allow adequate closure of the fascia transversalis anterior to the peritoneum emerges as a cardinal feature. Marcy and Bassini stress the fascia transversalis repair, Halsted emphasized it, and Andrews' diagram suggests it. Ferguson did not examine the entire posterior wall but tightened the internal ring lateral to the emergent cord. All are agreed that the deep ring is patulous in indirect herniation, and consequently the fascia transversalis must be repaired. In the English literature, Lockwood in 1893 clearly emphasized the fascia transversalis and Bassini's "triple layer." Lockwood obtained good results by repairing this important layer [36, 37]. Third, preservation of the obliquity of the canal is suggested by Marcy and Bassini and by the later Halsted and Bloodgood papers.

Fourth, double breasting (imbrication) of aponeurosis gives improved results and is recommended by Andrews. Lastly, all the authors stress careful technique. Avoidance of tissue trauma, hematoma, and infection leads to impressively better results. Sepsis is an important antecedent of recurrence.

After the nineteenth-century advances of Marcy and Bassini and the important contribution to surgical technique by Halsted, little of major importance was contributed until the 1920s. Countless modifications of Marcy's and Bassini's operations were made and reported frequently. The Bassini operation reemerged as the Shouldice repair in 1950s (Fig. 1.22). Earl Shouldice (1890–1965) also promulgated the benefits of early ambulation and opened the Shouldice clinic, a hospital dedicated to the repair of hernias to the abdominal wall. A huge experience accumulated with an annual throughput of 7000 herniorrhaphies per year, enabled the surgeons at the Shouldice clinic to study the pathology in primary and recurrent hernias and to emphasize adjuncts to successful outcomes. Continuous monofilament wire was used in preference to other suture materials and the hernioplasty incorporated repair of the internal ring, the posterior wall of the inguinal canal, and the femoral region. The cremaster muscle and fascia with vessels and genital branch of genitofemoral nerve were removed, and the posterior wall after division was repaired by a four-layer imbrication method using the iliopubic tract as its main anchor point. The landmark publication

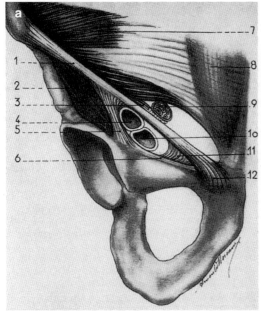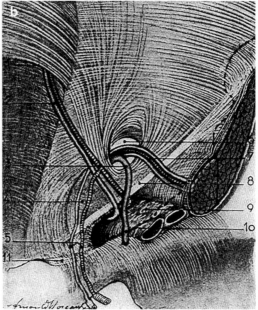

Fig. 1.23 (a) Fruchaud's concept of the myopectineal orifice ("l'orifice crural classique") incorporating the inguinal and the femoral canals. An external view showing the two canals separated by the inguinal ligament and internal dissection (b) demonstrating how the muscles of the groin form a tunnel down to the myopectineal orifice [51]

with long-term follow-up was produced by Shearburn and Myers in 1969, and from this time until the introduction of mesh, the Shouldice operation became the gold standard for inguinal hernia repair [38].

The Extraperitoneal–Preperitoneal Approach to the Groin

Alternatives to the anterior (inguinal) approach to the internal ring include the transabdominal (laparotomy) [3, 39] and the extraperitoneal (preperitoneal) [40]. Marcy recognized the advantages of the transabdominal intraperitoneal approach to the ring in 1892:

> It may rarely happen to the operator who has opened the abdomen for some other purpose to find the complication of hernia. When the section has been made considerably large, as in the removal of a large tumour; the internal ring is within reach of the surgeon. Upon reflection, it would naturally occur to any operator that under these conditions it is better to close the internal ring, and reform the smooth internal parietal surface from within by means of suturing. My friend, Dr N. Bozeman of New York, easily did this at my suggestion in a case of ovariotomy more than 10 years ago.

Marcy attributed the transabdominal technique to the French in 1749 [41]. Lawson Tait recommended midline abdominal section for umbilical and groin hernia in 1891 [42]. LaRoque, in 1919, recommended transabdominal repair of inguinal hernias through a muscle-splitting incision about 1 in. (2.5 cm) above the ring. The peritoneum was opened,

the sac dissected and then inverted into the peritoneal cavity by grasping its fundus and pulling it back into the peritoneal cavity. The sac was excised and a repair of the deep ring effected [39] (Fig. 1.23). LaRoque believed that the transabdominal approach provided absolute assurance of high ligation of the hernia sac and wrote three papers with accumulative experience of almost 2000 inguinal hernia repairs [43].

Battle, a surgeon at St Thomas' Hospital, London and the Royal Free Hospital, described his approach to repair of a femoral hernia in 1900. Battle pointed out the difficulties of diagnosing femoral hernia and the difficulties, principally the age, sex, and comorbidity, of managing patients with femoral hernia. He approached the hernia sac from above through an incision splitting the external oblique above the inguinal ligament. After dealing with the peritoneal sac, Battle repaired the femoral canal, constructing a "shutter" of the aponeurosis of external oblique which he sutured to the pectineus fascia and the pectineal ligament across the abdominal opening of the femoral canal [44, 45]. The Battle operation like many operations for groin hernia has now passed into oblivion.

The extraperitoneal–preperitoneal approach owes its origin to Cheatle (1920) who initially used a midline incision but subsequently (1921) changed to a Pfannenstiel incision [40, 45]. Cheatle explored both sides, and inguinal and femoral protrusions were reduced and amputated. If needed, for strangulation or adhesions, the peritoneum could easily be opened. The fascia transversalis was visible and easily repaired. Cheatle advised against this approach for direct hernia because the direct region was usually obscured and distorted by the retraction of the rectus muscles. However, Cheatle's landmark contribution had a minimal impact at the time and remained little used for many years [43].

A.K. Henry, a master anatomist, rediscovered and popularized the extraperitoneal approach in 1936 [46]. At this time he was the Director of the Surgical Unit, Kasr-el-Aini Hospital, and professor of clinical surgery in the University of Cairo although he later returned to the Hammersmith Hospital and subsequently became professor of anatomy at the Royal College of Surgeons in Ireland. The full impact of the Cheatle/Henry operation was not recognized until after the Second World War, when McEvedy [47] adopted a unilateral oblique incision retracting the rectus muscle medially to approach a femoral hernia. In the USA, Musgrove and McCready (1949) adopted the Henry approach to femoral hernia [48]. Mikkelsen and Berne (1954) reported inguinal and femoral hernias repaired by this technique and commended the excellent access obtained even in the obese. Furthermore femoral, inguinal, and obturator hernias were all repairable through this "extended suprapubic approach" [49].

Two Europeans: Lytle and Fruchaud

In the immediate aftermath of the Second World War two European surgeon anatomists, Lytle and Fruchaud, are important contributors. Lytle was principally concerned with the anatomy and shutter mechanism of the deep inguinal ring. He dissected the deep ring and in a remarkable film demonstrated its prophylactic mechanism in indirect herniation. He was concerned to preserve the mechanism of the ring and at the same time to reinforce its patulous medial margin in indirect herniation. He emphasized that maneuvers which damaged the lateral "pillars of the ring" inevitably compromised the physiological shutter mechanism. In a subsequent study he clearly described the embryological anatomy of the ring and how it could be repaired in the fascia transversalis layer, without losing its function [50] (Fig. 1.24).

A remarkable Frenchman, Henri Fruchaud, published two books in Paris in 1956: L'Anatomie Chirurgicale de la Region de l'Aine (Surgical Anatomy of the Groin Region) [51] and Le Traitement Chirurgical des Hernies de l'Aine (Surgical Treatment of Groin Hernias) [52]. Fruchaud combined traditional anatomical studies of the groin, the work of Cooper, Bogros, and Madden, with his own extensive anatomical and surgical experience. He invented an entirely new concept— "the myopectineal orifice"—which combined the traditionally separate inguinal and femoral canals to form a unified highway from the abdomen to the thigh. The abdominocrural tunnel of fascia transversalis extended through this myopectineal orifice, through which all inguinal and femoral hernias pass, as do the iliofemoral vessels. Based on this anatomical concept

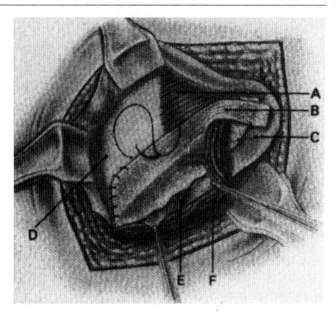

Fig. 1.24 The Lichtenstein's tension-free hernioplasty [150]

Fruchaud recommended complete reconstruction of the endofascial wall (fascia transversalis) of the myopectineal orifice. This unifying concept forms the basis for all extraperitoneal mesh repairs, open or laparoscopic, of groin hernias (Fig. 1.25). Fruchaud's two books were never published in English and therefore his findings remained relatively obscure and did not have the full impact and recognition until the laparoscopic era of hernia repair [53]. The concept of Fruchaud has been expanded by Stoppa in France and Wantz in the USA into the "giant reinforcement of the peritoneal sac" repairs of inguinal hernias [54, 55].

Inguinal Hernias in Soldiers in Georgian England

Hernias in England during the Georgian period of the early eighteenth century were prevalent amongst servicemen, typically recruited from amongst the malnourished. Civilian medical practice had deemed the rupture incurable taking a palliative approach. For the military, this was unacceptable; wastage rates due to ruptures were high and servicemen were valuable commodities. Treatment (experimentation) was a contentious activity relying on the whim of patronage and wartime budgets. Two clinical trials with war office funding were carried out between 1721 (Grenton) and 1770 (Lee) and were eventually exposed as ineffectual and "polemic doggerel and quackery."

The four major characteristics of eighteenth-century hernia treatment in Britain were as follows:

1. It was considered an unmanly ailment that questioned the virility and general health of the afflicted.

Fig. 1.25 Drs. Shulman, Lichtenstein, and Amid, pioneers at the Lichtenstein Clinic

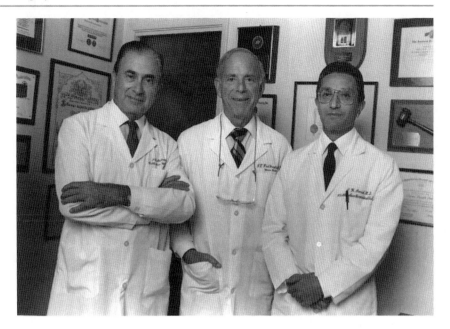

2. Hernia was a chronic disorder only to be managed by palliative nonoperative procedures.
3. Most hernias were inguinal.
4. Afflicted males were poor and usually laborers.

In 1776 Dr George Carlisle reported biographical and autopsy details of an ex-serviceman, John Hollowday, who died of natural causes aged approximately 80 with a massive inguinoscrotal hernia stretching down to his knees. Such a hernia was apparently not an uncommon finding in ex-military men, and Hollowday had initially concealed the hernia "to avoid the scoffs of his companions." The hernia increased in size until Hollowday was adjudged unfit to serve, and he was admitted as an outpensioner to the Royal Hospital Chelsea in 1725 while still in his mid-thirties. Neglected hernias such as these can now only be found in third-world countries such as Africa.

Radical cures for hernia in the eighteenth century included escharotics (a caustic seal of the inguinal rings with scar tissue), castration (skin was used to close the opening), and trusses (after reduction of the hernia) which were of multiple types and military trusses were mass produced. To treat this massive problem of hernia, a rupture hospital (voluntary) was opened in Greenwich in 1756 but which only stayed open until 1765.

The exact number and rate of hernia occurrences in the Georgian British Army is unknown. However, the periodically malnourished, diseased, and constipated; occasionally physically overworked; and perpetually unfit British troops manning camps and barracks ringing with hacking smokers' coughs and a distinctive short consumptive bark may be a gross characterization, but we should not detract from the fact that the underlying causes of hernia were endemic characteristics of eighteenth-century soldiers and soldiering. To counter this debilitating disorder, the army required an efficacious cure that conventional therapeutics could not deliver. But, even though patronage was directly responsible for the establishment of a preferred treatment in a military hospital, the management of rupture slipped back into the margins of military and medical consciousness. The cure for inguinal hernia had to wait for at least another 100 years.

Winston Churchill's Hernia Repair

Schein and Rodgers reported an interesting vignette of Winston Churchill's hernia repair in 1947 [56]. On an early summer morning, June 11th in a small private nursing home on Berwick Street, London, within walking distance of Harley Street, the 73-year-old Winston Churchill had his inguinal hernia repaired by Thomas Dunhill who was only 2 years younger than his patient. Both elderly gentlemen, the patient and his surgeon, were rather short in stature, gray haired, and balding, but the patient was corpulent and stocky, and his surgeon was lean and agile.

Dunhill was described by his colleagues as "modest, courteous, professionally correct and of complete intellectual integrity." He was a master surgeon being appointed to the Royal household in 1928, and in 1930 as honorary surgeon to King George V and later to King Edward VIII and King George VI. In 1935 on his 60th birthday, Dunhill retired from the staff of St Bartholomew's Hospital and engaged in a flourishing private practice at No 54 Harley Street. He was born and educated in Australia and after qualifying in medicine came to London as first assistant to

Professor George Gask at the new professorial unit at the University of London at St Bartholomew's Hospital. In 1939 he was awarded an honorary FRCS England, the first time this title had been bestowed on a surgeon who was in active practice.

Winston Churchill first became aware of his hernia on September 5th, 1945, writing to his wife Clementine that he had recently ruptured himself and developed a painless swelling and would have to be fitted with a truss. He was consulted by Lord Moran, long-time president of the Royal College of Physicians who in turn consulted Brigadier Edwards the consulting surgeon for the army in Italy who advised that Churchill should buy a truss in Milan.

For almost 2 years, nothing was heard about Churchill's hernia until in June 1947; in Moran's diaries, it is reported that the hernia was now much larger, it had been increasingly difficult to control with a truss, and it was hardly ever out of his mind. Thomas Dunhill has been selected as the prospective surgeon.

Churchill's habits of smoking cigars and alcohol consumption were well known, and he undoubtedly suffered from chronic obstructive airways disease and obesity. The operation would therefore have been challenging.

On the morning of the operation, Churchill was found in bed reading loudly from Thomas Babbington McCauley's essays. The operation was performed under general anesthesia, presumably ether, and lasted for more than 2 h. The type of hernia and the method of repair were unknown, but the method was probably a type of Bassini procedure. Postoperative recovery was uneventful with the patient experiencing little discomfort.

Dunhill's herniorrhaphy proved successful and durable for Churchill's groin remained asymptomatic for the next 17.5 years until his death. Dunhill stopped operating in 1949 when he had only three patients left, "The King (George VI), Queen Mary, and Winston Churchill."

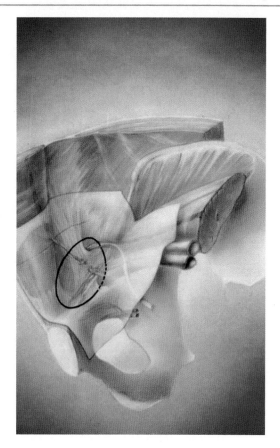

Fig. 1.26 Myopectineal orifice of Fruchaud

ideas but even so the first edition of his book "Hernia Repair Without Disability" written in 1970 sold rather poorly and never went beyond the first printing [43]. Subsequent additions, however, required numerous reprints to meet demand paralleling the increase in popularity and worldwide success of the mesh-patch repair devised by Lichtenstein.

Tension-Free Hernia Repair

Irving Lichtenstein is the seminal thinker who introduced tension-free prosthetic repair of groin hernias into everyday, commonplace, outpatient practices. As well as being an office procedure under local anesthetic, Lichtenstein pioneered the idea that hernia surgery is special, that it must be performed by an experienced surgeon and cannot be relegated to the unsupervised trainee doing "minor" surgery. The key feature of Lichtenstein's technique is the "tensionless" operation. With his coworkers, Shulman and Amid, he has developed a simple prosthetic operation, which can be performed on outpatients [57, 58] (Fig. 1.26). As a pioneer, Lichtenstein worked hard to promulgate his

Laparoscopic Repair

Laparoscopic repair continues to develop its place in the surgical armamentarium of inguinal hernia. The use of the laparoscope has been extended to repair incisional, ventral, lumbar, and paracolostomy hernias. This latter technique is rapidly gaining in popularity.

The first attempt to treat an inguinal hernia with the laparoscope was made by P. Fletcher of the University of the West Indies in 1979 [59]. He closed the neck of the hernia sac. The first report of the use of a clip (Michel) placed laparoscopically to close the neck of the sac was made by Ger in 1982, who reported a series of thirteen patients: all the patients in this series were repaired through an open incision except the thirteenth patient who was repaired under laparoscopic guidance with a special stapling device. The 3-year follow-up of that patient revealed him to be free of an identifiable recurrence. Ger continued his efforts to repair these hernias laparoscopically. He reported the closure of the neck of the hernia sac using a prototypical instrument called the "herniostat" in beagle dogs [60]. The results in these models appeared to be promising. In that same article, he reported the potential benefits of the laparoscopic approach to groin hernia repair as (1) creation of puncture wounds rather than formal incisions, (2) need for minimal dissection, (3) less danger of spermatic cord injury and less risk of ischemic orchitis, (4) minimal risk of bladder injury, (5) decreased incidence of neuralgias, (6) possibility of an outpatient procedure, (7) ability to achieve the highest possible ligation of the hernial sac, (8) minimal postoperative discomfort and a faster recovery time, (9) ability to perform simultaneous diagnostic laparoscopy, and (10) ability to diagnose and treat bilateral inguinal hernias. These potential advantages and advances in the laparoscopic repair of hernias continue to be the recognized goals that each method is attempting to achieve.

Bogojavalensky, a gynecologist, presented the first known use of a prosthetic biomaterial in the laparoscopic repair of inguinal and femoral hernias in 1989 [61]. He placed a roll of polypropylene mesh into indirect hernias of female patients. The neck of the internal inguinal ring was then closed with sutures. Popp repaired a coincidental direct hernia that was found at the time of a uterine myomectomy [62]. He recognized the need to provide coverage of a wider area than that of the defect itself. To accomplish this, he placed a 4×5-cm oval dehydrated dura mater patch over the defect. This was secured to the peritoneum with catgut sutures that were tied extracorporeally. Popp expressed concerns that the intra-abdominal repair of inguinal hernia could lead to adhesive complications and suggested that a preperitoneal approach might be preferable.

Schultz published the first patient series of laparoscopic herniorrhaphy in 1990 [63]. Rolls of polypropylene were stuffed into the hernial orifice, which was then covered by two or three flat sheets of polypropylene mesh (2.5×5 cm) over the defect. These rolls of mesh were not secured to either the fascia or peritoneum. To achieve access to the hernia defect, he incised the peritoneum. Following the placement of the rolls, he closed the peritoneum with clips. This probably represents the earliest attempt at a type of transabdominal preperitoneal (TAPP) repair that is commonly used today. Corbitt modified this technique by inverting the hernia sac and performing a high ligation with sutures or with an endoscopic stapling device [64]. Despite the initial success of these early reports, because of recurrence rates approaching 15–20%, these techniques were

abandoned [65]. The lack of extensive dissection with the above methods, however, remained appealing. A similar concept was applied in the intraperitoneal onlay patch (IPOM) technique. Salerno, Fitzgibbons, and Filipi investigated this type of repair in the porcine model [66]. They placed rectangular pieces of flat polypropylene mesh to cover the myopectineal orifice and secured it with a stapling device. The success of these repairs led them to apply this method in clinical trials.

At about the same time, Toy and Smoot reported upon their first ten patients that were repaired with the IPOM technique [67]. They secured an expanded polytetrafluoroethylene patch (ePTFE) to the inguinal floor with staples that were introduced by a prototypical-stapling device of their own design, the "Nanticoke Hernia Stapler." They successfully used this fixation device in 20–30 patients without adverse results. A subsequent report of their first 75 patients was published in 1992 [68]. In this later series, the same prosthetic biomaterial (7.5×10 cm) was attached with the Endopath EMS® stapler. After a follow-up of up to 20 months, the recurrence rate was 2.4%. They noted a significant decrease in postoperative pain and an earlier return to normal activity as compared to the open repair of the hernia defect. Others reported similar results [69].

Fitzgibbons later abandoned the IPOM repair except for simple indirect inguinal hernias [70]. One patient developed a postoperative scrotal abscess that may or may not have been related to the placement of the mesh in that position. This patient was noted to have firm attachment of the appendix to the site of the polypropylene mesh. He also noted that, in follow-up of these patients, the patch material could be pulled into the hernial defect because it was affixed to the peritoneum alone rather than fascia. Because of these adverse events, he believed that the TAPP approach, which had been reported by Arregui [71] for inguinal hernia repair, was more appropriate. In this repair, the peritoneum is incised and dissected away from the transversalis fascia to expose the inguinal floor. The mesh material is then secured to that fascia which was believed to ensure superior fixation and tissue ingrowth. Both the TAPP and IPOM techniques require the entry into the abdominal cavity.

In a continuing effort to prevent bowel contact to the prosthesis, Popp described a method to dissect the peritoneum away from the abdominal wall prior to the incision of the peritoneum in the TAPP repair in 1991 [72]. Saline was inserted into the preperitoneal space with a percutaneous syringe. This "aquadissection" was found to be helpful in the dissection of this area to create a space in which to operate within the preperitoneal space. This early concept probably led to the idea that the entire dissection could be accomplished from within the preperitoneal space, thereby eliminating the need to enter the abdominal cavity.

Additional variations that did not gain acceptance were the "ring plasty" and a preperitoneal iliopubic tract repair. The former method was simply a sutured repair that approximated the deep structures of the lateral iliopubic tract to the proximal arching musculotendinous fibers of the transversus abdominis muscle [73, 74]. The latter technique was also a "tissue" repair but secured the iliopubic tract to the transversus abdominis muscle [75, 76]. This repair incorporated the use of an inlay of a prosthetic material but still had the disadvantage of being a repair under tension. These methods may have limited usage in rare circumstances.

In these earlier years, the predominant laparoscopic method of inguinal herniorrhaphy was the TAPP approach using either a polypropylene mesh or an expanded polytetrafluoroethylene material [72, 74, 77]. In 1992, Dulucq [78, 79] was the first surgeon to perform "retroperitoneoscopy" to effect a repair of an inguinal hernia without any direct entry into the abdominal cavity. In 1993, Phillips and Arregui separately described a technique that did not utilize a peritoneal incision in the repair of the inguinal floor [80, 81]. The dissection of the preperitoneal space was accomplished under direct visualization of the area via a laparoscope placed into the abdominal cavity. The laparoscope was then moved into the newly dissected preperitoneal space to complete the repair. Ferzli and McKernan later popularized the technique of Dulucq preferring the term "totally extraperitoneal" [82, 83]. Using the "open" entry into the preperitoneal space, the dissection of the space was carried out under direct visualization. This totally extraperitoneal (TEP) repair was identical to that of the TAPP but appeared to incur less risk of injury to the intra-abdominal organs.

Currently, the majority of laparoscopic inguinal hernia repairs are approached by either the TAPP or TEP method and utilize a polypropylene mesh biomaterial. The majority of the surgeons that perform the TEP repair utilize the commercially available dissection balloons to create the space within the preperitoneal area to perform the repair.

In a multicenter report, the recurrence rate of these repairs was 0.4% in 10,053 repairs with a median follow-up of 36 months [84]. The surgeons that continue to perform the laparoscopic herniorrhaphy believe that the goals that were anticipated by Ger have been realized.

The improvement in recovery in laparoscopic cholecystectomy patients and results that were seen in herniorrhaphy patients encouraged attempts to repair ventral and incisional hernias in 1991. The initial report by LeBlanc involved only five patients using an ePTFE patch biomaterial [85]. Although the overlap of the hernia defect by the prosthesis was only 1.5–2 cm, these patients were free of recurrence after 7 years of follow-up. The fixation used was that of the "box-type" of hernia stapler without the use of sutures. Sutures were used only to aid in the positioning of the patch. These sutures were removed from the prosthesis at the completion of the stapling of the patch. With further patients and follow-up, no recurrences were noted [86]. Barie proposed the use of a polyester material covered on the visceral side with a mesh of absorbable polyglactin [87].

Park modified the technique for the repair of large ventral hernias by utilizing the transfascial fixation of the ePTFE or Prolene® mesh with transabdominally placed Prolene® sutures passed through a Keith needle [88]. In their series of thirty cases, only one recurrence was noted. This repair used a fascial overlap of 2 cm. Holzman placed a Marlex® prosthesis with a 4 cm. overlap onto normal fascial edges and secured them with an endoscopic stapler [89]. He found this technique to be safe and effective. In separate investigations, Holzman, Park, and others compared the open versus laparoscopic methods and found that the laparoscopic repair was associated with fewer postoperative complications, a shorter hospital stay and lower recurrence rates than open prosthetic repair [89–93]. The largest study published to date confirms that the laparoscopic repair of incisional and ventral hernias can be accomplished with reproducibility and with excellent results [94]. Additionally, the long-term follow-up of LeBlanc's patients has proven that this is a durable procedure when the tenets that are noted below are applied.

1. A minimum prosthetic overlap of 3 cm.
2. Helical tacks placed 1–1.5 cm intervals.
3. Transfascial sutures placed at 5 cm intervals [85, 86].

Others, however, do not share this view. Some surgeons, notably in Spain, prefer the use of the "double-crown" technique [95, 96]. In this technique no sutures are used. Instead, two concentric rows of helical tacks are placed. The first is at the periphery of the biomaterial as in the sutured technique, and the second is inside of this one, near the hernia defect itself. The initial reports seem to have similar results as that of the authors using the transfascial sutures, but only a longer interval of follow-up will prove or disprove of either one or both of these approaches are the best.

Chronology of Hernia Surgery

Ancient	
1500 BC	Inguinal hernia described in an Egyptian papyrus. An inguinal hernia is depicted on a Greek statuette from this period [2]
900 BC	Tightly fitting bandages are used to treat an inguinal hernia by physicians in Alexandria. A Phoenician statue depicts this [2]
400 BC	Hippocrates distinguished hernia and hydrocele by transillumination [2]
AD 40	Celsus described the older Greek operations for hernia [97]
AD 200	Galen introduced the concept of "rupture" of the peritoneum allowed by failure of the belly wall tissues [2]
AD 700	Paul of Aegina distinguished complete and incomplete hernia. He recommended amputation of the testicle in repair [2]
Medieval	
1363	Guy de Chauliac distinguished inguinal and femoral hernia [4]
1556	Franco recommended dividing the constriction at the neck of a strangulated hernial sac [5]
1559	Stromayr published Practica Copiosa, differentiating direct and indirect hernia and advocating excision of the sac in indirect hernia [6]
Renaissance	
1700	Littre reported a Meckel's diverticulum in a hernial sac [98]
1724	Heister distinguished direct and indirect hernia [99]
1731	De Carengeot described the appendix in a hernial sac [100]
1757	Pott described the anatomy of hernia and of strangulation [9]
1756	Cheselden described successful operation for an inguinal hernia [7]
1785	Richter described a partial enterocele [101]
1790	John Hunter speculated about the congenital nature of complete indirect inguinal hernia [102]
1793	De Gimbernat described his ligament and advocated medial rather than upward division of the constriction in strangulated femoral hernia. This avoided damage to the inguinal ligament and the serious bleeding, which sometimes followed [103]
1804	Cooper published his three-part book on hernia—The plates are a tour de force; they are almost life sized and depict anatomy as never before. Cooper defined the fascia transversalis; he distinguished this layer from the peritoneum and demonstrated that it was the main barrier to herniation. He carefully delineated the extension of the fascia transversalis behind the inguinal ligament into the thigh as the femoral sheath and the pectineal part of the inguinal ligament—Cooper's ligament [10, 104, 105]
1811	Colles, who had worked as a dissector for Cooper, described the reflected inguinal ligament [106]
1816	Hesselbach described the anatomy of his triangle [107]
1816	Cloquet described the processus vaginalis and observed it was rarely closed at birth. He also described his "gland," so important in the differential diagnosis of lumps in the groin [108]
1846	Anesthesia discovered
1870	Lister introduced antiseptic surgery and carbolized catgut [11]
1871	Marcy, who had been a pupil of Lister, described his operation [17]
1874	Steele described a radical operation for hernia [109]
1875	Annandale successfully used an extraperitoneal groin approach to treat a direct and an indirect inguinal and a femoral hernia on the same side in a 46-year-old man. Annandale plugged the femoral canal with the redundant inguinal hernial sacs [110]
1876	Czerny pulled the sac down through the external ring, ligated it at its neck, excised it, and allowed it to retract back into the canal [14]
1881	Lucas-Championniere opened the canal and reconstructed it by imbrication of its anterior wall [111]
1886	MacEwan operated through the external ring; he rolled up the sac and used it to plug the canal [15]
1887	Bassini published the first description of his operation [91]
1889	Halsted I operation described [27]
1890	Coley's operation—placing the internal oblique anterior to the cord which emerged at the pubic end of the repair. This was the most pernicious and least effective corruption of Bassini's operation [33]
1891	Tait advocated median abdominal section for hernia [42]
1892	Wolfler designed the anterior relaxing incision in the rectus sheath to relieve tension on the pubic end repair and prevent recurrence at that site [29]
1893	Lockwood emphasized the importance of adequate repair of the fascia transversalis [36]
1895	W.J. Mayo—a radical cure for umbilical hernia [112]
1895	Andrews introduced imbrication or "double breasting" of the layers [35]
1898	Lotheissen used Cooper's ligament in repair of femoral hernia [113]
1898	Brenner described "reinforcing" the repair by suturing the cremaster between the internal oblique arch and the inguinal ligament. The fascia transversalis is not inspected. A serious corruption of the Marcy–Bassini strategy [114]

(continued)

(continued)

1899	Ferguson advised leaving the cord undisturbed—a more serious corruption of Bassini [34]
1901	McArthur darned his inguinal repair with a pedicled strip of external oblique aponeurosis [115]
1902	Berger turned down a rectus flap to repair inguinal hernia [116]

Modern Aseptic 1903

1903	Halsted II operation. Halsted abandoned cord skeletonization to avoid hydrocele and testicular atrophy and adopted Andrews' imbrication and the Wolfler–Berger technique of a relaxation incision and a rectus sheath flap [117]
1906	Russell—the "saccular theory" of hernias, postulating that all indirect inguinal hernias are congenital [118]
1907	Kocher revised operation for indirect hernia without opening the canal. The sac was dissected, invaginated, and transposed laterally [16]
1909	McGavin used silver filigree to repair inguinal hernias [119]
1909	Nicol reported pediatric day-case inguinal herniotomy in Glasgow [120]
1910	Kirschner used a free transplant of fascia lata from the thigh to reinforce the external oblique [121]
1918	Handley reconstructed the canal using a darn/lattice technique [122]
1919	LaRoque—transperitoneal repair of inguinal hernia through grid iron (muscle-splitting) incision [39]
1920	Cheatle—extraperitoneal approach to the groin through a midline incision [40]
1921	Gallie used strips of autologous fascia lata to repair inguinal hernia [123]
1923	Keith—classic review of the causation of inguinal hernia. He remarked that aponeurosis and fascia are living structures and speculated that a tissue defect could be responsible for the onset of hernias in middle age [124]
1927	Keynes—surgeon to the London Truss Society—advocated elective operation using fascial graft techniques [125]
1936	Henry—extraperitoneal approach to groin hernia [46]
1940	Wakeley—a personal series of 2,020 hernias [126]
1942	Tanner popularized rectus sheath "slide" [31]
1945	Lytle reinterpreted the importance of the internal ring [127]
1945	Mair introduced the technique of using buried skin to repair an inguinal hernia [128]
1952	Douglas—first experimental studies of the dynamics of healing (aponeurosis) showed that aponeurotic strength was slow to recover and only reached an optimum at 120 days [129]
1953	Shouldice—a series of 8,317 hernia repairs with overall recurrence rate to 10 years of 0.8%. Emphasis on anatomic repair and early ambulation [130]
1955	Farquharson—an experience of 485 adults who had their hernias repaired as day cases [131]
1956	Fruchaud—the concept of the myopectineal orifice and fascia transversalis tunnel for all groin hernias [51]
1958	Marsden—a 3-year follow-up of inguinal hernioplasties. An important contribution to the evaluation of results [132]
1958	Usher—the use of knitted polypropylene mesh in hernia repair [133]
1960	Anson and McVay—classic dissections and evaluation of musculoaponeurotic layers based on a study of 500 body halves [134]
1962	Doran described the pitfalls of hernia follow-up and set out criteria for adequate evaluation [135]
1970	Lichtenstein showed the interdependence of suture strength and absorption characteristics with wound healing. Demonstrated experimentally the critical role of nonabsorbable or very slowly absorbable sutures in aponeurotic healing [136]
1972	Doran—critical review of short-stay surgery for inguinal hernia in Birmingham [137]
1973	Glassow reported 18,400 repairs of indirect hernia with a recurrence rate less than 1% [138]
1979	Laparoscopic hernia repair first attempted [59]
1981	Read demonstrated a tissue defect, metastatic emphysema, in smokers with direct herniation [139]
1981	Chan described patients developing hernia while undergoing continuous ambulatory peritoneal dialysis [140]
1983	Schurgers demonstrated an open processus vaginalis in a man 5 months after commencement on peritoneal dialysis [141]
1984	Gilbert described the umbrella plug for inguinal hernia repair [142]
1985	Read postulated an etiological relationship between smoking, inguinal herniation, and aortic aneurysm [143]
1986	Lichtenstein described the tension-free repair of inguinal hernias [144]
1989	Gullmo demonstrates the value of herniorrhaphy in patients with obscure symptoms in the groin or pelvis and to exclude primary or recurrent hernia [145]
1990	Robbins and Rutkow introduced the concept of a preformed mesh plug introduced into the hernia defect covered by a loose-lying mesh patch [146]
1990	Schultz first used a synthetic prosthetic biomaterial in the laparoscopic repair of an inguinal hernia [63]
1991	LeBlanc performs laparoscopic incisional hernia repair [147]
1992	Dulucq repairs an inguinal hernia laparoscopically without direct entry into the abdominal cavity [78]
1993	Environmental factors in hernia causation redefined [148]
1994	O Jeremy A Gilmore describes the surgical treatment of 1,400 sportsmen with groin disruption detailing the pathophysiology and treatment [149]

References

1. Primatesta P, Goldacre MJ. Inguinal hernia repair: incidence of elective and emergency surgery, readmission and mortality. Int J Epidemiol. 1996;25:835–9.
2. Read RC. The development of inguinal herniorrhaphy. Surg Clin North Am. 1984;64:185–96.
3. Stoppa R, Wantz GE, Munegato G, Pluchinotta A. Hernia Healers: an illustrated history. France: Arnette; 1998.
4. De Chauliac G. La Grande Chirurgie composee en 1363. Revue avec des notes, une introduction sur le moyenage. Sur la vie et les oeuvres de Guy de Chauliac par E. Nicaise. Paris: Felix Alcan; 1890.
5. Franco P. Traite des hernies contenant une ample declaration de toutes leurs especes et outres excellentes parites de la chirurgie, assauoir de la Pierre, des cataracts des yeux, et autres maladies, desquelles comme la cure est perilluese, aussi est elle de' peu d'hommes bien exercee. Lyon: Thibauld Payan; 1561.
6. Stromayr. Practica Copiosa-Lindau 1559. In: Rutkow IM, editor. Surgery. An illustrated history. St Louis: Mosby; 1993
7. Cheselden W. The Anatomy of the Human Body. 12th ed. London: Livingston, Dodsley, Cadell, Baldwin and Lowndes; 1784.
8. Le Dran HF. The operations in surgery. London: Dodsley and Lay; 1781. p. 59–60.
9. Pott P. Treatise on ruptures. London: Hitch and Howes; 1757.
10. Cooper A. The anatomy and surgical treatment of inguinal and congenital hernia I. London: T Cox; 1804.
11. Lister J. Note on the preparation of catgut for surgical purposes. Br Med J. 1908;1:125–6.
12. Devlin HB. History of surgical procedures. Sonderdruck aus Hygiene in Chirurgischen Alltag. Berlin: De Gruyter; 1993.
13. Wood J. On rupture, inguinal, crural and umbilical. London: JW Davies; 1863.
14. Czerny V. Studien zur Radikalbehandlung der Hernien. Wien Med Wochenschr. 1877;27:497–500.
15. MacEwen W. On the radical cure of oblique inguinal hernia by internal abdominal peritoneal pad and the restoration of the valved form of the inguinal canal. Ann Surg. 1886;4:89–119.
16. Kocher T. Chirurgische operationslehre. Jena: Verlag von Gustav Fischer; 1907.
17. Marcy HO. The cure of hernia. J Am Med Assoc. 1887;8:589–92.
18. Bassini E. Nuova technica per la cura radicale dell'ernia. Atti del Associazione Medica Italiano Congresso. 1887;2:179–82.
19. Bassini E. Nuova technica per la cura dell'ernia inguinale. Societa Italiana di Chirurgica. 1887;4:379–82.
20. Bassini E. Ueber die Behandlung des Leistenbruches, vol. 40. Berlin: Archiv fur Klinische Chirurgie; 1890. p. 429–76.
21. Read RC. Marcy's priority in the development of inguinal herniorrhaphy. Surgery. 1980;88:682–5.
22. Haidenthaller J. Die Radicaloperationen der Hernien in der Klinik des Hofraths Professor Dr Billroth, 1877–1889. Archiv fur Klinische Chirurgie. 1890;40:493–555.
23. Marcy HO. A new use of carbolized catgut ligatures. Boston Med Surg J. 1871;85:315–6.
24. Catterina A. Bassini's operation. London: Lewis; 1934.
25. Catterina A. L'operatione di Bassini der la cura radicale dell'ernia inguinale. Bolognia, Italia: L. Capelli; 1932.
26. Wantz GE. The operation of Bassini as described by Attilio Catterina. Surg Gyn Obst. 1989;168:67–80.
27. Halsted WS. The radical cure of hernia. Bull Johns Hopkins Hosp. 1889;1:12–3.
28. Halsted WS. An additional note on the operation for inguinal hernia. In: Halsted WS, editor. Surgical papers, vol. 1. Baltimore: John Hopkins Press; 1924. p. 306–8.
29. Wolfler A. Zur radikaloperation des Freien Leistenbruches. Beitr. Chir (Festchr Geuidmet Theodor Billroth). Stuttgart: Hoffman; 1892. p. 552–603.
30. Reinhoff Jr WF. The use of the rectus fascia for closure of the lower or critical angle of the wound in the repair of inguinal hernia. Surgery. 1940;8:326–39.
31. Tanner NC. A slide operation for inguinal and femoral hernia. Br J Surg. 1942;29:285–9.
32. Bull WT. Notes on cases of hernia which have relapsed after various operations for radical cure. NY Med J. 1891;53:615–7.
33. Coley WB. The operative treatment of hernia with a report of 200 cases. Ann Surg. 1895;21:389–437.
34. Ferguson AH. Oblique inguinal hernia. Typical operation for its radical cure. J Am Med Assoc. 1899;33:6–14.
35. Andrews WE. Imbrication of lap joint method: a plastic operation for hernia. Chicago Med Rec. 1895;9:67–77.
36. Lockwood CB. The radical cure of femoral and inguinal hernia. Lancet. 1893;2:1297–302.
37. Lockwood CB. The radical cure of hernia, hydrocele and varicocele. Edinburgh and London: Young; 1898.
38. Shearburn EW, Myers RN. Shouldice repair for inguinal hernia. Surgery. 1969;66:450–9.
39. LaRoque GP. The permanent cure of inguinal and femoral hernia. A modification of the standard operative procedures. Surg Gyn Obst. 1919;29:507–11.
40. Cheatle GL. An operation for radical cure of inguinal and femoral hernia. Br Med J. 1920;2:68–9.
41. Marcy HO. Note on mortality after operation for large incarcerated hernia. Ann Surg. 1900;31:65–74.
42. Tait L. A discussion on treatment of hernia by median abdominal section. Br Med J. 1891;2:685–91.
43. Rutkow IM. A selective history of groin herniorrhaphy in the 20th century. Surg Clin North Am. 1993;73:395–411.
44. Battle WH. Abstract of a clinical lecture on femoral hernia. Lancet. 1901;1:302–5.
45. Cheatle GL. An operation for inguinal hernia. Br Med J. 1921;2:1025–6.
46. Henry AK. Operation for femoral hernia by a midline extraperitoneal approach: with a preliminary note on the use of this route for reducible inguinal hernia. Lancet. 1936;2:531–3.
47. McEvedy PG. Femoral hernia. Ann R Coll Surg Engl. 1950;7:484–96.
48. Musgrove JE, McReady FJ. The Henry approach to femoral hernia. Surgery. 1949;26:608–11.
49. Mikkelsen WP, Berne CJ. Femoral hernioplasty: suprapubic extraperitoneal (Cheatle-Henry) approach. Surgery. 1954;35:743–8.
50. Lytle WJ. The deep inguinal ring, development, function and repair. Br J Surg. 1970;57:531–6.
51. Fruchaud H. L'Anatomie Chirurgicale de L'Aine. Paris: C. Dion & Co; 1956.
52. Le FH. traitement chirurgicale des hernies de l'aine chez l'adulte. Paris: G Dion; 1956.
53. Stoppa R, Wantz GE. Henri Fruchaud (1894-1960): a man of bravery, an anatomist, a surgeon. Hernia. 1998;2:45–7.
54. Stoppa R, Warlaumont CR, Verhaeghe PJ, Odimba BKFE, Henry X. Comment, pourquoi, quand utiliser les prostheses de tulle de Dacron pour traiter les hernies et les eventrations. Chirurgie. 1982;108:570–5.
55. Wantz GE. Atlas of hernia surgery. New York: Raven; 1991.
56. Schein M, Rodgers PN. Winston S Churchill's (1874-1965) inguinal hernia repair by Thomas P Dunhill (1878-1957). J Am Coll Surg. 2003;197:313–21.
57. Amid PK, Shulman AG, Lichtenstein IL. Critical suturing of the tension free hernioplasty. Am J Surg. 1993;165:369–72.
58. Lichtenstein IL, Shulman AG, Amid PK, Montilier MM. The tension-free hernioplasty. Am J Surg. 1989;157:188–93.

59. Ger R. The management of certain abdominal herniae by intra-abdominal closure of the neck of the sac. Ann R Coll Surg Engl. 1982;64:342–4.

60. Ger R, Monro K, Duvivier R, et al. Management of inguinal hernias by laparoscopic closure of the neck of the sac. Am J Surg. 1990;159:370–3.

61. Bogojavalensky S. Laparoscopic treatment of inguinal and femoral hernia (video presentation). 18th Annual Meeting of the American Association of Gynecological Laparoscopists. Washington DC; 1989.

62. Popp LW. Endoscopic patch repair of inguinal hernia in a female patient. Surg Endosc. 1990;5:10–2.

63. Schultz L, Graber J, Pietrafitta J, et al. Laser laparoscopic herniorrhaphy: a clinical trial, preliminary results. J Laparoendosc Surg. 1990;1:41–5.

64. Corbitt J. Laparoscopic herniorrhaphy. Surg Laparosc Endosc. 1991;1:23–5.

65. Corbitt J. Laparoscopic herniorrhaphy: a preperitoneal tension-free approach. Surg Endosc. 1993;7:550–5.

66. Salerno GM, Fitzgibbons RJ, Filipi C. Laparoscopic inguinal hernia repair. In: Zucker KA, editor. Surgical laparoscopy. St Louis: Quality Medical Publishing; 1991. p. 281–93.

67. Toy FK, Smoot RT. Toy-Smoot laparoscopic hernioplasty. Surg Laparosc Endosc. 1991;1:151–5.

68. Toy FK, Smoot RT. Laparoscopic hernioplasty update. J Laparoendosc Surg. 1992;2(5):197–205.

69. Spaw AT, Ennis BW, Spaw LP. Laparoscopic hernia repair: the anatomical basis. J Laparoendosc Surg. 1991;1:269–77.

70. Fitzgibbons RP. Laparoscopic inguinal hernia repair. In: Zucker KA, editor. Surgical laparoscopy update. St Louis: Quality Medical Publishing; 1993. p. 373–934.

71. Arregui ME. Preperitoneal repair of direct inguinal hernia with mesh. Indianapolis, Indiana: Presented at Advanced Laparoscopic Surgery: The International Experience; 1991.

72. Popp LW. Improvement in endoscopic hernioplasty: transcutaneous aquadissection of the musculo fascial defect and preperitoneal endoscopic patch repair. J Laparoendosc Surg. 1991;1(2):83–90.

73. Dion YM, Morin J. Laparoscopic inguinal herniorrhaphy. Can J Surg. 1992;35:209–12.

74. Kavic MS. Laparoscopic hernia repair. Surg Endosc. 1993;7:163–7.

75. Gazayerli MM. Anatomic laparoscopic repair of direct or indirect hernias using the transversalis fascia and iliopubic tract. Surg Laparosc Endosc. 1992;2:49–52.

76. Gazayerli MM, Arregui ME, Helmy HS. Alternative technique: laparoscopic iliopubic tract (IPTR) inguinal hernia repair with inlay buttress of polypropylene mesh. In: Ballabtyne GH, Leahy PF, Modlin IR, editors. EDS laparoscopic surgery. Philadelphia: WB Saunders; 1993.

77. Campos L, Sipes E. Laparoscopic hernia repair: use of a fenestrated PTFE graft with endo-clips. Surg Laparosc Endosc. 1993;3(1):35–8.

78. Dulucq JL. Treatment of inguinal hernia by insertion of a subperitoneal patch under pre-peritoneoscopy. Chirurgie. 1992; 118(1–2):83–5.

79. Dulucq JL. Treatment of inguinal hernias by insertion of mesh through retroperitoneoscopy. Post Grad Surg. 1992;4(2):173–4.

80. Phillips EH, Carroll BJ, Fallas MJ. Laparoscopic preperitoneal inguinal hernia repair without peritoneal incision: technique and early clinical results. Surg Endosc. 1993;7:159–62.

81. Arregui ME, Navarrette J, Davis CJ, et al. Laparoscopic inguinal herniorrhaphy: techniques and controversies. Surg Clin North Am. 1993;73(3):513–27.

82. Ferzli GS, Massad A, Albert P. Extraperitoneal endoscopic inguinal hernia repair. J Laparoendosc Surg. 1992;2(6):281–6.

83. McKernan JB, Laws HL. Laparoscopic repair of inguinal hernias using a totally extraperitoneal prosthetic approach. Surg Endosc. 1993;7:26–8.

84. Felix E, Scotts S, Crafton B, et al. Causes of recurrence after laparoscopic hernioplasty. Surg Endosc. 1998;12:226–31.

85. LeBlanc KA, Booth WV, Whitaker JA, Bellanger DE. Laparoscopic incisional and ventral herniorrhaphy: our initial 100 patients. Am J Surg. 2000;180(3):193–7.

86. LeBlanc KA. Current considerations in laparoscopic incisional and ventral herniorrhaphy. JSLS. 2000;4:131–9.

87. Barie PS, Mack CA, Thompson WA. A technique for laparoscopic repair for herniation of the anterior abdominal wall using a composite mesh prosthesis. Am J Surg. 1995;170:62–3.

88. Park A, Gagner M, Pomp A. Laparoscopic repair of large incisional hernias. Surg Laparosc Endosc. 1996;6(2):123–8.

89. Holzman MD, Parut CM, Reintgen K, et al. Laparoscopic ventral and incisional hernioplasty. Surg Endosc. 1997;11:32–5.

90. Park A, Birch DW, Lovrics P, et al. Laparoscopic and open incisional hernia repair: a comparison study. Surgery. 1998;124:816–22.

91. Carbajo MA, Martin del Olmo JC, Blanco JI, de la Cuesta C, Toledano M, Martin F, Vaqueto C, Inglada L. Laparoscopic treatment vs. open surgery in the solution of major incisional and abdominal wall hernias with mesh. Surg Endosc. 1999;13:250–2.

92. Ramshaw BJ, Escartia P, Schwab J, Mason EM, Wilson RA, Duncan TD, Miller J, Lucas GW, Promes J. Comparison of laparoscopic and open ventral herniorrhaphy. Am Surg. 1999;65:827–32.

93. DeMarie EJ, Moss JM, Sugerman HJ. Laparoscopic intraperitoneal polytetrafluoroethylene (PTFE) prosthetic patch repair of ventral hernia. Surg Endosc. 2000;14:326–9.

94. Heniford BT, Park A, Ramshaw BJ, Voeller G. Laparoscopic ventral and incisional hernia repair in 407 patients. J Am Coll Surg. 2000;190(6):645–50.

95. Carbajo MA, Martin del Olmo JC, Blanco JI, de la Cuesta C, Martin F, Toledano M, Pernac C, Vaquero C. Laparoscopic treatment of ventral abdominal wall hernias: preliminary results in 100 patients. JSLS. 2000;4:141–5.

96. Morales-Conde S. Personal communication. 2001.

97. Celsus AC. Of medicine. In: James Grieve, editor. Translated. London; 1756.

98. Littré A. Observation sur une nouvelle espece de hernie. Paris: Histoire de l'Academie des Sciences (1700); 1719. p. 300–10.

99. De Garengeot RJC. Traite des Operations de Chirurgie. 2nd ed. Paris: Huart; 1731. p. 369–71.

100. Heister L. A general system of surgery in three parts (translated into English from the Latin). London: Innys, Davis, Clark, Manby and Whiston; 1743.

101. Richter A. Abhandlung von den Brüchen. Göttingen: I.C. Dietrich; 1785.

102. Hunter J. Palmer's edition of Hunter's works. Vol. 4. London; 1837. p. 1.

103. De Gimbernat A. Nuevo metodo de operar en la hernia crural. Madrid: Ibarra; 1793.

104. Cooper A. The anatomy and surgical treatment of inguinal and congenital hernia I. London: T. Cox; 1804.

105. Cooper A. The anatomy and surgical treatment of hernia II. London: Longman, Hurst, Rees and Orme; 1807.

106. Colles AA. Treatise on surgical anatomy. Dublin: Gilbert and Hodges; 1811.

107. Hesselbach FK. Neueste Anatomisch-Pathologische Untersuchungen über den Ursprung und das Fortschreiten der Leisten- und Schenkelbrüche. Warzburg: Baumgartner; 1814.

108. Cloquet J. Recherches anatomiques sur les hernies de l'abdomen. These Paris. 1817;133:129.

109. Steele C. On operations for the radical cure of hernia. Br Med J. 1874;2:584.

110. Annandale T. Reducible oblique and direct inguinal and femoral hernia. Edinb Med J. 1876;21:1087–91.

111. Lucas-Championniere J. Chirurgie operatoire: cure radicale des hernies; avec une etude statistique de deux cents soixante-quinze

operations et cinquante figures intercalees dans le texte. Paris: Rueff; 1892.

112. Mayo WJ. An operation for the radical cure of umbilical hernia. Ann Surg. 1901;31:276–80.

113. Lotheissen G. Zur Radikaloperation der Schenkel-hernien. Centralblatt für Chirurgie. 1898;21:548–9.

114. Brenner A. Zur radical operation der Leisten-hernien. Zentralbl Chir. 1898;25:1017–23.

115. McArthur LL. Autoplastic suture in hernia and other diastases. J Am Med Assoc. 1901;37:1162–5.

116. Berger P. La hernie inguino-interstitielle et son traitement par la cure radicale. Rev Chir. 1902;25:1.

117. Halsted WS. The operative treatment of hernia. Am J Med Sci. 1895;110:13–7.

118. Russell H. The saccular theory of hernia and the radical operation. Lancet. 1906;3:1197–203.

119. McGavin L. The double filigree operation for the radical cure of inguinal hernia. Br Med J. 1909;2:357–63.

120. Nichol JH. The surgery of infancy. Br Med J. 1909;2:753–4.

121. Kirschner M. Die praktischen Ergebnisse der freien Fascien-Transplantation. Archiv für Klinische Chirurgie. 1910;92:889–912.

122. Handley WS. A method for the radical cure of inguinal hernia (darn and stay-lace method). Practitioner. 1918;100:466–71.

123. Gallie WE, Le Mesurier AB. Living sutures in the treatment of hernia. Can Med Assoc J. 1923;13:468–80.

124. Keith A. On the origin and nature of hernia. Br J Surg. 1924;11: 455–75.

125. Keynes G. The modern treatment of hernia. BMJ. 1927;1:173–9.

126. Wakeley C, Childs P. Spigelian hernia: hernia through the linea semilunaris. Lancet. 1951;1:1290–1.

127. Lytle WJ. Internal inguinal ring. Br J Surg. 1945;32:441–6.

128. Mair GB. Preliminary report on the use of whole skin grafts as a substitute for fascial sutures in the treatment of herniae. Br J Surg. 1945;32:381–5.

129. Douglas DM. The healing of aponeurotic incisions. Br J Surg. 1952;40:79–82.

130. Shouldice EE. Obesity and ventral hernia repair. Modern Medicine of Canada; 1953. p. 89.

131. Farquharson EL. Early ambulation with special reference to herniorrhaphy as an out-patient procedure. Lancet. 1955;2:517–9.

132. Marsden AJ. Inguinal hernia: a three year review of two thousand cases. Br J Surg. 1962;49:384–94.

133. Usher FC. Further observations on the use of Marlex mesh. A new technique for the repair of inguinal hernias. Am Surg. 1959; 25:792–5.

134. Anson BJ, Morgan EH, McVay CB. Surgical anatomy of the inguinal region based upon a study of 500 body halves. Surg Gyn Obst. 1960;111:707–25.

135. Doran FSA, Lonsdale WN. A simple experimental method of evaluation for the Bassini and allied types of herniorrhaphy. Br J Surg. 1949;36:339–45.

136. Lichtenstein IL. Hernia repair without disability. St Louis: C.V. Mosby; 1970.

137. Doran FSA, White M, Drury M. The scope and safety of short stay surgery in the treatment of groin herniae and varicose veins. Br J Surg. 1972;59:333–9.

138. Glassow F. Short stay surgery (Shouldice technique) for repair of inguinal hernia. Ann R Coll Surg Engl. 1976;58:133–9.

139. Read RC. Can relaxing rectus sheath incision predispose to recurrent direct inguinal hernia? Arch Surg. 1981;116:1493.

140. Chan MK, Baillod RA, Tanner RA, et al. Abdominal hernias in patients receiving continuous ambulatory peritoneal dialysis. Br Med J. 1981;283:826.

141. Schurgers ML, Boelaert JRO, Daneels RF, Robbens EJ, Vandelanotte MM. Genital oedema in patients treated by continuous ambulatory peritoneal dialysis: an unusual presentation of inguinal hernia. Br Med J. 1983;388:358–9.

142. Gilbert AI. Inguinal hernia repair: biomaterials and sutureless repair. Perspect Gen Surg. 1991;2:113–9.

143. Cannon DJ, Casteel L, Read RC. Abdominal aortic aneurysm, Leriche's syndrome, inguinal herniation and smoking. Arch Surg. 1984;119:387–9.

144. Lichtenstein IL. Hernia repair without disability. 2nd ed. St Louis/ Tokyo: Ishiyaku Euroamerica; 1986.

145. Gullmo A. Herniography. World J Surg. 1989;13:560–8.

146. Robbins AW, Rutkow IM. The mesh-plug hernioplasty. Surg Clin North Am. 1993;73:501–11.

147. LeBlanc KA, Booth WV. Laparoscopic repair of incisional abdominal hernias using expanded polytetrafluoroethylene: preliminary findings. Surg Laparosc Endosc. 1993; 3(1): 39–41.

148. Carbonell JF, Sanchez JLA, Peris RT, Ivorra JC, Delbano MJP, Sanchez C, Araez JIG, Greus PC. Risk factors associated with inguinal hernias: a case control study. Eur J Surg. 1993; 159: 481–6.

149. Gilmore OJA. Groin disruption in sportsmen. In: Kurzer M, Kark AE, Wantz GE, editors. Surgical management of abdominal wall hernias. London: Martin Dunnitz; 1999. p. 151–7.

150. Lichtenstein IL. Herniorrhaphy—a personal experience with 6321 cases. Am J Surg. 1987;153:553–9.

Vishy Mahadevan

The anatomy of the abdominal wall has been well documented in several standard anatomical reference texts. Detailed information is readily available from these sources. The lined drawings in this chapter have been adapted from a small selection of publications in the anatomical and surgical literature, with particular emphasis being made in these illustrations, to applied surgical anatomy and surgically significant anatomical variations and anomalies.

Certain pathological processes may, on occasion, distort the underlying anatomy, and the surgeon must be cognizant of, and take into account, these alterations in order to ensure successful outcome from hernia surgery. Optimally, the surgeon should tailor each operation to the specific anatomy encountered in the individual patient.

The impetus to revisit and redefine the anatomy of the anterior abdominal wall and in particular the anatomy of the inguinal region, was driven chiefly by a desire to identify the reasons for the observed shortcomings of the traditional Bassini operation undertaken for the repair of inguinal hernias. This detailed reexamination of abdominal wall anatomy (both topographical and functional) has resulted in a significant enhancement in our understanding of the development of hernias and has also resulted in the generation of much practical advice for surgeons in the surgical management of hernias, in particular when faced with variant forms of hernia that diverge from standard descriptions.

Under normal circumstances the complex musculoaponeurotic elements within the abdominal wall are designed to retain the contents of the peritoneal cavity. There are, however, a number of finite and predetermined areas of relative deficiency or weakness in the musculoaponeurotic layers, and it is at these sites that there is a particular tendency for hernias to present. Most notable among these areas of deficiency is the groin region in relation to the inguinal and femoral canals. Other sites of potential weakness include the umbilicus, epigastrium, lumbar triangle (of Petit), obturator canal, sciatic foramina, perineum, pelvic sidewall, and the spigelian line. The list is long, and it is likely that a given clinician may not necessarily encounter some of the rarer types of abdominal wall hernias during a professional lifetime.

The work of Anson and McVay on the inguinal canal appeared in 1938 [1], and since then they and their associate Zimmerman have published extensively. Other notable contributors to the field of abdominal wall anatomy include Askar, Condon, Fruchaud, Griffith, Harkins, Kark, Lytle, Madden, Mizrachy, Nyhus, Ruge, Skandalakis, and Van Mameren.

External Anatomy: Surface Markings and Surface Features

Since the vast majority of abdominal wall hernias involve the *anterior* abdominal wall, it is the latter that will be the principal focus of this chapter. The geographical outline of the anterior abdominal wall is approximately hexagonal. It is bounded superiorly by the arched costal margin (with the xiphisternum at the summit of this arch) (Fig. 2.1). The lateral boundary on either side is defined, arbitrarily, as the midaxillary line (between the lateral part of the costal margin and the summit of the iliac crest). Inferiorly, on either side, the anterior abdominal wall is bounded, in continuity, by the anterior half of the iliac crest, inguinal ligament, and pubic crest, with the two pubic crests meeting at the pubic symphysis. Situated vertically in the midline of the anterior abdominal wall is the linea alba. In the muscular or thin individual, the linea alba is manifest as a shallow furrow, being more evident above the level of the umbilicus. No such furrow is evident in the obese or rounded abdomen. The umbilicus lies, normally, at the junction of the upper three-fifths and lower two-fifths of the linea alba. In the healthy young adult, the rectus abdominis muscle is evident as a prominence on

V. Mahadevan (✉)
Department of Education, The Royal College
of Surgeons of England, London, UK
e-mail: vmahadev@rcseng.ac.uk

A.N. Kingsnorth and K.A. LeBlanc (eds.), *Management of Abdominal Hernias*,
DOI 10.1007/978-1-84882-877-3_2, © Springer Science+Business Media London 2013

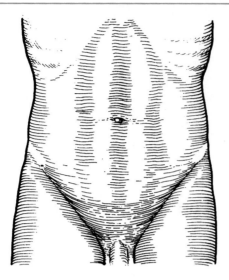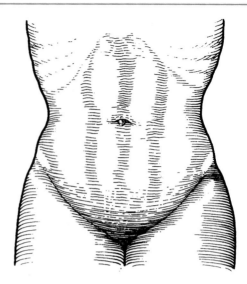

Fig. 2.1 Topographical anatomy of the abdomen—the distinctly different male and female characteristics are important in hernia surgery. The boundaries of the abdomen, the costal cartilages above and the crests of the iliac and pubic bones, and the inguinal ligament inferiorly are illustrated. The umbilicus, the rectus muscle, and the semilunar lines are important surface landmarks

either side of the vertical midline. The rectus muscle is particularly prominent inferolateral to the umbilicus: this rectus mound below the level of the umbilicus is of surgical importance. With aging and obesity, the lower abdomen tends to sag. The rectus mound, however, remains obvious and visible to the subject, even into old age.

The linea semilunaris (semilunar line) is easily observed in the abdominal wall of a fit and muscular individual, though not readily seen in the lax or obese abdomen. It indicates the outer margin of each rectus sheath and is a longitudinally disposed shallow groove with a gentle convexity facing laterally. It is most distinct in the upper abdomen where it commences at the tip of the ninth costal cartilage. At first it descends almost vertically, but inferior to the umbilicus, it turns medially with a gentle curve to terminate at the pubic tubercle. It is along this line that the internal oblique aponeurosis splits into two laminae which run on either side of the rectus abdominis to enclose the muscle in the upper two-thirds of the abdomen. The area corresponding to the inferior third of the semilunar line is also referred to as the Spigelian fascia and is one of the many documented sites of herniation (Chap. 18). In the lower abdomen the relative configurations of the linea semilunaris and the rectus sheath differ between the sexes. This is chiefly due to the wider pelvis and greater pubic prominence which characterizes the female form (Fig. 2.1).

The anterior superior iliac spine (ASIS) is the abrupt anterior extremity of the iliac crest. It is visible in the thin individual and readily palpable in all. The pubic tubercle can be felt as a bony nodule on the anterior aspect of the pubic crest, 2–3 cm lateral to the pubic symphysis. A line joining the ASIS to the pubic tubercle denotes the location of the inguinal ligament. The base of the triangular superficial inguinal

ring is superomedial to the pubic tubercle. Inferolateral to the pubic tubercle is the femoral ring (the proximal, open end of the femoral canal, and through which a femoral hernia enters the femoral canal).

The deep inguinal ring (internal inguinal ring) may be represented on the surface by identifying a point 2 cm vertically above the midpoint of the inguinal ligament (a point halfway between the ASIS and pubic tubercle).

The inguinal canal may be indicated on the surface as an oblique band, 1–1.5 cm wide, running above and parallel to the medial half of the inguinal ligament.

The anterior abdominal wall is a many-layered structure (see Fig. 2.23), a feature which is readily discernible in a transverse section through the abdomen of a cadaver as well as in an axially viewed CT or MR image of the abdominal wall (see Figs. 2.46 and 2.47). A detailed and critical appreciation of these multiple layers, their relationship to each other, their individual textures and consistencies, and variations in consistency of a given layer in different parts of the anterior abdominal wall are all crucial not only to our understanding of the development of abdominal wall hernias but also to the rational and optimal surgical management of the condition.

From the surface inwards, the multiple layers which make up the anterior abdominal wall are, successively:
- Skin
- Superficial fascia comprising two layers, an outer fatty layer known as Camper's fascia and an inner fibrous (fibroelastic) layer known as the membranous layer of superficial fascia or eponymously as Scarpa's fascia
- Musculoaponeurotic plane (which is structurally complex and made up of several layers)
- Transversalis fascia (part of the endoabdominal fascia)

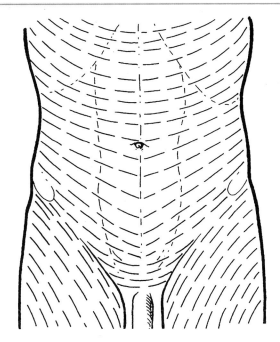

Fig. 2.2 Tension lines of the skin. Incisions at right angles to these lines tend to splay and lead to unsightly scars. This adverse phenomenon is enhanced if the incision also crosses a joint crease. Vertical incisions in the groin for hernia repair are particularly unsightly

- Layer of extraperitoneal fat (or properitoneal fat)
- Parietal peritoneum

Skin

The skin over the anterior abdominal wall is thin compared with that of the back. It is relatively mobile over the underlying layers except in the vicinity of the umbilicus where it is tethered to subjacent layers and consequently relatively immobile.

The surgeon must be aware of the elastic and connective tissue lines in the skin if optimal cutaneous healing is to be obtained. Natural elastic traction lines in the skin of the anterior abdominal wall (known as relaxed skin tension lines or Kraissl's lines) are disposed transversely. Above the level of the umbilicus these tension lines run almost horizontally, while below this level they run with a slight inferomedial obliquity (Fig. 2.2). Incisions made along, or parallel, to these lines tend to heal without much scarring, whereas incisions made at right angles to these lines gape and tend to splay out and eventually result in heaped-up scars. The longitudinal contraction of the healing wound, particularly when the wound crosses a skin delve or body crease, can result in unsightly scars and wound contracture, and for these reasons vertical incisions over the groin should be avoided. However, rapid abdominal access requires adequate vertical incisions, and they continue to remain useful in everyday general surgical and gynecological practice, particularly in emergency surgery (Fig. 2.2).

The Subcutaneous Layer

Beneath the skin there is the subcutaneous areolar tissue and fascia. Superiorly over the lower chest and epigastrium, this layer is generally thin and less organized than in the lower abdomen where it becomes bilaminar—a superficial fatty stratum (Camper's fascia) and a deeper, stronger, and fibroelastic layer termed membranous layer of superficial fascia (or Scarpa's fascia). Scarpa's fascia is well developed in infancy, forming a distinct layer which must be separately incised when the superficial inguinal ring is approached in childhood herniotomy.

It is to be noted that traced laterally around the abdominal wall, Scarpa's fascia can be made out distinctly only as far as the midaxillary line. Posterior to that line Scarpa's fascia thins out rapidly, and no Scarpa's fascia is evident in the posterior abdominal wall. Traced superiorly, Scarpa's fascia is seen to cross over onto the anterior chest wall, superficial to the costal margin, as a very thin layer, known as the retromammary fascia. This retromammary extension, which can be traced as far superiorly as the 2nd intercostal space, is easier to demonstrate in the premenopausal adult female.

Even in the adult, Scarpa's fascia is more prominent, of firmer consistency and more readily demonstrable in the lower abdomen than in the upper abdomen. It is generally more membranous, contains elastic tissue, and is almost devoid of fat. Traced inferiorly, the abdominal subcutaneous fat merges imperceptibly with the subcutaneous fat of the thigh. Scarpa's fascia, by contrast, crosses into the thigh anterior to the inguinal ligament and fuses with the deep fascia of the thigh (fascia lata) at the groin crease (flexure skin crease of the hip joint) below the level of the inguinal ligament, as far medially as the pubic tubercle and laterally as far as an area just inferior to the ASIS. Medially, Scarpa's fascia is prolonged into the anterior part of the perineum (urogenital region of the perineum) as the superficial perineal fascia (Colles' fascia) (Fig. 2.3). In the male, this extension is prolonged into the scrotum and also around the penile shaft. The proximal part of this fascia which is prolonged over the penile shaft is anchored to the front of the pubis and is referred to as the suspensory ligament of the penis.

The superficial fascia in the upper medial thigh has important anatomic features for the hernia surgeon. It is interrupted by the passage, from superficial to deep, of the great saphenous vein and other structures, at the saphenous opening or fossa ovalis. Attenuated connective tissue, the cribriform fascia, packs and "closes" the saphenous opening. Although the cribriform fascia lies in the same plane as the deep fascia, it has many of the structural characteristics of the superficial fascia: it is loose and fatty in texture and is easily distorted by the dilatation of any of the structures in its neighborhood, for example, a varicose saphenous vein,

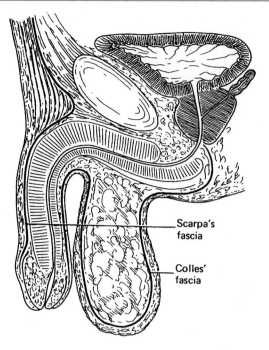

Fig. 2.3 The membranous layer of superficial fascia (Scarpa's fascia) is stronger over the lower abdomen where it forms a distinct layer that requires division in groin hernia operations

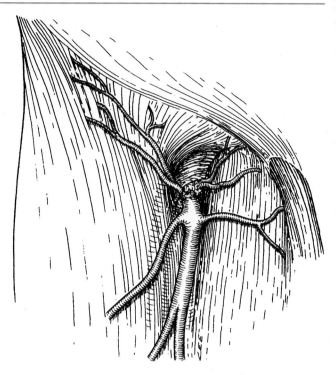

Fig. 2.4 In the upper thigh the long saphenous vein goes from superficial to deep to join the femoral vein which is contained in the femoral sheath, an extension of the extraperitoneal fascia

enlarged lymph nodes and lymphatics, and a femoral hernia. The cribriform fascia is the anterior boundary of the femoral canal at this site (Fig. 2.4).

After deciding on the site of an incision in the abdominal wall, the surgeon will encounter a reasonably constant pattern of blood vessels. Superficially these vessels anastomose to make a network in the subcutaneous tissue. The lower intercostal arteries (7th to 11th), the subcostal artery, the musculophrenic, and the right and left superior epigastric arteries (continuations of the internal thoracic from the subclavian) supply the abdominal wall cephalad to the umbilicus. Caudal to the umbilicus, the superior epigastric vessels anastomose with the inferior epigastric vessels inside the rectus sheath either within the substance of the rectus abdominis muscle or deep to the muscle. The inferior epigastric artery arises from the external iliac artery just proximal to the inguinal ligament. The inferior epigastric artery and accompanying veins form the lateral margin of Hesselbach's triangle [2]. The neck of an indirect inguinal hernia is lateral to these vessels while that of a direct inguinal hernia is medial to the vessels.

In addition to the serially arranged vessels, there are three small superficial branches of the femoral artery in the upper thigh (the corresponding and accompanying veins drain to the great saphenous vein) which spread out from the groin over the lower abdomen. These vessels are the superficial circumflex iliac passing laterally and upward overlying the inguinal canal, the superficial epigastric coursing upward and medially toward the umbilicus, and the superficial external pudendal artery making its way medially to supply the skin of the penis and scrotum. This vessel anastomoses with the spermatic cord vessels to the scrotal contents. All these arteries are frequently encountered in inguinal and femoral hernioplasty; all anastomose adequately both with the serial intercostal and lumbar arteries and across the midline. In most instances they can be divided with impunity, but sometimes they are an important auxiliary blood supply to the testicle (Fig. 2.5). The veins draining the lower abdomen enter the femoral vein via the great saphenous vein through the saphenous opening or directly into the external iliac vein. From the upper abdomen venous blood eventually drains into the subclavian veins either via tributaries of the internal thoracic veins or via tributaries of the axillary veins.

The finer details of the vascular supply of the anterior abdominal wall are beyond the scope of this chapter but are of paramount importance in the context of tissue transfer in plastic and reconstructive surgery [3].

Superficial Nerves

The cutaneous nerves to the anterior abdominal wall are arranged and distributed segmentally, as in the anterior chest wall. The lower five intercostal nerves and the subcostal nerve (12th thoracic nerve) having run in their respective intercostal spaces cross the costal margin obliquely to enter

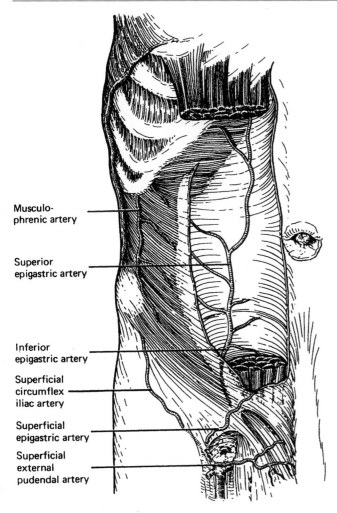

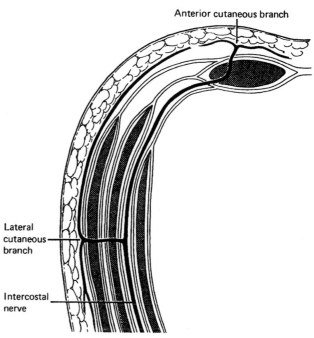

Fig. 2.6 The lower abdomen is segmentally supplied by the intercostal nerves. Each nerve has a lateral cutaneous branch which gives anterior and posterior divisions in the subcutaneous tissue. When a local anesthetic is administered, it is important to block the anterior division of the lateral cutaneous branch of these nerves

Fig. 2.5 The vasculature of the abdomen and groin is of particular interest to the surgeon. Fortunately the vessels all anastomose freely, so surgery does not need to be locked into vascular anatomy, except for the anastomosis of the pudendal with the cord vessels over the pubis. Care should be taken not to dissect the superficial tissues medial to the pubic tubercle to avoid threat to the pudendal anastomosis and the testicle

the neurovascular plane of the anterior abdominal wall (i.e., the plane between the internal oblique and transversus abdominis) to supply the abdominal parietes. While still in the intercostal space, each gives off a lateral cutaneous branch which enters the overlying digitation of the external oblique muscle; this branch divides into a small posterior nerve which extends back to supply the skin over the latissimus dorsi and a larger anterior nerve which supplies the external oblique muscle and the overlying subcutaneous tissue and skin (Fig. 2.6). The main stem of the intercostal nerve continues forward in the neurovascular plane and enters the rectus sheath from behind by piercing the posterior lamella of the internal oblique aponeurosis. It gains the surface by passing through the rectus abdominis muscle which it supplies before emerging through the anterior rectus sheath a centimeter or so from the midline.

The most caudal of the abdominal wall nerves are derived from the ventral ramus of the first lumbar spinal nerve; they are the iliohypogastric and ilioinguinal nerves. The ilioinguinal nerve is generally the smaller of the two—although occasionally, it may be the larger of the two. Rarely the ilioinguinal nerve is very small and may even be absent. The anterior cutaneous branch of the iliohypogastric nerve emerges through the aponeurosis of the external oblique, 1 or 2 cm above the superficial inguinal ring and innervates the skin in the suprapubic region. The ilioinguinal nerve enters the inguinal canal at its lateral extremity (and not through the deep inguinal ring) and running through the canal usually inferolateral to the spermatic cord (or uterine round ligament) it becomes superficial by emerging through the superficial inguinal ring to supply the anterior one-third of the scrotal skin (vulval skin in the female) and a small area of the medial upper thigh and suprapubic skin (Fig. 2.7).

The genitofemoral nerve is derived from the ventral rami of the first and second lumbar spinal nerves and completes the innervation of the anterior abdominal wall and groin areas. At first it passes obliquely forward and downward through the substance of the psoas major. It emerges from the muscle and crosses its anterior surface behind the posterior parietal peritoneum, running posterior to the ureter. It divides at a variable distance from the deep inguinal ring into a genital and a femoral branch.

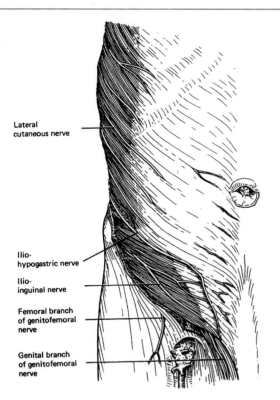

Fig. 2.7 The groin area is innervated principally by branches of the first lumbar nerve—the iliohypogastric and ilioinguinal nerves. These nerves innervate the skin area over the iliac crest (the lateral branch of the iliohypogastric nerve), the suprapubic region (the anterior branch of iliohypogastric nerve), and the front and side of the scrotum and upper medial thigh (the ilioinguinal nerve after it emerges from the inguinal canal)

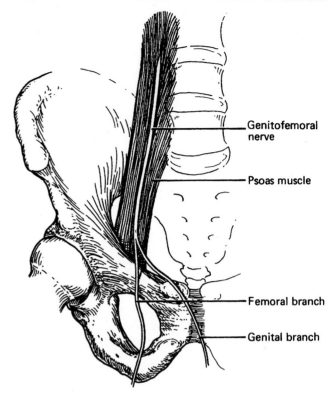

Fig. 2.8 The genitofemoral nerve, from L1 and L2, innervates the femoral sheath and the skin over it. It should be blocked prior to surgery for a femoral hernia under local anesthetic

The genital branch, a mixed motor and sensory nerve, crosses the femoral vessels and enters the inguinal canal at or just medial to the deep inguinal ring. The nerve penetrates the fascia transversalis of the posterior wall of the inguinal canal either through the deep ring or separately medial to the deep ring. The nerve traverses the inguinal canal lying between the spermatic cord above and the upturned edge of the inguinal ligament inferiorly; the nerve is vulnerable to surgical trauma as it progresses along the floor of the canal (the gutter produced by the upturned internal edge of the inguinal ligament). The genital branch supplies motor innervation to the cremaster muscle and sensory innervation to the fascial coverings of the spermatic cord (or coverings of the uterine round ligament in the female). It may supply the skin of the scrotum.

The femoral branch enters the femoral sheath overlying the femoral artery and supplies a small area of skin over the upper part of the femoral triangle (Fig. 2.8).

The posterior two-thirds of the scrotum are supplied by S2 and S3 through the perineal and posterior femoral cutaneous nerves. The anterior scrotal cutaneous supply is frequently disrupted in inguinal hernioplasty (Fig. 2.9) no doubt due to injury to the ilioinguinal nerve (caused inadvertently or otherwise).

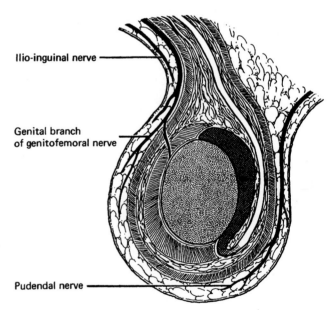

Fig. 2.9 The skin of the anterior scrotum is supplied by the ilioinguinal nerve, L1, and the genital branch of the genitofemoral nerve, L1. These nerves are often disrupted in hernioplasty

The sensory nerve supply of the upper anterior and anterolateral thigh is derived from the lateral cutaneous nerve of the thigh, the femoral branch of the genitofemoral nerve, the ilioinguinal nerve, and the genital branch of the

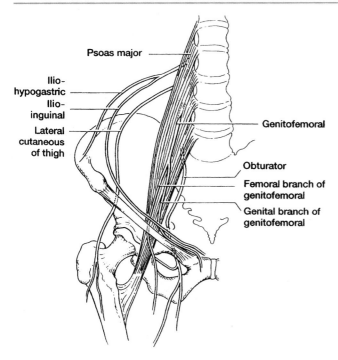

Fig. 2.10 The nerves of the lower abdomen, the groin and upper thigh. The lateral cutaneous nerve of the thigh and the femoral branch of the genitofemoral nerve are at special risk in extraperitoneal operations on groin hernia

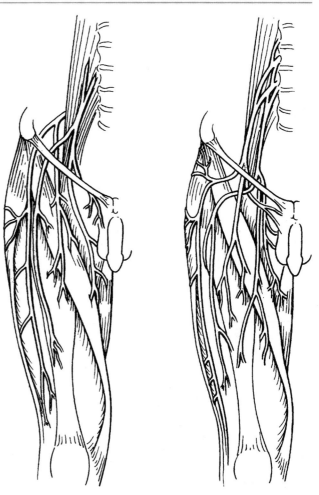

Fig. 2.11 The variable anatomy of the lateral cutaneous nerve of thigh and the femoral branch of the genitofemoral nerve. Both these nerves are in close proximity to the inguinal ligament as they progress to the thigh [4]

genitofemoral nerve (Figs. 2.10 and 2.11). There is overlap between the territories of these nerves, and their pathways also show considerable variation.

The lateral cutaneous nerve of the thigh arises from the ventral rami of the second and third lumbar nerves. It emerges from the lateral border of the psoas major and crosses the ventral aspect of iliacus obliquely, running toward the anterior superior spine. It lies in the adipose tissue between the iliopsoas fascia and the peritoneum.

Usually the lateral cutaneous nerve of the thigh forms one single trunk, but it may divide into two branches at a variable distance proximal to the inguinal ligament (Fig. 2.11) [4]. The nerve then crosses into the anterior thigh by passing deep to the lateral portion of the inguinal ligament. It may then lie superficial to the sartorius muscle or may pass through the sartorius before becoming superficial to supply the skin of the lateral side of the thigh. The variability of the course of the nerve in the abdomen is considerable and the distance between nerve and the deep inguinal ring also variable [5]. The nerve may traverse the anterior abdominal wall cranial to the inguinal ligament or through the attachment of the ligament to the ASIS.

The nerve supply of the scrotum and its contents is complex [6]. The autonomic supply of the testis is from T10 to T12, via nerves which accompany the spermatic vessels. These autonomic nerves are motor to the vasculature and to

the smooth muscle of the tunica albuginea. However, they also have free, sensory, endings in the interstitial spaces of the testis and convey noxious stimuli which may present as referred pain in the lower abdomen (T10–T12 segments). The autonomic supply of the vas and epididymis are distinct from those of the testis; pain from these structures is felt in the L1 segment, lower than testicular pain, in the distributions of the genitofemoral nerve.

The somatic nerve supply is by the ilioinguinal and genitofemoral nerves, L1 and L2, and by the sacral nerves, S2 and S3. The genital branch of the genitofemoral nerve supplies the cord, the cremaster, the tunica vaginalis, and, along with the L1 component of the ilioinguinal nerve, the anterior third of the scrotal skin.

When viewed from behind as during endoscopic hernia surgery, the area lateral to the cord vessels and above the inguinal ligament where the femoral branch of genitofemoral nerve and lateral cutaneous nerve of the thigh lie has been dubbed the "triangle of pain" by laparoscopic surgeons

Fig. 2.12 (**a**) Laparoscopic view of the nerves immediately proximal to the inguinal ligament after reflection of the parietal peritoneum. These nerves lie in the adipose tissue just deep to the peritoneum and superficial to the iliopsoas muscle: the "triangle of pain." (**b**) Laparoscopic view of the deep inguinal ring and adjacent structures, the "triangle of doom" [29]

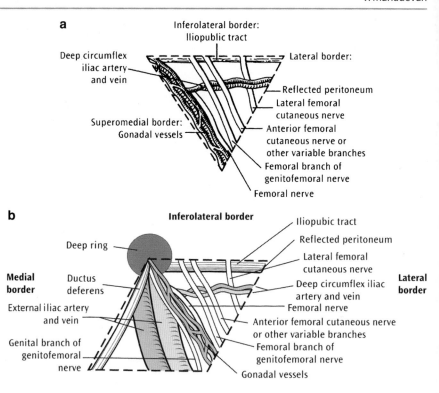

because of the hazard of nerve injury by entrapment with staples. In this area thick globular adipose tissue can surround and conceal the nerves. On a deeper plane the femoral nerve crosses this triangle with the genitofemoral and lateral cutaneous nerve superficial to it (Fig. 2.12). This entire area is spoken of as the "quadrangle of doom." All of the nerves that can be injured during laparoscopic inguinal hernia repair are located in this anatomic region.

Musculoaponeurotic Plane

The musculoaponeurotic "plane" is architecturally complex and composed of several layers.

A long and thick strap-like muscle, the rectus abdominis, lies on either side of the vertical midline. Lateral to the rectus abdominis on each side, the musculoaponeurotic plane comprises a three-ply arrangement of concentric muscular sheets. The largest and most superficial of the three is the external oblique muscle. The intermediate muscular sheet is the internal oblique muscle, while the deepest (innermost) sheet is the transversus abdominis. Of these three layers, the internal oblique and transversus abdominis curve posteriorly to attach to the lumbar fascia at the very lateral edge of the quadratus lumborum muscle on the posterior abdominal wall. The external and internal obliques and the transversus abdominis may be spoken of, collectively, as the anterolateral abdominal musculature.

Anteromedially, each of the above-mentioned three muscular sheets becomes an aponeurosis (a flattened tendinous sheet). These aponeuroses envelop the ipsilateral rectus abdominis muscle in a highly specific and well-defined manner, and having done so, they interdigitate in the vertical midline with their counterpart aponeuroses from the contralateral side to form the linea alba. The aponeurotic envelope surrounding the rectus abdominis muscle is referred to as the rectus sheath.

A description of the rectus abdominis (and pyramidalis) muscles shall be followed by a detailed consideration of the three muscles which make up the anterolateral abdominal musculature.

The Rectus Abdominis Muscle

The rectus muscle is flat and strap-like and extends from the level of the pubis to the thorax. The muscle is separated from its fellow of the opposite side by the linea alba. Each rectus abdominis muscle arises by two short tendons: the larger and lateral tendon from the pubic crest and the smaller and medial tendon from the upper and anterior surfaces of the pubic symphysis. (Some of the fibers from the medial tendon mingle with those of the medial tendon of the other side.) The two tendons, lateral and medial, unite a short distance above the pubis to give rise to a single muscle belly which broadens as it runs upward and crosses the costal

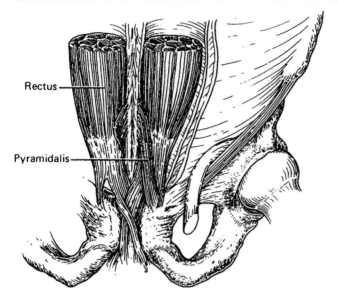

Rectus

Pyramidalis

Fig. 2.13 The rectus muscle arises by two tendons—the larger and lateral from the crest of the pubis and the smaller and medial from the pubis of the opposite side and from the ligamentous fibers of the symphysis. The pyramidalis is variable; it arises from the ligamentous fibers of the symphysis and adjacent pubis and is inserted into the linea alba

margin to attach to the anterior surfaces and inferior margins of the 7th, 6th, and 5th costal cartilages, and by a small slip, to the xiphisternum.

The upper part of the muscle belly usually shows three transverse tendinous intersections; one at the level of the xiphisternum, one at the level of the umbilicus and one halfway between the other two. Sometimes a further incomplete intersection is present below the umbilical level. The intersections extend into the thickness of the muscle for a variable distance but never penetrate the entire thickness of the muscle. They are always intimately adherent to the anterior lamina of the sheath of the muscle, but have no attachment to the posterior sheath.

The pyramidalis muscle is triangular in shape, arising by its base from the ligaments on the anterior surface of the symphysis pubis and being inserted into the lower linea alba 2–3 cm above the pubic symphysis. The muscle is absent in 10% of subjects (Fig. 2.13), and in any case is not thought to be of any functional consequence.

The External Oblique Muscle

The external oblique muscle arises, typically, by eight slips; from the external surface and inferior border of each of the lower eight ribs. The upper four slips interdigitate with the origins of the serratus anterior and the lower four with those of the latissimus dorsi muscle. The fibers pass downward and forward from their costal origins; the posterior fibers are nearly vertical and are inserted into the anterior half of the

external lip of the iliac crest. The uppermost fibers run almost horizontally toward the ventral midline. The intervening fibers from above downward display a progressively increasing obliquity as they run toward the ventral midline. All the superior and intermediate fibers end in the strong external oblique aponeurosis. The muscle may be said to have three borders: a posterior border which is muscular and upper and lower borders which are both aponeurotic.

The posterior border of the external oblique is free, so to speak, and forms the anterior boundary of the lumbar triangle (of Petit). The posterior boundary of the lumbar triangle is the anterolateral edge of the latissimus dorsi muscle, and the inferior boundary is the iliac crest. The "floor" of this triangle is formed by the internal oblique and the underlying transversus abdominis. Both sheets are relatively thin at this level, and it is through this triangle that a lumbar hernia may present as a lump in the flank.

Superiorly the external oblique aponeurosis is relatively thin and passes medially to be attached to the xiphoid process. Inferiorly the aponeurosis is very strong. The inferior margin of the aponeurosis forms the inguinal ligament, which is attached superolaterally to the ASIS and inferomedially to the pubic tubercle. Medially, the aponeurosis of the external oblique contributes to the anterior rectus sheath and thence interdigitates with its fellow of the opposite side at the linea alba and in front of the pubis. The external oblique aponeurosis is broadest inferiorly, narrowest at the umbilicus and broad again in the epigastrium.

The aponeurosis of the external oblique muscle fuses with the aponeurosis of the internal oblique in the anterior wall of the rectus sheath. This line of fusion which is considerably medial to the semilunar line, has an oblique and somewhat curved trajectory, being more lateral above and more medial below. In fact, the external oblique aponeurosis contributes very little to the lower portion of the anterior rectus sheath. This latter point is of importance in inguinal hernioplasty (Fig. 2.14) [7].

There is a natural defect in the external oblique aponeurosis just above the pubic crest. This aperture known as the superficial inguinal ring (external inguinal ring) is triangular in shape and in the male, transmits the spermatic cord from the abdomen to the scrotum. In the female the round ligament of the uterus emerges through this opening before blending with the subcutaneous tissue in the ipsilateral labium majus. The superficial inguinal ring is not a "ring"; it is a triangular cleft with its long axis obliquely disposed in a superolateral direction from the pubic tubercle. It is approximately parallel to the inguinal ligament. The base of the triangle is formed by the crest of the pubis, and the apex is laterally directed toward the ASIS. The superficial inguinal ring represents the interval between that part of the external oblique aponeurosis which inserts into the pubic symphysis and pubic crest on the one hand, and the inguinal ligament on

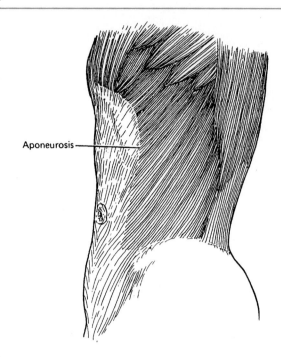

Aponeurosis

Fig. 2.14 The external oblique muscle and its aponeurosis invests the abdomen. The aponeurosis of this muscle forms the anterior wall of the rectus sheath by fusing with the underlying aponeurosis of the internal oblique. However, this line of fusion, in the lower abdomen especially, is considerably medial to the semilunar line. This is an anatomical point of importance in inguinal hernioplasty, as it allows a "slide operation" on the internal oblique without compromising the anterior rectus sheath

the other, which inserts into the pubic tubercle. The aponeurotic margins of the ring are described as the superior and inferior crura. The spermatic cord, as it comes through the superficial inguinal ring, rests on the inferior crus which is a continuation of the floor of the inguinal canal (the enrolled inferomedial end of the inguinal ligament).

The dimensions of the superficial inguinal ring, or aponeurotic cleft, are of surgical importance and are far from being of standard size and predictable extent. It may sometimes fit snugly around the spermatic cord. At other times it may extend upward and laterally beyond the ASIS. In 80% of cases the cleft is confined to the lower half of the area between the midline and the anterior superior spine, but in the remaining 20% it extends more laterally. In about 2% of individuals, one or more accessory clefts are seen. When present, they are usually superolateral to the main cleft. The accessory cleft may transmit the iliohypogastric nerve (Fig. 2.15) [8].

The relationship between the apex of the cleft and the inferior (deep) epigastric vessels (indicating the lateral margin of Hesselbach's triangle) is of crucial importance in closing the inguinal canal anteriorly and containing a potential direct inguinal hernia. Whereas the canal is usually described as closed anteriorly by the external oblique aponeurosis, in only 11% of cases does the apex of the cleft lie less than

halfway along a line from the pubic tubercle to the inferior epigastric artery, in 52% the cleft extends to the level of the epigastric vessels, and, most importantly, in 37% the apex of the cleft is lateral to the epigastric vessels (Fig. 2.16) [8].

The crura of the superficial ring are joined together by intercrural fibers derived from the outer investing fascia of the external oblique aponeurosis. The size and strength of these intercrural fibers vary. In 27% of specimens these fibers do not cross from crus to crus and, therefore, do not reinforce the margins of the cleft (Fig. 2.17) [8].

The inferior border of the external oblique aponeurosis is rolled inward to form a gutter. **This enrolled edge** is termed the inguinal ligament (Poupart's ligament). It is attached superolaterally to the ASIS and inferomedially to the pubic tubercle. Both bony landmarks are readily palpable. Reciprocal to the gutter-shaped, concave upper surface, the inguinal ligament presents a rounded inferior border toward the thigh. Attached to this rounded distal surface of the inguinal ligament is the deep fascia of the thigh, the fascia lata. The medial end of the inguinal ligament at the pubic tubercle gives rise to the lacunar ligament (Gimbernat's ligament) which extends upward and backward to reach the pectineal line on the superior ramus of the pubis. The crescentic, free, lateral edge of the lacunar ligament forms the medial boundary of the femoral ring. From its attachment on the pectineal line, the lacunar ligament sends a strong extension which runs superolaterally and has a firm attachment along the iliopectineal line. This extension is termed the pectineal ligament (of Astley Cooper). Finally, from the pubic tubercle, certain fibers of the inguinal ligament run superiorly and medially behind the spermatic cord to interdigitate at the linea alba with corresponding fibers from the contralateral side. This superomedial extension of the inguinal ligament is termed the reflected part of the inguinal ligament. The inguinal ligament shows a gentle curvature, with its concavity directed superomedially toward the abdomen (Fig. 2.18) and the reciprocal convexity directed inferolaterally toward the thigh.

The lateral extensions of the inguinal ligament as the lacunar (Gimbernat's) and the pectineal (Cooper's) ligaments give a fan-like expansion of the inguinal ligament at its medial end. This expansion has important surgical implications.

The lacunar ligament is a triangular continuation of the medial end of the inguinal ligament. Its apex is at the pubic tubercle, its superior margin is continuous with the inguinal ligament, and its posteromedial margin is attached to the iliopectineal line on the superior ramus of the pubis. Its lateral crescentic edge is free and is an important firm structure which forms a medial margin of the femoral ring (the proximal end of the femoral canal). The ligament lies in an oblique plane, with its upper (abdominal) surface facing superomedially and being crossed by the spermatic cord, and its lower (femoral) surface looking inferolaterally. With the external

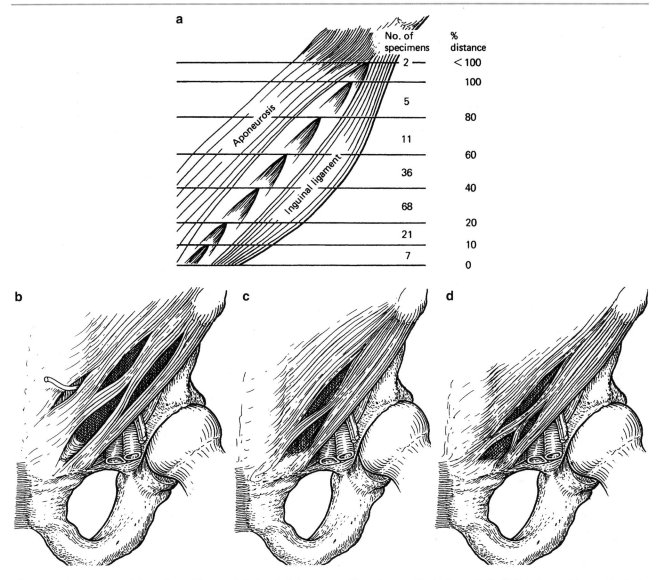

Fig. 2.15 The anatomy and dimensions of the superficial inguinal ring are very variable. The "ring" is a triangular cleft separating the insertions of the external oblique aponeurosis into the pubic crest and the pubic tubercle. Its base is medial and inferior and its apex superior and lateral. In 80% of subjects the apex lies in the medial half of the lower abdomen, but in the remaining 20% the apex approaches the anterior superior iliac spine (**a**). In 2% of subjects, there are accessory clefts superior to the main cleft (**b–d**). One of these clefts may transmit the iliohypogastric nerve (**b**) [8]

oblique aponeurosis and the inguinal ligament, the superior surface forms a groove for the cord as it emerges from the inguinal canal (Fig. 2.19).

The reflected part of the inguinal ligament (Colles') is a broad band of rather thin fibers which arise from the crest of the pubis and the medial end of the iliopectineal line and pass anterosuperiorly behind the superior crus of the superficial inguinal ring to the linea alba. The reflected part of the inguinal ligament is very variable in its extent, but it is an important structure closing the potential space in the posterior wall of the inguinal canal between the iliopectineal line and the lateral margin of the rectus muscle (Fig. 2.20).

The Internal Oblique Muscle

The internal oblique muscle arises from the lateral two-thirds of the abdominal surface of the inguinal ligament, the intermediate line on the anterior two-thirds of the iliac crest, and from the whole length of the lumbar fascia. The general direction of the fibers (above the level of the ASIS) is upward and medial. The posterior fibers are inserted into the inferior borders of the cartilages of the lower four ribs. The intermediate fibers pass upward and medially and end in a strong aponeurosis which extends from the inferior borders of the seventh and eighth costal cartilages and the xiphisternum to

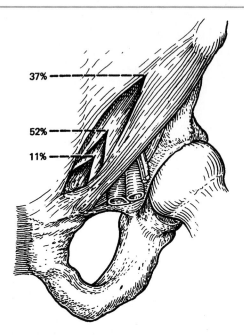

Fig. 2.16 The size of the superficial inguinal ring, the cleft in the external oblique, is crucial in closing the inguinal canal anteriorly. In 11% of subjects the cleft extends less than 50% of the length of the inguinal canal, in 52% it extends as far as the deep epigastric vessels, and in 37% the cleft extends lateral to the deep epigastric vessels [8]

the linea alba along the entire length of the latter. The lowermost fibers arise from the inguinal ligament and arch downward and medially. These fibers along with the lowest fibers of the transversus muscle pass in front of the rectus abdominis muscle, contribute to the anterior rectus sheath, and insert on to the pubic crest and the iliopectineal line behind the lacunar ligament and reflected part of the inguinal ligament (Fig. 2.21).

A recent publication has questioned the traditional description of the lowest fibers of internal oblique (and transversus abdominis) arising from the upper surface of the inguinal ligament [9]. According to Acland, the lowest fibers of internal oblique and transversus abdominis arise not from the inguinal ligament but from a thickened ridge of iliopsoas fascia.

The internal oblique is not invariable in its anatomy in the inguinal region. Its origin may commence in front of the internal ring or at a variable distance lateral to the ring. The muscle may then insert either onto the pubic crest and tubercle or into the lateral margin of the rectus sheath a variable distance above the pubis. With regard to the behavior of the internal oblique in the region of the groin, there are thus four possible combinations of origin and insertion. The contribution of the internal oblique to groin anatomy and in particular to the "**defenses**" of the inguinal canal is very variable. There are a number of well-recognized variations in the anatomy of the internal oblique in the groin (see p. 46) (Fig. 2.22).

The detailed anatomy of the semilunar line and rectus sheath, and that of the insertion of the lowermost fibers of the internal oblique into the pubic bone, is of surgical significance and warrants more detailed consideration.

At the lateral margin of the rectus muscle the aponeurosis of the internal oblique splits into two lamellae—the superficial lamella passes anterior to the rectus, and the deep lamella goes posterior to the rectus. The superficial lamella fuses with the aponeurosis of the external oblique to form the anterior rectus sheath. The deep lamella fuses with the aponeurosis of the underlying transversus abdominis muscle. The detailed anatomy varies but has importance in the causation of umbilical and epigastric hernias. In the lower part of the abdomen, in an area inferior to a point about midway between the umbilicus and the pubis, the aponeurosis does not split into lamella but courses entirely in front of the rectus to fuse with the overlying aponeurosis of the external oblique (Fig. 2.23).

The internal oblique muscle in its lateral fleshy part is not uniform in structure; it is segmented or banded. The muscular bands terminate just lateral to the border of the rectus muscle and are most marked in the inguinal and lower abdominal region. The bands are generally arranged like the blades of a fan with the interspaces increasing as the medial extremities are reached [10, 11]. The bands may be separable up to the point where they fuse with the aponeurosis lateral to the rectus muscle. In a fifth of cases there are potential parietal deficits between these bands. Spigelian hernias occur through these defects in the region of the semilunar line; these defects being more pronounced in the lower abdomen.

At the lowermost part of the internal oblique muscle, adjacent to its origin from the inguinal ligament, the spermatic cord passes through or adjacent to the inferomedial margin of the muscle. Laterally the cord lies deep to the fleshy muscular fibers, then as it emerges alongside the muscle, it acquires a coat of cremaster muscle from the muscle.

The fascicles of the lower part of the internal oblique muscle follow a transverse or oblique direction. Medial to the cord the muscle fibers replaced an aponeurosis which continues inferomedially to reach the pubis. There are variations both in the medial and the inferior extent of the muscle fibers of the internal oblique.

The fleshy muscle extends to the inferior margin in only 2% of cases; in 75% the extent is a centimeter or so above the margin, and in 20% there is a broad aponeurotic leaf superior to the spermatic cord. Likewise the fleshy muscle extends as far as the emergent cord in 20%, medial to the cord but not as far medially to the rectus margin in 75%, and medial to the lateral margin of the rectus in 2%.

In clinical practice a direct inguinal hernia is never encountered when the lower margin of the internal oblique is fleshy *and* when the fleshy fibers extend medial to the

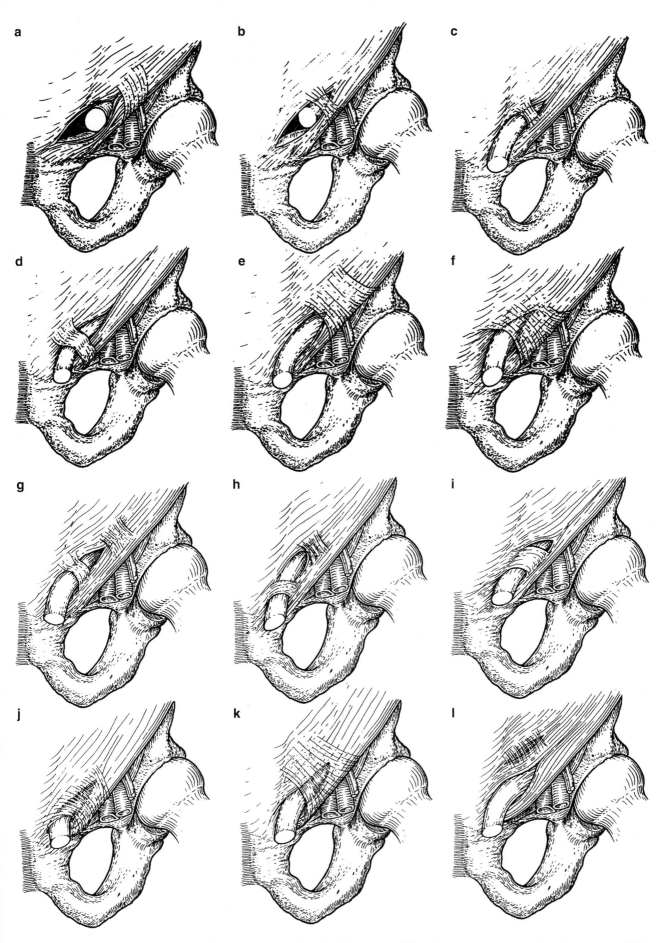

Fig. 2.17 (a–l) Variations in the structure of the superficial inguinal ring. The intercrural fibers between the two crura of the ring are very variable; in 27% of subjects these intercrural fibers do not cross from one crus to the other [8]

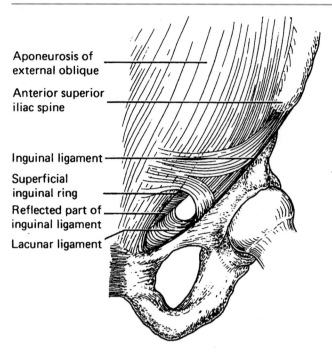

Fig. 2.18 The inguinal ligament is the lower margin of the external oblique muscle. Medially it is attached like a fan to the iliopectineal line (Cooper's ligament) and the tubercle of the pubis

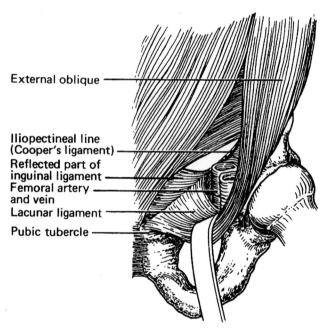

Fig. 2.19 The upper abdominal surface of the attachment of the inguinal ligament to the pubic tubercle is the floor of the inguinal canal which the cord rests on as it emerges from the canal

superficial ring. Direct herniation is most frequently found at operation when the internal oblique muscle is replaced with flimsy aponeurosis in the roof of the inguinal canal (Fig. 2.24) [8].

In 52% of cases the lowermost arching fibers of the internal oblique are continuous above with the remainder of the internal oblique muscles, but in the remainder a variety of spaces between banding occur. In the medial and lower musculoaponeurotic part, defects superior to the spermatic cord may compromise the shutter mechanism of the canal and lead to direct inguinal herniation. Similarly, Spigelian hernia defects can develop between the muscle bands, enter the inguinal canal, and present as direct inguinal hernia (Fig. 2.25) [12].

Rarely (0.15% of hernia cases), the spermatic cord is seen to come through the fleshy part of the lower muscle belly. In this rare situation, the muscle may be said to have an origin from the inguinal ligament medial to the emergent cord. In these cases there is prominent banding of the muscle in the lower abdomen; effectively, there is a band caudal to the cord (Fig. 2.26).

The Transverse Abdominal Muscle

The transversus abdominis is the third and deepest of the three abdominal muscle layers. The muscle arises in continuity from the inner surface of the costal margin, from the lumbar fascia, from the iliopsoas fascia along the internal lip of the anterior two-thirds of the iliac crest, and from the lateral half or so of the superior surface of the inguinal ligament. The iliopsoas fascia is continuous posterosuperiorly with the anterior layer of the lumbar fascia (which is effectively the posterior aponeurosis of the muscle extending the latter's origin to the vertebral column) and the costal cartilages of the lower six ribs interdigitating with the origin of the diaphragm (Fig. 2.27).

Traced anteromedially, the muscle fibers end in a strong aponeurosis which is inserted into the linea alba, the pubic crest and the iliopectineal line. For the most part the muscle fibers run transversely, but the lowest of the muscle fibers take on a downward and medial curve so that the lower margin of the muscle forms an arch over the inguinal canal. The lower fibers of the muscle give way to the aponeurosis which gains insertion into the pubic crest and the iliopectineal line. The insertion of the transverse muscle is broader than that of the internal oblique and consequently its aponeurosis extends further along the iliopectineal line (Fig. 2.28).

In the epigastrium and in the lower abdomen, down to a point midway between the umbilicus and the pubis, the transverse aponeurosis fuses with the posterior lamella of the aponeurosis of the internal oblique to form the posterior rectus sheath. In the lowermost abdomen, the aponeurosis passes in front of the rectus muscle and fuses with the deep surface of the aponeurosis of the internal oblique which in turn fuses with the deep aspect of the external oblique muscle to form the anterior rectus sheath (Fig. 2.29).

The transversus abdominis muscle is made up, proportionately, of more aponeurotic tissue and less muscle tissue

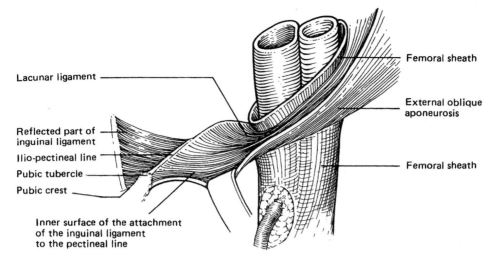

Lacunar ligament

Reflected part of
inguinal ligament

Ilio-pectineal line

Pubic tubercle

Pubic crest

Inner surface of the attachment
of the inguinal ligament
to the pectineal line

Femoral sheath

External oblique
aponeurosis

Femoral sheath

Fig. 2.20 Medially the posterior wall of the inguinal canal is reinforced by the reflected part of the inguinal ligament, a strong triangular fascia arising from the pubic crest anteriorly to the attachments of the internal oblique and transversus muscles and passing medially to the linea alba into which it is inserted

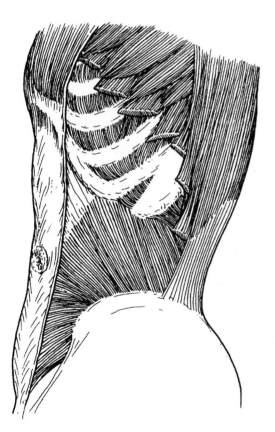

Fig. 2.21 The internal oblique muscle arising from the lateral half of the inguinal ligament and the iliac crest to be inserted into the lower costal cartilage and, via its aponeurosis, continuous with its fellow muscle contralaterally

than either the external or internal oblique muscles. In one study [8], it was observed that in 67% of cases fleshy muscle covered only the upper part of the inguinal region. In only 14% of cases were any fleshy fibers found in the lowermost fibers arching over the inguinal canal. Similarly, in 71% of subjects the red fibers did not extend medial to the inferior epigastric vessels. The aponeurotic portion of the muscle shows its greatest anatomical variation in the inguinal region, where it is most important in hernia repair.

The lower border of the transversus abdominis aponeurosis is called the "arch." Above the arch the transversus aponeurosis forms a continuous strong sheet, with no spaces between its fibers. Below the arch the posterior wall of the inguinal canal is closed by transversalis fascia alone. This is a weak area through which direct herniation can occur. The aponeurotic arch is easily identifiable as a "white line" of aponeurosis at operation (Figs. 2.28 and 2.30).

The Conjoint Tendon

The transverse fibers of the transversus muscle proceed horizontally to their insertion in the rectus sheath and the linea alba, while the lower fibers course downward and medially—sometimes to fuse with the overlying fibers of the internal oblique as they insert onto the pubic crest and the iliopectineal line.

Only when the aponeuroses of the transversus and the internal oblique are fused, some distance lateral to the rectus sheath is the term *conjoint tendon* appropriate and accurate. Thus the conjoint tendon represents the fused aponeuroses of the internal oblique and transversus muscles and which in turn is inserted onto the anteromedial 2 cm of the iliopectineal line. The transversus muscle contributes 80% of the substance of the conjoint tendon. The conjoint tendon is lateral to the rectus muscle and lies directly deep to the superficial inguinal ring. It passes down to its insertion on the pubis, deep to the inguinal and lacunar ligaments. The spermatic

Fig. 2.22 The origin and insertions of the internal oblique muscle and aponeurosis in the inguinal region are variable. The origin of the red muscle fibers is from the lateral inguinal ligament; this origin may extend as far medially as the deep ring (**a**), or the muscle may arise more laterally (**b**). The insertion of the aponeurosis is also variable; it may be inserted into the pubic crest and pubic tubercle (**c**) or solely into the rectus sheath (**d**). This gives four variants of the lower margin of the internal oblique in the inguinal canal: A–C, A–D, B–C, and B–D

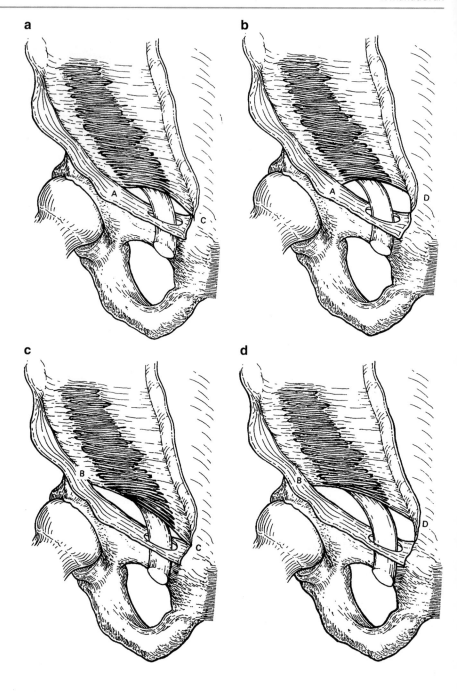

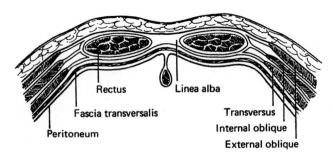

Fig. 2.23 Structure of the posterior rectus sheath in the upper abdomen. The internal oblique divides into two lamellae which enclose the rectus. The line of the fascia transversalis is deliberately emphasized

cord (or uterine round ligament) lies anterior to the conjoint tendon as it passes through the superficial inguinal ring.

The conjoint tendon has a very variable structure, and in 20% of subjects it does not exist as a discrete anatomic structure. It may be totally absent or only partially developed, or it may be replaced by a lateral extension of the tendon of origin of the rectus muscle, or it may extend lateral to the deep inguinal ring so that no interval is present between the lower border of the transversus and the inguinal ligament. A shutter mechanism for the conjoint tendon can only be demonstrated when laterally the transversus and internal oblique muscles that give rise to the conjoint tendon are seen to extend onto and are attached to the iliopectineal line [13]. The extent of

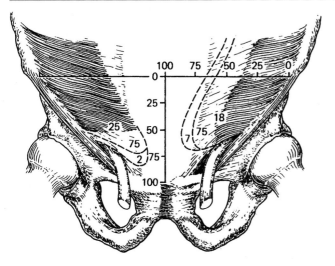

Fig. 2.24 Extent of the muscular fibers of the internal oblique. In only 2% of subjects the muscle extends inferiorly to the inguinal canal (*left* of diagram). Similarly the medial extent of the fleshy muscle fibers varies (*right* of diagram). The contribution of the internal oblique to the "defenses" of the inguinal canal is very variable [8] (from Anson et al.; with permission)

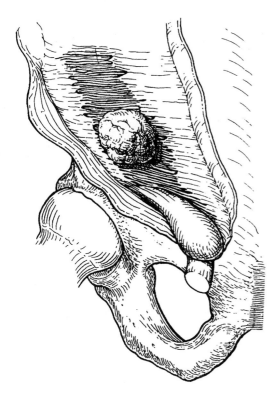

Fig. 2.25 A hernia can occur between bands of the internal oblique muscle. Although this hernia is in effect a variant Spigelian hernia, it presents as a direct hernia into the inguinal canal

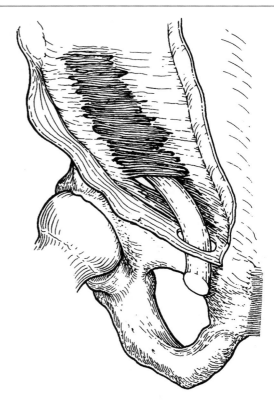

Fig. 2.26 Rarely fibers of the internal oblique muscle may extend medial to the deep ring, both above and below the ring, so that the cord is seen to pass between bands of the muscle

it extends as far laterally as the inferior epigastric vessels. In a minority of cases, bands of aponeurosis arise from the main aponeurotic arch and are inserted independently into the ilio-pectineal line. Sometimes, therefore, the lateral margin of the rectus sheath is formed only from the lowermost fibers of the transversus aponeurosis which curve inferiorly to become attached to the pubis—this is called the falx inguinalis.

A few fibers of the lowermost lateral margin of the rectus tendon may be fused with the fascia transversalis in their attachment to the iliopubic ligament—this has been called Henle's ligament (Fig. 2.31).

To understand the importance of the attachment of the internal oblique and transversus aponeuroses to the ilio-pectineal line, the posterior aspect of the inguinal canal must be visualized from inside the abdomen. If there is full attach-ment of the conjoint tendon to the iliopectineal line, the pos-terior wall of the inguinal canal may be said to be completely reinforced by aponeurosis. Absence of this attachment there-fore renders the posterior wall devoid of reinforcement. In this situation there is clearly the potential for a direct hernia or a large indirect hernia to develop.

Of all the anatomic layers, the external oblique is the least variable; in the inguinal region, it is invariably aponeurotic. The internal oblique and transversus layers are very variable; they may be fleshy almost to the midline, aponeurotic or banded fan-like with the space between the musculoaponeu-rotic bands occupied only by the flimsiest fascia. If these

this insertion is very variable. In 8% of cases this attachment does not extend lateral to the rectus muscle, leaving the pos-terior wall of the inguinal canal (fascia transversalis) in such individuals, unsupported. In 31% the attachment extends to the midpoint of the posterior wall between the pubic tubercle medially and the inferior epigastric vessels laterally; in 40%

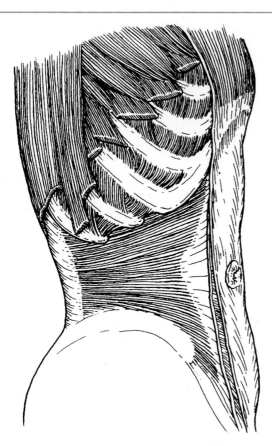

Fig. 2.27 The transversus muscle is the deepest of the anterolateral abdominal wall muscles; it arises from the iliopsoas fascia and inner lip of the iliac crest in its anterior two-thirds. The muscle extends to the inner surfaces of the lowest six costal cartilages, and its aponeurosis extends to the linea alba

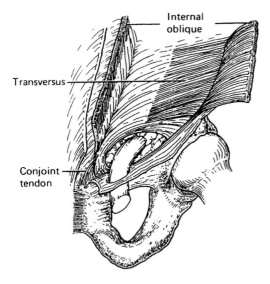

Fig. 2.28 The transversus muscle fibers run transversely, except in the lower abdomen where they form a strong aponeurosis (tendon) which is inserted to the pubic crest and the iliopectineal line. The insertion of the transversus tendon is broader than that of the internal oblique. The extent to which this tendon extends along the iliopectineal line determines its contribution to reinforcing the posterior wall of the inguinal canal. In surgical jargon the lowest fibers of the transversus aponeurosis cross over the cord to form the "roof" of the canal. These white aponeurotic fibers are referred to as the "arch" by some surgeons

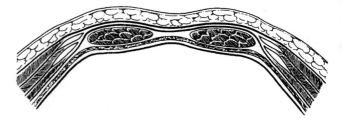

Fig. 2.29 Composition of the posterior rectus sheath in the lower abdomen. In the lower abdomen, inferior to the arcuate line of Douglas, the rectus sheath becomes deficient posteriorly. This is due to the fact that below the level of the arcuate line, all three aponeuroses (ext. oblique, int. oblique, and transversus abdominis) run in front of the rectus abdominis. The fascia transversalis, however, runs behind the rectus abdominis and in this location is denser and stronger than it is elsewhere

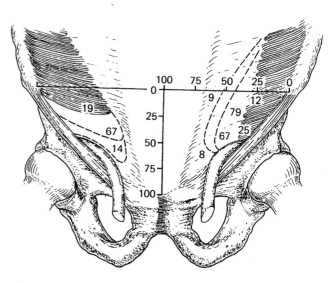

Fig. 2.30 The extent of fleshy red muscle in the transversus muscle is much less than in the internal oblique. Only in 14% of subjects is the lower margin of this muscle in the roof of the inguinal canal composed of red muscle (*left* of diagram). The medial extent of red fibers is similarly restricted; in 71% of subjects muscle fibers do not extend medially to the inferior epigastric vessels (*right* of diagram) [8] (from Anson et al.; with permission)

local weaknesses in the internal oblique and transversus are superimposed, herniation is facilitated.

Zimmerman et al. have drawn attention to the frequency with which defects occur in the internal oblique and transversus muscles in this area. In 45% of their dissections there was a defect in one or other of these two layers and in 6% the defects were present in both layers and superimposed in the region of the lower linea semilunaris. These defects predispose to spontaneous ventral hernias either of preperitoneal fat or more extensive hernias with peritoneal sacs [13].

Having considered the individual muscles in detail, it is now opportune to define the inguinal canal as an oblique slit, entirely within the layers of the abdominal wall, situated above and parallel to the inguinal ligament. It extends from the deep inguinal ring superolaterally to the superficial inguinal ring inferomedially. Its anterior wall is the deep

Fig. 2.31 The extent to which the tendon of transversus abdominis contributes to the posterior wall of the inguinal canal. In each illustration the arrow indicates the lateral most extension of the tendon and the corresponding percentage of subjects [8]

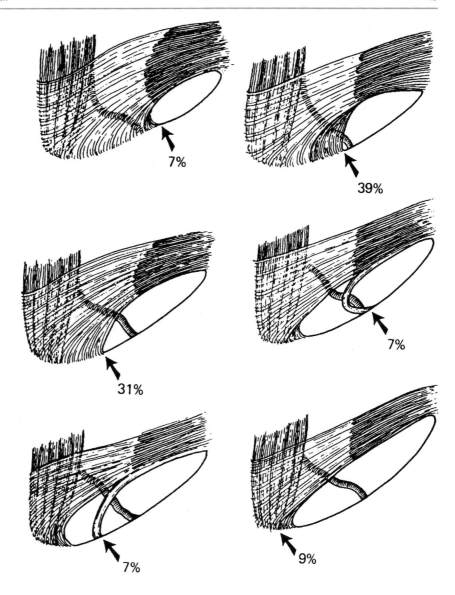

surface of the external oblique aponeurosis; its inferior boundary (floor) is the upper surface of the inguinal ligament, and its posterior wall is the fascia transversalis medial to the deep inguinal ring. This posterior wall is reinforced from its anterior aspect by the conjoint tendon. The roof (upper boundary of the inguinal canal) is formed by the inferior edges of the lowest fibers of internal oblique and transversus abdominis as they arch across from lateral to medial above the deep inguinal ring.

The Linea Alba and the Rectus Sheath and its Contents

The linea alba is a longitudinally disposed, midline interdigitation (decussation) of the aponeuroses of the three-ply muscles of one side (external oblique, internal oblique, and transversus abdominis) with those of the other. It is a pale band of dense fibrous tissue which extends from the xiphoid process above to the pubic symphysis below. The linea alba, interposed between the right and left rectus sheaths, is wide, thick, and tough above the level of the umbilicus. It is broadest at the umbilicus, and below the umbilicus it becomes progressively narrower until it is little more than a thin strip between the two rectus muscles at the suprapubic level. The linea alba is pierced by several small blood vessels and by the umbilical vessels in the fetus.

The anterior rectus sheath forms the most important portion of the abdominal wall aponeuroses. When the anterior sheath is gently dissected, during a paramedian incision, for example, it is shown to be made of three laminae. The most superficial fibers are directed downward and laterally; these are derived from the contralateral external oblique. The next layer is derived from the ipsilateral external oblique and has fibers which are oriented at right angles to those of the first layer, that is, they run downward and medially. Finally, the third component of the anterior rectus sheath is formed from the anterior lamina of the ipsilateral internal oblique muscle, whose fibers generally run in the same direction as, and parallel to, the fibers of the external oblique of the opposite side. This gives the anterior rectus sheath a triple crisscross pattern similar to plywood [14, 15]. In the lower abdomen the fusion of the external oblique aponeurosis to the internal oblique aponeurosis is very medial, an important anatomical arrangement that allows a tendon slide to be used to release the tension of the internal oblique in direct inguinal hernia repair without compromising the integrity of the anterior rectus sheath [14].

The most important feature from a surgical perspective is that the fibers of the rectus sheath run from side to side. **Vertical incisions divide fibers by running across them while horizontal incisions lie parallel to the line of the fibers in the rectus sheath and do not divide them**.

The posterior rectus sheath has a similar trilaminar crisscross pattern above the umbilicus, where it is composed of the posterior lamina of the internal oblique and the aponeuroses of the transversus abdominis muscle from either side.

Four or five centimeters below the level of the umbilicus, there is an abrupt change in the rectus sheath arrangement. Below this level all three aponeuroses (external oblique, internal oblique, and transversus abdominis) run altogether in front of the rectus abdominis muscle. Thus, below this level there is no aponeurotic contribution to the posterior wall of the rectus sheath; only fascia transversalis. This change in the relationship of the aponeuroses to the rectus abdominis muscle is manifest as the arcuate line (semicircular fold of Douglas) that is evident when the rectus abdominis is viewed from behind (Figs. 2.32 and 2.33). Below the arcuate line there is no aponeurosis in the **posterior wall of the rectus sheath**.

Within each rectus sheath are the rectus abdominis muscle, the pyramidalis muscle, the terminal portions of the lower six thoracic nerves, and the superior and inferior epigastric vessels (Fig. 2.34).

Innervation and Blood Supply of the Muscles of the Anterior Abdominal Wall

The muscles of the anterior and anterolateral abdominal wall are supplied segmentally by the 7th to 11th intercostal nerves and the subcostal nerve. These nerves (accompanied by their corresponding posterior intercostal vessels) cross the costal margin obliquely to run in the neurovascular plane of the anterior abdominal wall, between the internal oblique and transversus abdominis muscles. The nerves supply these muscles and divide into lateral and anterior branches. The former penetrate the overlying internal oblique to supply the external oblique muscle, while the anterior branches con-

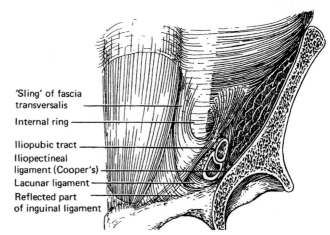

Fig. 2.32 The fascia transversalis, part of the endoabdominal fascia, lies on the deep surface of the transversus muscle. In the upper abdomen this fascia is thin and featureless; however, in the lower abdomen and pelvis the fascia transversalis has an important role. It is thickened and includes specialized bands and folds. It forms the posterior wall of the inguinal canal, and at the deep ring it has a condensation medial to the cord. This condensation is part of a U-shaped sling through which the cord passes. This sling hitches the cord up laterally when the transversus muscle contracts. Just above the inguinal ligament, the fascia transversalis is thickened as the iliopubic tract or Thomson's band [30]

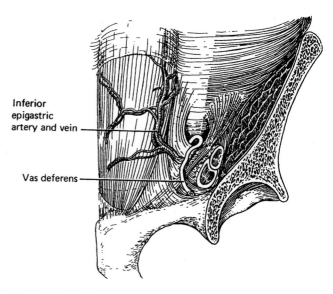

Fig. 2.33 Seen from behind, the view from within the abdomen, the inferior epigastric vessels are deep, on the abdominal side, of this curtain of fascia transversalis. The vas deferens and cord structures ascend to and hook over the sling of fascia transversalis at the deep ring

tinue medially in the neurovascular plane, before entering the rectus abdominis muscle through its posterior surface. The supraumbilical part of rectus abdominis is supplied segmentally by the 7th, 8th, and 9th intercostal nerves.

Having supplied all these muscles segmentally, the nerves eventually reach the surface either as lateral or anterior cutaneous nerves (as previously described).

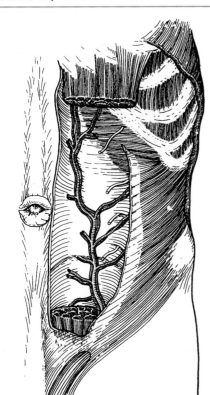

Fig. 2.34 Rectus sheath and linea alba. The contents of the rectus sheath are the rectus and pyramidalis muscles, the superior and inferior epigastric vessels, and the terminal branches of the lower six thoracic nerves

The lowest fibers of the internal oblique and transversus abdominis (i.e., those that contribute to the shutter mechanism of the inguinal canal) are supplied by the iliohypogastric and ilioinguinal nerves (L1 fibers).

The posterior intercostal arteries supply the three-ply muscles in the lateral part of the anterior abdominal wall, and in this function are reinforced by the lumbar arteries (direct branches of the abdominal aorta). The rectus abdominis muscle by contrast is supplied by the ipsilateral superior and inferior epigastric vessels which anastomose with each other within the rectus sheath.

Function of the Anterior Abdominal Wall

Although the anterior abdominal wall is composed of symmetrical halves, right and left, these halves function together in a coordinated and synergistic manner. The individual muscles cannot work separately and independently. The upper part of the anterior abdominal wall is the actively mobile respiratory zone, where the rectus sheath—the (anterolateral) flank muscles and the rectus muscle through its tendinous attachments to the rectus

sheath—functions collectively as an accessory respiratory muscle. The lower part has no tendinous intersections and is a relatively fixed lower belly support zone. This anatomical and physiological configuration has been demonstrated using a transillumination silhouette technique by Askar [14].

The Fascia Transversalis: The Space of Bogros

The fascia transversalis lies immediately deep to the transversus abdominis muscle and for the most part, is intimately adherent to the deep surface of the muscle. It is continuous from side to side and extends from the rib cage above to the pelvis inferiorly.

In the upper abdominal wall the fascia transversalis is thin, but in the lower abdomen and especially in the inguinofemoral region, the fascia is thicker and has specialized bands and folds within it. In the groin region, where the fascia transversalis is an important constituent of the posterior wall of the inguinal canal and where it forms the femoral sheath distal to the inguinal ligament, the anatomy and function of the fascia transversalis is of particular importance to the surgeon. As originally stated in his exquisite and detailed account of the fascia transversalis in the groin [16], Sir Astley Cooper described the fascia transversalis as consisting of two layers. The anterior strong layer covers the deep aspect of the transversalis muscle where it is intimately blended with the tendon of the transversus muscle. It then extends across the posterior wall of the inguinal canal medial to the deep ring aperture and is attached to the inner margin of the medial end of the inguinal ligament. The posterior (deeper) layer of fascia transversalis is a filmy layer, and lies between the anterior substantial layer of fascia transversalis and the peritoneum. The extraperitoneal fat lies behind this filmy layer: between it and the peritoneum (Fig. 2.35). The (deep) inferior epigastric vessels run between the two layers of fascia transversalis.

These two distinct layers of fascia transversalis are readily identified laparoscopically and must be opened separately to allow access to the avascular preperitoneal space (of Bogros) when undertaking an extraperitoneal repair of a groin hernia either endoscopically or by open surgery. The deeper layer extends down behind the inguinal canal and fuses with the pectineal ligament (of Cooper) before continuing downward into the pelvis. The deeper layer fuses with the spermatic cord at the deep ring and continues along the cord as part of the internal spermatic fascia [16–18]. The existence of the bilaminar structure of the fascia transversalis at the deep ring was confirmed by Lytle [19] and by Cleland et al. [20], but its nature disputed by the later anatomists Anson and McVay [8], and its relevance and importance questioned by experienced surgeons [21].

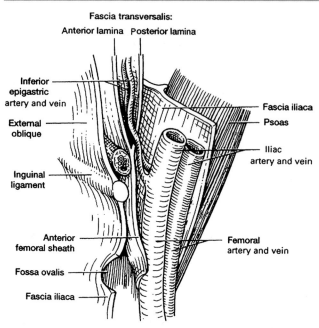

Fig. 2.35 The bilaminar fascia transversalis in the groin [18, 29]

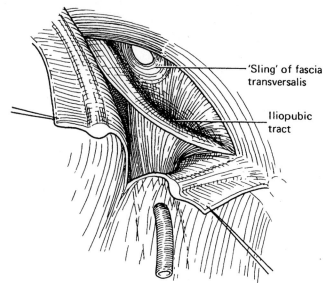

Fig. 2.36 Dissected further anteriorly, if the inguinal ligament is divided, the fascia transversalis can be seen to be continuous with the femoral sheath. The thickening at the junction of fascia transversalis with the femoral sheath is the iliopubic tract. The internal oblique muscle, which arises from the lateral inguinal ligament, acts as a shutter or "lid" on the deep inguinal ring

The dissection of both layers of fascia transversalis from the cord structures at the deep inguinal ring is an important component of hernioplasty; it allows dissection of an indirect peritoneal sac and the divided peritoneal stump to retract at the deep ring in a classic Bassini and Shouldice operation for indirect hernias.

In the lower abdomen it is attached laterally to the internal lip of the iliac crest, along which line it becomes continuous with the fascia over the iliacus and psoas muscles. From these lateral attachments the fascia extends medially as a continuous curtain, which is interrupted only by the transit of the spermatic cord at the deep inguinal ring. The fascia transversalis invests the cord structures as they pass through it with a thin layer of fascia, the internal spermatic fascia. On the medial margin of the deep ring the fascia transversalis is condensed into a U-shaped sling, with the cord supported in the concavity of the ring and the two limbs extending superiorly and laterally to be suspended from the posterior aspect of the transversus muscle. The curve of the "U" lies at or just below the "arched" lower border of the aponeurosis of the transverse muscle.

This U-shaped fold, the fascia transversalis sling, is the functional basis of the inguinal "shutter" mechanism; as the transverse muscle contracts during coughing or straining, the column/pillars of the ring are pulled together, and the entire sling drawn upward and laterally. This motion increases the obliquity of exit of the spermatic cord structures through the ring and provides protection from forces tending to cause an indirect hernia (Figs. 2.32 and 2.33) [19]. The reconstruction of this sling medially with preservation of the function of the ring laterally is the rationale of

anterior inguinal hernioplasty. In front of the ring lies the lower border of the transverse muscle and the internal oblique muscle. Each of these structures supports the internal ring, and together they provide a very effective valve when the intra-abdominal pressure rises.

The "shutter" action of the internal ring, the fascia transversalis sling, can be demonstrated readily at operation under local anesthetic. If the patient is asked to cough, the ring is suddenly pulled upward and laterally behind the lower margin of the transverse muscle. In the adult with an obliterated processus vaginalis, a flat lid of peritoneum covers the ring internally for the spermatic vessels, and the vas deferens lies extraperitoneally. The spermatic vessels pass down almost vertically retroperitoneally on the psoas muscle. As they enter the narrow gutter of the groin, they are joined by the vas deferens: the spermatic cord thus formed, turns obligingly upward, and then hooks around the fascia transversalis sling to enter the deep ring, acquiring an investment of internal spermatic fascia as it traverses the ring (Fig. 2.36).

The inferior border of the internal ring abuts on a condensation of the fascia transversalis, the iliopubic tract, or bandelette ilio-pubienne of Thomson. This narrow fascial band extends from the ASIS laterally to the pubis medially. The band is a condensation (and integral part) of the fascia transversalis; it lies on a plane somewhat deeper than the inguinal ligament which can be readily demonstrated as distinct from it, at operation. The iliopubic tract bridges the femoral canal medially and then curves inferiorly and posteriorly to spread out fanwise to its attachment to a broad area of the superior

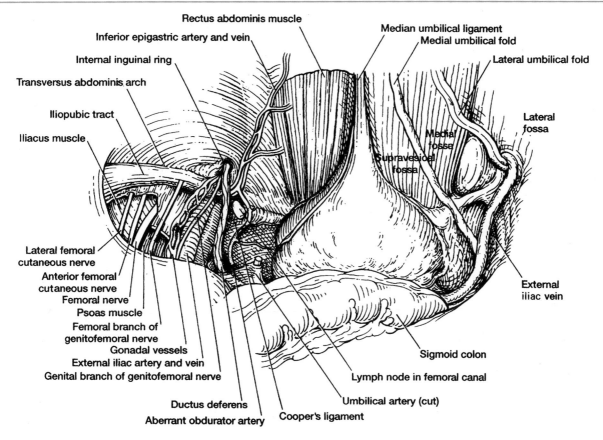

Rectus abdominis muscle
Inferior epigastric artery and vein
Internal inguinal ring
Transversus abdominis arch
Iliopubic tract
Iliacus muscle
Median umbilical ligament
Medial umbilical fold
Lateral umbilical fold
Lateral fossa
Medial fossa
Supravesical fossa
Lateral femoral cutaneous nerve
Anterior femoral cutaneous nerve
Femoral nerve
Psoas muscle
Femoral branch of genitofemoral nerve
Gonadal vessels
External iliac artery and vein
Genital branch of genitofemoral nerve
External iliac vein
Sigmoid colon
Lymph node in femoral canal
Umbilical artery (cut)
Ductus deferens
Aberrant obdurator artery
Cooper's ligament

Fig. 2.37 The posterior view of the lower abdomen. The peritoneum is intact on the right side, illustrating the fossae demarcated by the umbilical ligaments. On the contralateral side the peritoneum has been removed to allow visualization of the extraperitoneal structures, the vessels and nerves [31, 32]

ramus of the pubis along the iliopectineal line just behind Cooper's ligament. The iliopubic tract thus forms the inferior margin of the defect in the fascia transversalis both in an indirect inguinal hernia and in a direct hernia. However, it is superior to the neck of the peritoneal sac of a femoral hernia (Figs. 2.32 and 2.37).

The fascia transversalis superior to the iliopubic tract extends over the posterior wall of the inguinal canal up to and posterior to the arch of the transverse muscle. Medially the fascia transversalis runs behind the aponeurosis of the transversus abdominis muscle and thereby blends with the posterior wall of the rectus sheath above the level of the arcuate line. Below the level of the arcuate line, it is directly related to the posterior surface of the rectus abdominis. Inferolaterally, it is directly posterior to the lowermost arching fibers of transversus abdominis muscle and conjoint tendon. The fascia transversalis in the posterior wall of the inguinal canal is supported to a variable extent by the aponeurosis of the transverse muscle as it arches down to its attachment to the pubis and iliopectineal line. Medial to the deep inguinal ring and deep to the fascia transversalis, lying in the extraperitoneal fat between the peritoneum and the fascia, the deep epigastric vessels follow an oblique course upward and medially to the

deep aspect of the rectus muscle. This triangular area, bounded by the deep epigastric vessels laterally, the lateral margin of the rectus muscle medially, and the inguinal ligament below, is known to surgeons as Hesselbach's triangle; this is the area through which a direct inguinal hernia protrudes.

More exactly, a direct hernia explodes through the fascia transversalis in the area bounded by the iliopubic tract inferiorly, the medial limb of the fascia transversalis sling laterally and the lower margin of the arch of the transversus aponeurosis superiorly.

Condon has investigated the anatomy of the fascia transversalis using a technique of transillumination of fresh tissue. He clearly shows these anatomic details and defines the margins of the aponeurotic deficiency in the posterior inguinal canal wall through which direct hernia protrudes. This area of fascia transversalis is buttressed anteriorly to a greater or lesser degree by the aponeurosis of the transverse muscle as it inserts to the iliopectineal line. At operation these features—the iliopubic tract, the deep ring, and the "line" of the arch of the transverse aponeurosis—are easily identifiable if the fascia transversalis is adequately dissected. Indeed, the identification of all these features is an essential prerequisite to adequate inguinal hernioplasty (Fig. 2.37) [22].

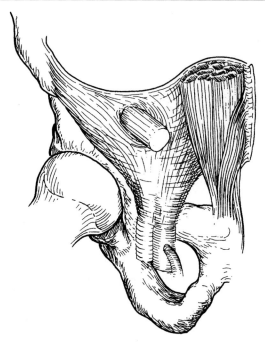

Fig. 2.38 From the front, as the surgeon visualizes the subject, the fascia transversalis in the groin resembles a funnel with a valved side vent. The femoral vessels come out of the funnel below and the cord structures out of the "side vent" which is "valved" by the sling of the fascia transversalis at the deep ring

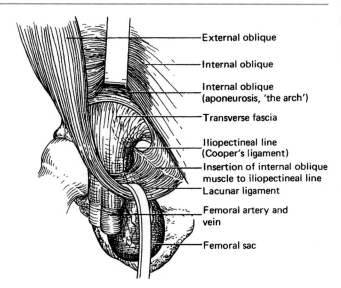

- External oblique
- Internal oblique
- Internal oblique (aponeurosis, 'the arch')
- Transverse fascia
- Iliopectineal line (Cooper's ligament)
- Insertion of internal oblique muscle to iliopectineal line
- Lacunar ligament
- Femoral artery and vein
- Femoral sac

Fig. 2.39 A dissection to demonstrate the anatomy of a femoral hernia. The femoral cone of fascia transversalis is stretched on its medial aspect; the hernial sac extends within this cone of fascia transversalis medial to the femoral vein and lateral to the lacunar ligament

The fascia transversalis in the groin is but a part of the fascial continuum which surgical anatomists refer to as the endoabdominal fascia. This fascia is distinct in the lower abdomen but is fused into the fascia on the deep surface of the transverse abdominal muscle superiorly. This composite layer, the transverse muscle and its fascia (the fascia transversalis), is the most important of the abdominal wall strata in solving the problem of inguinofemoral hernia, as the integrity of this layer prevents herniation. Defects in it, congenital or acquired, are the etiology of all groin hernias.

The fascia transversalis descends behind the inguinal ligament into the thigh as the sheath of the femoral vessels—this is a funnel-like sheath. Inferior to the inguinal ligament, the fascia transversalis attaches to the iliopectineal line medially and posteriorly to the femoral vessels. This funnel of fascia transversalis extends into the thigh as far as the fossa ovalis in the deep fascia. This anatomic arrangement allows for a small "space" medial to the femoral vein through which some lymphatics pass. When a femoral hernia develops, this "space" is expanded (Figs. 2.38 and 2.39).

What, then, is the anatomy of the peritoneum relative to the layering of the abdominal wall we have considered previously? In the lower abdomen the peritoneum is thrown up into fivefolds which converge as they pass upwards to the umbilicus. The median umbilical fold extends from the apex of the bladder to the umbilicus and contains the remnant

urachus. To either lateral side the medial umbilical fold contains the obliterated umbilical artery, and more laterally the inferior epigastric vessels raise the lateral umbilical fold. These folds create depressions or fossae in the anterior abdominal peritoneum: the supravesical fossae right and left, and the medial and the lateral inguinal fossae right and left. A further depression on either side is below and medial to the lateral inguinal fossa and separated from it by the inguinal ligament. This overlies the femoral ring and is called the femoral fossa.

Hernias egress through these fossae—the femoral through the femoral fossa, the indirect inguinal through the lateral inguinal fossa and the direct through the medial fossa. Internal supravesical hernias can occur in the supravesical fossa (Fig. 2.37).

The landmarks are the peritoneal folds, particularly the medial umbilical ligament (containing the obliterated umbilical artery) and the lateral umbilical fold (containing the inferior epigastric vessels). The peritoneum overlying the deep inguinal ring is identified with the testicular vessels and vas deferens clearly visible beneath the peritoneum. The peritoneum is separated from the underlying fascia transversalis by adipose tissue except medial to the deep ring where the peritoneum is more firmly fixed to the subjacent fascia transversalis. Below, posterior to, the inguinal ligament, the genital branch of the genitofemoral nerve is seen joining the cord structures at the deep ring.

The lateral cutaneous nerve of the thigh and the femoral branch of the genitofemoral nerve lie rather deeper in the fatty tissue overlying the iliopsoas muscle. Blood vessels are also found in the adipose tissue beneath the peritoneum, in the extraperitoneal plane branches of the deep circumflex iliac vessels laterally and of the obturator vessels inferiorly and medially. There is an extensive venous circulation (anastomosis) in the extraperitoneal tissues between the inferior epigastric vein and obturator veins. This venous anastomosis lies between the two lamina of the fascia transversalis in the space of Bogros [17]. This space is continuous from side to side and with the pelvic space, the cave of Retzius. The space of Bogros is important for extraperitoneal repair of hernia and is the repository of bleeding in pelvic trauma.

The Peritoneum: The View from Within

Hernia sacs are composed of peritoneum, and they may contain intra-abdominal viscera. From within they consist of the peritoneum, then a loose layer of extraperitoneal fat, then the deep membranous lamina of fascia transversalis, then the vessels such as the epigastric vessels in the space of Bogros, then the stout anterior lamina of fascia transversalis, and then the muscles and aponeuroses of the abdominal wall [23]. The preperitoneal space lies in the abdominal cavity between the peritoneum internally and transversalis fascia externally. Within this space lies a variable quantity of adipose tissue, loose connective tissue, and membranous tissue and other anatomical entities such as arteries, veins, nerves, and various organs such as the kidneys and ureters. The clinically significant parts of the preperitoneal space include the space associated with the structural elements related to the myopectineal orifice of Fruchaud, the prevesical space of Retzius, the space of Bogros, and retroperitoneal periurinary space [24]. The myopectineal orifice of Fruchaud represents the potentially weak area in the abdominal wall, which permits inguinal and femoral hernias. The preperitoneal space lies deep to the supravesical fossa, and the medial inguinal fossa is the prevesical space of Retzius. The space of Retzius contains loose connective tissue and fat but more importantly vascular elements such as an abnormal obturator artery and vein. Bogros' space, which is a triangular area between the abdominal wall and peritoneum, can be entered by means of an incision through the roof and floor of the inguinal canal through which the posterior preperitoneal approach for hernia repair can be achieved. In the groin these muscles and aponeuroses are variously absent over the inguinal and crural canals. The myopectineal orifice of Fruchaud (Fig. 2.40) [25, 26] denotes a well-defined area through which all groin herniae present. Such a unifying concept of a single groin aperture is relevant for mesh repairs, whether repair is achieved by anterior open operation or by posterior endoscopic operation. The boundaries of the myopectineal orifice of Fruchaud are as follows: superiorly the "arch" of the transversus muscle, laterally the iliopsoas muscle, medially the lateral border of rectus

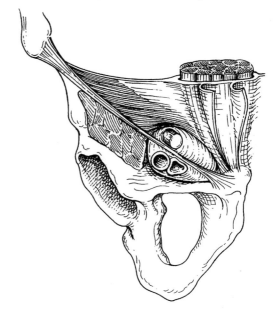

Fig. 2.40 The "myopectineal orifice of Fruchaud": the area of the groin limited above by the arching fibers of internal oblique and transversus abdominis, and below by the superior ramus of the pubis. It is crossed obliquely by the rigid inguinal ligament above which is the inguinal canal and below which lies the femoral canal [26]

abdominis muscle, and inferiorly the superior ramus of the pubis [27]. The space is utilized in both the transabdominal preperitoneal and the totally extraperitoneal laparoscopic approaches to the repair of inguinal and femoral repairs. A thorough understanding of the limits of this myopectineal orifice is necessary to accomplish an effective repair of the inguinal floor using laparoscopic methods.

Between the peritoneum and the fascia transversalis, there is a loose layer of extraperitoneal fat, used as an important landmark in many surgical operations. Hernial protrusions progress from within outward through deficiencies in the musculoaponeurotic lamina of the abdominal wall; they carry this extraperitoneal fat with them along the track of the hernia sac. Abundance of this fat at the fundus of an indirect inguinal hernia gives rise to the surgical misnomer a "lipoma of the cord"—in reality this no more than extraperitoneal fat around the fundus of a peritoneal hernia sac (Fig. 2.41).

The Umbilicus

Between the sixth and tenth week of gestation, the abdominal viscera enlarge rapidly and to such an extent that they can no longer be contained within the proportionately smaller coelomic cavity. Consequently, developing viscera (derived exclusively from the midgut) are temporarily extruded through the broad umbilical deficit into the exocoelom which occupies the base of the umbilical cord. At about the tenth week the abdominal cavity has enlarged

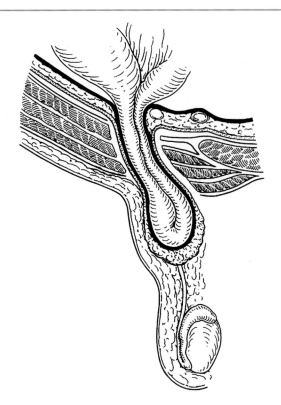

Fig. 2.41 As the peritoneum forms an indirect inguinal hernia it carries with it a covering of extraperitoneal fat. This extraperitoneal fat is referred to by many surgeons as "lipoma of the cord"

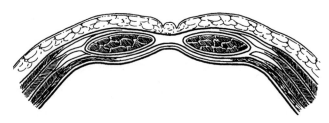

Fig. 2.42 Cross section through the umbilicus and adjacent anterior abdominal wall. The aponeuroses of the anterolateral abdominal muscles of the two sides are fused with each other in the umbilical cicatrix

sufficiently to reaccommodate the extruded viscera, and by the time of birth all the intestines are contained within the abdominal cavity proper. At birth the abdominal wall is complete except for the space occupied by the umbilical cord. Running in the cord are the urachus (from the apex of the urinary bladder), the umbilical arteries coursing up from the pelvis, and the umbilical vein directed to the liver. After the cord is ligated, the stump sloughs off, and the resultant granulating surface cicatrizes and epithelializes from its periphery.

In the normal umbilicus there is a single layer of fused fibrous tissue consisting of the superficial fascia, the medial edge of the rectus sheath and linea alba, and the fascia transversalis. The peritoneum is adherent to the deep aspect of this (Fig. 2.42).

The Spermatic Cord

The spermatic cord is composed of (a) arteries: the testicular artery, the artery to the vas deferens, and the cremasteric artery; (b) veins: the testicular veins form the pampiniform plexus of veins within the spermatic cord; (c) lymphatics; (d) nerves: the genital branch of the genitofemoral nerve and autonomic nerves; (e) vas deferens; and (f) the processus vaginalis.

The spermatic cord, as it emerges through the abdominal wall from the deep inguinal ring, receives investments of fascia. The fascia transversalis forms a thin, funicular coat called the internal spermatic fascia: the internal oblique invests it with a tracing of muscle fibers, the cremaster muscle, and most superficially it is coated with external spermatic fascia derived from the external oblique aponeurosis at the margins of the superficial inguinal ring. Each of these fascial layers requires opening to identify the processus vaginalis or sac of an indirect hernia. Until birth the processus vaginalis, although minute and narrow, remains, nevertheless, as an uninterrupted diverticulum from the abdominal peritoneum through the length of the cord to the testis, where it opens out to become the tunica vaginalis of the testis. Normally, the processus vaginalis becomes obliterated in most males soon after birth, except for the portion of the processus that surrounds the testis. This unobliterated part is known as the tunica vaginalis testis. More recently the persistence of the processus vaginalis into adult life has been confirmed when hydrocele or hernia has complicated peritoneal dialysis in renal failure patients. The theories and mechanism of testicular descent and the development of the processus vaginalis (Fig. 2.43) are described in detail in Chap. 9.

An indirect inguinal hernial sac is a similar peritoneal diverticulum which extends into the spermatic cord and occupies the same position as the primitive processus vaginalis. Often indirect hernias also have extraperitoneal fat at their fundus.

Comparative Anatomy

A cool environment for spermatogenesis is a necessity in warm-blooded birds and mammals. Birds, which have high blood temperatures and are invariably cryptorchid, keep their testes cool by an air stream around the abdomen. In some sea-living mammals—whales and sea cows—the testes remain intra-abdominal, but presumably the constant contact with cold water is effective in keeping them cool.

The necessity to have the testes reside in a colder scrotum leads to problems, not only in humans but in domestic and farm animals; the topic of hernia and undescended testicles appears in veterinary textbooks where it has a practical and economic importance of its own. Inguinal hernias are fairly common in pigs and horses but less common in bovine

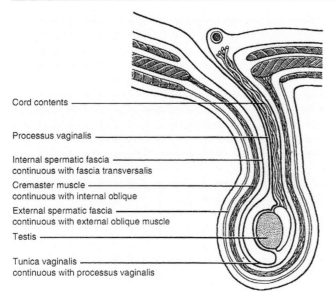

Cord contents

Processus vaginalis

Internal spermatic fascia
continuous with fascia transversalis

Cremaster muscle
continuous with internal oblique

External spermatic fascia
continuous with external oblique muscle

Testis

Tunica vaginalis
continuous with processus vaginalis

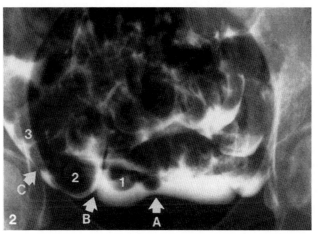

Fig. 2.44 Normal herniography. *A*, median umbilical fold; *B*, medial umbilical fold; *C*, lateral umbilical fold; *1*, supravesical fossa; *2*, medial inguinal fossa; *3*, lateral inguinal fossa

Fig. 2.43 Section through the spermatic cord and testis. The importance of the layers is demonstrated. The external spermatic fascia is derived from the fascia over the external oblique muscle at the superficial ring, the cremaster arises from the internal oblique muscle, and the internal spermatic fascia is the continuation of the fascia transversalis over the cord structures. Each of these layers needs division in inguinal hernia repair

species. The economic consequence of an inguinal hernia in a stallion is considerable; the hernia may become incarcerated during mating, and this may hinder full consummation. A similar problem is documented in stud bulls. Hernias are relatively common in dogs, but are rather rare in cats. Dogs, both male and female, may develop inguinal hernias, but the males are more likely to have intestine caught within the hernial sac. When a female dog develops a hernia, the usual content is one of the uterine horns and the broad ligament; this can present the danger of strangulation if the animal becomes pregnant (the content of a congenital hernia in a girl is most likely an ovary and a fallopian tube). In the dog, most veterinary surgeons treat the hernia by orchidectomy (a proposition which is sometimes put forward for the handling of the same situation in the elderly human).

Bats have testicles which are normally intra-abdominal and descend into the scrotum only at the time of mating. In these animals there is a low incidence of hernia and of a patent processus vaginalis. The testicles in bats descend to the scrotum and ascend to the abdomen, although there is no patent processus vaginalis. In small boys with retractile testicles which disappear up to the external inguinal ring, a hernia is rarely present.

Radiological Anatomy

Precise knowledge of the radiological anatomy is the key to success in the diagnosis and evaluation of groin masses which defy clinical diagnosis. Several diagnostic modalities

are available including conventional radiography, ultrasound, CT, and Magnetic resonance imaging (MRI) scanning [28]. Herniography can be used in the diagnosis of hernia for patients with equivocal findings or those presenting with groin pain (see Chap. 13). The technique involves intraperitoneal administration of 50 mL of nonionic contrast medium; a standard series of views of both groins is obtained during straining with the patient prone and in a slightly elevated position, as follows: posteroanterior, posteroanterior with caudocranial angulation of the tube (15°), two oblique views, and a lateral view. A normal herniogram shows the median medial and lateral umbilical folds and the supravesical, medial inguinal, and lateral inguinal fossae (Fig. 2.44). A disadvantage of herniography is its invasiveness and its inability to depict pathological conditions other than hernias.

Ultrasonography with a high-frequency (7.5–10 MHz), short-focus transducer can depict the muscle and fascial layers of the abdominal wall and groin region. In these patients 5- or even 3.5-MHz transducers may be used which however result in low-resolution images. The entire anterior abdominal wall including the oblique muscles, transversus muscle, rectus abdominis, and peritoneum can be visualized separately and clearly (Fig. 2.45). A major advantage is the ability to perform the examination in supine and upright positions as well as at rest and during straining, the so-called dynamic scanning technique. Yet another advantage is that ultrasound examination is noninvasive and allows comparison between the symptomatic and the asymptomatic side. The disadvantage however is its operator dependency and the considerable variation in imaging quality associated with the body habitus of the subject.

Computed tomography (CT) is usually performed in the inguinal region during breath-hold without straining. The anatomy of the anterior abdominal wall can be delineated clearly (Fig. 2.46). Because the inferior epigastric vessels

Fig. 2.45 Extended field-of-view ultrasound image demonstrating part of the anterior abdominal wall. *A*, external oblique muscle; *B*, internal oblique muscle; *C*, transversus muscle; *D*, rectus abdominis muscle

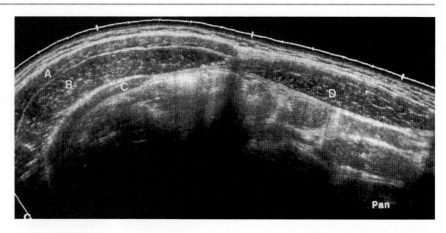

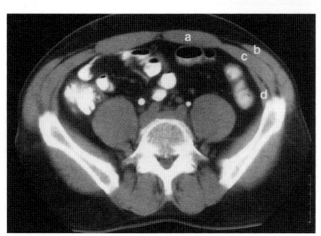

Fig. 2.46 A CT scan demonstrating normal anatomy of the muscles of the abdominal wall. *a*, Rectus abdominis muscle; *b*, external oblique muscle; *c*, internal oblique muscle; *d*, transversus muscle

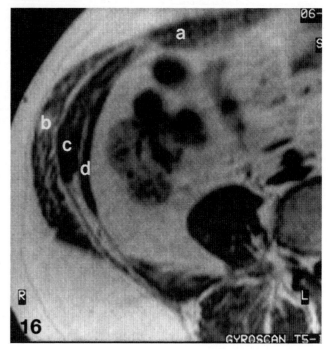

Fig. 2.47 Transverse T2-weighted MR image depicting the muscles of the anterior abdominal wall; *a*, rectus abdominis muscle; *b*, external oblique muscle; *c*, internal oblique muscle; *d*, transversus muscle; *R*, lateral; *L*, medial

forming the lateral umbilical folds can be clearly identified, CT is very reliable in helping differentiate between direct and indirect inguinal hernias.

MRI has the advantage of being able to obtain images in any plane either by direct scanning in different planes or by making multi-planar reconstructions on a work station. MRI can also be performed during straining to gain dynamic images. The layers of the anterior abdominal wall (including transversalis fascia, extraperitoneal fat, and peritoneum) can be delineated with precision using MRI (Fig. 2.47). CT scanning and MRI imaging have approximately the same order of sensitivity and specificity in diagnosing groin hernias.

References

1. Anson BJ, McVay CB. The anatomy of the inguinal region. Surg Gynecol Obstet. 1938;66:186–94.
2. Hesselbach FK. Neueste Anatomisch-Pathologische Untersuchungen uberden Ursprung und das Fortschreiten der Leisten und Schenkelbruche. Warzburg: Baumgartner; 1814.
3. Rozen WM, Ashton MW, Taylor GI. Reviewing the vascular supply of the anterior abdominal wall: redefining anatomy for increasingly refined surgery. Clin Anat. 2008;21:89–98.
4. Ruge, 1908 Cited in Rauber's Lehrbuch der Anatomie des Menschen, Kopsch FR Abt 5; Nervansystem 388; 1920.
5. Horner CH et al. Cited in Van Mameren H, PMNYH Go. Anatomy and variations of the internal inguinal region. In: Schumpelick V, Wantz GE, editors. Inguinal hernia repair. Basel: Karger; 1994.
6. Yeates WK. Pain in the scrotum. Br J Hosp Med. 1985;133:101–4.
7. McVay CB. The anatomy of the relaxing incision in inguinal hernioplasty. Q Bull North West Univ Med School. 1962; 36: 245–52.
8. Anson BJ, Morgan EH, McVay CB. Surgical anatomy of the inguinal region based upon a study of 500 body halves. Surg Gynecol Obstet. 1960;111:707–25.
9. Acland RD. The inguinal ligament and its lateral attachments: correcting an anatomical error. Clin Anat. 2008;21:55–61.

10. Spangen L. Spigelian hernia. Acta Chir Scand Suppl. 1976; 462: 1–47.
11. Zimmerman LM, Anson BJ. Anatomy and surgery of hernia. 2nd ed. Baltimore: Williams and Wilkins; 1967. p. 216–27.
12. Ulbak S, Ornsholt J. Para-inguinal hernia: an atypical spigelian variant. Acta Chir Scand. 1983;149:335–6.
13. Zimmerman LM, Anson BJ, Morgan EH, McVay CB. Ventral hernia due to normal banding of the abdominal muscles. Surg Gynecol Obstet. 1944;78:535–40.
14. Askar O. Surgical anatomy of the aponeurotic expansions of the anterior abdominal wall. Ann R Coll Surg Engl. 1977;59: 313–21.
15. Rizk NN. A new description of the anterior abdominal wall in man and mammals. J Anat. 1980;131:373–85.
16. Cooper A. The anatomy and surgical treatment of inguinal and congenital hernia I. London: T. Cox; 1804.
17. Bendavid R. The space of Bogros and the deep inguinal circulation. Surg Gynecol Obstet. 1992;174:355–8.
18. Read RC. Cooper's posterior lamina of transversalis fascia. Surg Gynecol Obstet. 1992;174:426–34.
19. Lytle WJ. The deep inguinal ring, development, function and repair. Br J Surg. 1970;57:531–6.
20. Cleland J, MacKay JY, Young RB. The relation of the aponeurosis of the transversalis and internal oblique muscles to the deep epigastric artery and the inguinal canal. Mem Memor Anat. 1889; 1:142.
21. Condon RE. The Anatomy of the inguinal region and its relation to groin hernia. In: Nyhus LM, Condon RE, editors. Hernia 4th ed. Philadelphia: Lippincott;1995.
22. Condon RE. Surgical anatomy of the transversus abdominis and transversalis fascia. Annals of Surgery. New York: Raven Press; 1971.
23. Condon RE. Reassessment of groin anatomy during the evolution of preperitoneal hernia repair. Am J Surg. 1996;172:5–8.
24. Kingsnorth AN, Skandalakis PN, Colborn GL, Weidman TA, Skandalakis LJ, Skandalakis JE. Embryology, anatomy and surgical applications of the preperitoneal space. Surg Clin North Am. 2000;80:1–24.
25. Fruchaud H. Anatomie chirurgicale des hernies de l'aine. Paris: G. Dion; 1956.
26. Wantz GE. Atlas of hernia surgery. New York: Raven Press; 1991.
27. Arregui ME. The laparoscopic perspective of the anatomy of the peritoneum, preperitoneal fascia, transversalis fascia and structures in the space of Bogros. Postgrad Gen Surg. 1995;6:30–6.
28. van den Berg JC, de Valois JC, Go PMNYH, Rosenbusch G. Radiological anatomy of the groin region. Eur Radiol. 2000;10:661–70.
29. Skandalakis LJ, Gadacz TR, Mansberger AR, Mitchell WE, Colborn GL, Skandalakis IE. Modern hernia repair. New York: Parthenon Publishing; 1996.
30. Lytle WJ. Internal inguinal ring. Br J Surg. 1945;32:441–6.
31. van Mameren H, Go PMNYH. Surgical anatomy of the interior of inguinal region: consequences for laparoscopic hernia repair. Surg Endosc. 1994;8(10):1212–5.
32. Horner CH et al. Cited in Van Mameren H, Go PMNYH. Anatomy and variations of the internal inguinal region. In: Schumpelick V, Wantz GE, editors. Inguinal hernia repair. Basel: Karger; 1994.

Epidemiology and Etiology of Primary Groin Hernias

Brian M. Stephenson

The population prevalence (the percentage of a population being studied that is affected with a particular disease at any given time) and the incidence (the rate of occurrence of new cases of a particular disease in a population being studied) of groin hernias have been studied extensively by a variety of authors in the last 100 years [1]. In developed countries the incidence of operations for groin hernia is approximately 2000 operations per million population per year [2]. Nationwide information on the relation between the number of procedures performed per year and the rates of incidence of groin hernia have been more difficult to establish. However, the 1981/1982 morbidity statistics from general practice (third national study) estimated that approximately the same number of *new* hernias was diagnosed annually by general practitioners as the number of patients consulting their doctors with *existing* hernias [3]. This clearly suggests that a large number of groin hernias are not referred for definitive surgical treatment and that the prevalence is far higher than the annual incidence of operation. A survey in Somerset and Avon Health Authority in the United Kingdom of a stratified random sample of 28,000 adults aged over 35 enquired about lumps in the groin and invited those indicating positive replies to attend for interview and examination. The results revealed that of the hernias discovered, one-third of patients had not consulted their primary care physician and of the two-thirds that had seen their primary care physician, less than half had been referred to a surgeon for a decision on definitive management. Interestingly of the third of patients who had not consulted their general practitioner, two-thirds said they would accept an operation if this was advised. Of the patients who eventually reached a surgeon, 20% were advised that operation was not required. These findings suggest that there is an unmet need for groin hernia surgery with many patients being denied access by their

family doctor. Once referred, surgeons seem to act as gatekeepers and may indeed "cherry-pick." Finally, there certainly appears to be a need for patient education in terms of the potential dangers of having a groin lump. Nevertheless, it is estimated that the number of groin herniorrhaphies done worldwide annually exceeds 20 million [4] and the lifetime risk of groin hernia is 27% for men and 3% for women [5].

Epidemiology

Prevalence and incidence data give no indication about the actual or potential demand for hernia surgery. Although incomplete and subject to many pitfalls in interpretation, UK data sources which relate to the need for hernia surgery include the English Hospital In-Patient Enquiry (HIPE) data, 1975–1985; the English Hospital Episodes System (HES) data, 1989/1990; and data on Surgical Activity in Independent Hospitals in the National Health Service (NHS) from local and national surveys [6].

There have been no true population or community-based studies of the incidence of groin hernia. The closest estimates for the true incidence of groin hernias (inguinal and femoral) can be obtained from the 1981/1982 Morbidity Statistics from General Practice [3]. These figures are however probably an underestimate because of an unquantifiable proportion of patients who fail to seek medical advice. Nevertheless, based on these figures the annual incidence of inguinal hernia in England will be of the order of 110,000 per year.

The published evidence comes from three main sources. Firstly, population prevalence and incidence: There have been few community-based estimates of the prevalence of groin hernias. None have estimated the incidence. Each has been performed in communities where access to surgery was and often still remains limited, for example, African populations. Further research defining the population incidence of groin hernias is required. Prevalence estimates are of local value only; they reflect not only the distribution and morbidity in the community but also the success of past local activity.

B.M. Stephenson (✉)
Department of General Surgery, Royal Gwent Hospital,
Newport, Wales, UK
e-mail: Brian.stephenson@wales.nhs.uk

A.N. Kingsnorth and K.A. LeBlanc (eds.), *Management of Abdominal Hernias*,
DOI 10.1007/978-1-84882-877-3_3, © Springer Science+Business Media London 2013

Secondly, "demand" incidence rates are based on the number of people who seek medical advice for their problem. However, numerous factors may influence this decision, and the data must therefore be treated with caution. Estimates of the incidence of inguinal and femoral hernias (Table 3.1) come from the 1981/1982 Morbidity Statistics from General Practice ("third national study") based on consultations with 143 volunteer general practice principals caring for 332,000 patients [3]. Figures 3.1 and 3.2 show incidence rates for inguinal and femoral hernia, each of which denotes a consultation where the patient was seeking medical advice concerning a groin hernia for the first time during the study year. Again, these data must be interpreted with caution because neither the doctors nor the patients may be representative of the general population, and the diagnoses were not validated. The age-specific incidence rates are given with 95% confidence intervals.

Demand for Groin Hernia Surgery in Adults

The overall rates for inguinal hernia repair (primary and recurrent) performed in NHS hospitals in England have not changed in the 15 years between 1975 and 1990 (Fig. 3.3). The total numbers for 1989/1990 were 64,998 primary inguinal hernia repairs and 3,480 recurrent inguinal hernia repairs (Table 3.2). Age-specific hernia rates have altered considerably since 1975 with a significant increase in the surgical rates for older men. For instance, the age-specific inguinal repair rate for the 65–74-year age group rose from 40 per 10,000 in 1975 to 70 per 100,000 in 1990. This probably reflects improvements in anesthetic delivery, including the wider use of locoregional anesthesia and monitored recovery programs. A more detailed analysis of age-specific inguinal hernia repair rates for males and females is shown in Fig. 3.4, which indicates the high rates in infants and men over the age of 55.

Of the approximately 65,000 inguinal and 6,000 femoral hernia repairs performed in NHS hospitals in England each year, 10% are emergency operations; these have remained constant for two decades. There has been an expansion in the private sector, which now accounts for 14% of all elective groin operations. Referring to the data in Figs. 3.4 and 3.5, it cannot be assumed that these repair rates approximate to the population incidence of inguinal and femoral hernias, because only 60% of groin hernias are referred to specialists for operation [3]. The implications for the English population will be 112,700 new cases per annum for inguinal hernias, and 6,900 for femoral hernias. Because a considerable proportion of patients are not undergoing groin hernia surgery, this may account for the surprisingly high number of trusses (40,000) sold annually [7, 8].

There is considerable variation in surgical rates for populations of health districts in England, and the weak correlations between these rates and supply factors (e.g., consultants per

Table 3.1 Incidence rates (95% confidence limits) of inguinal and femoral hernia per 10,000 persons at risk

Age (years)	Males	Females
Inguinal hernias		
0–4	58 (44.9,74.8)	13 (6.9,22.2)
5–14	7 (2.8,14.4)	3 (0.6,8.8)
15–24	7 (2.8,14.4)	3 (0.6,8.8)
25–44	20 (12.2,30.9)	4 (1.1,10.2)
45–64	70 (55.5,88.2)	6 (2.2,13.1)
65–74	88 (71.5,108.2)	7 (2.8,14.4)
75	150 (128.2,175.5)	17 (9.9,27.2)
Femoral hernias		
0–4		
5–14		
15–24		
25–44	1 (0.02,5.6)	2 (0.2,7.2)
45–64	1 (0.02,5.6)	2 (0.2,7.2)
65–74	1 (0.02,5.6)	2 (0.2,7.2)
75	9 (4.1,17.1)	7 (2.8,14.4)

Data from Royal College of General Practitioners [3]

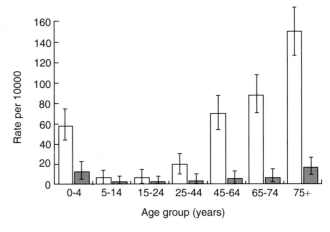

Fig. 3.1 Incidence rates of inguinal hernia per 10,000 persons at risk. *White* males; *shaded* females. Data from Royal College of General Practitioners [3]

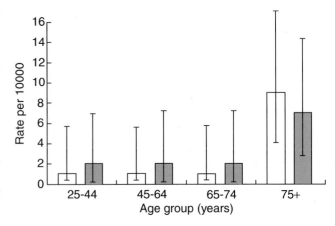

Fig. 3.2 Incidence rates of femoral hernia per 10,000 persons at risk. *White* males; *shaded* females. Data from Royal College of General Practitioners [3]

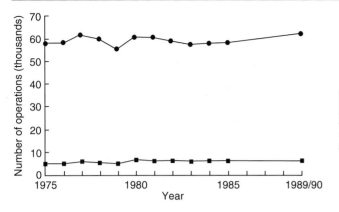

Fig. 3.3 Trends in number of inguinal hernia repairs, NHS hospitals in England, 1975–1989/1990. *Filled circle* males; *filled square* females. Data from Williams et al. [9]

Table 3.2 Number and percentage of single procedure inguinal hernia operations performed in NHS hospitals, England, 1989/1990

Inguinal hernia	Total no. of operations	No. (%) done as single procedure
Primary	64 998	54 090 [80]
Recurrent	3480	2790 [77]

Data from Williams et al. [9]

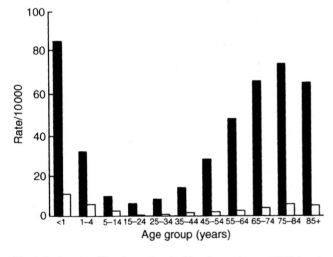

Fig. 3.4 Age-specific primary inguinal hernia repair rates, NHS hospitals, England, 1989/1990. *Shaded* males; *white* females. Data from Williams et al. [9]

1,000 population) and demand factors (e.g., waiting lists) suggest that a considerable proportion of the variation is accounted for by differences in medical decision making [9].

Demand incidence is based on surgical procedures. In a stable catchment population, the number of people who seek surgery during a defined period can be established.

Of more importance is the demographic structure of the population being studied, which may vary widely between regional populations. The demand for emergency treatment of strangulated inguinal hernia is better defined, being

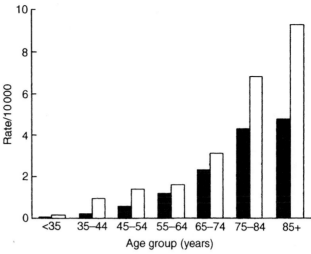

Fig. 3.5 Age-specific surgery rates for femoral hernia per 10,000 for males and females, NHS hospitals, England, 1989/1990. *Shaded* males; *white* females. Data from Williams et al. [9]

estimated at 3.25–7.16 per 100,000 per annum, in Western Europe [10, 11]. However, deficiencies of available data arise from three facts: Firstly, they are based on health service use rather than healthcare needs; secondly, patterns of morbidity have an uncertain relationship to indications for treatment; and thirdly, patients will seek treatment only if they are fully informed of the significance of potential morbidity and the consequences of treatment as opposed to nontreatment.

Inguinal hernias are more common than femoral hernias, occurring in ratios of 8:1 or 20:1 depending on the surgical series, and are more common in males, where the inguinal to femoral ratio may be up to 35:1. Seventy percent of inguinal hernias are indirect and 30% direct. Inguinal and femoral hernias may also coexist: 2% of males with inguinal hernias also have a femoral hernia, *and* 50% of men with femoral hernias have a coexisting inguinal hernia. This distribution of groin hernias is illustrated by Fig. 3.6 taken from a large series of 4,173 hernias operated on in Truro, England by Barwell between 1974 and 1992 [9, 12]. Nilsson from Sweden reports similar figures [13].

Age-standardized hernia surgery rates vary considerably throughout the world. For instance, the hernia surgery rate per 100,000 population per year in England and Wales is 200, Norway 200, the USA 280, and Australia 180. The actual approximate number of operations performed per year in respective countries is 5,500 in Scotland, 10,000 in Finland, 25,000 in Belgium, 30,000 in Holland, 100,000 in England and France, and 180,000 in Germany [14–17]. In the USA, where at least 550,000 inguinal hernia operations are carried out per year, the annual costs estimated in 1987 were 2.8 billion US dollars or 3% of the total healthcare budget! These figures are obtained from the National Center for Health Statistics (NCHS) through its National Hospital Discharge Survey, which has compiled data on the

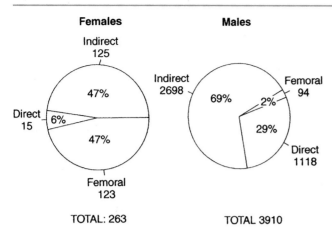

Fig. 3.6 Groin hernia diagnoses in males and females (Truro 1974–1992). Data from Williams et al. [9]

number of operations performed annually in the USA, from a 5–8% sample of patient records [18]. In the UK, hernia surgery rates peak in the 55–85-year age group, at 600 operations per 100,000 population per year, and the incidence of strangulated hernia is 13 per 100,000 population, with a peak in the 80-year-old age group. A graphical analysis of hospital discharge data and demographic information guided by three hypotheses on urgency of surgery, age, and evidence of discordance between population prevalence of disease and rates of surgery has suggested that in the last 10 years in Scotland, the rates of operation have increased in the over 65-year-olds, but the rate of elective surgery has decreased in the more socioeconomically deprived areas [19]. It could be concluded from this data that more hernia surgery is being carried out in an aging population and the need for patient education is of particular importance, in terms of health gains, in lower socioeconomic or uninsured population groups. Certainly in developing countries, large hernias in the younger population place a significant economic burden on society that is difficult to quantify [20].

In the USA the high rates of hernia surgery may have contributed to the reduction in mortality associated with strangulation. For instance, the mortality for hernia and intestinal obstruction obtained by analysis of statistics data from the NCHS shows a fall in the number of deaths per year per 100,000 population in patients over the age of 15 years, from 5 in 1968 to 3.1 in 1978, and stabilizing at 3.0 in 1988. This was in spite of the fact that hernia patients with intestinal obstruction were on average 15 years older in 1988 than in 1968. In 1971 Medicare discharges for inguinal hernia without intestinal obstruction showed 94% of patients having surgery, with a probability of death at 0.005 (5 per 100,000 population) [21]. Despite this low figure, uninsured patients still seem five times more likely to present with complicated hernias implying preventative measures still need to be addressed even in well-developed countries [22].

Inguinal Hernias in Adults

Inguinal hernias are more common in males than females, in a ratio of 8:1 or 20:1 in different series. However, there is considerable incidence of underreporting of inguinal hernia, as illustrated by two validity checks in the US National Health Surveys. In both studies half the hernias recorded during the previous year were unreported on interview, and in another study in Baltimore positive reports were received from only 21% of men found to have hernias on clinical examination.

Incidence estimates in the literature vary widely and depend on the source of the data. Approximately 94% of hernias among males are estimated to be in the inguinal region. Ninety-five percent of inguinal hernia operations are on males. Three times more females undergo femoral hernia operations than males. By the age of 75 years, 10–15% of males have already received inguinal hernia surgery. In the period 1975–1990, mortality from inguinal hernia surgery in the UK fell by 22% and for femoral hernia by 55%. In the USA, for inguinal hernia with obstruction, 88% underwent surgery with a mortality rate of 0.05% [21].

In a study of World War I British recruits, aged between 18 and 41 years, there was a marked variation in the reported incidence of inguinal hernia. In Scotland 31 per 1,000 were found, whereas in London and the southeast of England, it was 17–56 per 1,000. In men aged 16–30 years the rate was 6 per 1,000 and in older men (aged 40–50) it was 24 per 1,000. In contrast, the overall rate in Stockport and Manchester was 125 per 1,000. Sir Arthur Keith, in 1924, estimated the prevalence at 25 per 1,000 males [23]. The figures for World War II recruits are equally mystifying: the prevalence was about 26 per 1,000 but ranged from 6 to 80 per 1,000 men. Despite these variations the overall incidence is probably much higher given that these figures were recorded in young fit servicemen [24].

Sixty-five percent of inguinal hernias in adult European males are indirect in type. Right-sided inguinal hernias in adult males are slightly more frequent than left-sided, 55% occurring on the right, regardless of whether the hernia is indirect or direct. Bilateral hernias are four times more often direct than indirect. In Western series the peak incidence of groin hernias is in the sixth decade [25].

A possible genetic link has been postulated in the Inuit living in the Western Arctic of Greenland. Hernia is common in males and thought to be due to a high prevalence of disorders associated with instability of mesenchymal tissues, such as spondylolisthesis, arthritis, and heart block. The Inuit have been living in almost complete genetic isolation for 150–200 generations and have a high incidence and frequency of the HLA-B27 allele. Such polymorphism could result in the observed frequency of hernia in this closed knit population [26].

Table 3.3 Percentage of age group with inguinal hernia

Age (years)							
	25–34	35–44	45–54	55–64	65–74	75	Total
No. examined	620	438	300	322	156	47	1,883
Current prevalence (excluding	11.9	15.1	19.7	26.1	29.5	34.1	18.3 successful repairs)
"Obvious" hernias[a]	1.0	4.8	9.0	14.3	19.2	29.8	7.6
Unoperated swellings	0.7	3.7	5.7	10.9	13.5	23.4	5.5
Recurrences	0.3	1.4	3.7	3.4	5.8	6.4	2.2
Palpable impulse only	11.0	10.3	10.7	11.8	10.3	4.3	10.7
Lifetime prevalence (including	15.2	19.4	28.0	34.5	39.7	46.8	24.3 successful repairs)
"Obvious" hernias[a]	4.7	9.6	18.3	24.2	30.8	44.7	14.5

Data from Abramson et al. [28]

[a]"Obvious" hernias included swellings and repaired hernias and excluded those presenting with a palpable impulse only. The current prevalence of obvious hernias may be less than the combined prevalences of unoperated swellings and recurrences, since a person may have for example an unoperated swelling in one groin and a recurrence in the other

The difference between the ratio of indirect to direct inguinal hernia in different geographical locations supports a polygenic predisposition to herniation. In Japan, hernias are seen twice as frequent in twins. In Ghana, West Africa, one in every five live births is a twin (twice the rate seen in non-Africans), a fact that may account for the higher incidence of hernias recorded in Ghanaian men [27]. Comparing the age structure of the patients with inguinal hernia operated in Accra (the capital of Ghana) with the age structure found in a field study shows that all age groups are equally represented in the Accra hospital population, whereas in rural Ghana the prevalence of groin hernia rises with increasing age [27].

It is impossible to compare these findings. Clearly the results of the two large-scale surveys of fit uncomplaining males, drawn from recruits of the British and American forces in two world wars, do not represent fair and unbiased sampling. The only field study is from southern Ghana and confirms that inguinal hernias are at least three times more common in Africans than Europeans.

The true prevalence of inguinal hernias can be estimated only by community-based epidemiological studies, the validity of which will depend on the diagnostic criteria used. The presence of a visible, palpable lump may be supplemented by such diagnostic criteria as cough impulse at the internal or external ring and the presence of an incision in the groin. The latter, of course, may represent another form of surgery, such as orchidopexy, rather than hernia. Moreover, recurrent inguinal hernias may not be adequately ascertained. These drawbacks are well illustrated by the two studies alluded to above, carried out on British Army recruits in the first and second World Wars. The prevalence of groin hernias in recruits aged 30–40 years in World War I was 1.6% as compared to 11% in World War II [9, 23].

Perhaps the most rigorous epidemiological study carried out was that of Abramson in Western Jerusalem between 1969 and 1971 [28]. Males from differing ethnic and social backgrounds were studied, although young males were largely excluded because of national service. The study involved interviewing subjects in their own homes where the response rate approached 90%. Of these, 91% participated in the second stage of the study, that is, of a physical examination. Both interviewers and examiners had been trained in the use of questionnaires and diagnostic criteria. The results are shown in Table 3.3. The prevalence increased with age in all cohorts studied with the majority diagnosed on the basis of a visible swelling [28]. An important finding from the Abramson study was the concordance between interview and examination findings: Only 50% of men reported a swelling in the groin on interview, which is in close agreement with the 50% underreporting revealed from validity checks by the US National Health Surveys [29]. It is obvious from these studies that questionnaire-based data must be augmented by clinical examination if the true prevalence is to be ascertained, although this may be confounded by problems with diagnostic criteria. Clearly data regarding the incidence statistics of hernia patients are difficult to ascertain accurately and are probably all underestimates.

Femoral Hernias in Adults

The prevalence and incidence of femoral hernias in the population cannot be determined accurately for a number of reasons. However, the demand incidence can be estimated from the General Practitioner Morbidity Survey of 1981/1982, which was summarized in Table 3.1. An incidence figure for England derived from these data is approximately 7,000 per year [3], but the 95% confidence intervals are very wide indeed (1,500–24,000).

Femoral hernias are less common than inguinal and account for only 10% of all groin hernias. They are more frequent in females than males with an average ratio of 2.5:1, but this is also age dependent (see Figs. 3.1 and 3.2). However, there is other data that disputes this statistic (see Chap. 17). Maingot states that femoral hernias in women are eight times more common than in men [30]. Glasgow, from the Shouldice Clinic in Toronto Canada, reports more males than females in his series, at a ratio of 5:3 [31]. However, it must be remembered that Glasgow's large series is of patients undergoing elective operation for inguinal hernia and many of the cases were found as *concomitant* femoral hernias in men undergoing elective inguinal hernia repair. Clearly this series, or similar ones, does not fairly represent everyday general surgical practice.

Over 30 years ago approximately 40% of femoral hernias in the UK were admitted acutely with complications such as strangulation or incarceration [32]. This is also still unfortunately true in many other developed countries at the time of writing [33, 34]. Women still however undergo three times as many inguinal as opposed to femoral hernia repairs. Femoral hernias are rare in those under 35, are most common in multiparous women, and surprisingly as common in men as in multiparous women. The ratio of inguinal to femoral hernias is between 10:1 and 8:1. In Accra, Ghana, femoral hernias are rare, accounting for only 1.2% of groin hernias, with an inguinal to femoral ratio of 77:1. In Kampala, Uganda, the ratio is very different, 22:1. It is interesting to observe that indirect inguinal hernias outnumber direct inguinal hernias in Accra and in Zaria, Nigeria, whereas in Kampala direct hernias are more frequent. In Kampala there are nine women with femoral hernias to one man, whereas in West African Hausa the male to female ratio of femoral hernias is 1.2:1 [35–39].

The surgical volume for rates of femoral hernia repair in NHS hospitals in England has remained stable between 1975 and 1990, with 5,083 primary femoral hernia repairs and 299 recurrent femoral hernia repairs being performed in 1989/1990. The age-specific data indicate an increasing rate of repair through the decades with a peak in our elderly female population (Fig. 3.5).

There is also considerable variation in surgical rates for both inguinal and femoral hernia repair in the districts of English Regional Health Authorities. The range for primary inguinal hernia repair is 0.57–24 per 10,000 and for primary femoral hernia repair 0.16–2.3 per 10,000. Such unexplainable wide variations reflect the diversity of clinical practice and the "demand and supply" of treatment options already noted [9].

Etiology of Primary Groin Hernia

The pathogenesis of groin herniation is multifactorial. Sir Astley Cooper's "predispositions" to hernia, in 1827, and the subsequent addition of chronic cough, obesity, constipation,

pregnancy, ascites, and prostatic hypertrophy are now only of historic interest. These factors may reveal a hernia but certainly did not cause it *ab initio*.

As indirect inguinal hernias are so common in infancy, the first surgical speculation was that they were due to a developmental defect. Indirect inguinal hernia arises from incomplete obliteration of the processus vaginalis, the embryological out pocketing of peritoneum that precedes testicular descent into the scrotum. The testes originate along the urogenital line in the retroperitoneum and migrate caudally during the second trimester of pregnancy to arrive at the internal inguinal ring at about 6 months of intrauterine life. During the last trimester they proceed through the abdominal wall via the inguinal canal and descend into the scrotum, the right slightly later than the left. The processus vaginalis then normally obliterates postnatally except for the portion surrounding and serving as a covering for the testes. Failure of this obliterative process results in congenital indirect inguinal hernia. The modern epidemiological support for this hypothesis has already been reviewed, while the differing familial and tribal incidences, and the coincidence of hernias in twins, are supportive.

John Hunter, in the late eighteenth century, researched the development and descent of the testis in men and domestic animals. He showed that in some inguinal hernias, the sac was continuous with the processus vaginalis [40]. The Parisian surgeon Cloquet, of nodal fame, observed that the processus vaginalis was frequently not closed at birth [41]. Indeed a complete (or scrotal) indirect hernia in an adult man has the same anatomy as that of the neonate—it is invested by all the three layers of the spermatic cord as it transverses the inguinal canal and its sac is continuous with the tunica vaginalis of the testis. Additional support for the congenital theory of indirect inguinal herniation is the finding at autopsy that 15–30% of adult males without clinically apparent inguinal hernias have a patent processus vaginalis at death [42]. A Bedouin mother and her four daughters with indirect inguinal hernia in whom there was no evidence of collagen diseases, normal hormone profile, and normal pelvic anatomy suggest that in adult females as well, there is genetic heterogeneity [43]. Such an occurrence in females may be associated with an alteration in the anatomy of the round ligament, which normally terminates in a hernia sac and is attached to the midportion of the fallopian tube near the ovary [44].

Review of the contralateral side in infantile inguinal hernias reveals a patent processus vaginalis in 60% of neonates and a contralateral hernia in 10–20%. In slightly older children (say 2 years or so) the rate of developing a metachronous contralateral inguinal hernia is of the order of 5–7% with those children having a left-sided one at a higher risk of later herniation than had the first hernia been on the other side [45, 46]. In addition, at 20 years of follow-up after an infantile hernia repair, 22% of men will develop a contralateral inguinal hernia, of which 41% occur if the initial hernia was on the left and 14% if the initial hernia was on the right.

The introduction of continuous ambulatory peritoneal dialysis (CAPD) in the management of renal failure has demonstrated that a persistent processus vaginalis, if subjected to intra-abdominal pressure, will dilate to give a hydrocele or hernia [47–49]. Indeed this has been documented as late as 2 years after commencing CAPD. In addition the development of an inguinal hernia in female CAPD patients adds further support to this premise [49–51].

Russell, an Australian pediatric surgeon, in 1906 advanced the "saccular theory" of the formation of hernia, a theory that "rejects the view that any hernia can ever be "acquired" in the pathological sense and maintains that the presence of a developmental peritoneal diverticulum is a necessary antecedent condition in every case … We may have an open funicular peritoneum and we may have them separately or together in infinitely variable gradations" [52]. In recent years, with the increasing use of "diagnostic" laparoscopy, some light has been shed on this debate. When the inguinal anatomy of 600 patients undergoing diagnostic laparoscopy for other reasons was carefully recorded, the prevalence of a sac or remnant of a patent processus vaginalis did not seem to increase with age [53]. However and interestingly, when these patients were followed for over 5 years, those in whom an asymptomatic patent processus vaginalis had been noted were four times more likely to have undergone a later hernia repair [54].

It would be apparent from the above that the problem of indirect inguinal hernia may not be simply one of a congenital defect, that is, there is more to the story than just a persistent patent processus vaginalis. The high frequency of indirect inguinal hernia in middle-aged and older people suggests a pathological change in connective tissue of the abdominal wall to be a contributory factor. Indeed, simple removal of the sac in adults results in an unacceptably high recurrence rate and clearly is inappropriate. Thus the susceptibility to herniation is based on *both* the presence of a congenital sac *and* failure of the transversalis fascia. In direct inguinal hernia there is no peritoneal sac and the prevalence parallels aging and other factors including smoking [55, 56]. Furthermore the absence of an adequate musculoaponeurotic support for the fascia transversalis and the medial half of the inguinal canal has been described in about a quarter of individuals [24]. In these men there is deficiency of the lower aponeurotic fibers of the internal oblique muscle, coupled with a narrow insertion of the transversus abdominis onto the superior pubic ramus [57, 58]. Because such a congenital anomaly would be symmetric, this explanation is consistent with the clinical finding that direct hernias are frequently bilateral and often surprisingly asymptomatic.

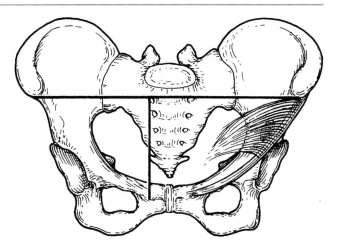

Fig. 3.7 The European pelvis is relatively wide with a less deep arch than the Negro pelvis. This ensures that the internal oblique muscle origin from the lateral inguinal ligament is broad, so that the internal oblique muscle "protects" the deep ring

The anatomic disposition of the pelvis, and particularly the height of the pubic arch, may also be a significant and possibly ethnic characteristic predisposing to inguinal hernia formation. The height of the pubic arch is measured as the distance of the pubic tubercle from the bispinous line between the innermost parts of the two anterior superior iliac spines. African (Negro) peoples have lower pubic arches than Europeans and a higher incidence of inguinal hernia. In West and East Africa the "lowness" of the pubic arch is greater than 7.5 cm in 65% of males; in Europeans and in Arabs the arch is less low, 65% of males having a height of between 5 and 7.5 cm (Fig. 3.7). In European females 80% have an arch between 5 and 7.5 cm, and they have the lowest incidence of groin hernias [39, 59, 60].

This "low" arch is associated with a narrower pelvis and with a narrower origin of the external oblique muscle from the lateral inguinal ligament. With these anatomic variations the inguinal canal is shorter with the deep inguinal ring left uncovered by the internal oblique. The canal may then be so short that no significant muscular "shutter mechanism" is apparent [59] as illustrated by Fig. 3.8. There is another much rarer form of direct hernia where a narrow peritoneal diverticulum comes directly through the conjoint tendon lateral to the rectus and pyramidal muscles to project at the superficial inguinal ring. In addition there are numerous unusual types of interparietal hernias where the sac may be mono- or bilocular and associated or not with a patent indirect sac.

It must be concluded that there are congenital, anatomical, and genetic factors that render individuals more likely to manifest direct as opposed to indirect inguinal hernias.

Over 80 years ago Sir Arthur Keith, a Scottish anatomist and anthropologist, observed: "There is one other matter, which requires further observation. We are so apt to look on

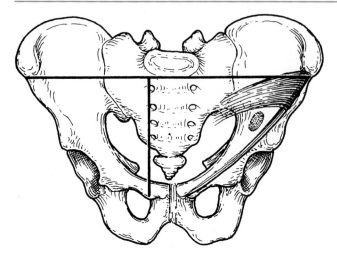

Fig. 3.8 The Negro pelvis is narrower than the European, which means that the lowness of the arch of the pelvis is greater in the Negro and the origin of the internal oblique relatively narrower. Hence the internal oblique will not cover the deep ring during straining, and the "shutter mechanism" of the inguinal canal is deficient. Negroes have a ten times greater incidence of indirect inguinal hernia than Europeans

tendons, fascial structures and connective tissues as dead passive structures. They are certainly alive, and the fact that hernias are so often multiple in middle aged and old people leads one to suspect that a pathological change in the connective tissues of the belly wall may render certain individuals particularly liable to hernia." He concluded his argument with a statement regarding "the importance of a right understanding of the etiology of hernia … If they occur only in those who have hernial sacs already formed during fetal life then we must either excise the sacs at birth or stand by and do nothing but trust to luck. But if … the occurrence of hernia is due to circumstances over which we have control then the prevention of hernia is a matter worthy of our serious study" [23].

Some 50 years later, Read, an American surgeon, made a crucial clinical observation which further advanced our thoughts as to the etiology of inguinal hernia. In 1970 he noted, when using an open preperitoneal approach to the inguinal region, that the rectus sheath is thinner and has a "greasy" feel in those patients who turned out to have direct inguinal defects. This observation was confirmed by weighing samples of a constant cross-sectional area; specimens from controls weighed significantly more than those from patients with indirect, pantaloon, and direct hernias (in that order). Bilateral hernias were associated with more severe atrophy. Adjustments for age and muscle mass confirmed the validity of this observation [56]. Further evidence in support of a collagen derangement in the transversalis fascia was presented by Peacock and Madden in 1974, who observed that satisfactory repair of adult inguinal herniation depended on the local extent of any collagen deficiency. And, if surgical technical failure can be excluded, the logical treatment of

recurrent herniation is a fascial graft or prosthetic repair [61]. This concept was enthusiastically promoted by Irving Lichtenstein, one of the earliest pioneers of prosthetic repair for *primary* inguinal hernia [62]. We now all know how this revolutionized modern hernia practice [17].

Hernias "Under the Microscope"

Let us start with some basic science that we may have forgotten! Surgical wound healing is a controlled cascade in which there are sequential cellular and molecular events allowing ordered tissue repair. After the initial wound there is a phase of healing characterized by hemostasis and inflammation followed by one of proliferation, which is predominantly one of increased fibroblastic activity with extracellular deposition and increased angiogenesis. Collagen is the end product of fibroblast activity, and while there are many types of collagen, type I and type III are those most implicated in wound healing. Subsequent remodeling involves collagen bundle organization to give rise to a mature scar. Now, before moving on, let us remind ourselves that the inguinal canal and transversalis fascia comprise tissues made up of collagen, elastic fibers consisting of elastin and microfibrils, and the glycosaminoglycan component of the extracellular matrix.

Following the earlier observations regarding the "greasy" feel of the rectus sheath [56], Read and coworkers showed that hydroxyproline, which comprises 80% of the dry weight of collagen, was strikingly decreased in the rectus sheath of inguinal hernia patients especially if the hernia was of a direct type [63, 64]. The extracted collagen revealed a reduced hydroxyproline:proline ratio. Intermolecular cross-linking is unaffected, but synthesis of hydroxyproline is inhibited, and there is variability in the diameter of the collagen fibrils in hernia patients [65]. Similar electron microscopic findings are also present in pericardial and skin biopsies from these patients [65] and have also been described in connective tissue tumors [66], pulmonary emphysema [67], and scurvy [68]. Based upon these observations and the results of later similar studies, the prosthetic repair of inguinal hernias was promoted as the new "gold standard" of surgery. These findings also changed the approach to the repair of ventral (including incisional) hernias such that the vast majority are now also augmented with prosthetic biomaterials.

The above observations led Read, in 1978, to the postulate that inguinal herniation is not a localized defect of the groin fascia but is in fact a manifestation of a generalized connective tissue disorder similar to emphysema, α1-antitrypsin deficiency, osteogenesis imperfecta, scurvy, varicose veins, and experimental nicotine deficiency [67]. This hypothesis was then tested with a computerized suction device to assess the biomechanical properties of the transversalis fascia and rectus abdominis so as to measure any functional connective tissue abnormalities in the groin [69]. The study was unable to demonstrate any differences in the properties of aponeurosis between hernia patients and controls. There was, however, a difference in collagen ultrastructure when it was examined under an electron microscope and in its physicochemical properties as observed by altered perceptibility and deficiency in hydroxyproline content. It appears thus that the fundamental problem in the aponeurosis of men with direct inguinal herniation is failure of hydroxylation of the collagen molecule.

Berliner in 1984 confirmed these findings by studying biopsies from three sites in patients with inguinal hernia [70]. Degenerative changes in the musculoaponeurotic fibers were found not only in the transversalis fascia/transversus abdominis of patients with direct inguinal hernias but also in the transversalis fascia at the superior aspect of the internal ring in patients with indirect inguinal hernia and also distant from the hernia site in grossly normal transversus abdominis aponeurosis. The main changes observed were reduction in elastic tissue with a paucity and fragmentation of elastic fiber similar to that seen in Marfan and Ehlers–Danlos syndrome (EDS). The implication from these findings is that collagen malsynthesis and enzymolysis mutually but not necessarily equally play a *major* role in the etiology of both direct *and* indirect inguinal hernia. Indeed, this was supported when the in vitro synthesis of types I and III collagens (and their procollagen mRNAs) was studied from isolated skin fibroblasts in patients with inguinal hernia. Fibroblasts incubated with radiolabeled tritiated proline secreted increased amounts of type III procollagen, suggesting that an altered fibroblast phenotype in patients with inguinal hernia could result in reduced collagen fibril assembly and defective connective tissue formation [71]. Further support for this suggestion comes from a case–control (fresh cadavers) study where *both* the total and type I collagen were decreased in fit young men with indirect inguinal hernias [72].

Could an uninhibited elastolytic enzyme system cause groin herniation—a similar mechanism to low serum levels of the protease inhibitor α1-antitrypsin globulin allowing endogenous enzymes to destroy alveoli? [73]. Experimental evidence certainly supports the biochemical hypothesis that the pulmonary connective tissue disorder in emphysema is an imbalance between proteolytic enzyme levels and their inhibitors. Evidence of raised elastolytic enzyme has been found in smokers, and in smokers with inguinal herniation there is a close association between raised elastolytic levels and raised white counts. Neutrophils carry proteolytic and elastolytic enzymes and are actively involved in the lung inflammatory response to cigarette smoke. Could they not also deliver the same proteolytic insult to the transversalis fascia? The neutrophil-derived enzyme metalloproteinase (MMP-2 and MMP-9) has been identified as one that breaks down collagen, elastin, and other components of the extracellular matrix.

They have been found in transversus abdominis biopsies of patients with direct but not indirect inguinal hernias. MMP-2 overexpression has been measured in fibroblasts of patients with direct hernias, and MMP-13 overexpression detected in recurrent inguinal hernias [74, 75]. While these studies are best described as observational they are important indicators of the pathological process at the cellular level. Although it is unclear whether a deteriorating groin expresses increased MMP levels, it is of interest to see that transforming growth factor beta1 (TGF-β1) is overexpressed in the transversalis fascia of young patients with direct hernias [76]. Such growth factors are known to play a role in tissue remodeling and are presumably doing so or attempting to counterbalance the microscopic problems of a failing groin.

On a "macroscopic" or clinical scale, is there evidence that collagen is at fault? The prevalence of inguinal hernia (41%) in 119 patients with infrarenal aortic aneurysms was significantly higher when compared with 81 patients with aortic–iliac occlusive disease (18.5%) and 293 patients with coronary artery disease (18.1%). In addition, the number of patients who had undergone a recent hernia repair (16%) or were still waiting for repair (19%) was very high [77]. Also following elective aortic reconstruction for aneurysmal or occlusive aortic disease, at 1 year follow-up, incisional hernias were found in 31% of patients with aneurysm and 12% with occlusive disease, and inguinal hernias were found in 19% of patients with aneurysm and 5% with occlusive disease further supporting the concept of a biochemical abnormality [78]. The smoking habits of the three groups were not different, and again the findings support the concept of systemic fiber degeneration [79]. Although the enzymatic elastase content of the wall of abdominal aortic aneurysms has been shown to be increased, the concept of high levels of circulating elastase has not been confirmed. Nevertheless, overall patients with aneurysmal disease have a fourfold increased risk of inguinal and incisional herniation [80, 81]. Similar findings have been found in patients examined by a magnetic resonance imaging of the abdominal wall following aortic surgery [82]. These findings indicate that 50% or more of patients with nonocclusive infrarenal aortic aneurysm suffer from inguinal hernia. Indeed, it has been suggested that an inguinal hernia in certain high-risk age groups be used as an index for ultrasonic screening for aneurysmal disease [83]. However as the ultrasonography would have to be performed and repeated over a substantial period of time, the results of a small ($n=70$) prospective study go some way to point out this is not going to be a useful screening tool [84].

A number of years ago the term "metastatic emphysema" was coined by Cannon and Read [67] for the concept of a generalized connective tissue disorder, which was maybe due to a leakage of proteases from the lungs of heavy smokers [85]. Read emphasized that the data indicate that more than

Fig. 3.9 Persistent
herniation in Ehlers–
Danlos syndrome. Note the
unusual skin appearance

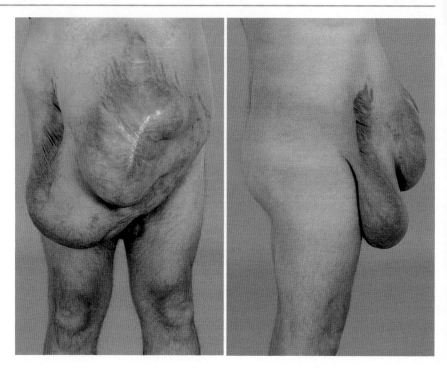

one factor can cause systemic metabolic disease of collagen leading to abdominal herniation including the imbalanced expression of different collagens. Subsequent results have confirmed this in the transversalis fascia of patients with inguinal hernia by direct measurement of the important collagens (types I and III) [72, 86]. Nevertheless we must be cautious in interpreting the experimental data about a proteolytic defect in inguinal hernia patients and then relating it to the proven association with abdominal aortic aneurysm. It is however tempting to relate this "metastatic emphysema theory of inguinal herniation" to Hunt's and Tilson's ideas that aortic aneurysm is a copper transport collagen disorder enhanced by cigarette smoking [87, 88].

With all the available data [89–91], it seems probable and indeed highly likely that primary inguinal hernias are a connective tissue disorder as opposed to recurrent ones, which are due to a combination of this underlying innate problem and a technical failure of wound healing/repair. This further supports the need for a well-dissected prosthetic repair in the first instance. Whether biological meshes will play a part in the elective repair of primary inguinal hernias, other than in a few very selected cases, remains to be seen [92].

A Curious Case of Recurrent Recurrence

A 45-year-old otherwise asymptomatic man developed an incisional hernia following a lower midline laparotomy for peritonitis from a perforated appendix. This was repaired but recurred and did so again when this recurrence was repaired with preperitoneal mesh. Wound healing seemed attenuated

and the hernia unmanageable. After a further repair using the component separation technique (again augmented with onlay mesh) failed, a diagnosis of EDS was contemplated and later established (Fig. 3.9).

This unusual inherited connective tissue disorder, also known as "cutis hyperelastica," is caused by a defect in the synthesis of collagen (type III). There are numerous recognized types of EDS [93] with the genetic mutations (autosomal dominant mode of inheritance) altering the structure, production, or processing of collagen or the proteins that interact with collagen to varying degrees. Even in established EDS, now known to be more prevalent than previously thought, the symptoms and presentation vary widely. Treatment is generally supportive and the prognosis dependent on the type of EDS.

Could "milder" defects in collagen synthesis/metabolism be even more prevalent in the population than otherwise contemplated with other factors such as smoking accelerating the general wear and tear process that we subject ourselves too? Interestingly inguinal hernia occurs more frequently in patients with milder EDS phenotypes.

Genetics in Pediatric Surgical Practice

Inguinal hernia may be associated with many different genetic syndromes including single gene and chromosomal disorders. Given the known constituents of the inguinal canal and transversalis fascia, one would expect such disorders to be associated with a higher risk of inguinal hernia [94]. Indeed genetic diseases of the microfibril (Marfan syndrome), elastin (Costello syndrome and Menkes disease), and collagen (EDS and osteogenesis imperfecta) are all associated with an increased risk of inguinal hernia.

While the vast majority of childhood inguinal hernias do not have a genetic basis warning signs that a hernia may have, a genetic basis includes a direct hernia, a recurrent hernia, or a hernia in girls as well as the more commonly recognized features associated with genetic disorders such as developmental delay.

The Genetics of Inheritance of the "Common" Indirect Inguinal Hernia

Although there is considerable evidence suggesting the role of genetic factors in the etiology of inguinal hernia, its mode of inheritance remains controversial [95]. A number of hypotheses have been suggested:

1. Autosomal dominant inheritance with incomplete penetrance [96]
2. Autosomal dominant inheritance with sex influence [97, 98]
3. X-linked dominant inheritance [99]
4. Polygenic inheritance [100, 101]

In a study from Budapest [100], the parents of 707 index patients with operated indirect congenital inguinal hernia born during the years 1962–1966 were studied for their frequency of indirect inguinal hernia. There was a 2 and 5.6 times higher incidence respectively in the fathers and mothers than in the general population, and the rate of affected siblings was higher than that of parents but was generally dependant on the sex of the index patient. In twins the hereditability was 0.77. These data suggested a multifactorial threshold model involving dominant variance.

A study of 280 families with congenital indirect inguinal hernia in the Shandong province of China has indicated that the mode of transmission in these families is autosomal dominant with incomplete penetrance and sex influence. There is preferential paternal transmission of the gene, suggesting a role for genomic imprinting in the etiology of indirect inguinal hernias [102]. In this study the probands (index cases) had all been operated on by 5 years of age, with the hernia occurring on the right side in 138 and on the left side in 84. This is consistent with the known embryological facts that the right testis descends later than the left and that the processus vaginalis is therefore obliterated later on the right side than on the left side; hence hernia is more frequent on the right than on the left side.

In a record linkage study from the UK reported in 1998, of the risk of congenital inguinal hernia in siblings, 1921 male and 347 female cases born during 1970–1986 and who were operated on for inguinal hernia at the ages of 0–5 years were matched against 12,886 male and 2,534 female controls [103]. The relative risk for inguinal hernia was found to be 5.8 for brothers of male cases and 4.3 for brothers of female cases, while the relative risk was 3.7 for sisters of male cases and 17.8 for sisters of female cases. This pattern of sex-dependant risk suggests a multifactorial threshold model for the disease. In essence as girls have a much lower incidence of inguinal hernia, those girls *who* do develop the disease might have a potentially larger contribution to susceptibility from genetic or intrauterine risk factors unrelated to their sex.

More recently a study from Hong Kong has examined the strength of a positive family history as a risk factor for developing an inguinal hernia [104]. As compared to controls and using multivariate logistic regression analyses, a positive family history was the *only* truly independent predictor for a hernia; indeed a man with a positive family history is eight times more likely to develop a primary inguinal hernia.

Indirect inguinal hernia arises from incomplete obliteration of the processus vaginalis, the embryological protrusion of peritoneum that precedes testicular descent into the scrotum. The testes originate along the urogenital line in the retroperitoneum and migrate caudally during the second trimester of pregnancy to arrive at the internal inguinal ring at about 6 months of intrauterine life. During the last trimester they proceed through the abdominal wall via the inguinal canal and descend into the scrotum, the right slightly later than the left. The processus vaginalis then normally obliterates postnatally except for the portion surrounding and serving as a covering for the testes. Failure of this obliterative process results in congenital indirect inguinal hernia.

It is plausible to speculate that morphogenesis may be determined by single genes and complicated by environmental factors. In the case of indirect inguinal hernia, an autosomal dominantly inherited gene with reduced penetrance and sex influence would therefore be susceptible to environmental factors influencing its expression as a clinical inguinal hernia. In most families, however, a monogenic mode of inheritance is not apparent. Therefore the maternal allele (of a/the gene?) may protect against failure of closure of the patent processus vaginalis.

In conclusion, the fact that most affected males have inherited an indirect inguinal hernia gene(s) from their father implicates a role of genomic imprinting (i.e., the paternal allele) in the etiology of the indirect inguinal hernia phenotype. Finally it may be of interest to note that certain chromosomal loci have been identified as genetic susceptibility targets in pigs at known "high risk" of developing inguinoscrotal hernias [105]. We all have to start somewhere!

Intra-abdominal Diseases Causing Hernias

Ascites due to liver, heart disease (failure), and more rarely abdominal or peritoneal carcinomatosis can present as recent onset groin and umbilical herniation. The mechanism is similar to that already described in CAPD patients, with increasing hydrostatic pressure dilating a preexisting sac irrespective of its earlier size. Intra-abdominal contents may then follow into this enlarged space. Clearly the sudden onset of a hernia in middle-aged or elderly patients should thus arouse diagnostic suspicion. It is a sound policy to subject hernial sacs to histological examination, especially in older patients, where ascites (blood stained or not) is found or when the sac is thickened or indurated. However, the routine histological examination of "normal" hernial sacs is not justified. Indeed the chance of unexpected "pathology" in an otherwise normal hernial sac has been estimated (!) to be 0.00098% [106]. Routine histology is certainly *unnecessary* and obviously uneconomical.

Interestingly the histological examination of sacs obtained from children with hernia, hydrocoele, or undescended testis revealed that in the inguinal hernia patients during childhood, smooth muscle was found within the wall of the sac but not in sacs associated with undescended testis. This suggests that this smooth muscle may have played a role in the prevention of obliteration and clinical outcome [107].

Thickening of a hernial sac *per se* is not necessarily due to significant pathology; peritoneum is active tissue and particularly in children and young adults can exhibit overexuberant tumor-like reaction to mechanical injury. This so-called mesothelial hyperplasia may follow wearing a truss or occur simply after repeated attacks of near-incarceration. Microscopically there are atypical mesothelial cells that are either free or attached to the wall of the sac. Mitoses and multinucleated cells are frequently seen but despite this mesothelial hyperplasia are reactive and certainly not neoplastic [108].

The development of an abdominal wall hernia may be a rare but initial sign of decompensated heart or liver disease. Whereas good surgical practice is to repair an uncomplicated hernia, the question of repair in cirrhotics raises other issues. Leonetti et al. [109] reported that repair of umbilical hernias in uncontrolled unshunted cirrhotics led to a mortality of 8.3%, a morbidity of 16.6%, and a recurrence rate of 16.6%. However umbilical herniorrhaphy in patients with a functioning peritoneovenous shunt was associated with minimal morbidity (7%). The authors suggested that peritoneovenous shunting should be a prerequisite to hernia repair [109]. While this may not now always be necessary, these patients clearly need medical optimization before surgery [110]. There is now little doubt that elective surgery has significantly [111, 112] improved the quality of life of these patients with mesh repairs well tolerated and outcomes similar to patients without cirrhosis [113].

Intra-abdominal pus can also collect in and distend an empty hernial sac, as with any peritoneal recess, at the initial peritonitis. It may also collect in a long-standing hernia even after successful emergency surgery (Fig. 3.10). In a review of 32 examples of this phenomenon, 19 were right inguinal, five right femoral, three left inguinal, one epigastric, and one

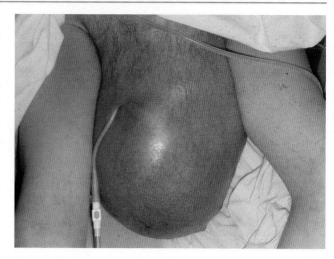

Fig. 3.10 Residual collection in a large long-standing hernia after emergency surgery for gastric perforation

umbilical. Acute appendicitis accounted for 16 examples, perforated peptic ulcers for three, one followed pneumococcal peritonitis in a 2-week-old male child, one an acute pyosalpinx, and one followed a biliary leak after removal of a common bile duct drain [114]. Every patient with this complication was originally diagnosed as having a strangulated hernia, which is not surprising. If pus is found in a hernial sac, abdominal exploration is usually mandatory with acute appendicitis being the commonest diagnosis, especially in right-sided hernias [115]. When confronted with a tender incarcerated hernia, the diagnosis remains primarily a clinical one, but appropriate and recently more immediately available radiological investigations can usefully augment ones suspicions allowing a tailored minimally invasive staged approach when appropriate [116, 117]. A tender inguinal mass may not represent a hernia as demonstrated by Fig. 3.11!

Inguinal Hernia and Appendectomy

Over a hundred years ago Hoguet first reported the development of inguinal hernia in patients who had undergone previous appendectomy [118]. He found eight right inguinal hernias in a series of 190 patients who had undergone appendectomy and suggested a causal relationship. Other authors have supported this contention [119–121].

Right inguinal hernias are more frequent when appendectomy is performed through a lower, "more cosmetic" incision, which is placed below the anterior superior iliac spine and in which the iliohypogastric nerve is injured. Electromyographic studies have shown conflicting results. While some investigators [121] have shown that denervation of the transversus abdominis muscle in the groin does occur and could therefore interfere with the shutter mechanism of the deep ring and be a factor in the subsequent development of inguinal hernia, other

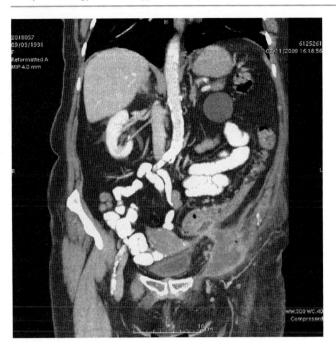

Fig. 3.11 A diverticular abscess presenting as a hernia. Fortunately a colocutaneous fistula did not develop in this frail 78-year-old lady

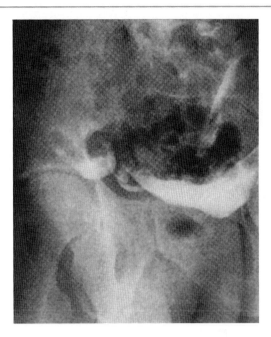

Fig. 3.12 Herniography on a 40-year-old man who had sustained a fracture of both pubic rami. The patient developed a "pantaloon" inguinal hernia

investigators have failed to detect any significant denervation of the musculature in and around the right groin [122].

Using the *standard* McBurney (introduced by Charles McBurney in 1894) appendectomy incision (at right angles to a line from the umbilicus to the anterior superior iliac spine, at a point at the junction of its lateral third and medial two-thirds and parallel to the iliohypogastric nerve which is rarely injured if the flank muscles are opened by splitting in their fiber line), there is no evidence that inguinal herniation is a consequence of appendectomy. In a series of 549 patients who had undergone inguinal hernia repair, the percentage incidence of previous appendectomy in right-sided hernias was $8.9 \pm 1.7\%$ and in left-sided inguinal hernias $11.2 \pm 2.1\%$ [123].

It is the *lower* and "more cosmetic" incisions, which carry a particular hazard to the iliohypogastric nerve and a propensity to subsequent inguinal herniation. The introduction of effective antibiotics and the consequent reduction in wound complications are also clearly important. If and when laparoscopic appendectomy is fully embraced as a standard approach (with reasons for and follow-up of converted cases) will we know if this technique also contributes to a lower incidence of subsequent inguinal herniation. The debate regarding open or laparoscopic appendectomy will no doubt continue for sometime before this becomes universal surgical practice even in the developed world [124].

Hernias Related to Trauma and Pelvic Fracture

Abdominal hernias related to trauma and blunt injuries are rare and are only reported following lower abdominal and pelvic injuries. To diagnose a traumatic hernia there must be immediate signs of local soft-tissue injury, bruising, hematoma, etc., and then there must be the early presentation of the symptoms of the hernia. The aponeuroses close to their pelvic attachments are most at risk.

Disruption of the inguinal canal and complete ruptures of the conjoint tendon are recorded but are very rare [125]. Ryan, from the Shouldice clinic, reported only five hernias related to pelvic fractures in 8,000 hernia repairs [126]. Figure 3.12 illustrates an unusual case of a patient whose hernia was related to a pelvic fracture: A 40-year-old man developed a "pantaloon" hernia after fracture of both rami of the pubis in a traffic accident. Such "traumatic" hernias are also recognized after pelvic diastasis in the absence of fracture and often present late and may contain bladder or small bowel alone (supravesical).

Hernias related to iatrogenic pelvic fractures, for example, an osteotomy for congenital dislocation of the hip, are well described in the literature. Ryan classifies these fracture-related hernias according to the mechanism of the fracture [126]:

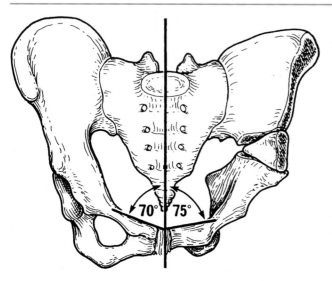

Fig. 3.13 Diagram to show how innominate osteotomy predisposes to inguinal herniation

1. Due to acute anteroposterior forces acting on the pelvis: In these instances there is tearing of the rectus abdominis origin from the pubic crest. The tearing is maximal on the side opposite to that on which maximum bony displacement had occurred. The damage to the muscle is usually more severe medially than laterally, leading to the development of a broad-necked sac just suprapubically from the midline extending laterally across the attachment of the rectus to the pubic crest.

2. Due to lateral or lateral/vertical forces: These fractures involve the superior pubic ramus with consequent tearing of the fascial and aponeurotic attachments of the inguinofemoral region. In these circumstances a direct inguinal hernia develops through the fascia transversalis immediately above the bony fracture line. A repair of the direct hernia corrects the situation.

3. Due to surgical innominate osteotomy: This hernia occurs in children with congenital dislocated hips. The hernia following innominate osteotomy is either a direct inguinal hernia, a prevascular femoral (Narath's) hernia, or a combination of the two [127].

Following innominate or Salter's osteotomy, there is a downward lateral and forward displacement of the lower fragment of the pelvis produced by a combination of hinging and rotation at the symphysis pubis [128]. This procedure leads to an increase in the distance between the edge of the rectus abdominis muscle and the inguinal and pectineal ligaments. There is a consequent weakening in the posterior wall of the inguinal canal. The angle between the midline (and, therefore, the lateral edge of the rectus muscle) and the superior ramus of the pubis is increased by a minimum of 5° when compared to the opposite side, and there is also an increase in the distance from the pubic tubercle to the anterior superior iliac spine. These changes alter the anatomy of the inguinofemoral

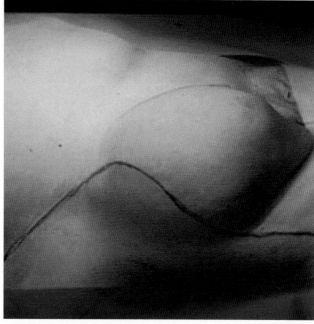

Fig. 3.14 An external femoral hernia (Hesselbach's) passing deep into the thigh below the inguinal ligament lateral to the femoral vessels. Note the previous incision for corrective hip surgery of uncertain nature

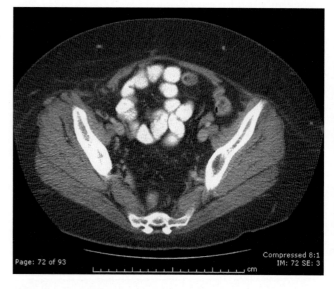

Fig. 3.15 An earlier anterior bone graft site complicated by groin herniation. The sac contained incarcerated omentum

region predisposing to hernia. It must be stressed that a consequent hernia is rare and undoubtedly compensatory remodeling of the soft tissues occurs as the child develops after the traumatic procedure (Fig. 3.13). Any earlier musculoskeletal surgery, iatrogenic or not, in the region of the groin can lead to the later unusual groin herniation (Fig. 3.14).

The use of autologous bone grafts from the iliac crest is also troublesome. When full thickness grafts are taken from the posterior iliac crest, the inferior lumbar triangle is enlarged

Table 3.4 Severity of abdominal wall injury

Description	Grade	Incidence (%)
Tissue bruising/contusion	I	54
Muscle(s) hematoma	II	28
Single-layer disruption	III	8
Complete-layer disruption	IV	8
IV with herniation	V	2
IV with evisceration	VI	0

Data from Dennis et al. [130] based on CT scans in 1,549 patients with blunt trauma

predisposing to herniation. These "iatrogenic" lumbar hernias cause backache and can be complicated by irreducibility and strangulation and should be repaired [129]. Bone grafts from the anterior iliac crest are similarly complicated by later herniation and require corrective surgery (Fig. 3.15).

Truly blunt traumatic abdominal wall hernias may occur after both low- (falls) or high-"energy" (motor vehicle accidents) impact injuries. Despite the use of early CT scanning, the mechanism of injury is vitally important, and a high index of suspicion is necessary when managing such patients. High-energy trauma cases may need urgent laparotomy for concomitant intra-abdominal injuries, whereas in low impact injuries local wound toilet, debridement, and immediate repair may suffice. In a review of 1,549 CT scans from a level I trauma center, abdominal wall injuries were graded as to their severity with respect to the documented disruption of the layers of the abdominal wall [130]. Overall abdominal wall injuries occurred in 9% of cases (Table 3.4) with those at risk of later herniation (not necessarily in the groin) estimated to be 16%. The role of subsequent follow-up CT scanning may well define the place of "early vs. late" repair of these injuries. To date the later repairs of such hernias should probably be undertaken through a preperitoneal approach so that the anatomy, or lack of it, can be best appreciated.

Exertion and Groin Herniation

There is no firm evidence that strong muscular or strenuous athletic exertion causes inguinal hernia in the absence of a fascial and/or muscular abnormality—either acquired connective tissue disease or congenital anomaly of the abdominal wall. Indeed, inguinal hernias (as opposed to sliding hiatal hernias) are rare in weight lifters [131]. However, in a study of inguinal hernia and a "single strenuous event," in which 129 patients with a total of 145 inguinal hernias were included, in 7% the hernia was subjectively attributable to a single muscular strain [132]. Indeed these authors suggested guidelines to assist in assessing "causation" in work-related compensation claims in such patients, which included the following four recommendations:

1. The patient should have made an official report of the incident of muscular strain.
2. Severe groin pain must have been experienced at the time of the strain.
3. The diagnosis of hernia should preferably have been made within 3 days of the incident (or certainly within 30 days).
4. There should be no previous history of inguinal hernia.

Interestingly, a recent similar study, using structured postal questionnaires, suggested that inguinal herniation may be attributed to a single event in a similar proportion of patients [133], but another report questions the appearance of a hernia (of any type) after such an event [134].

At the moment, the relative importance of genetic, anatomic, and environmental (smoking and heavy manual work) factors cannot be construed in each case. Manual work or strain is never, or very rarely, the *sole* cause of inguinal herniation; it may however reveal an underlying previously asymptomatic one of which our patient was "clearly" unaware of.

Recent research suggests that persistent straining and heavy work is relevant (but not causal) to the development of groin hernia. Recent European research has stressed these environmental factors rather than congenital defects in hernia development [135, 136]. In man and many mammalian quadrupeds, there is an abstinence of the posterior rectus sheath below the arcuate line (of Douglas) and an "ineffectual" transversalis fascia in the groin. Gravitational stresses, while in the erect posture, amplify this hindrance of weakness, which is an evolved anatomical defect [137]. The etiology of groin hernia also has importance in terms of prevention; smoking is a causal agent but possibly less so in women [138].

In medicolegal terms, the situation remains somewhat confused—an accident or heavy strain at work is generally construed as a causal factor in the onset of a hernia, and in British courts damages are usually awarded. Our current understanding of the etiology of inguinal hernias casts doubt on judicial reasoning in many cases. The legal foundation for compensating a workman who develops a hernia after an accident at his workplace is the commission of a tort or breach of contract by his employer. The heads of damages awarded are for pain or suffering, loss of amenities (usually sex life), pecuniary loss, medical expenses, and loss of later earning capacity. The role of a preexisting disability, patent processus vaginalis or metastatic emphysema, will need offsetting against these "damages." This is definitely a task for the judiciary, being largely unrelated to the observations of natural science [139]. Nevertheless in preparing a medicolegal report, surgeons and other medical experts must carefully examine all the contemporaneous medical records to support a claim. If there is insufficient evidence to support a claim, they have a duty to the court to nullify the plaintiff's claim and associated litigation [134, 140]. Finally the risk of a "work-related" hernia causes many patients to seek surgical correction of a hernia that is discovered in a preemployment physical examination (especially in the United States). These hernias must be repaired regardless of the paucity of symptoms due to the medicolegal risks to both employer *and* surgeon.

Conclusions

The incidence of primary groin hernia varies in different communities. The exact incidence in adult males is very difficult to estimate, but 16% of adult males will undergo operation. The incidence of inguinal hernia is higher in African people, who tend to have a narrower male pelvis than Europeans. Of interest is that the incidence of herniation varies considerably even between different African tribes.

Genetic and acquired factors clearly interact to allow a hernia to develop. However, we are forced to the conclusion that it is the failure of the fascia transversalis to withstand the stresses and strains of an upright posture that is crucial to the development of an inguinal hernia. A preformed, congenital, peritoneal processus or sac is an important prerequisite of indirect hernias in children and of an indirect sac in adults.

Connective tissue defects and imbalances are demonstrated in adult males with inguinal herniation and are causally related to smoking. Persistently heavy labor is also associated with herniation.

References

1. Rutkow IM. Epidemiologic, economic, and sociologic aspects of hernia surgery in the United States in the 1990s. Surg Clin North Am. 1998;78:941–51.
2. Bay-Nielsen M, Kehlet H. Establishment of a national Danish Hernia data-base: preliminary report. Hernia. 1999;3:81–3.
3. Royal College of General Practitioners, OPCS 1981–82. Morbidity statistics from general practice. Third National Study, London: HMSO; 1986.
4. Bay-Nielsen M, Kehlet H, Strand L, Malmstrom J, Andersen FH, Wara P, et al. Prospective nationwide quality assessment of 26,304 herniorrhaphies in Denmark. Lancet. 2001;358:1124–8.
5. Primatesta P, Goldacre MJ. Inguinal hernia repair: incidence of elective and emergency surgery, readmission and mortality. Int J Epidemiol. 1996;25:835–9.
6. Williams BT, Nicholl JP, Thomas KJ, Knowlenden J. Differences in duration of stay for surgery in the NHS and private hospitals in England and Wales. Br Med J. 1985;290:978–80.
7. Cheek C, Black NA, Devlin HB, Kingsnorth AN, Taylor RS, Watkins J. Systematic review on groin hernia surgery. Ann R Coll Surg Engl. 1998;80 Suppl 1:S1–80.
8. Law NW, Trapnell JE. Does a truss benefit a patient with inguinal hernia. Br Med J. 1992;304:1092.
9. Williams M, Frankel S, Nanchalal K, Coast J, Donovan J. Hernia repair: epidemiologically based needs assessment. Bristol: Health Care Evaluation Unit, University of Bristol Print Services; 1992.
10. Andrews NJ. Presentation and outcome of strangulated external hernia in a district general hospital. Br J Surg. 1981;68:329–32.
11. Coulter A, McPherson K. Socioeconomic variations in the use of common surgical operations. Br Med J. 1985;291:183–7.
12. Barwell NJ, Schumpelick V, Wantz GE, editors. Inguinal hernia repair. Basel: Karger; 1995.
13. Nilsson F, Anderberg B, Bragmark M, Eriksson T, Fordell R, Happaniemi S, et al. Hernia surgery in a defined population: improvements possible in outcome and cost-effectiveness. Amb Surg. 1993;1:150–3.
14. Schumpelick V, Treutner KH, Arit G. Inguinal hernia repair in adults. Lancet. 1994;344:375–9.
15. Hair A, Duffy K, McLean J, Taylor S, Smith H, Walker A, et al. Groin hernia repair in Scotland. Br J Surg. 2000;87:1722–6.
16. Schoots IG, van Dijkman D, Butzelaar RMJM, van Geldere D, Simons MP. Inguinal hernia repair in the Amsterdam region 1994–1996. Hernia. 2001;5:37–40.
17. Penttinen R, Grunroos JM. Mesh repair of common abdominal hernias: a review on experimental and clinical studies. Hernia. 2008;12:337–44.
18. Rutkow IM, Robbins AW. Demographic, classificatory, and socioeconomic aspects of hernia repair in the United States. Surg Clin North Am. 1993;73:413–26.
19. Seymour DG, Garthwaite PH. Age deprivation and rates of inguinal hernia surgery in men. Age Aging. 1999;28:485–90.
20. Sanders DL, Porter CS, Mitchell KC, Kingsnorth AN. A prospective cohort study comparing the African and European hernia. Hernia. 2008;12:527–9.
21. Milamed DR, Hedley-White J. Contributions of the surgical sciences to a reduction of the mortality rate in the United States for the period 1968 to 1988. Ann Surg. 1994;219:94–102.
22. London JA, Utter GH, Sena MJ, Chen SL, Romano PS. Lack of insurance is associated with increased risk for hernia complications. Ann Surg. 2009;250:331–7.
23. Keith A. On the origin and nature of hernia. Br J Surg. 1924;11:455–75.
24. Zimmerman LM, Anson BJ. Anatomy and surgery of hernia. 2nd ed. Baltimore: Williams & Wilkins; 1967. p. 216–27.
25. Iles JDH. Specialisation in elective herniorrhaphy. Lancet. 1965;1:751–5.
26. Harvald B. Genetic epidemiology of Greenland. Clin Genet. 1989;36:364–7.
27. Belcher DW, Nyame DK, Wurapa FJ. The prevalence of inguinal hernia in adult Ghanaian males. Trop Geogr Med. 1978;30:39–43.
28. Abramson JH, Gofin J, Hoppe C, Makler A. The epidemiology of inguinal hernia. A survey in western Jerusalem. J Epidemiol Community Health. 1978;32:59–67.
29. National Centre For Health Statistics. Health interview responses compared with medical records, Health Statistics from the US. National Health Survey Series D. Washington DC: US Dept of Health, Education and Welfare; 1961.
30. Maingot R. Abdominal operations. 4th ed. New York: Appleton; 1961. p. 939.
31. Glassow F. Femoral hernia in men. Am J Surg. 1971;121:637–40.
32. Quill DS, Devlin HB, Plant JA, Denham KR, McNay RA, Morris D. Surgical operation rates: a twelve year experience in Stockton-on-Tees. Ann R Coll Surg Engl. 1983;65:248–53.
33. Suppiah A, Gatt M, Barandiaran J, Heng MS, Perry EP. Outcomes of emergency and elective femoral hernia surgery in four district general hospitals: a 4-year study. Hernia. 2007;11:509–12.
34. Dahistrand U, Wollert S, Nordin P, Sandblom G, Gunnarsson U. Emergency femoral hernia repair: a study based on a national register. Ann Surg. 2009;249:672–6.
35. Ashley GT. Hernia in East Africa—an anatomical analysis of 700 cases. East Afr Med J. 1954;31:315–9.
36. Badoe EA. External hernia in Accra-some epidemiological aspects. Afr J Med Sci. 1973;4:51–8.
37. Kreymer M. Inguinal hernien bei centralafrikan-ern. Munchen Med Wochenschr. 1968;110:1750–5.
38. Onukak EE, Grundy DJ, Lawrie JH. Hernia in Northern Nigeria. J R Coll Surg Edinb. 1983;28:147–50.

39. Yordanov YS, Stroyanov SK. The incidence of hernia on the Island of Pemba. East Afr Med J. 1969;46:687–91.

40. Hunter J. Palmer's edition of Hunter's works. London; 1837. vol. iv, p.1.

41. Cloquet J. Recherches anatomiques sur les hernies de l'abdomen. Thesis, Paris, 1817, 133:129.

42. Hughson W. The persistent or preformed sac in relation to oblique inguinal hernia. Surg Gynecol Obstet. 1925;41:610–4.

43. Grover VK, Nur AMA, Usha R, Farag TI, Sabry MA. Indirect inguinal hernia among Bedouins. J Med Genet. 1996;33:887.

44. Ando H, Kaneko K, Ito F, Seo T, Ito T. Anatomy of the round ligament in female infants and children with an inguinal hernia. Br J Surg. 1997;84:404–5.

45. Ron O, Eaton S, Pierro A. Systematic review of the risk of developing a metachronous contralateral inguinal hernia in children. Br J Surg. 2007;94:804–11.

46. Zamakhshardy M, Ein A, Ein SH, Wales PW. Predictors of metachronous inguinal hernias in children. Pediatr Surg Int. 2009;25:69–71.

47. Chan MK, Baillod RA, Tanner RA, et al. Abdominal hernias in patients receiving continuous ambulatory peritoneal dialysis. Br Med J. 1981;283:826.

48. Engeset J, Youngson GG. Ambulatory peritoneal dialysis and hernial complications. Surg Clin North Am. 1984;64:385–92.

49. Schurgers ML, Boelaert JRO, Daneels RF, Robbens EJ, Vandelanotte MM. Genital oedema in patients treated by continuous ambulatory peritoneal dialysis: an unusual presentation of inguinal hernia. Br Med J. 1983;388:358–9.

50. Cooper JL, Nicholls AJ, Simms IM. Genital oedema in patients treated by continuous ambulatory peritoneal dialysis: an unusual presentation of inguinal hernia. Br Med J. 1983;286:1923–4.

51. Sherlock DJ, Smith S. Complications resulting from a patent processus vaginalis in two patients on continuous ambulatory peritoneal dialysis. Br J Surg. 1984;71:477.

52. Russell H. The saccular theory of hernia and the radical operation. Lancet. 1906;3:1197–203.

53. Van Wessem KJ, Simons MP, Plaisier PW, Lange JF. The aetiology of indirect inguinal hernias: congenital and/or acquired? Hernia. 2003;7:76–9.

54. Van Veen RN, van Wessem KJ, Halm JA, Simons MP, Plaisier PW, Jeekel J, et al. Patent processus vaginalis in the adult as a risk factor for the occurrence of indirect inguinal hernia. Surg Endosc. 2007;21:202–5.

55. Edwards H. Discussion on hernia. Proc R Soc Med. 1943;36:186–9.

56. Read RC. Attenuation of the rectus sheath in inguinal herniation. Am J Surg. 1970;120:610–4.

57. McVay CB. The normal and pathologic anatomy of the transversus abdominis muscle in inguinal and femoral hernia. Surg Clin North Am. 1971;51:1251–61.

58. McVay CB. The anatomic basis for inguinal and femoral hernioplasty. Surg Gynecol Obstet. 1974;139:931–45.

59. Dutta CR, Katzarski M. The anatomical basis for the inguinal hernia in Ghana. Ghana Med J. 1969;8:185–6.

60. Zinanovic S. The anatomical basis for the high frequency of inguinal and femoral hernia in Uganda. East Afr Med J. 1968;45:41–6.

61. Peacock EE, Madden JW. Studies on the biology and treatment of recurrent inguinal hernia: 11 Morphological changes. Ann Surg. 1974;179:567–71.

62. Lichtenstein IL, Shore JM. Exploding the myths of hernia repair. Am J Surg. 1976;132:307–15.

63. Wagh PV, Read RC. Defective collagen synthesis in inguinal herniation. Am J Surg. 1972;124:819–22.

64. Wagh PV, Leverich AP, Read RC, Sun CN, White JH. Direct inguinal herniation in man: a disease of collagen. J Surg Res. 1974;17:425–33.

65. White HJ, Sun CN, Read RC. Inguinal hernia: a true collagen disease. Lab Invest. 1977;36:359.

66. Allegra SR, Broderick PA. Desmoid fibroblastoma. Intracytoplasmic collagen synthesis in a peculiar fibroblastic tumour: light and ultrastructural study of a case. Hum Pathol. 1973;4:419–29.

67. Cannon DJ, Read RC. Metastatic emphysema. A mechanism for acquiring inguinal herniation. Ann Surg. 1981;194:270–6.

68. Levene CL, Ockleford CD, Harber CL. Scurvy: a comparison between ultrastructural and biochemical changes observed in cultural fibroblasts and the collagen they synthesize. Virchows Arch B Cell Pathol. 1977;23:325–38.

69. Pans A, Pierard GE, Albert A. Adult groin hernias: new insight into their biomechanical characteristics. Eur J Clin Invest. 1997;27:863–8.

70. Berliner SD. An approach to groin hernia. Surg Clin North Am. 1984;64:197–213.

71. Friedman DW, Boyd CD, Norton P, Greco RS, Boyarsky AH, Mackenzie JW, et al. Increases in Type III collagen gene expression and protein expression in patients with inguinal hernias. Ann Surg. 1993;218:754–60.

72. Casanova AB, Trindade EN, Trindade MRM. Collagen in the transversalis fascia of patients with indirect inguinal hernia: a case–control study. Am J Surg. 2009;198:1–5.

73. Laurell CB, Ericksson S. The electrophoretic alpha-1-globulin pattern of serum alpha-1-anti trypsin deficiency. Scand J Clin Lab Invest. 1963;15:132–40.

74. Bellon JM, Bajo A, Ga-Honduvilla N, Gimeno MJ, Pascual G, Guerrero A, et al. Fibroblasts from the transversalis fascia of young patients with direct inguinal hernias show constitutive MMP-2 overexpression. Ann Surg. 2001;233:287–91.

75. Zheng H, Si Z, Kasperk R, Bhardwaj RS, Schumpelick V, Klinge U, et al. Recurrent inguinal hernia: disease of the collagen matrix? World J Surg. 2002;26:401–8.

76. Pascual G, Corrales C, Gomez-Gil V, Bujan J, Bellon JM. TGF-beta1 overexpression in the transversalis fascia of patients with direct inguinal hernia. Eur J Clin Invest. 2007;37:516–21.

77. Lehnert B, Wadouh F. High coincidence of inguinal hernias and abdominal aortic aneurysms. Ann Vasc Surg. 1992;6:134–7.

78. Adye B, Luna G. Incidence of abdominal wall hernia in aortic surgery. Am J Surg. 1998;175:400–2.

79. Cannon DJ, Casteel L, Read RC. Abdominal aortic aneurysm, Leriche's syndrome, inguinal herniation and smoking. Arch Surg. 1984;119:387–9.

80. Liapis CD, Dimitroulis DA, Kakisis JD, Nikolaou AN, Skandalakis P, Daskalopoulos M, et al. Incidence of incisional hernias in patients operated on for aneurysm or occlusive disease. Am Surg. 2004;70:550–2.

81. Takagi H, Sugimoto M, Kato T, Matsuno Y, Umemoto T. Postoperative incision hernia in patients with abdominal aortic aneurysm and aortoiliac occlusive disease: a systematic review. Eur J Vasc Endovasc Surg. 2007;33:177–81.

82. Musella M, Milone F, Chello M, Angelini P, Jovino R. Magnetic resonance imaging and abdominal wall hernias in aortic surgery. J Am Coll Surg. 2001;1993:392–5.

83. Pleumeekers HJ, De Gruijl A, Hofman A, Van Beek AJ, Hoes AW. Prevalence of aortic aneurysm in men with a history of inguinal hernia. Br J Surg. 1999;86:1155–8.

84. Anderson O, Shiralkar S. Prevalence of abdominal aortic aneurysms in over 65-year-old men with inguinal hernias. Ann R Coll Surg Engl. 2008;90:386–8.

85. Read RC. Metabolic factors contributing to herniation: a review. Hernia. 1998;2:51–5.

86. Klinge U, Zheng H, Si ZY, Bhardwaj R, Klosterhalfen B, Schumpelick V. Altered collagen synthesis in fascia transversalis of patients with inguinal hernia. Hernia. 1999;4:181–7.

87. Hunt DM. Primary defect in copper transport underlies mottled mutant in mouse. Nature. 1974;249:852–4.

88. Tilson MD, Davis G. Deficiencies of copper and a compound with iron exchange characteristics of pyridinoline in skin from patients with abdominal aortic aneurysms. Surgery. 1983;94:134–41.

89. Bendavid R. The unified theory of hernia formation. Hernia. 2004;8:171–6.

90. Klinge U, Binnebosel M, Mertens PR. Are collagens the culprits in the development of incisional and inguinal hernia disease? Hernia. 2006;10:472–7.

91. Franz MG. The biology of hernia formation. Surg Clin North Am. 2008;88:1–15.

92. Hiles M, Record Ritchie RD, Altizer AM. Are biologic grafts effective for hernia repair: a systematic review of the literature. Surg Innov. 2009;16:26–37.

93. Beighton P, De Paepe A, Steinmann B, Tsipouras P, Wenstrup RJ. Ehlers-Danlos syndromes; revised nosology. Am J Med Genet. 1998;77:31–7.

94. Barnett C, Langer JC, Hinek A, Bradley TJ, Chitayat D. Looking past the lump: genetic aspects of inguinal hernia in children. J Pediatr Surg. 2009;44:1423–31.

95. West LS. Two pedigrees showing inherited predisposition to hernia. J Hered. 1936;27:449–55.

96. Smith MP, Sparkes RS. Familial inguinal hernia. Surgery. 1965;57:807–12.

97. Morris-Stiff G, Coles G, Moore R, Jurewicz A, Lord R. Abdominal wall hernia in autosomal dominant polycystic kidney disease. Br J Surg. 1997;84:615–7.

98. Weimer BR. Congenital inheritance of inguinal hernia. J Hered. 1949;40:219–20.

99. Montagu AMF. A case of familial inheritance of oblique inguinal hernia. J Hered. 1942;33:355–6.

100. Czeizel A, Gardonyi J. A family study of congenital inguinal hernia. Am J Med Genet. 1979;4:247–54.

101. Savatguchi S, Matsunaga E, Honna T. A genetic study on indirect inguinal hernia. Jpn J Hum Genet. 1975;20:187–95.

102. Gong Y, Shao C, Sun Q, et al. Genetic study of indirect inguinal hernia. J Med Genet. 1994;31:187–92.

103. Jones ME, Swerdlow AJ, Griffith M, Goldacre MJ. Risk of congenital inguinal hernia in siblings: a record linkage study. Paediatr Perinat Epidemiol. 1998;12:288–96.

104. Lau H, Fang C, Yuen WK, Patil NG. Risk factors for inguinal hernia in adult males: a case–control study. Surgery. 2007;141:262–6.

105. Grindflek E, Moe M, Taubert H, Simianer H, Lien S, Moen T. Genome-wide linkage analysis of inguinal hernia in pigs using affected sib pairs. BMC Genet. 2006;7:25.

106. Kasson MA, Munoz E, Laughlin A, Margolis IB, Wise L. Value of routine pathology in herniorrhaphy performed upon adults. Surg Gynecol Obstet. 1986;163:518–22.

107. Tanyel FC, Dagdeviren A, Muftuoglu S, Gursoy MH, Yuruker S, Buyukpamukcu N. Inguinal hernia revisited through comparative evaluation of peritoneum, processus vaginalis and sacs obtained from children with hernia, hydrocele, and undescended. J Paediatr Surg. 1999;34:552–5.

108. Rosai J, Dehner LP. Nodular mesothelial hyperplasia in hernia sacs. A benign reactive condition simulating a neoplastic process. Cancer. 1975;35:165–75.

109. Leonetti JP, Aranha GV, Wilkinson WA, Stanley M, Greenlee HB. Umbilical herniorrhaphy in cirrhotic patients. Arch Surg. 1984;119:442–5.

110. Carbonell AM, Wolfe LG, DeMaria EJ. Poor outcomes in cirrhosis-associated hernia repair: a nationwide cohort study of 32,033 patients. Hernia. 2005;9:353–7.

111. Gray SH, Vick CC, Graham LA, Finan KR, Neumayer LA, Hawn MT. Umbilical herniorrhaphy in cirrhosis: improved outcomes with elective repair. J Gastrointest Surg. 2008;12:675–81.

112. Patti R, Almasio PL, Buscemi S, Fama F, Craxi A, Di Vita G. Inguinal hernioplasty improves the quality of life in patients with cirrhosis. Am J Surg. 2008;196:373–8.

113. Ammar SA. Management of complicated umbilical hernias in cirrhotic patients using permanent mesh: a randomized trial. Hernia. 2010;14:35–8.

114. Cronin K, Ellis H. Pus collections in hernial sacs. Br J Surg. 1959;46:364–7.

115. Thomas WEG, Vowles KDL, Williamson RCN. Appendicitis in external herniae. Ann R Coll Surg Engl. 1982;64:121–2.

116. Greenberg J, Arnell TD. Diverticular disease presenting as an incarcerated inguinal hernia. Am Surg. 2005;71:208–9.

117. Bunting D, Harshen R, Ravichandra M, Ridings P. Unusual diagnoses presenting as incarcerated inguinal hernia: a case report and review of the literature. Int J Clin Pract. 2006;60:1681–2.

118. Hoguet JP. Right inguinal hernia following appendectomy. Ann Surg. 1911;54:673–6.

119. Arnbjornsson E. Development of right inguinal hernia after appendectomy. Am J Surg. 1982;143:174–5.

120. Gue S. Development of right inguinal hernia following appendectomy. Br J Surg. 1972;59:352–3.

121. Arnbjornsson E. A neuromuscular basis for the development of right inguinal hernia after appendicectomy. Am J Surg. 1982;143:367–9.

122. Gilsdorf JR, Friedman RH, Shapiro P. Electromyographic evaluation of the inguinal region in patients with hernia of the groin. Surg Gynecol Obstet. 1988;167:466–8.

123. Leech P, Waddell G, Main RG. The incidence of right inguinal hernia following appendicectomy. Br J Surg. 1972;59:623.

124. Jorgensen LN, Wille-Jorgensen P. Open or laparoscopic appendicectomy? Colorectal Dis. 2009;11:795–6.

125. Clain A. Traumatic hernia. Br J Surg. 1964;51:549–50.

126. Ryan EA. Hernias related to pelvic fractures. Surg Gynecol Obstet. 1971;133:440–6.

127. Narath A. Ueber eine Eigenartige Form von Hernia Cruralis (prevascularis) in Anschlusse an die umblitige Behandlung angeborener Huftgelenkverrenkung. Arch Klin Chir. 1899;59:396–424.

128. Salter RB. Innominate osteotomy in the treatment of dislocation and subluxation of the hip. J Bone Joint Surg. 1961;43-B:518–39.

129. Castelein RM, Saunter AJM. Lumbar hernia in an iliac bone graft defect. Acta Orthop Scand. 1985;56:273–4.

130. Dennis RW, Marshall A, Deshmukh H, Bender JS, Kulvatunyou N, Lees JS, et al. Abdominal wall injuries occurring after blunt trauma: incidence and grading system. Am J Surg. 2009;197:413–7.

131. Davis PR. The causation of herniae by weight lifting. Lancet. 1969;ii:155–7.

132. Smith GD, Crosby DL, Lewis PA. Inguinal hernia and a single strenuous event. Ann R Coll Surg Engl. 1996;78:367–8.

133. Sanjay P, Woodward A. Single strenuous event: does it predispose to inguinal herniation? Hernia. 2007;11:493–6.

134. Pathak S, Poston GJ. It is unlikely that the development of an abdominal wall hernia can be attributable to a single strenuous event. Ann R Coll Surg Engl. 2006;88:168–71.

135. Carbonell JF, Sanchez JLA, Peris RT, Ivorra JC, Delbano MJP, Sanchez C, et al. Risk factors associated with inguinal hernias: a case control study. Eur J Surg. 1993;159:481–6.

136. Flich J, Alfonso JL, Delgrado F, Prado MJ, Cortina P. Inguinal hernias and certain risk factors. Eur J Epidemiol. 1992;8:277–82.

137. McArdle G. Is inguinal hernia a defect in human evolution and would this insight improve concepts for methods of surgical repair. Clin Anat. 1997;10:47–55.

138. Liem MS, van der Graaf Y, Zwart RC, Geurts I, van Vroonhoven TJ. Risk factors for inguinal hernia in women: a case–control study. The Coala Trial Group. Am J Epidemiol. 1997;146:721–6.

139. Kemp DA (ed) Kemp and Kemp. The quantum of damages. Revised edn, vol. 1. London: Sweet & Maxwell; 1975.

140. Hendry PO, Paterson-Brown S, de Beaux A. Work related aspects of inguinal hernia: a literature review. Surgeon. 2008;6:361–5.

Logistics

4

Giampiero Campanelli, Marta Cavalli, Valentina Bertocchi, and Cristina Sfeclan

Introduction

Over the last 25 years ambulatory surgery rates have steadily increased in many countries, and inguinal hernia repair is a common accepted outpatient procedure.

> Ambulatory surgery refers to surgical or diagnostic interventions, currently performed with traditional hospitalisation, that could, in most cases, be accomplished with complete confidence without a night of hospitalization. Among other things these procedures require the same technically sophisticated facilities as when done on an inpatient basis, rigorous pre-operative selection procedures and post-operative follow-up of several hours. Terms used to express the concept are: ambulatory surgery, major ambulatory surgery, day surgery, ambulatory anaesthesia. Modern day surgery is not simply a shortened hospital stay or an architectural model. Rather, it is a complex, multifaceted concept involving institutional, organizational, medical, economic and qualitative consideration [1].

Day surgery can be performed in:

- Freestanding on campus: Department with free management and administration engaged in a hospital site, with own operating theater, division, and staff.
- Freestanding off campus: Department located out of a hospital site, with free management and administration,

with own operating theater, division, and staff, but with a formal agreement with a health center with an emergency room in case of complication or emergency.
- Division: Integrated unit in a hospital, multidisciplinary or unidisciplinary. Operating room is shared with other divisions according as agreed turns.
- Beds: Beds in an ordinary division dedicated to day surgery. Operating room is shared with other division according as agreed turns [2].

Day surgery rather than inpatient surgery must be regarded as the standard for all elective surgery: it should be considered the principal option and no longer an alternative form of treatment [3].

However, not all patients can be treated on a day surgery basis: it is not the operation that is ambulatory; it is the patient. It is of paramount importance that all patients are carefully selected, taking social, medical (comorbidity), and surgical criteria into account.

Day surgery procedure must be performed by highly qualified professionals, with considerable experience in traditional inpatient surgery, to reduce the number of complications and/or unplanned readmission and to achieve greater efficiency.

Surgical principles, basis for conventional surgery too, for example, avoiding unnecessary tissue traction or tissue tension, aiming to a complete hemostasis, and choosing minimally invasive procedures, are essential for the promotion of an uneventful recovery and a reduction of the number of unplanned admission [4].

Advantages of Day Surgery

In a self-contained day unit, the day surgery patient is the center of attention and receives more personalized care than if an inpatient and among more seriously ill patients [5].

A daily hospitalization avoids problems that may arise from prolonged stay, like exposure to infection [6, 7] or variation in the usual drug therapy (e.g., diabetic inpatient is

G. Campanelli (✉) • M. Cavalli
Surgical Department - Università Insubria, Istituto Clinico Sant'Ambrogio, via Faravelli 16, 20149 Milano, Italy
e-mail: giampiero.campanelli@grupposandonato.it; marta_cavalli@hotmail.it

V. Bertocchi
Surgical Department - Università Insibria, Ospedale di Circolo di Varese, Viale Borri 57, 21100 Varese, Italy
e-mail: valentinabertocchi@virgilio.it

C. Sfeclan
Surgical Department, University of Pharmacy and Medicine of Craiova, Istituto Clinico Sant'Ambrogio, Via Faravelli 16, 20149 Milano, Italy
e-mail: sfeclancristina@gmail.com

A.N. Kingsnorth and K.A. LeBlanc (eds.), *Management of Abdominal Hernias*,
DOI 10.1007/978-1-84882-877-3_4, © Springer Science+Business Media London 2013

often unnecessarily switched from their oral drugs to insulin or drug doses may be missed, delayed, or duplicated by hospital staff) [8].

Day surgery is not associated with complication rates in excess of those encountered following inpatient surgery. Readmission rates [9, 10] and contacts with the primary and community healthcare teams [11] are no greater than for the same procedures undertaken as an inpatient. There is less postoperative pain and also a reduction in the risk of thromboembolism associated with early ambulation [12], and it is less stressful for patient. Patients satisfaction rates following day surgery are high [13].

Because the risk of last-minute cancelation is minimal in dedicated day surgery facilities, hospital can manage elective surgery more efficiently. This allows more accurate scheduling than for inpatient work and makes more effective use of staff and facilities alike [14].

Day surgery is cost-effective compared with inpatient surgery as hospitalization time is reduced, night and weekend staffing is not required, the hotel element of treatment is removed, and capital facilities and staff are used more intensively and effectively [15].

Hernia Repair

As early as 1955, the advantages of inguinal hernia repair as day surgery were already described in the literature [16], and nowadays they are confirmed in several studies, many retrospective [17–21], and some randomized [22–26].

EHS guidelines for inguinal hernia repair report day surgery as safe, effective, and in addition cheaper [27].

In a large American cohort study, the cost of inguinal hernia repair in a clinic setting was found to be 56% higher than those for day surgery [28].

Also in Germany, this procedure is generating less costs [29].

In addition to these few randomized studies, there are a multitude of cohort studies concerning patients successfully operated on as day surgery, under general, regional, or local anesthetics, and with both classical operation techniques as well as open tension-free repairs and endoscopic techniques. A large study conducted in Denmark noted the hospital readmission rate of 0.8% [29, 30].

Although a tension-free repair under local anesthetic seems to be the most suitable operation, the published series showed that other surgical and anesthesiological techniques can also be effectively used as day surgery. Only the extensive open preperitoneal approach (Stoppa technique) has not been described in the context of day surgery [27].

When day surgery was in its infancy, there was a strict selection of patient with a low risk of complication (ASA I-II, age limit, length of operation <1 h, no serious obesity,

etc.). Such a strict selection is becoming less common and, in principle, a primary inguinal hernia repair as day surgery can be considered for every patient who has satisfactory care at home [31–33].

On a worldwide basis there is a clear increase in the percentage of inguinal hernia repairs in ambulatory surgery [32, 34].

There is a considerable variation between different countries, which cannot be clarified solely by the degree of acceptability of day surgery among patients and surgeons but, to a significant extent, is also determined by healthcare financing system. In the last year (2000–2004), 35% of inguinal hernia operation carried out in the Netherlands and 33% in Spain were done on a day surgery basis; there is room for this number to be increased. In the Swedish National Registry, 75% of inguinal hernia repair are performed in day care [27]. In 2005 in Italy 50% of inguinal hernia repair in adult were done in day surgery [35].

In literature there is no high evidence about abdominal wall hernia in ambulatory surgery rather than inguinal hernia, but some successful personal experience for umbilical, epigastric, or incisional hernia repair in outpatient setting are reported [36–38].

Pathway

First Access in Hospital

Surgeon, during the first examination in the consulting room, requires more test (e.g., ecotomogrophy or CT) if necessary, makes a diagnosis, and if necessary, gives a surgical indication. In this case, he makes the first choice about the kind of recovery (ambulatory surgery, extended recovery, short stay, or ordinary hospitalization) according to social, medical, and surgical criteria.

Social Criteria

To ensure that patients are discharged to safe and acceptable home conditions, they are required to be accompanied by a responsible, physically able adult who can care for them overnight. Patients and their carer must understand the planned procedure and postoperative care and be willing to accept responsibility for providing further supervision of the patient. Easy access to a telephone is important so that emergency help can be summoned, if required [39].

Medical Criteria

Selection of patient should be based on their overall physiological status and not limited by arbitrary limits such as age, weight, or ASA status. For every patient who is not completely healthy, the nature of any preexisting condition, its stability, and functional limitation should be all evaluated. Treatment should obviously be optimized; if it is not, the patient is not adequately prepared for any form of elective surgery. A pragmatic question to ask is whether the management or outcome would be improved by pre- or postoperative hospitalization. If not, the patient should undergo treatment on an ambulatory basis [39].

Surgical Criteria

Procedure suitable for ambulatory surgery has the following characteristics:

- Postoperative care might be specific but is neither invasive nor prolonged and will not lead to unexpected admission to hospital.
- The risk of severe pre- and postoperative blood loss is low.
- The duration of the procedure is less than 90 min.
- Postoperative pain is easily controlled [4].

Almost all primary inguinal or femoral hernia repairs with normal size or little recurrent hernia near the internal inguinal ring (suitable to be repair with a Gilbert plug), approachable with open or laparoscopic technique, can be performed in outpatient setting [40].

Huge, old, unreducible, primary, or recurrent (or multiple recurrent) inguinal or femoral hernia should have the option to be access at least to an extended recovery.

Little epigastric or umbilical hernia suitable for a primary repair or for a little mesh repair can be performed in ambulatory surgery.

All ventral defect requiring large mesh repair must to be hospitalized for a short stay or longer.

Preoperative Screening and Selection

Advanced assessment provides a valuable opportunity to have more knowledge about whole health condition of patient, correct abnormalities, and drug therapy.

The patient during a day hospital admission is submitted to some routine screening test, including blood test, ECG, and chest X-rays (the last one depends on hospital policy, e.g., it is required just for adult with more than 65 years old or in smoker or in patient with lung disease history) and to an interview with a surgeon, in order to report a complete clinic history, answer patient' questions, and obtain written informed consent to surgery, and with an anesthetist. The patient will be supplied with a written booklet with informations about preparation at home, surgery, and postoperative care.

At the end of the day, hospital surgeon and anesthetist decide if the patient is suitable to surgery and to the kind of recovery proposed. Otherwise the patient can be switched to a different kind of hospitalization.

The patient will be advised by hospital secretariat by phone about the day of the surgery.

Table 4.1 The modified Aldrete scoring system

Discharge criteria from PACU	Score
Activity: able to move voluntary or on command	
Four extremities	2
Two extremities	1
Zero extremities	0
Respiration	
Able to deep breath and cough freely	
Dyspnea, shallow or limited breathing	
Apneic	
Circulation	
Blood pressure +/−20 mm of pre-anesthetic level	2
Blood pressure +/−20–50 mm of pre-anesthetic level	1
Blood pressure +/−50 mm of pre-anesthetic level	0
Consciousness	
Fully awake	2
Arousable on calling	1
Not responding	0
O_2 saturation	
Able to maintain O_2 saturation >92% on room air	2
Needs O_2 inhalation to maintain O_2 saturation >90%	1
O_2 saturation <90% even with O_2 supplementation	0

Day of Surgery

Patient is admitted to the hospital the same day of the surgery. A nurse and a surgeon receive the patient and check his preparation (drug therapy, depilation, fast), do the last blood test if necessary, and mark the correct side of the hernia.

Operating Theater

The patient is taken to the operating theater according as the list written the day before, reporting full name of the patient, date of birth, unit and number of the bed, diagnosis, surgical procedure, kind of anesthesia, surgeon team, any antibiotic, or thromboembolism prophylaxis or annotation.

During surgery, at least one senior surgeon, one resident, one anesthetist, one scrub nurse, and one nurse have to be present in the operating room.

After surgery the patient is transferred to postanesthesia care unit (PACU). To discharge safely from there, the Aldrete scoring system can be used [41]. When the patient achieves a score of ≥9, he can be discharge from the PACU to day surgery unit (Table 4.1).

The fast tracking is a clinical pathway that involves transferring the patient from the operating room to the day surgery unit and bypassing the PACU. The use of ultrashort-acting drugs, proper selection of patients, and elimination of postoperative complication (pain and postoperative nausea and vomiting) will enable patients to achieve an Aldrete score of 9 or 10 in the operating room and therefore bypass the PACU. A minimal score of 12 (with no score <1 in any individual category)

Table 4.2 White et al. scoring system

Discharge criteria	Score
Level of consciousness	
Awake and oriented	2
Arousable with minimal stimulation	1
Responsive only to tactile stimulation	0
Physical activity	
Able to move all extremities on command	2
Some weakness in movement of extremities	1
Unable to voluntarily move extremities	0
Hemodynamic stability	
Blood pressure <15% of baseline mean artery pressure value	2
Blood pressure 15–30% of baseline mean artery pressure value	1
Blood pressure >30% below baseline mean artery pressure value	0
Respiratory stability	
Able to breathe deeply	2
Tachypnea with good cough	1
Dyspnea with weak cough	0
Oxygen saturation status	
Maintains value >90% on room air	2
Requires supplemental oxygen (nasal prongs)	1
Saturation <90% with supplemental oxygen	0
Postoperative pain assessment	
None, or mild discomfort	2
Moderate to severe pain controlled with IV analgesics	1
Persistent severe pain	0
Postoperative emetic symptoms	
None, or mild nausea with no active vomiting	2
Transient vomiting or retching	1
Persistent moderate to severe nausea and vomiting	0
Total possible score	14

Table 4.3 Chung et al. postanesthesia discharge scoring system (PADS)

Postanesthesia discharge scoring system	Score
Vital signs	
Vital signs must be stable and consistent with age and preoperative baseline	
Blood pressure and pulse within 20% of preoperative baseline	2
Blood pressure and pulse 20–40% of preoperative baseline	1
Blood pressure and pulse $w > 40\%$ of preoperative baseline 0	0
Activity level	
Patient must be able to ambulate at preop level	
Steady gait, no dizziness, or meets preop level	2
Requires assistance	1
Unable to ambulate	0
Nausea and vomiting	
Patient should have minimal nausea and vomiting before discharge	
Minimal: successfully treated with os medication	2
Moderate: successfully treated with intramuscular medication	1
Severe: continues after repeated treatment	0
Pain	
Patient should have minimal or no pain before discharge	
The level of pain that the patient has should be acceptable to the patient	
Pain should be controllable by oral analgesics	
The location, type, and intensity of pain should be consistent with anticipated postop discomfort	
Pain acceptable	2
Pain not acceptable	1
Surgical bleeding	
Postoperative bleeding should be consistent with expected blood loss for the procedure	
Minimal: does not require dressing change	2
Moderate: up to two dressing changes required	1
Severe: more than three dressing changes required	0

would be required for a patient to be fast tracked after general anesthesia in White et al. scoring system [42, 43] (Table 4.2).

Discharge

Discharge of patients home from the DSU requires strict adherence to validate criteria to ensure patient safety and avoid unplanned readmission. Discharge assessment has to be performed by the surgeon and anesthetist; this one just in case of regional or general anesthesia is performed in the same day of discharge. Chung et al. [44] devised the postanesthesia discharge scoring system (PADS), which was later modified to eliminate the fluid intake and output parameter [45]: patients who achieve a score of 9 or greater and have an adult escort are considered fit for discharge (Table 4.3).

Voiding seems not to be a requirement before discharge from DS as it could delay the discharge of 5–10% of patients who have no risk factors of urinary retention after ambulatory surgery [46].

But hernia surgery is considered, with anorectal surgery, old age, male sex, and spinal anesthesia, risk factor for postoperative urinary retention [47]. So, we usually prefer to wait for spontaneous voiding before discharge.

Of course patient must accept discharge in readiness, and he is required to be accompanied by a responsible, physically able adult who can accompany him at home and care for him overnight. Patients and their carer must understand the planned procedure and postoperative care.

At the discharge the patient receives a discharge letter, where it is described the reason for the admission to the hospital, preoperative test results, procedure underwent and kind of anesthesia, instruction for drugs and dressing, and date for a clinical check.

Follow-Up

The patient comes back to the hospital for a clinical check some days after surgery, as well as described in the discharge letter.

Periodic follow-up by phone is organized for long-term results.

References

1. Opening Statement of founding members of the International Association for Ambulatory Surgery (IAAS) in 1995.
2. Modelli organizzativi e sedi di svolgimento. In: Celli G, Campanelli G, Corbellini L, B de Stefano, Fortino A, Francucci M, Mastrobuono I, Torre M. Proposta per l'organizzazione, lo sviluppo e la regolamentazione delle attività chirurgiche a ciclo diurno. Ministero della Sanità, Commissione di studio sulla day-surgery e la chirurgia ambulatoriale istituita con decreto Ministeriale del 12 settembre 2000; 2001. p. 21–23.
3. NHS Modernisation Agency. The 10 high impact changes for service improvement and delivery. London, UK: Department of Health Publications; 2004.
4. De Jong D, Rinkel RNPM, Marin J, van Kesteren PJM, Rangel R, Imhof S, Henry Y, Baart JA, de Gast A, Ekkelkamp S, van der Horst CMAM, de la Rosette JJMCH, Laguna Pes MP. Day surgery procedures. In: Lemos P, Jarrett P, Philip B, editors. Day surgery: development and practice. London: First International Edition; 2006. p. 91–2.
5. Davis JE. The major ambulatory surgical center and how it is developed. Surg Clin North Am. 1987;67:671–92.
6. Baxter B. Day case surgery. In: Clarke P, Jones J, editors. Brigden's operating department practice. Edinburgh: Scotland. Churchill Livingstone; 1998. p. 24–31.
7. Cole BOI, Hislop WS. A grading system in day surgery: effective utilisation of theatre time. J R Coll Surg Edinb. 1998;43:87–8.
8. Sorabjee JS. Day care surgery—the physicians viewpoint. Bombay Hosp J. 2003;45:2.
9. Handerson J, Goldacre MJ, Griffith M, et al. Day case surgery: geographical variation, trends and readmission rates. J Epidemiol Community Health. 1989;43:302–5.
10. Cahill CJ, Tillin T, Jarrtt PEM. Wide variations in day case practice and outcomes in Southern England—a comparative audit in 15 hospitals. In: Abstracts of the 1st International Congress on AmbulatorySurgery. Brussels, Belgium; 1995.
11. Lewis C, Bryson J. Does day case surgery generate extra workload for primary and community health service staff? Ann Roy Coll Surg Engl. 1998;80:200.
12. Australian Day Surgery Council. Day surgery in Australia. Revised, edition. Melbourne, Australia: Royal Australasian College of Surgeons; 2004. First published; 1981.
13. Commission A. Measuring quality: the patients view of day surgery. London, UK: HMSO; 1991.
14. Department of Health. Day surgery: operational guide. Waiting, booking and choice. London, UK: Department of Health Publications; 2002.
15. Jarrett PEM, Staniszewski A. The development of ambulatory surgery and future challenges. In: Lemos P, Jarrett P, Philip B, editors. Day surgery: development and practice. London: First International Edition; 2006. p. 24–6.
16. Farquharson EL. Early ambulation; with special reference to herniorrhaphy as an outpatient procedure. Lancet. 1955;269:517–9.
17. Goulbourne IA, Ruckley CV. Operations for hernia and varicose veins in a day-bed unit. Br Med J. 1979;2:712.714.
18. Michelsen M, Walter F. Comparison of outpatient and inpatient operations for inguinal hernia (1971 to 1978). Zentralbl Chir. 1982;107:94–102.
19. Dhumale R, Tisdale J, Banwell N. Over a thousand ambulatory hernia repairs in a primary care setting. Ann R Coll Surg Engl. 2010;92:127–30.
20. Acevedo A. León J Ambulatory hernia surgery under local anesthesia is feasible and safe in obese patients. Hernia. 2010;14(1):57–62.
21. Kurzer M, Kark A, Hussain ST. Day-case inguinal hernia repair in the elderly: a surgical priority. Hernia. 2009;13(2):131–6. Epub 2008 Nov 26.
22. Pineault R, Contandriopoulos AP, Valois M, Bastian ML, Lance JM. Randomized clinical trial of one-day surgery. Patient satisfaction, clinical outcomes, and costs. Med Care. 1985;23(2):171–82.
23. Prescott RJ, Cutherbertson C, Fenwick N, Garraway WM, Ruckley CV. Economic aspect of day care after operations for hernia or varicose vein. J Epidemiol Community Health. 1978;32:222–5.
24. Ruckley CV, Cuthbertson C, Fenwick N, Prescott RJ, Garraway WM. Day care after operations for hernia or varicose veins: a controlled trial. Br J Surg. 1978;65:456–9.
25. Ramyl VM, Ognonna BC, Iya D. Patient acceptance of outpatient treatment for inguinal hernia in Jos, Nigeria. Cent Afr J Med. 1999;45:244–6.
26. Ramyil VM, Iya D, Ogbonna BC, Dakum NK. Safety of daycare hernia repair in Jos, Nigeria. East Afr Med J. 2000;77(6):326–8.
27. Simons MP, Aufenacker T, Bay-Nielsen M, Bouillot JL, Campanelli G, Conze J, de Lange D, Fortelny R, Heikkinen T, Kingsnorth A, Kukleta J, Morales Conde S, Nordin P, Schumpelick V, Smedberg S, Smietanski M, Weber G, Miserez M. European Hernia Society guidelines on the treatment of inguinal hernia in adult patients. Hernia. 2009;13:343–403.
28. Mitchell JB, Harrow B. Costs and outcomes of inpatient versus outpatient hernia repair. Health Policy. 1994;28:143–52.
29. Weyhe D, Winnemoller C, Hellwig A, Meurer K, Plugge H, Kasoly K, Laubenthal H, Bauer KH, Uhl W. (Section sign) 115 b SGB V threans outpatient treatment for inguinal hernia. Analysis of outcome and economics. Chirurg. 2006;77:844–55.
30. Engbaek J, Bartholdy J, Hjortsø NC. Return hospital visits and morbidity within 60 days after day surgery: a retrospective study of 18736 day surgical procedures. Acta Anaesthesiol Scand. 2006;50:911–9.
31. Davies KE, Houghton K, Montgomary JE. Obesity and day-case surgery. Anaesthesia. 2001;56:1112–5.
32. Jarrett PE. Day care surgery. Eur J Anaesthesiol Suppl. 2001;23:32–5.
33. Prabhu A, Chung F. Anaesthetic strategies towards development in day care surgery. Eur J Anaesthesiol Suppl. 2001;23:36–42.
34. De Lathouwer C, Poullier JP. How much ambulatory surgery in the World in 1996-1997 and trends? Ambul Surg. 2000;8:191–210.
35. Databank of Ministero della Salute, http://www.sanita.it. Healthcare Department of Italy.
36. Moreno-Egea A, Cartagena J, Vicente JP, Carrillo A, Aguayo JL. Laparoscopic incisional hernia repair as a day surgery procedure: audit of 127 consecutive cases in a university hospital. Surg Laparosc Endosc Percutan Tech. 2008;18(3):267–71.
37. Donati M, Gandolfo L, Privitera A, Brancato G, Donati A. Day hospital for incisional hernia repair: selection criteria. Acta Chir Belg. 2008;108(2):198–202.
38. Engledow AH, Sengupta N, Akhras F, Tutton M, Warren SJ. Day case laparoscopic incisional hernia repair is feasible, acceptable, and cost effective. Surg Endosc. 2007;21(1):84–6. Epub 2006 Nov 16.

39. Gudimetla V, Smith I. Pre-operative screening and selection of adult day surgery patients. In: Lemos P, Jarrett P, Philip B, editors. Day surgery: development and practice. London: First International Edition; 2006. p. 126.

40. Campanelli G, Pettinari D, Nicolosi FM, Cavalli M, Avesani EC. Inguinal hernia recurrence: classification and approach. Hernia. 2006;10(2):159–61.

41. Aldrete JA. The post-anesthesia recovery score revisited. J Clin Anesth. 1995;7:89–91.

42. Awad I, Chung F. Discharge criteria and recovery in ambulatory surgery. In: Lemos P, Jarrett P, Philip B, editors. Day surgery: development and practice. London: First International Edition; 2006. p. 242.

43. White P, Song D. New criteria for fast-tracking after outpatient anesthesia: a comparison with the modified Aldrete's scoring system. Anesth Analg. 1999;88:1069–72.

44. Chung F, Chan V, Ong D. A post-anesthetic discharge score system for home readiness after ambulatory surgery. J Clin Anesth. 1995;7:500–6.

45. Chung F. Recovery pattern and home-readiness after ambulatory surgery. Anesth Analg. 1995;80:896–902.

46. Pavlin DJ, Rapp SE, Polissar NL, et al. Factors affecting discharge time in adult outpatients. Anesth Analg. 1998;87:816–26.

47. Lau H, Larn B. Management of post-operative urinary retention: a randomized trial of in-out patient versus overnight catheterization. ANZ J Surg. 2004;74:658–61.

Luke Vale

Introduction

Hernia repair is one of the most frequently performed surgical procedures in the developed world with over 700,000 being performed each year in both the USA and Europe. Few surgical procedures have been as intensively evaluated as surgical methods for hernia repair. In recent years, there have been many high quality randomized controlled trials and several rigorous systematic reviews and meta-analyses (the recent European Hernia Society guideline provides, at the time of writing, one of the most up to date of reviews and meta-analyses) [1]. Almost uniquely for surgical interventions, there also have been a considerable number of economic evaluations performed. Some of these have been conducted as part of randomized controlled trials, and there have been several attempts to systematically review them [2–4]. In this chapter, evidence has been drawn from one of these evaluations [3], which was used to inform policy recommendations made by the National Institute for Health and Clinical Excellence (NICE) [5] and the European Hernia Society guidelines [1].

The condition has received so much attention from the research community because hernia repair is such a common procedure (although as is illustrated below, the cost per patient is relatively modest). Also until the early 1990s, the method of open repair of groin hernias changed little since the introduction of Bassini's method in the late nineteenth century. Since then, new techniques have been introduced for the repair of inguinal hernias and the evidence for and against these approaches.

Given the large number of hernia repairs carried out per year, the annual cost of surgery in the UK in 2001/2002 was estimated to be £56 million (Table 5.1) [3], and by 2006–2007, the costs to secondary care services in the UK were between £92 million and £113 million (Table 5.1). Both these cost estimates exclude any management costs of subsequent symptoms, so are likely to be an underestimate of the true cost.

The primary purpose of surgery is to prevent the hernia recurring; recurrence is likely to lead to further surgery, which may be technically more difficult the second time. After surgery, patients may suffer pain or numbness, the significance of which depends on whether it is short term or persistent [6–8]. There are also rare but potentially serious intraoperative risks of the surgical procedure themselves [9]. Furthermore, because of the materials and instrumentation required, the procedure costs may be considerable. This means that a decision maker (be it a clinician, a patient, or a manager) has to make judgments between the trade-off between different measures of effectiveness (e.g., what reduction in a risk of recurrence would be needed to compensate for an increase in persisting pain?) and also about whether any improvements in effectiveness are worth any increase in costs.

In the next section of this chapter, an introduction to economics and economic evaluation is provided. This introduction has been illustrated by the results of the economic evaluation conducted to inform the NICE guidance [5]. In subsequent sections, attention is then turned to a number of specific issues that the economic perspective can inform. These include economic issues around factors that affect a patient's experience of care, focusing on day case surgery, type of anesthesia, and the use of disposable equipment. The impact of a surgeon experience is also considered. This chapter concludes with a summary of the key results presented.

An Introduction to Economics

In order to judge how to act on the evidence on relative effectiveness of alternative methods of hernia care in the face of scarce resources, decision makers need to consider further evidence. Nearly every health-care intervention has an impact not only on health and social welfare but also on the resources

L. Vale (✉)
Institute of Health and Society, Newcastle University,
Newcastle upon Tyne, United Kingdom
e-mail: luke.vale@newcastle.ac.uk

A.N. Kingsnorth and K.A. LeBlanc (eds.), *Management of Abdominal Hernias*,
DOI 10.1007/978-1-84882-877-3_5, © Springer Science+Business Media London 2013

Table 5.1 Estimated NHS cost of hernia repair for England, 2001–2002

Name of operation	Finished episodes (*N*)	Cost per episode (£)	Cost to the NHS (£ million)[a]
2001–2002			
Laparoscopic	2,172[b]	£1,078	£2.3
Open mesh	50,805[b]	£987	£50.1
Open non-mesh	3,534	£942	£3.3
Total			£55.8 (95 CI £30.6–98.8)
2006–2007			
Inpatient procedures	35,350	£1,400–1,700	£49.5–60.1
Day case procedures	47,790	900–1,100	£43.0–52.6
Total			Range: £92.5–112.7

[a]Costs to NHS are rounded to the nearest £100,000
[b]Based on the assumption that 4.1% of the 52,977 mesh repairs are laparoscopic repair and the remainder are open mesh

used in the production of care. As resources have alternative beneficial uses, information is needed on the health benefits and also the extent of resource use (or cost) so that the best decisions about alternative courses of action can be made. One method for generating information about which alternative courses of action is best is economic evaluation. In simple terms, the objective of economic evaluation is to provide information to assist decision makers in the allocation of available scarce resources available so that benefits can be maximized.

The rationale underpinning economic evaluation is that in any health-care system, there are never enough resources to meet all potential uses. As a result, decisions must be made about what activities will be funded, to what levels, and which activities will not. The decision to use resources one way means that the opportunity to use them in other desirable ways is given up. The cost of this decision is the benefits (health gain, etc.) that could have been obtained had the resources been used another way. The "opportunity cost" of a decision to use resources in one way is equivalent to the benefits forgone in the best alternative use of these resources [10–12]. One of the goals of health-care decision-making is to maximize benefits and minimize opportunity costs. To achieve this, information is required on both resource use (i.e., costs) and benefits (i.e., effectiveness) from alternative courses of action. Linking estimates of relative costs and effectiveness of alternative procedures makes it possible to determine whether a new procedure is:

- Less costly and at least as effective as its comparators (ideally, one of which is the status quo), in which case the new procedure would be judged, unequivocally, to be a better use of health-care resources (in economics language, dominant).
- More costly and more effective than the next best comparator, in which case a judgment would have to be made about whether the extra cost of the new procedure is worth

incurring given the gains in health achieved (in economic language, a judgment is needed about whether the intervention is efficient).

Data on effectiveness and costs can be brought together in a matrix format (Fig. 5.1) to aid in the judgment about whether a new procedure is preferable to a comparator. In Fig. 5.1, it can be seen that, relative to a comparator, the new procedure could achieve (1) greater effectiveness, (2) the same level of effectiveness, or (3) less effectiveness. Of course, a fourth option is possible whereby, after reviewing the literature or performing a study, there is not enough evidence to make a judgment on whether the new procedure is more or less effective.

There may be situations where effectiveness is measured in multidimensional terms, in which case a composite assessment of the value of these outcomes in the form of quality adjusted life years (QALYs) or willingness to pay (WTP) may be useful [10, 12]. Both QALYs and WTP are composite measures which can potentially combine several outcomes into a single score. QALYs, which are commonly used in economic evaluation, combine an assessment of quality of life with an estimate of length of life. Another approach that economists use is WTP. WTP is useful when individuals have preferences not just for health-related quality of life but also about different ways care might be provided, for example, in addition to it being less costly to a health service, patients may prefer day case surgery to surgery that requires an overnight stay. Both the QALY and WTP approaches may help to highlight the choices and trade-off that exist between different measures of effectiveness. For example, is a reduction in pain following laparoscopic surgery worth an increased risk of recurrence when compared with open repair of inguinal hernia?

Table 5.2 shows the estimated clinical outcomes for a comparison of laparoscopic vs. open mesh inguinal hernia repair. In this table, both short- (serious perioperative

Fig. 5.1 Matrix combining costs and effectiveness

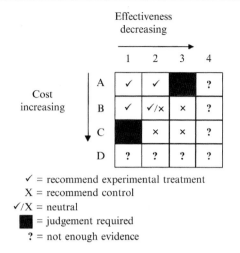

Effectiveness decreasing

Cost increasing

Compare with control treatment, experimental treatment is:

1. more effective
2. of equal effectivenss
3. less effective
4. insufficient evidence to judge

A. less costly
B. of equal cost
C. more costly
D. insufficient evidence to judge

✓ = recommend experimental treatment
X = recommend control
✓/X = neutral
■ = judgement required
? = not enough evidence

Table 5.2 Comparison of laparoscopic repair to open flat mesh for a five-year time horizon[a]

Favors TAPP and TEP	Favors open flat mesh
More time at usual activities after five years	*Potentially more serious complications*
TAPP: 2.90 (95% CI 1.67–4.17) more days	TAPP: 7.9 more serious complications per 1,000 patients
TEP: 3.93 (95% CI 2.82–4.95) more days	TEP: 0.2 more serious complications per 1,000 patients
Fewer people with numbness	
TAPP: 20.1 fewer patients per 1,000. (95% CI 6.8–38.2)	
TEP: 18.5 fewer patients per 1,000. (95% CI −3.9 to 35.7)	
Fewer people have long-term pain	
TAPP: 4.8 (95% CI 0.8–11.4) fewer people per 1,000	
TEP: 13.4 (95% CI 2.7–29.2) fewer people per 1,000	
Similar risk of recurrence for TAPP and TEP compared to OFM over five years	
TAPP: 2 more recurrences per 100 patients. (95% CI −2 to 3)	
TEP: 1 more recurrence per 100 patients. (95% CI −1 to 11)	

[a]These data were estimated from an economic model used to inform NICE Guidance [5]

complications, return to usual activities) and longer-term outcomes (persisting pain, numbness, and recurrences) are presented. If effectiveness is assessed in terms of a single clinical measure such as return to usual activities then compared with open mesh, laparoscopic repair would be considered more effective (column 1, in Fig. 5.1). However, if effectiveness was assessed solely in terms of serious complications, then laparoscopic repair would be less effective (column 3 in Fig. 5.1).

Considering all the measures together means that a decision maker has to weigh up whether the reductions in return to usual activities, pain, and numbness are worth the increases in recurrence rates and serious complications. Both the QALY and WTP method make explicit valuations about the importance of each outcome and combine these data to produce a single composite measure of effectiveness. The QALY estimates presented in Table 5.3 were calculated in the economic model used by NICE in their 2005 guidance on surgery for inguinal hernia [5]. This model used data from the best meta-analyses available at the time. QALYs were estimated by combining information on the risk of a person suffering an event (e.g., long-term pain), occurring at a given point in time with information on the health state utility associated with suffering that event. Health state utilities varied between "1" which is assigned to full health and "0" which is assigned to dead. The health state utilities used were calculated from responses to the EQ-5D questionnaire completed by patients in the MRC Laparoscopic Groin Hernia Trial [13]. The EQ-5D is a generic health status, and responses are then assigned a utility score on the basis of a tariff scale. The tariff scale used was developed from a series of time trade-off questions completed by a sample of the UK general public [14]. WTP can be determined either by directly asking respondents how much they are willing to pay for a good or service [15] or indirectly using a discrete choice experiment (DCE), an approach increasingly used in economics, to value benefits [16, 17]. The idea behind a DCE is that any good, such as a method of surgery, can be described by its characteristics (e.g., the risk of recurrence, risk of short-term pain, and type of anesthesia) and, second, the extent to which an individual values that good or service depends upon the levels of these characteristics [18, 19]. The technique involves presenting choices to individuals that vary with respect to the levels of the characteristics. Statistical methods are then used to model preferences for a change in the level of a given characteristic compared with a change in the level of another characteristic. For example, how important would a 1% reduction in recurrence rates be compared to

Table 5.3 Estimated QALYs and WTP[a] estimates for laparoscopic compared with open mesh inguinal hernia repair

Procedure	QALYs	WTP (£)	WTP (risk of serious complications for laparoscopic procedures is equal to risk for open mesh)
TAPP	4.44	−£3,233	£1,270
TEP	4.45	£1,363	£1,441
Open mesh	4.42	£1,301	£1,301

[a]These data were derived from a discrete choice experiment [20]. Similar data from a WTP experiment is not available

an increase in the risk of serious complications or an increase in the out-of-pocket expenses or taxes that a patient would need to pay.

Table 5.3 reports the QALY and WTP estimates for each treatment laparoscopic and open mesh methods of inguinal hernia repair. Both these estimates are derived from the effectiveness data reported in Table 5.2 above.

Regardless of the measure used to aggregate benefits, TEP is associated with more benefits on average than the open mesh procedures (it is in the first column of Fig. 5.1). When benefits are measured in terms of QALYs, TAPP is on average more effective than open mesh (column 1 of Fig. 5.1) but less effective than TEP (column 3 of Fig. 5.1). However, when benefits are measured in terms of WTP, the TAPP procedure is the least effective treatment (it is in column 3 of Fig. 5.1 for comparisons with both TEP and open mesh). The reason for this is the importance people place on avoiding rare but serious complications following surgery. Each 0.01% reduction in the chance of a serious complication was estimated to be worth £672, but because the serious complications happen so rarely and typically resolved relatively quickly, their impact on QALYs is negligible. Assuming that the risks for laparoscopic surgery are the same as those for open surgery, then the WTP for both laparoscopic approaches increases, although the value for TAPP is still less than open mesh. While TEP, because it is associated with less pain, has the highest WTP.

The Cost-Effectiveness of Hernia Repair Surgery

Although economic methods can be used to help understand the benefits of care, Fig. 5.1 illustrates what economics most obviously adds to an evaluation, which is the consideration of the resource consequences of any proposed changes in the way health care is delivered. Thus, in terms of cost, a new procedure could (A) be less costly, (B) result in no difference in costs, or (C) be more costly (again, there is the possibility of there being not enough evidence to judge, as represented by row D).

For any procedure, the optimum position on the matrix is square A1, where one treatment, for example, an open mesh procedure, would both save costs and have greater effectiveness relative to an alternative treatment. In Fig. 5.1 squares A1, A2, and B1, the new procedure is more efficient and is assigned a ✓ response to the question of whether it is to be preferred to an alternative surgical approach. In squares B3, C2, and C3, the new procedure is less efficient and thus receives a × response. Generally, cells A1, A2, and B1 (as well as B3, C2, and C3) represent the situation where economic evaluation can tell us how to achieve a given outcome at less cost or how to spend a limited amount of funds more effectively. However, it is uncommon that an economic evaluation shows that an intervention clearly falls in squares A1, A2, or B1 (or conversely B3, C2, or C3). This is partly because economic evaluations tend to focus on comparisons where one procedure is likely to be more effective but more costly than an alternative approach but because we rarely know for certain how one treatment compares to another (in clinical effectiveness studies, the same is true, and this uncertainty is often described in a confidence interval surrounding a difference in effectiveness).

Comparison of Open Mesh with Non-mesh Repair

The comparison of open mesh repair with open non-mesh repair provides an example of where one intervention provides more benefits at lower cost (Table 5.4). This table describes the balance of evidence for the comparison of open mesh repair with open non-mesh repair. The evidence presented in this table was derived from a series of systematic reviews comparing mesh vs. non-mesh procedures but has "lumped" different procedures into broad classes [3]. This probably represents a bias against the best performing non-mesh procedures, for example, the Shouldice technique [1], but the broad result is still likely to apply.

Table 5.4 shows the balance of evidence is in favor of open flat mesh. Although open non-mesh is associated with a lower operation cost, the increased cost of treating recurrences more than cancels this out even over a relatively short time horizon of 5 years. As the time horizon over which a patient is followed-up for costs and benefits increases, then the result becomes stronger if it is believed that non-mesh procedures will continue to be associated with higher recurrence rates.

As noted above, it is more likely that when comparing alternative methods of hernia repair that we would find ourselves in squares A3 and C1 of Fig. 5.1. In these squares, a judgment would be required as to whether the more costly procedure is worthwhile in terms of the additional effectiveness gained. It is, however, also possible that we fall in square B2 where there is no meaningful difference in either costs or effectiveness. It is also possible, especially for new surgical

Table 5.4 Balance sheet for the comparison of open flat mesh to open non-mesh for a five-year time horizon[a]

Favors open mesh	Favors open non-mesh
Lower costs over five years	*Lower operation costs*
Mean saving £101; 95% CI £58 to £101	
More time at usual activities after five years	
7.84 (95% CI 6.70 to 9.50) more days	
Fewer people have recurrences	
5 (95% CI 2 to 12) fewer people per 100	
Fewer people have long-term pain	
6.1 (95% CI 0.3 to 19.5) fewer people per 1,000	
Similar risk of numbness for OM compared to ONM over five years	
Same risk of numbness per 1,000 patients. (95% CI −20.7 to 330)	

[a]These data were estimated in an economic model conducted for NICE in 2005 [3] but have not previously been presented

innovations, that there is not enough evidence on effectiveness, costs, or both to judge whether the new procedure is to be preferred. In this situation, we fall into one of the squares marked with a ? response. This would be a common situation for comparisons involving new innovations simply because their evidence on effectiveness and costs just has not had time to be generated.

In situations represented by cells A3 and C1, the question of the additional cost of achieving the health gains becomes important. Some information can be provided by measurement of the effectiveness in natural or clinical outcomes such as hernia recurrences. In such situations, the economic evaluation may take the form of a cost-effectiveness analysis, where costs are equated to a single natural or clinical outcome, or a cost-consequence analysis where costs are equated to several outcomes (e.g., recurrences, pain numbness, serious complications, and time to recovery).

Comparison of Laparoscopic with Open Repair

Table 5.5 shows the results of two different cost-effectiveness analyses comparing laparoscopic, open mesh, and open non-mesh methods of inguinal hernia repair over a 5-year time horizon. In the first analysis, costs have been equated against recurrences avoided as the measure of effectiveness, and in the second, they have been compared with time away from usual activities (other measures of effectiveness such as risk of suffering persisting pain could have been used to produce cost-effectiveness analyses, but for simplicity, only two outcomes have been focused upon). The difficulty with these analyses is in deciding which one is the most appropriate for decision-making. For open non-mesh, this is straightforward as open non-mesh is always dominated by the open mesh regardless of which measure of effectiveness is focused

because open mesh is both more effective across all measures and less costly. Similarly TAPP is on average both less effective and more costly than at least one other procedure. In comparison to open mesh, TEP is associated with a relatively modest additional (incremental) cost per additional day at usual activities (in terms of return to usual activities, TEP is in cell C1 in Fig. 5.1), but on average, it is more costly and results in slightly more recurrences than open mesh. Consequently when effectiveness is determined by recurrence rates alone, TEP is in cell C3 in Fig. 5.1, the worst possible location.

The choices and trade-off between costs and different outcome can be highlighted in a cost-consequence analysis. Table 5.4 has already shown the cost-consequence analysis for the comparison of open mesh with open non-mesh, and Table 5.6 shows the comparison of open mesh with the laparoscopic procedures. In the comparison of laparoscopic with open mesh repair, it can be seen that decisions to increase the use of laparoscopic repair depend upon whether the benefits of laparoscopic repair (reduced persisting long-term pain and numbness and earlier return to usual activities) are worth the extra cost, the increased risk of serious complication, and the uncertainty about differences in rates of recurrence.[1]

As noted above, approaches such as QALYs and WTP can be used to consider the relative importance of these different outcomes. When QALYs are used in an economic evaluation, then that evaluation takes the form of a cost-utility analysis, and when WTP methods are used to value benefits, the economic evaluation becomes a cost-benefit analysis. Valuing results in terms of QALYs or WTP allows the incremental value of the benefits gained to be calculated along with an incremental value of the cost incurred to achieve such a gain. With the benefits valued in such a manner, decision makers can compare the benefits gained by the new procedure, for example, laparoscopic repair, with those that would be gained by some alternative uses of the resources which the new procedure would require (Table 5.7).

When benefits are measured in QALYs, then the incremental cost per QALY is less than the typical threshold values for society's WTP for a QALY (which is between £20,000 and £30,000) that groups such as the NICE in England generally consider acceptable [20]. The results of the cost-benefit analysis suggest that TEP is an average very slightly less efficient than open mesh. Given that the incremental net benefit compared with open mesh is small and that there is uncertainty surrounding this estimate, the most sensible conclusion from the cost-benefit analysis is that both the open

---

[1] In this analysis, the statistical precision of estimates has also been presented. Ideally this statistical precision should also be included for other forms of economic evaluation but has been omitted thus far to simplify presentation of key issues.

Table 5.5 Examples of cost-effectiveness analyses for comparisons of different methods of inguinal hernia repair[a]

Procedure	Costs		Return to usual activities (RUA)				Recurrence		
	Cost (£)	Incremental cost (£)	RUA (days)	Reduction in recovery time	Incremental cost per additional day at UA	Recurrences (%)	Reduction in recurrences (%)	Incremental cost per recurrence avoided
Open mesh (OM)	£1,009		11.06			0.07		
Open non-mesh (ONM)	£1,110	£101	18.90	−7.84	OM dominates ONM	0.02	−0.05	OM dominates ONM
TEP	£1,114	£105	7.13	3.93	£27	0.04	−0.01	OM dominates TEP
TAPP	£1,190	£76**	8.16	−1.03	TEP dominates TAPP	0.04	−0.02	OM dominates TAPP

[a]These data were all derived from the same analysis used to inform the 2005 NICE guidelines. *RUA* return to usual activities; *UA* usual activities

Table 5.6 Balance sheet for the comparison of laparoscopic repair to open flat mesh for a 5-year time horizon[a]

Favors TAPP and TEP	Favors Open Mesh
More time at usual activities after five years	*Lower costs over five years*
TAPP: 2.90 (95% CI 1.67–4.17) more days	TAPP: mean saving £181; (95% CI £148 to £214)
TEP: 3.93 (95% CI 2.82–4.95) more days	TEP: mean saving £105; (95% CI £66 to £213)
Fewer people with numbness	*Potentially more serious complications*
TAPP: 20.1 fewer patients per 1,000. (95% CI 6.8–38.2)	TAPP: 7.9 more serious complications per 1,000 patients
TEP: 18.5 fewer patients per 1,000. (95% CI −3.9–35.7)	TEP: 0.2 more serious complications per 1,000 patients
Fewer people have long-term pain	
TAPP: 4.8 (95% CI 0.8–11.4) fewer people per 1,000	
TEP: 13.4 (95% CI 2.7–29.2) fewer people per 1,000	
Similar risk of recurrence for TAPP and TEP compared to OM over five years	
TAPP: 2 more recurrences per 100 patients. (95% CI −2 to 3)	
TEP: 1 more recurrence per 100 patients. (95% CI −1 to 11)	

mesh and TEP procedure are equally likely to be cost-effective (in Fig. 5.1, we are in cell C3 but tending toward cell B2, as the differences in costs and benefits are modest).

Presenting the Uncertainty Surrounding Estimates of Efficiency

Thus far, only point estimates of the efficiency of the different surgical techniques have been presented. In reality, these estimates presented are imprecise, and one of the limitations

of many of the existing economic evaluations was the failure to adequately consider this imprecision. Statistical methods can be used to quantify the imprecision surrounding estimates of cost, effects, and relative efficiency and can provide confidence intervals around the mean differences between interventions in terms of costs and benefits [21]. Unfortunately the calculation of a confidence interval around an incremental cost-effectiveness ratio is not straightforward although methods for use in economic evaluations conducted as part of RCTs are available and are now in routine use[2] [22]. When decision analytic modeling is employed for economic evaluation, alternative methods are used to deal with uncertainty. Decision analytic models require many individual parameters to be estimated from the available literature. A degree of uncertainty will surround the specific point estimates obtained for all these parameters, and to reflect the joint uncertainty surrounding all parameter estimates used in the model, probabilistic sensitivity analysis is used [22]. For analyses conducted as part of an RCT or using modeling, the results of both cost-utility and cost-effectiveness analysis data are typically presented in the form of cost-effectiveness acceptability curves (CEACs) which show the probability that an intervention would be cost-effective at different levels of society's WTP for a unit of outcome, for example, a recurrence avoided or a QALY gained. In a cost-benefit analysis, the results are simply presented as the likelihood that a procedure, for example, laparoscopic repair, is associated with greater net benefits.

Figure 5.2 shows the CEAC for the comparison of TAPP, TEP, open mesh, and open non-mesh. What this figure shows is that regardless of how much society would be willing to pay for a QALY, the open non-mesh approach has a

---

[2] The two most popular methods, Fieller's approach and the nonparametric bootstrap approach, are discussed by Briggs (2004).

Table 5.7 A cost-utility analysis and cost-benefit analysis comparing laparoscopic with open mesh methods of inguinal hernia repair

		Cost (£)	QALYs	Incremental cost (£)	Incremental QALY	Incremental cost per QALY (£)
Cost-utility analysis	*OM*	£1,009	4.42			
	TEP	£1,113	4.45	£105	0.02	£4,928
	TAPP	£1,190	4.44	£76	0.01	Dominated by TEP
		Cost (£)	*Total benefits (£)*	*Incremental cost (£)*	*Incremental benefits (£)*	*Incremental net benefit (£)*
Cost-benefit analysis	OM	£1,009	£1,301			
	TEP	£1,113	£1,363	£105	£61	−£44
	TAPP	£1,190	−£3,233	£76	−£4,596	−£4,672

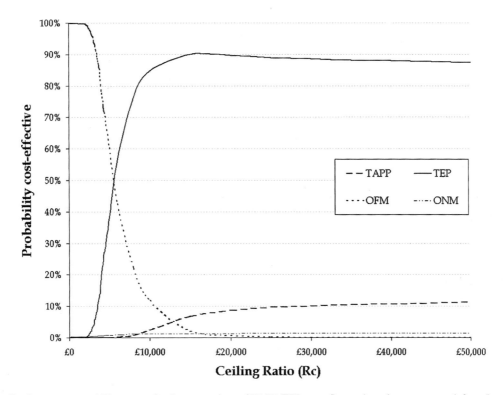

Fig. 5.2 Cost-effectiveness acceptability curves for the comparison of TAPP, TEP, open flat mesh, and open non-mesh for a 5-year time horizon

very low likelihood of ever being considered cost-effective. TEP is more likely to be considered cost-effective than TAPP at all threshold values for society's WTP for an additional QALY. A decision about cost-effectiveness depends on the level of society's WTP for an additional QALY. If society were willing to pay only very little, then open mesh repair would be most likely to be considered cost-effective. If society is willing to pay more than £15,000 per QALY, the likelihood that open mesh is cost-effective is very low. These data can be contrasted with those from the cost-benefit analysis that show that both TEP and open mesh have approximately a 50% likelihood of being considered

efficient and TAPP has a 0% chance of being considered economically worthwhile.

Summary of Cost-Effectiveness Data

From the economic data presented, it is clear that while the open non-mesh procedure is an efficacious method of treating hernias (i.e., the procedure works), it is outperformed by the laparoscopic and open mesh approaches and is therefore highly unlikely to be considered cost-effective. These data were produced using UK data, and while effectiveness data may be transferable between countries, it is less likely that cost data would be. When the economic model used to generate the data presented was being developed, advice was sought from a variety of clinical advisors. One of these noted that even though much of the synthetic mesh used was manufactured within their own country, it was all exported, and any mesh used had to be reimported at considerable expense. This was further compounded by the fact that while the operation cost was state funded, the patient had to pay for any mesh used. The consequence of this was that in this particular country, approaches using mesh (or disposable equipment) were not generally considered cost-effective compared with non-mesh repair.

The conclusion from the comparison of open mesh and laparoscopic approaches is less clear. The laparoscopic approaches are likely to be more costly, may carry more risk, and may be slightly less effective in terms of hernia repair [1, 2] than open mesh approaches. They are, however, associated with less persisting pain/numbness and an earlier recovery. Conclusions about relative efficiency are heavily influenced by the relative importance placed on the different outcomes. When a QALY framework is used, the TEP approach appears be more likely to be considered cost-effective. However, in the cost-benefit analysis when benefits were valued using a DCE, both TEP and open mesh procedures were both equally likely to be considered efficient. Regardless of the method used to value benefits, the TAPP approach was highly unlikely to be considered worthwhile.

In the next sections, consideration is given to a series of factors that might influence both the costs and cost-effectiveness of alternative procedures.

Day Case Surgery

For many surgical procedures, one of the main determinants of costs and cost-effectiveness is length of hospitalization. There is some evidence from systematic reviews to suggest that laparoscopic approaches may reduce length of hospitalization [2], although the studies included in the review were heterogeneous as they were conducted in many different countries and hospitals, with differing discharge policies. Internationally, there is considerable variation in practice with reported rates of day case surgery between 2000 and 2004 varying from 75% in Sweden to 33% in Spain [1]. The causes of these differences are multifactorial and include differences in health-care financing arrangements and to a lesser extent, surgeon and patient preferences and expectations.

Both laparoscopic and open procedures can be performed as day case procedures [1], and in these circumstances, differences in length of stay between procedures will be small and of limited practical significance and hence economic value. More important will be changes in the proportion of patients managed as day cases, but the savings from this are

difficult to estimate. Typically, within economic evaluations, an average cost per a day in hospital might be used to value reductions in length of stay. Such an approach assumes that each day in hospital has the same value. This approach is useful, but it should not be accepted without question because it assumes that the intensity of care provided is the same on every day a person is in hospital. It is likely, however, that care will be more intensive immediately after a procedure than in subsequent days. Reducing length of stay removes the days where the least intensive days of care are provided.

The implications of this depend upon what will be done with the freed-up resource. If beds remain empty and there are no changes in staffing levels, then the opportunity cost of reducing length of stay may be close to zero. If the freed-up bed space is used to provide care to another group of patients, then the opportunity cost is the benefit received by this other group of patients. There may be other economically important effects that flow from using the freed-up space to provide additional care. For example, this group of patients may receive additional (costly) treatments that they would not otherwise receive. Changing the patient mix on the ward may also increase the intensity of work by staff. If staff are working at less than sustainable capacity, then the increase in day cases means that staff will work more efficiently, but if the change is not sustainable, either the staff mix must change (at probable extra cost); otherwise, care will suffer (i.e., benefits will be reduced) and absenteeism and staff turnover will increase (increasing cost but also further reducing benefits). In the longer term, more substantial savings from adopting day care may be realized if inpatient wards are closed, staff reassigned or made redundant, and the provision of dedicated day case facilities increased.

The precise nature of these effects will vary from hospital to hospital. Therefore, savings will also vary because the opportunity cost of the freed-up resources will vary. In such circumstances, published economic evaluations may inform local decision makers but require interpretation to understand precisely what the implications are for the local circumstances.

In some countries, especially the United States, these economic forces forged the development of surgical centers, which perform day case surgical procedures exclusively. These have been very successful both in the delivery of cost-effective care and providing high quality of care. In many cases, significant reductions in overall costs have been realized.

Type of Anesthesia

Recent guidelines have recommended that for open repair patients with a primary reducible unilateral inguinal hernia, local anesthesia should be used. This is because local

Table 5.8 Benefit estimates obtained from the DCE

Characteristic	Levels considered in the DCE[a]	Characteristic unit	WTP (£) per unit
Type of anesthetic	0 = general, 1 = local	Categorical	£327.65
Risk of serious complications (%)	0.1%, 0.5%, 1%	0.01%	£668.33
Days in pain following surgery (days)	3 days, 7 days, 14 days	1 Day	£120.20
Cost (£)	£500, £1,000, £1,500	£1	N/A[b]
Chance of long-term pain at 1 year (%)	3%, 5%, 13%	1%	£85.35
Chance of recurrence (%) within 4 years	4%, 16%, 20%	1%	£101.88
Constant			N/A

[a]The levels presented are those used to develop the discrete choices presented to patients. The statistical model fitted to the responses allows inferences to be made for the range of plausible values that a characteristic, for example, chance of recurrence, might take

[b]Patients' preferences for avoiding having to incur a cost were used to calculate the WTP for a 1-U change in each of the other characteristics

anesthesia is safer and associated with shorter short-term recovery, less postoperative pain, less micturition difficulties, and fewer anesthesia-related complaints [1]. Local anesthesia may also be associated with less cost although this will depend primarily on whether an anesthetist needs to be present during the procedure and, to a lesser extent, the cost savings that result from equipment and medications not needed. In terms of incremental cost per QALY (which ignores patient preferences for the process of care) and with other things being equal, open repair under local anesthesia will be more efficient than open repair under general anesthesia.

Clinically some patients, such as the increasing numbers of patients who are morbidly obese, will not be suitable for local anesthesia [1]. Furthermore, patients may have strong preferences for the type of anesthesia they receive. This may reflect anxiety, fear (or prior experience) of intraoperative pain, and the overall experience of consciousness while undergoing surgery.

One of the characteristics included in the DCE used in the cost-benefit analysis was type of anesthesia that a patient received (the choice was between general and local anesthesia). Table 5.8 shows the WTP estimates obtained from the DCE for a change of 1 U in each characteristic included as part of the DCE. For example, on average a patient would be willing to pay £120 for a 1-day reduction in pain following surgery or £102 for a 1% reduction in the risk of recurrence.

On average, patients would pay £328 to obtain a general anesthetic rather than a local anesthetic. Indeed these data suggest a very strong patient preference against local anesthesia,[3] such that the preferences for general anesthesia are greater than the cost difference between open mesh and laparoscopic repair. Using a cost-benefit analysis framework, it is likely that the laparoscopic repair under general anesthetic would on average be considered more efficient than open mesh repair performed under local anesthetic. The implication of these results is that the increased use of local anesthesia for open repair may not be efficient, at least for all patients.

More importantly, the wider perspective of benefits provided by the DCE illustrates the importance of making care patient centered and the need to consider the trade-offs between safety, clinical effectiveness, cost, and patient preference, which might not always be immediately obvious.

Choice Between Disposable and Reusable Laparoscopic Equipment

Laparoscopic equipment costs are strongly influenced by whether disposable or reusable equipment is used. Disposable equipment can include all of the main surgical items required, or it may be limited to specific items like trocars, staplers, diathermy scissors, or ports. Wellwood and colleagues (1998) reported that the cost difference between laparoscopic surgery and open surgery would fall to £75 (range −£31 to £181) when a policy of largely reusable equipment was adopted. If a policy of largely disposable equipment was adopted, the difference in cost would increase to £523 (range £419 to £626) [23]. The MRC Groin Hernia Trial reported that the total cost of laparoscopic repair would be £1,113 for a policy of using reusable equipment and £1,294 for a policy of using disposable equipment. While the precise magnitude of the extra costs of using disposable equipment is not known for the economist, the issue is whether these additional costs are worth any additional benefits that they might provide.

A number of benefits have been suggested for disposable equipment, notably decreased risk of infection, but this and other benefits have not been demonstrated. However, the DCE suggests that patients very strongly prefer avoiding even very small risks of serious complications. Should a reduction in the risk of serious complications of around 1 in 10,000 exists, then the use of disposable equipment in place

---

[3]The DCE study was carried out at two centers in London and Glasgow. The sample of patients was identified from hospital records as having had an hernia repair in the past. In total, 658 patients were identified, the majority of those had been involved in the two UK-based trials.[13,24] The response rate to the questionnaires was 49% (320/658), which is usual in these types of studies.[19]

of reusable equipment would be efficient. It is worth noting that it would be difficult to statistically demonstrate a difference in serious complications of this magnitude because of the size of the sample needed. Furthermore, the economic evaluations conducted to date exclude the costs of litigation and compensation (or the costs of insuring against these costs) that might be incurred if serious complication occurred. Assuming the additional costs of disposable equipment are £180 (based upon the MRC Groin Hernia Trial data) [13], then the net cost of using disposable equipment would be same as the cost of using reusable equipment if the cost of litigation and compensation for a serious complication were in excess of £1.8 million. A judgment would be needed as to whether such a value is plausible.

There is also some uncertainty about how much more costly disposable equipment actually is compared with reusable equipment. The economic data reported above is dated, and the relative differences between disposable and reusable equipment may no longer be applicable. Furthermore, the costs paid for disposable equipment will vary markedly between centers as a result of any deals and negotiations that might exist as well as the purchasing power of the organization (typically larger organizations can negotiate better deals than smaller ones). Finally, there may be operational reasons for a hospital to use disposable equipment. For example, it might simplify the organization of surgery, which in turn may reduce the opportunity costs of using disposable equipment. Overall, it is a matter of judgment whether there is any meaningful difference in the short- or long-term complications and whether any other benefits of using disposable equipment that are of sufficient magnitude to outweigh the likely extra cost.

The Impact of Surgeon Experience on Cost-Effectiveness

Laparoscopic repair is technically more difficult than open repair and so takes longer to learn and tends to be performed by more experienced surgeons. It is therefore associated with a learning curve [24]. During the period that the surgeon is "learning," their outcomes may be worse, and their cost greater than those observed for experienced surgeons. There is some limited evidence that the operation time for inexperienced operators (up to 20 procedures) is approximately 70 min for TAPP and 95 min for TEP. For experienced operators (between 30 and 100 procedures), the estimated operation times are 40 min for TAPP and 55 min for TEP.

Operation length is only a very crude proxy as it does not reflect any impact of experience on effectiveness or safety. Some data on the impact of experience on effectiveness was provided by the trial by Neumayer and colleagues. This trial found that the recurrence rates were higher for laparoscopic

compared with open mesh repair [25]. One suggested explanation of this was the inexperience of some surgeons. This seemed to be supported by the findings of long-term follow-up of patients recruited by the most experienced surgeon in the MRC trial: at 5 years, there were equal numbers of recurrence in the two groups [26]. Post hoc analyses in Neumayer and colleagues' trial suggested that the excess of recurrences in the laparoscopic group was explained by the performance of surgeons who had performed fewer than 250 laparoscopic procedures. Among the 20/78 surgeons who had performed more than this number, the recurrences in the two trial groups were similar.

Allowing for both longer operating times and an increase in recurrence rates would tend to make laparoscopic repair less cost-effective in comparison to open mesh repair and improve the cost-effectiveness of TAPP compared with TEP. However, in terms of the incremental cost per QALY, it is unlikely that any of these differences are sufficient to change any conclusions. Understandably patients would probably prefer to be treated by experienced surgeons, but given that surgeons need to be trained, this will not always be possible. What the results do suggest is that for a society, the extra costs of training and care and the loss of benefit experienced by some patients are likely to be worth the additional benefits (and reductions in cost) obtained in the longer term.

Conclusions

Economics and economic evaluation are increasingly being seen as a prerequisite for informing health-care decision-making. This is because it provides an explicit framework for valuing benefits and for bringing information on health outcomes, other benefits, and costs together to the best ways to use the scarce resources available.

The different methods of hernia repair have been shown to be efficacious surgical techniques, and although in comparison to many other health-care interventions, the cost per procedure is relatively modest, the large number of procedures performed each year and development of newer techniques since the 1990s highlight the need for evaluations. It is therefore not surprising that hernia repair and particularly inguinal hernia repair have been subject to such intensive evaluation, including numerous economic evaluations.

- For inguinal hernia repair, mesh approaches appear superior for many patients than non-mesh approaches. The comparison of laparoscopic and open mesh approaches is not as straightforward. Laparoscopic approaches are associated with quicker recovery, less persisting pain, and numbness but are more costly, associated with more serious complications, and potentially slightly more recurrences. In terms of health outcomes, the economic methods of benefit assessment suggest that laparoscopic approaches are associated with more benefits, but this crucially depends upon the importance placed on avoiding rare serious complications.

- Both the cost-utility analysis and cost-benefit analysis suggest that laparoscopic approach (primarily TEP) might be considered an efficient use of resources compared with open mesh approaches. However, because not all surgeons are proficient in the laparoscopic approach, the differences in cost are similar, and there are trade-offs between different measures of effectiveness; patient and surgeon choice is important.
- There is some evidence that patients have a strong preference against local anesthesia even though there may be clinical and cost arguments in its favor.
- Laparoscopic approaches can use varying amounts of disposable equipment, but the economic arguments in favor of using disposable equipment have not been demonstrated in published economic evaluations. Nevertheless, local circumstances may provide compelling practical reasons for using disposable equipment.
- Both laparoscopic and open approaches can be performed as day case surgery, but rates of day case surgery vary between countries. Increasing rates of day case surgery should free up resources for other desirable uses. The full implications of increasing rates of day case surgery need careful consideration, as there may be wider effects on both costs and benefits.

References

1. European Hernia Society Guidelines. Treatment of inguinal hernia in adult patients. 2009. http://www.herniaweb.org.
2. Vale L, Grant A, Ludbrook A. Assessing the costs and consequences of laparoscopic versus open methods of groin hernia repair: a systematic review. Surg Endosc. 2003;17:844–9.
3. McCormack K, Wake B, Perez J, Fraser C, Cook J, McIntosh E, Vale L, Grant A. Systematic review of the clinical effectiveness and cost-effectiveness of laparoscopic surgery for inguinal hernia repair. Health Technol Assess. 2005;9(14):1–203. iii-iv.
4. Gholghesaei M, Langeveld H, Veldkamp R, Bonjer H. Costs and quality of life after endoscopic repair of inguinal hernia vs. open tension-free repair: a review. Surg Endosc. 2005;19:816–21.
5. National Institute for Clinical Excellence. Laparoscopic Surgery for inguinal hernia repair. Technology Appraisal 83. 2004. http://www.nice.org.uk/pdf/TA083guidance.pdf. National Institute for Clinical Excellence.
6. BayNielsen M, Perkins F. Pain and functional impairment 1 year after inguinal herniorrhaphy: a nationwide questionnaire study. Ann Surg. 2001;233:1–7.
7. Callesen T, Bech K, Kehlet H. Prospective study of chronic pain after groin hernia repair. Br J Surg. 1999;86:1528–31.
8. Courtney CA. Outcome of patients with severe chronic pain following repair of groin. Br J Surg. 2002;89:1310–4.
9. Felix EL, Harbertson N, Vartanian S. Laparoscopic hernioplasty: significant complications. Surg Endosc. 1999;13:328–31.
10. Drummond MF, O'Brien B, Stoddart GL, Torrance GW. Methods for the economic evaluation of health care programmes. Oxford: Oxford University Press; 1997.
11. Auld C, Donaldson C, Mitton C, Shackley P. Economic evaluation. In: Detels R, Holland W, Omenn G, editors. Oxford textbook of public health. Oxford: Oxford University Press; 2001.
12. Fox Rushby J, Cairns J, editors. Economic evaluation. Understanding public health. Maidenhead: Open University Press; 2005.
13. MRC Laparoscopic Groin Hernia Trial Group. Cost-utility analysis of open versus laparoscopic groin hernia repair: results from a multicentre randomized clinical trial. Br J Surg. 2001;88:653–61.
14. Kind P, Hardman G, Macran S. UK Population Norms for EQ-5D. Centre for Health Economics Discussion Paper; 1999. p. 172.
15. Donaldson C, Mason H, Shackley P. Contingent valuation in health care. In: Jones A, editor. The Elgar companion to health economics. Cheltenham: Elgar; 2006.
16. Ryan M. Methodological issues in the monetary valuation of benefits in healthcare. Expert Rev Pharmacoecon Outcomes Res. 2003;3:717–2739.
17. Ryan M, et al. Using discrete choice experiments in health economics. In: Jones A, editor. The Elgar companion to health economics. Bodmin: MPG Books; 2006.
18. Louviere J, et al. Stated choice methods: analysis and application. Cambridge: Cambridge University Press; 2000.
19. Ryan M, Gerard K. Using discrete choice experiments to value health care programmes: current practice and future research reflections. Appl Health Econ Health Policy. 2003;2:55–64.
20. National Institute for Health and Clinical Excellence Guide to the Methods of Technology Appraisal http://www.nice.org.uk/about-nice/howwework/devnicetech/technologyappraisalprocessguides/guidetothemethodsoftechnologyappraisal.jsp
21. Briggs A, O'Brien B. The death of cost-minimization analysis. Health Econ. 2001;10:179–84.
22. Briggs A. Statistical approaches to handling uncertainty in health economic evaluation. Eur J Gastroenterol Hepatol. 2004;16:551–61.
23. Wellwood J, Sculpher M, Stoker D, Nicholls G, Geddes C, Whitehead A, Singh R, Spiegelhalter D. Randomised controlled trial of laparoscopic versus open mesh repair for inguinal hernia: outcome and cost. Br Med J. 1998;317:103–10.
24. Lau H. Learning curve for unilateral endoscopic totally extraperitoneal (TEP) inguinal hernioplasty. Surg Endosc. 2002;16:1724–8.
25. Neumayer L, Giobbie-Hurder A, Jonasson O, Fitzgibbons Jr R, Dunlop D, Gibbs J, et al. Open mesh versus laparoscopic mesh repair of inguinal hernia. N Engl J Med. 2004;350:1819–27.
26. Wright D, Paterson C, Scott N, Hair A, O'Dwyer PJ. Five-year follow-up of patients undergoing laparoscopic or open groin hernia repair: a randomized controlled trial. Ann Surg. 2002;235(3):333–7.

Principles in Hernia Surgery

6

David H. Bennett

Abdominal wall hernia surgery is no different from any other surgical procedure in that the rules of appropriate patient selection and preparation apply. The mortality from hernia surgery relates either to operating prior to optimization of the patient or to complications of the surgery itself. An analysis of the Scottish Audit of Surgical Mortality noted inadequate resuscitation, failure to use HDU, and inadequate perioperative monitoring as adverse factors contributing to death [1]. Most hernias never require emergency surgery, and 4 or 5 h of careful resuscitation may be beneficial in the most ill patients [2]. Analysis of the Swedish Hernia registry revealed a sevenfold increase if the surgery was performed as an emergency and a 20-fold increase if bowel resection was undertaken [3]. The same principles apply for elective hernia surgery: -full assessment and optimization of the patient prior to embarking on surgery. An analysis of 175 patients with ages greater than 66 years, of whom 58% were ASA III or higher, revealed that elective or urgent operation can be carried out with zero mortality, provided prompt diagnosis and management of primary systemic diseases are performed.

Careful consideration should be given to the type of anesthesia employed with general, regional, or local anesthesia all available. However, it should be remembered that in some cases, general anesthesia may be safer than epidural anesthesia. Severe systemic disease that limits activity but is not incapacitating is not a contraindication for elective groin repair.

General Principles

There are three principles which dictate the management of abdominal wall hernias:

D.H. Bennett (✉)
Department of Surgery, Royal Bournemouth Hospital,
Dorset, United Kingdom
e-mail: david.bennett@rbch.nhs.uk

1. Identification of the hernia sac and dissection of the sac neck. It is important to identify the sac neck as this defines the fascial edges which will form the basis of subsequent repair. In large incisional hernias the neck may be many centimeters distant from the apparent extent of the sac itself.

2. Reduction of the contents. For elective inguinal hernia surgery, indirect sacs are often reduced at the time of operation, and there is no necessity to open the sac. For incarcerated or strangulated hernias, the sac should be opened, and the contents inspected for viability prior to reduction. In the case of large sacs containing large amounts of bowel and/or organs, the possibility of loss of domain should be considered. The forcible reduction of sac contents into an abdominal cavity which has lost capacity can result in the development of abdominal compartment syndrome. In the case of large incisional hernias, following opening of the sac, there may be a significant amount of redundant sac which must be excised prior to the repair.

3. Repair of the fascial defect. Over the last 10 years, the concept of "tension-free repair" has become established, and one of the commonest causes of recurrence post repair is excessive tension on the fascial edges. In parallel with this philosophy has been the development of prosthetic material to aid this approach. The primary goal of repair is therefore to achieve apposition of the fascial edges with reinforcement of the muscle layers with prosthetic material, if appropriate.

It should be noted that only tendinous/aponeurotic/fascial structures can be successfully sutured together; suturing fleshy muscle to tendon or fascia does not provide a permanent union of these structures nor does it restore normal anatomy. The development of prosthetic reinforcement has led to a new range of procedures for hernia repair including the laparoscopic approach. The use of prosthetic material in the repair of hernias of all etiologies is now commonplace, its use exceeding 90% in the USA.

A.N. Kingsnorth and K.A. LeBlanc (eds.), *Management of Abdominal Hernias*,
DOI 10.1007/978-1-84882-877-3_6, © Springer Science+Business Media London 2013

Hemostasis

Although hernia surgery is sometimes considered to be "minor surgery," the principles of careful hemostasis and tissue handling are just as important as in any other operation if hematoma formation and sepsis are to be avoided. There are significant vessels in the subcutaneous fat, especially veins, which are prone to bleed and should either be appropriately controlled with electrocautery or the time taken to ligate them with an absorbable suture. For ligatures, metric 3.5 (3/0)-braided polyglycolic acid (Dexon) or metric 3.5 (3/0)-braided polyglactin (vicryl) is recommended.

If local anesthesia with adrenaline is used, extra care with hemostasis is advised as hematomas are more likely. If the dissection is extensive or there is a large "dead space" in which hematoma or serum can collect, a closed suction drain can be used. During the open repair of large incisional hernias, suction drains are frequently employed, both in the retromuscular plane to reduce seroma formation if a prosthetic mesh has been used and in the subcutaneous residual cavity left following reduction of a large hernia sac. Suction drains are rarely used when a hernia has been repaired laparoscopically.

Sepsis

The presence of infection in hernias can be divided into superficial and deep sepsis. When present, deep sepsis in the presence of a synthetic prosthetic mesh is a significant complication which may require the explant of the prosthesis. The prophylactic use of antibiotics has not been shown to reduce the risk of either superficial or deep infection in inguinal hernia repair. In a Cochrane review totaling almost 9,000 patients, the incidence of infection was 3.9% and 4.5% in the prophylaxis and control groups, respectively [4]. Analysis of the Swedish hernia registry revealed just over 20% of patients undergoing elective inguinal hernia surgery received prophylactic antibiotics. The European Hernia Society published recommendations on the use of antibiotics in inguinal hernia surgery in 2008 [5]. It was noted that, in clinical settings with low rates (5%) of wound infection, there is no indication for the routine use of antibiotic prophylaxis in elective open groin hernia repair in low-risk patients. The consensus group also concluded that in endoscopic hernia repair, antibiotic prophylaxis is probably not indicated. Finally, it was concluded that in the presence of risk factors for wound infection based on patient (recurrence, advanced age, immunosuppressive conditions) or surgical (expected long operating times, use of drains) factors, the use of antibiotic prophylaxis should be considered. As with all surgical procedures, one must nevertheless utilize scrupulous surgical technique if infection is to be avoided. The skin may be covered at the site of operation with sterile adherent film, which is not removed until the wound is closed. This is particularly popular during laparoscopic incisional hernia repair.

It had been recommended in the past that sutures should not be used to close the skin, for by their very nature they have the potential to introduce bacteria into the subcutaneous tissue along their tracks [6]. However, current practice reveals many methods are used to close the skin incision. These include the use of skin staples, subcuticular sutures, skin closure tapes, and skin adhesives. There is no evidence that any one technique is significantly superior to the others such that a recommendation can be made. It falls upon each surgeon to maintain vigilance of his or her practice and base the skin closure upon the best results that are obtainable.

The rates of infection following laparoscopic hernia repair are compatible with those of open inguinal hernia repair, which is of the order of 1% [7]. Infection following inguinal hernia repair is an important complication as it increases the risk of hernia recurrence by a factor of four [8,9]. If an infection develops following a laparoscopic incisional hernia repair, in the majority of cases the prosthetic material will need to be removed, resulting in the original fascial defect requiring repair again. An open primary suture technique may be employed with or without reinforcement with a biological (fully absorbable) mesh.

Wound Healing

Important variables in hernia repair are the rate at which the aponeurosis regains strength and the stability of the healing process. This is becoming more important as the newer meshes are incorporating a component which is absorbable over time and relies on the increase in wound strength with time to compensate for the absorption of the synthetic material. Many of the factors that regulate wound healing are under the control of the surgeon, and an appreciation of their effects and their clinical significance is important in the care of the patient and the type of prosthetic reinforcement selected.

The pioneering work on the maturation and development of tensile strength in wounds was reported by Howes and his group in 1933. They reported the healing of experimental skin, fascia, muscle, and gastric wounds in dogs. They observed a lag phase extending from wounding until the 5th or 6th day. During the lag phase, the wound appeared quiescent, the wound strength did not increase, and wound apposition was maintained by the sutures only (Fig. 6.1) [10,11]. This was followed by a phase of fibroplasia, during which wound strength increased rapidly, reaching a maximum around the 14th to 16th day.

Howes also went on to describe a third phase—the maturation phase—which he did not study, attributing restoration of the mechanical strength to the fibroblastic phase. However,

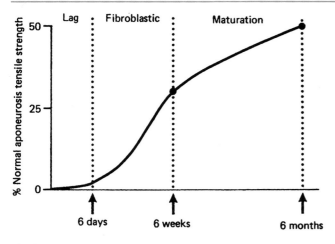

Fig. 6.1 Phases of wound healing. During the initial lag phase the wound is quiescent and during the fibroplastic phase wound strength increases rapidly over a few days; however, it is in the third, maturation, phase that significant and permanent strength gain occurs

we now know that this third phase is crucial to the healing of aponeurotic wounds.

Douglas (1952) studied the rate of tensile strength gain of incisions in the lumbodorsal aponeurosis of rabbits. He demonstrated that the rate of increase of tensile strength was slow, 50% of the original strength was gained at 50 days, and only 80% achieved after 1 year [12,13]. Similarly, Mason and Allen (1941) had observed healing tendons. They noted that if the tendon was rested, the rate of gain of strength during the maturation phase was slower than if active motion was permitted [14], an observation supporting early ambulation after hernia surgery.

In humans, the lag (or latent) phase extends from the time of incision to the fourth to sixth day. During this phase the inflammatory reaction prepares the wound for subsequent healing by removing debris, necrotic tissue, and bacteria. At the same time there is mobilization and migration of fibroblasts and epithelial cells and accumulation of non-collagenous proteins and glycoproteins. During the lag phase, fibrin alone holds the wound edges together, and wound security is a property of the suture material not the tissue. Similarly, the initial cellular penetration of any prosthetic material occurs at this time.

At about day 4–6 post incision, proliferating fibroblasts begin to synthesize collagen, mucopolysaccharides, and glycoproteins, the fibroblastic stage of repair. The collagen quickly aggregates into fibers commensurate with the most rapid increase in the tensile strength of the wound. It is at this stage that incorporation of the prosthetic meterial into the tissues occurs. The meshes with the largest pores (macroporous) experience a greater degree of collagen deposition during this time interval than the microporous meshes. Prior to this stage, even the microporous interstices are filled with fluid rather than cells. The newer microporous meshes are manufactured

into such a form that the fibroblasts and macrophages appear earlier in the healing phase, thereby providing greater collagen and tissue attachment earlier [15].

As the fibrotic phase runs down, the phase of maturation begins. During this phase, further wound strength gain is due to intra- and intermolecular collagen remodeling and crosslinking. This remodeling continues for 6–12 months, and it has been postulated that failure of this remodeling process may account for the late appearance of incisional hernias in healed laparotomy incisions [16–18].

The principles of wound healing remain the same regardless of whether the incision is for a primary laparotomy, a primary hernia, or an incisional hernia. Incised fascial and aponeurotic edges heal faster and are ultimately stronger than invaginated or infolded aponeurotic or fascial wounds. This is because incision of tissues initiates the normal cascade of healing mechanisms, which ultimately leads to formation of organized collagen and mature strong connective tissue. Invagination causes disorganized healing and defects in collagen formation which can become apparent as areas of weakness with potential for recurrence. Similarly, interrupted suture closure causes areas of local ischemia and uneven distribution of tension along the incision, resulting in the multiple small incisional hernias sometimes seen occurring through the suture holes. Aponeuroses have only weak powers of regeneration, the abdominal wall taking up to 120 days before it reaches 80% or more of its original strength [19]. In principle, continuous suturing of aponeurosis and fascial planes by evenly distributing the tension gives better ultimate healing than interrupted suture closure.

It is likely that a connective tissue abnormality underlies the majority of hernia occurrences and, over the last 15 years, reinforcement of the native abdominal wall with prosthetic material has been employed to prevent hernia recurrence [20]. The normal process of wound healing in the presence of a prosthetic material involves coagulation, inflammation, angiogenesis, and epithelialization. This is then followed by fibroplasia, matrix deposition, and, finally, scar contraction. The cellular components involved in this process are initially platelets followed by monocytes, macrophages, leukocytes, fibroblasts, endothelial cells, and smooth muscle cells. A variety of growth factors and cytokines are activated which coordinate the process [21]. The prosthetic material subsequently undergoes maturation with the scar contraction that occurs in all wounds and accounts for the shrinkage of meshes. If an explanted mesh is placed in a collagenase solution and the scar tissue dissolved from the mesh interstices, the mesh returns to its original size.

The rate of wound healing and the ultimate tensile strength of wounds are adversely affected by severe protein deficiency, vitamin C deficiency, prolonged hypovolemia, increased blood viscosity, intravascular coagulation, cold vasoconstriction, and chronic stress. Hypoxia, some drugs, irradiation,

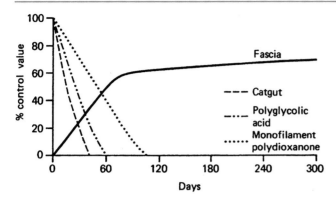

Fig. 6.2 Relationship of wound strength gain to the rate of wound healing in aponeurotic wounds. Absorbable sutures do not survive long enough to ensure wound stability. Polydioxanone occupies an intermediate position between the traditional catgut and the absorbable polymers on the one hand and the nonabsorbables on the other

and other factors can be critical in wound healing. For the surgeon, the most important variables are suture strength to maintain wound apposition until collagen synthesis is well advanced and exercise of the healing incision which speeds the entire process [14,22–24].

Currently, the rate of wound healing has become less of a factor due to the introduction of prosthetic meshes and modern suture materials (in open repairs) or fixation devices (in laparoscopic repairs). Surgeons who routinely employ prosthetic implants for their hernia procedures do not wait for the maturation phase of wound healing to be completed before encouraging patients to resume normal activities. Most patients would be expected to have returned to normal daily activities 2–3 weeks after elective open or laparoscopic inguinal hernia surgery.

Sutures

"The material used for sutures is probably not very important" observed Aird, in 1957 (Fig. 6.2) [25]. It is more than 50 years since this quote and during this time the dynamics of wound healing has been defined and a revolution has overtaken sutures [26] and methods of hernia surgery. With regard to sutures, the current surgeon chooses a suture according to objective biological data and marries biological science to surgical craft. Naturally occurring sutures—silk, linen, and catgut—are obsolete in hernia surgery; synthetic fibers are today's choice [27].

In the past, the choice of suture material was based on availability and experience and, indeed, until recently surgeons have concentrated on the mechanical properties of the suture with scant attention to the interaction of the suture and host tissue. Three principles should be taken into account when considering the mechanical and biological relations of suture and tissue [28].

1. Sutures should be at least as strong as the normal tissue through which they are placed.
2. If the tissue reduces suture strength with time, the relative rates at which the suture loses strength and the wound gains strength are important.
3. If the suture alters the biology of wound healing, the impact of this alteration is important.

Applying these principles to wound healing, the surgeon requires information about the normal strength of the tissue, the rate of gain of strength of the wounded tissue, the strength of the suture, the rate at which the suture loses strength when placed in tissue, and the interaction of suture and tissue. Only after considering these factors can the surgeon proceed to account for the handling and knotting properties, the "memory," ease of sterilization, and shelf life of the suture.

Sir Berkeley Moynihan, at the inaugural meeting of the Association of Surgeons in 1920, set out the essential conditions for sutures and ligatures which must remain within the wound [29]. Such material should ideally (a) achieve its purpose,—be sufficient to hold parts together, close a vessel, etc.; (b) disappear as soon as its work is accomplished; (c) be free from infection; and (d) nonirritant. These principles are still important today.

Sutures are either absorbable or nonabsorbable and are made from natural or synthetic products, distinctions that are increasingly blurred by modern polymer chemistry.

Tissues that are mainly formed of collagen/fascia/aponeurosis tend to heal slowly, so that only 50% of their original tensile strength has been recovered at 3 months; thus most older absorbable sutures, whether natural or synthetic, do not generally persist long enough for the adequate structural integrity to be restored. However, the healing curve of these tissues, a curve that reflects the laying down of collagen, is initially steep, so that fascia or aponeurotic incisions of the abdominal wall closed with absorbable sutures or, more particularly, the modern synthetics may just have enough strength to withstand disruption unless there are major forces, such as coughing applied to them. In contrast, tissues which do not contain much structural collagen heal and gain their initial tensile strength much more rapidly, the intestine being a particular example of this [30].

The suture material must retain its strength for long enough to maintain tissue apposition and allow sound union of tissues to occur. In aponeurotic wounds, a nonabsorbable or very slowly absorbable suture material must therefore be employed. The inherent disadvantageous properties of nonabsorbable suture materials—proneness to sepsis, adverse tissue reaction, and sinus formation—have led some surgeons to seek compromises for hernia repair.

Table 6.1 lists the properties of natural and synthetic suture material.

Table 6.1 Sutures (in the sizes available for hernia surgery)

Suture	Raw material	Type	In vivo tensile strength retention	Trade name
Plain	Sheep submucosa	Absorbable	67% lost in 5–6 days	
Chromic	Sheep submucosa	Absorbable	67% lost in 10–14 days	
Poliglecaprone 25	Copolymer of glycolide and E-caprolactone	Absorbable	70–80% lost in 14 days	Monocryl®
Polyglycolic acid	Polyglycolic acid	Absorbable		Dexon®
Polyglactin 910	Copolymer of lactide and glycolide	Absorbable	60% lost in 21 days	Vicryl®
Polyglactin 910 coated with polyglactin 370	Copolymer of lactide and glycolide coated with same combined with calcium stearate	Absorbable	60% lost in 21 days	Coated Vicryl®
Polydioxanone	Polyester of poly (p-dioxanone)	Absorbable	50% lost in 28 days	PDSII®
Silk	Silkworm larvae	Nonabsorbable	Lost in 1 year	Panacryl®
Nylon	Polyamide polymer	Nonabsorbable	15–20% per year is lost	Ethilon®
Stainless steel	Stainless steel	Nonabsorbable	Fatigue fractures at 1 year	
Braided Nylon	Polyamide polymer	Nonabsorbable	15–20% per year is lost	Nurolon®
Polypropylene	Polymer of propylene	Nonabsorbable	Two years or longer	P rolene®
Polyester	Polyethylene terephthalate	Nonabsorbable	Lasts indefinitely	Mersilene®
Coated polyester	Polyethylene terephthalate coated with polybutilate	Nonabsorbable	Lasts indefinitely	Ethibond® extra
Expanded polytetra-fluoroethylene	Polytetrafluoroethylene	Nonabsorbable	Lasts indefinitely	Gore-tex®

Synthetic Absorbable Sutures

The first polymer possessing reasonable physical and biological properties was synthesized in the 1960s by Du Pont Research Laboratories. It was a braided polyester suture made of poly-L-lactide. The first commercially available absorbable synthetic suture was also a braided polyester, polyglycolic acid (PGA, Dexon), introduced in 1971. In 1974 another braided polyester suture polyglactin 910 (Vicryl), a copolymer of lactide and glycolide, was introduced [31].

The basic ingredients of these polymers and their eventual breakdown products are lactic acid, glycolic acid, or a combination of the two. Compared with catgut and collagen, these biodegradable polymer sutures have some interesting properties. Catgut and collagen are digested by cellular enzymes and, therefore, excite an intense cellular reaction, which prolongs the lag phase in wound healing. The new polyester sutures degrade by hydrolysis and do not excite cellular activity; indeed they will hydrolyze similarly in vitro if placed in buffer solution at body temperature. Consequently they do not delay wound healing. They are also much more uniform and predictable in their dimensions and tensile strength than the biologically made natural fibers formerly used because they are synthetic materials produced under tight manufacturing control.

The polymer sutures however do have disadvantages. While they possess greater and more predictable strength than catgut and collagen, they are also much harsher and stiffer fibers. These sutures have to be braided to provide good handling characteristics and carefully tied to avoid slippage on the first throw when tied. Their stiffness means only extremely fine monofilaments can be used in surgery, their usefulness confined to microsurgery and ophthalmology.

In order to overcome the abrasive quality of these fibers and to improve tying, coated polymer sutures have been introduced. The coating decreases the "drag" through tissues and allows sliding of knots for better control.

Polydioxanone (PDS) is a newer more flexible polyester suture, introduced in 1981. Its greater flexibility, compared with PGA and polyglactin 910, allows it to be used as a monofilament. Like all polyesters it degrades by hydrolysis and excites little tissue reaction; however, its rate of degradation is much slower than that of PGA or polyglactin 910. Polydioxanone suture was completely absorbed from rat muscle by 180 days versus 60–90 days for polyglactin 910 and 120 days for PGA suture. In vivo polydioxanone retains its strength for longer than other synthetic absorbable sutures: 58% versus 1–5% at 4 weeks and 14% versus 0% at 8 weeks [32,33].

The place of synthetic absorbable sutures in hernioplasty is unclear. There were early favorable reports of the use of

PGA sutures (Dexon) for laparotomy closure. Irvine et al. (1976) [34] compared PGA, polyglactin, and polypropylene in a randomized clinical trial and reached the conclusion that there was little to choose between these sutures. The trial was small: 161 cases randomized equally to each suture, a layered closure used—the wound failure rate was 5.8% for polyglactin, 9.6% for PGA, and 8.8% for polypropylene. Wound failure rate was closely related to wound infection [34]. When PGA was compared with nylon mass closure rate, the rate of wound failure was 12.5% in the PGA group, compared with 4.7% in the nylon group. It was concluded that closure of abdominal wounds with absorbable sutures does not appear to be justified [35]. Polyglactin and particularly polydioxanone sutures have prolonged tissue integrity compared with PGA and may therefore be more satisfactory for laparotomy closure—indeed, polydioxanone has been shown to be comparable to a nonabsorbable suture [36]. Current practice would suggest most laparotomy incisions are primarily closed with nylon or polydioxanone. In the case of prosthetic mesh fixation in open inguinal hernia surgery, a longer-lasting absorbable suture, particularly polyglactin or a monofilament such as prolene, is utilized. In the case of laparoscopic inguinal hernia surgery, the initial method of fixation was nonabsorbable metal tacks. However, this practice has been superseded by the use of absorbable tacks, fibrin glue, or, indeed, no fixation at all.

Nonabsorbable Sutures

For closure of aponeurosis/fascial planes, a nonabsorbable monofilament flexible material with good knotting properties has been considered the gold standard. Stainless steel wire provides the greatest strength and knot security and is routinely used in sternotomy closure. However, the poor handling characteristics of wire limit its usefulness in hernia surgery, despite its additional advantage of minimal tissue reaction. For many years, silk was the standard nonabsorbable suture material and has enjoyed the widest use. Silk was recommended by Halsted and by Whipple [35,37].

In terms of strength and knot security however, silk is distinctly inferior to many other materials, and the tissue reaction to silk correlates to the incidence of granuloma and sinuses in clinical use. Cotton was introduced in 1940 during World War II when silk was relatively unobtainable. Its strength is similar to silk, but its handling characteristics are inferior—again it has a high incidence of granuloma and sinus formation. Linen is similar to cotton in many properties.

Nylon was developed by the Du Pont Company and introduced as an alternative to silk in 1943. Compared with silk, nylon has distinct advantages: it can be used as a monofilament, it loses less strength when wet (15% versus 25%), it is stronger, and it causes less tissue reaction. However, it is not as flexible, it is more difficult to handle and to knot, and the knots have a tendency to slip. Monofilament nylon undergoes both plastic (irreversible) and elastic (reversible) elongation when subjected to tension. When nylon is stretched using a force of 5 kg, the total elongation produced is 22.5%, of which 6.9% is irreversible. When aponeurotic incisions are closed with nylon and then the sutures are tightened to 5 kg to produce "compression" of the wound, the suture stretches by 27.7% [38]. This plastic irreversible elongation has an importance in closing fascial incisions: unless the nylon is tightened adequately, its elongation when the patient breathes and moves will lead to loss of apposition of the wound edges and ultimately to wound failure.

Monofilament polypropylene is an alternative to nylon. It has greater flexibility and easier handling characteristics. It also knots better than nylon [39,40]. The "memory" characteristic does, however, make this material difficult to use in certain circumstances.

Braided nonabsorbable sutures have distinctly better handling and knotting characteristics than monofilaments, but they give the least good results for suturing aponeurosis and repairing hernias. The specific problems are infection, and the persistent sinuses that develop and so braids should be abandoned. If infection occurs in a wound repaired with a nonabsorbable braid, there is no alternative to removing he suture. With monofilaments, infection can be controlled and suture removal is not always required. Others have confirmed the unsuitability of braided nonabsorbable sutures in hernia repair [41].

Mechanical Factors in Abdominal Wound Closure

Wounds are not set in their dimensions but undergo change as they heal. Not only do the wounds themselves change but the cavities or tissues they contain alter, and these alterations critically vary the dimensions of the wound.

The events of wound healing lead to edema of the wound and then to the development of a healing ridge and fibroblast proliferation as collagen placement gets under way. Edema of the wound by increasing wound bulk increases the tension in each suture bite. If suture bites are initially tight, this increase in tension may lead to (a) suture breakage, (b) knot failure, or (c) cutting out. These three consequences may also develop from changes in body compartments beneath suture lines. In the abdomen, extreme examples of this phenomenon occur. In voluntary inspiration, pregnancy, and abdominal distension, mean alterations of girth of 6%, 18%, and 27% have been measured, while simultaneously the mean xiphoid to pubis distance increases by 12%, 15%, and 37%, respectively (Table 6.2). In these circumstances an abdominal wound will increase in length by an estimated 30% overall.

Table 6.2 Increases in girth and xiphoid–pubis distance caused by abdominal distension (from Jenkins 1976, with permission)

Percentage increase in distension			
Abdominal distension associated with:	Type of measurement	Mean value	Extreme value
Voluntary inspiration ($n-18$)	Girth	6	11
	Xiphoid–pubis	12	18
Cesarean section ($n-27$)	Girth	18	94
	Xiphoid–pubis	15	36
Gut obstruction or paralytic ileus ($n-5$)	Girth	27	53
	Xiphoid–pubis	37	67

The alterations in wound length that occur during healing have a critical impact on the technique of suturing an abdominal wound. Jenkins has analyzed this geometrically [42] and concluded that the ratio of suture length (SL) to wound length (WL) is critical aponeurosis repair.

An SL:WL ratio of 4:1 is optimum; if the SL:WL ratio decreases below 2.5:1, the risk of wound disruption increases geometrically. Wound disruption is inevitable as the SL:WL ratio approaches 1:1. This mathematical analysis (Jenkins' rule) is confirmed when tested in clinical practice. These findings have been corroborated by Israelsson 30 years later [43,44]. In two studies examining cohorts of over a 1,000 patients from 1989–1991 to 1991–1993, respectively, Israelsson showed that a suture length to wound length of less than 4 was the greatest risk factor for wound failure and predictor of later incisional hernia with lesser risks associated with age, obesity, and wound infection. The surgeon was also an important risk factor in that incisional hernia rates varied from 5 to 26% between individuals. Interestingly in overweight patients (BMI > 25), there was no increase in wound infection rate if the suture length to wound length was between 4.0 and 4.9 although incisional hernias developed in these patients in 15% of cases after 12 months.

Surgical practice, however, continues to rely largely on tradition rather than high-quality level 1 evidence when choosing the ideal method of abdominal fascial closure [45]. Hodgson and colleagues carried out a systemic review and meta-analysis to determine which suture material and which technique reduces the odds of incisional hernia. They studied only randomized controlled trials with a Jadad quality score of >3 (Jadad Quality Scale is the only validated instrument available to assess the quality of randomized control trials.) There were two independent reviewers masked to the study site, authors, journal, and date. The results showed:

1. There was a low occurrence of incisional hernia with non-absorbable sutures.
2. Suture technique favored nonabsorbable, continuous suturing.
3. Sinus tract formation and wound pain were lower with absorbable sutures.

4. There was no difference in dehiscence rates or wound infection rates with respect to method of closure or material used.

Abdominal fascial closure with a continuous nonabsorbable suture had a significantly lower rate of incisional hernia. The ideal suturing technique is continuous. The data for this study drew information from 13 randomized trials including a total of 5,145 patients and utilizing nine different suture materials with a continuous or an interrupted technique, mostly in vertical midline incisions. This meta-analysis provides the most powerful evidence yet for informing surgeons on the optimal technique for abdominal fascial closure.

Over the last decade, there has been a significant expansion in the number of techniques described to repair hernias, and it is beyond the scope of this chapter to describe each one in turn. The pure tissue hernia repair is rapidly becoming outdated and currently probably only applies to small (<2 cm diameter) primary umbilical and paraumbilical hernias. The European Hernia Society (EHS) issued a recommendation in 2008 that all male adult (<30 years) patients with a symptomatic inguinal hernia should be operated on using a mesh technique. The open Lichtenstein and endoscopic inguinal hernia techniques were recommended as the best evidence-based options for the repair of a primary unilateral hernia. If a non-mesh repair was to be used, the Shouldice technique was recommended. For the repair of recurrent hernias after conventional open repair, endoscopic inguinal hernia techniques were recommended [5].

However, the situation for anterior abdominal wall hernias is not so clear cut. It should be noted that the surgical literature has become very difficult to interpret during this time due to the lack of consistency in the terms used to describe anterior abdominal wall defects. In an attempt to make comparisons possible, the EHS held a consensus meeting in 2008. While a definitive EHS classification of incisional hernias was not realized, a classification for primary abdominal wall hernias and a division of subgroups of incisional abdominal wall hernias were formulated. This classification should provide enough information to establish incisional hernia registries and may be used to compare studies on treatment and outcome of incisional hernia repair [46].

Certain principles should be adhered to when implanting any prosthetic mesh. It is important to provide secure fixation of the prosthesis so that it does not move and to ensure there will be no or minimal deformation of the mesh during the healing process. Synthetic mesh should not be placed in an infected field as the mesh will act as a foreign body and chronic sepsis will ensue, often requiring explantation of the mesh. Newer "biological" meshes are being developed which are completely absorbed, and these can be utilized in an infected field, often in combination with wound management systems such as negative pressure dressings.

Knots

The knot is the weakest part of a suture and knot efficiency is a crucial component of the suture technique. Conventional knots cause a 40% decrease in the strength of most suture materials except for nylon (and probably polypropylene). Self-locking knots permit the end of a continuous suture to slide inside the knot, thus absorbing some of the energy which would otherwise be transmitted to the knot and cause it to break [47]. Additionally, self-locking knots are less bulky than conventional knots, thus diminishing the risk of infection and sinus formation [48,49]. To avoid a traditional knot at the commencement of a wound closure, loop sutures have been developed, the needle simply being passed through the loop to anchor the initial stitch. A suture with miniature barbs along its length has also been developed which does not need to be knotted at all.

Suture Manipulation

Generally, little thought is given to the handling of the suture material during its use and implantation into the tissues. Most of the modern synthetics can tolerate considerable manipulation as they are placed. One should be cognizant of the fact that some of these materials can be frayed and weakened when they are secured in the jaws of a needle holder, forceps, or hemostat. Sometimes the surgeon does not recognize this newly created weakness. This can result in an early fracture of the suture material which, in effect, results in a cut suture that is no longer intact. This can result in failure of healing of the tissues that are held with that suture. Similarly, this can result in a hernia recurrence if that suture is the method of fixation of a prosthetic material. Therefore it is incumbent upon the surgeon to be careful in handling any portion of a suture that will remain within the tissues so that this will not become a problem that is manifest by a new or recurrent hernia.

Skin Closure

Sutures, penetrating the skin and then tied on the surface, have been the traditional closure method for wounds. Alternatives include subcuticular sutures; skin clips, which do not penetrate the full skin thickness; plastic tape adherent to the skin; and fibrin glue.

The requirements for adequate skin closure are that the skin should be held together in apposition for sufficient time to allow the skin to grow together. To promote rapid healing, the edges should not move in relation to each other and tension should be minimal to prevent necrosis. Careful suturing should prevent the introduction of sepsis. Lastly, but perhaps of overriding importance to the patient, a good cosmetic result is needed.

Clean or contaminated surgery demands different regimens for wound management. One of the oldest surgical principles is that a frankly contaminated wound should be left open. The wound which is expected to be compromised by early (reactionary) hemorrhage is managed by delayed primary suture. If localized infection is anticipated, interrupted sutures may allow early controlled drainage. These have been the traditions of wound care. Elective hernia operations nowadays are clean operations—we are searching for quick uncomplicated healing with the best functional and cosmetic results. Hence we should review our methods of skin closure and optimize skin healing as far as possible.

Conventional skin suturing techniques do have certain disadvantages—the needle passing through the skin on either side carries fragments of both epidermis and skin organisms down its track and into the depths of the subcutaneous tissue. This causes an increased wound infection rate than when skin closed by a sutureless technique is used. The complications of suture track infection are greater when a multistrand suture is used and when the tension upon the wound edges is too great. Poor technique in inserting the sutures and subsequent edema after suturing lead to localized ischemia and a poor cosmetic result.

Clips avoid the problem of introducing deep infection into the wound. Michel-type clips may produce localized tension and cause local pressure necrosis. Unless they are removed within 24–48 h, this local ischemia can cause tissue necrosis and a permanently poor cosmetic result. Consequently, these are seldom used in modern surgical theaters. Currently available disposable applicators for the introduction of wire clips with a rectangular configuration of the closed clip give excellent results although the skin puncture sites may detract from the overall cosmetic appearance. Closure with adherent skin tape gives excellent healing [50–52].

A randomized controlled clinical trial comparing skin closure using vertical mattress sutures of monofilament nylon and steel clips in laparotomy incisions has confirmed the significant advantage of avoiding skin sutures. In a consecutive series of 341 wounds (182 skin sutured and 159 closed with clips), the infection rate in the sutured wounds was 17% versus 6.3% in those closed with clips ($P < 0.01$) [53]. Subcuticular absorbable sutures are probably the most favored with surgeons, nurses, and patients. In a randomized control trial, four different methods of thigh incision closure after removal of the saphenous vein for coronary artery bypass grafting were used [6]. Continuous nylon vertical mattress sutures, continuous subcuticular absorbable PGA sutures, metal skin clips, and adhesive sutureless closure (Opsite) were compared. Assessment of the healing showed subcuticular PGA to be more effective than skin clips or vertical mattress nylon sutures. The final cosmetic result showed

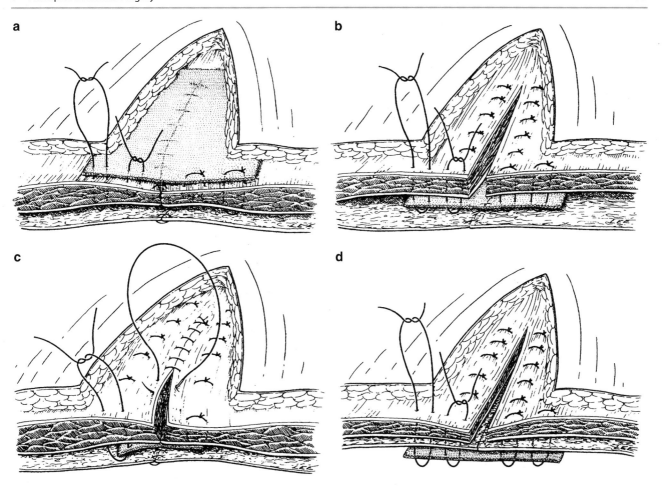

Fig. 6.3 Prosthetic repairs of abdominal wall defects. The prosthesis can be placed extraparietally or subcutaneously (**a**); subaponeurotically, extraperitoneally, or preperitoneally leaving any aponeurotic defect open superficial to the prosthesis (**b**); subaponeurotically with closure of the defect (**c**); or intraperitoneally (**d**)

subcuticular PGA to be superior to mattress sutures or skin clips and as effective as sutureless adherent closure. Subcuticular absorbable sutures do not require removal; this is an economic saving [54]. Subcuticular skin closure for open inguinal hernia repair using polydioxanone or polyglactin 910 is recommended. The result with these sutures is excellent, and no suture removal is required. Wound healing is quick and neat and, most importantly, the lack of through-skin sutures has removed much of the postoperative pain and reduced infection rates to 2–3%. Closure of laparoscopic trocar sites may be performed with subcuticular polyglactin 910, polydioxanone, fibrin glue, and/or skin tapes.

Techniques of Placement of Prosthetic Materials

There are a number of open techniques which have been described to repair abdominal wall defects with prosthetic mesh, the variation in the technique relating to the anatomical plane in which the mesh is placed [55–58]: (a) extra-aponeurotic—subcutaneous (on-lay technique); (b) and (c) subaponeurotic and extraperitoneal or preperitoneal (sublay technique); and (d) subaponeurotic and intraperitoneal (Fig. 6.3). Additionally, intraperitoneal (or subaponeurotic) placement of the mesh can be supported by an extra-aponeurotic buttress (Fig. 6.4). It should be remembered that the use of mesh in open hernia surgery is an adjunct to the application of first principles, i.e., apposition of the aponeurotic edges should be the primary goal, and if specialist approaches such as the component separation technique are employed, fascial apposition is usually achievable.

The laparoscopic approach is somewhat different in that in most cases it does not close the fascial layer but bridges the fascial defect with a prosthetic mesh. In this technique it is vital to establish a significant overlap of the mesh beneath the native fascia. Laparoscopically, the prosthetic mesh will always be in the subaponeurotic plane. In an inguinal hernia

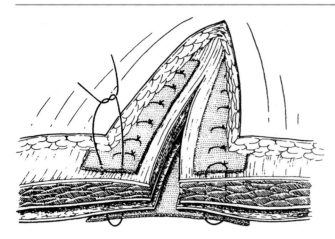

Fig. 6.4 Intraperitoneal placement can be reinforced by an extra-aponeurotic stent

repair, the mesh is placed in the preperitoneal space using either a transabdominal or totally extraperitoneal approach. The laparoscopic repair of incisional and ventral hernias will, on the other hand, generally place the prosthesis in the intraperitoneal position. However, as the technique has developed, the prosthetic mesh may now be placed preperitoneally, via a transabdominal approach, for some anterior abdominal wall hernias (e.g., Spigelian hernias and incisional hernias through Pfannenstiel incisions).

There are now numerous varieties of prosthetic pre-shaped or preformed devices that have been designed for the repair of inguinal hernias. In some cases, these have been used for the repair of incisional or ventral hernias as well. These are too numerous and their methodologies so variant that they are discussed in detail in Chap. 7. One point that should be emphasized, however, is that all of these products are inserted with an individual technique specific for that prosthetic device. Deviation from this methodology may subject the patient to an increased incidence of complications or recurrence.

Summary: Recommendations

- The patient must be appropriately prepared for theater and adequately resuscitated, if necessary, before any operation is undertaken.
- The fascial edges should be defined, and the hernia sac contents reduced.
- The fascial edges should be apposed by a method which maintains tissue strength in excess of 3 months (unless a laparoscopic intraperitoneal technique is employed).
- If a primary closure is performed, a monofilament nonabsorbable synthetic suture such as polypropylene or nylon is preferred.

- The knot should be tied carefully and instrumentation of the suture material itself avoided.
- If the subcutaneous fatty later is closed, an absorbable suture which causes little reaction is recommended—polyglactin 910 or polydioxanone is suitable.
- Closed suction drains may be used where there is a possibility of seroma or hematoma formation.
- For skin closure, the technique should leave no skin markings from sutures, cause a minimal reaction, and have a low incidence of infection and sinus formation. Recommended techniques include polyglactin 910 or polydioxanone sutures, skin tape, or fibrin glue.
- The use of an appropriate mesh prosthesis for the majority of hernia surgery is recommended.

References

1. Mcgugan E, Burton H, Nixon S, Thompson A. Deaths following hernia surgery: room for improvement. J R Coll Surg Edinb. 2000;45(3):183–6.
2. Buck N, Devlin HB, Lunn JN. The report of a confidential enquiry into perioperative deaths. London: Nuffield Provincial Hospital Trust and the King Edward's Hospital Fund for London; 1987.
3. Nilsson H, Stylianidis G, Haapamäki M, Nilsson E, Nordin P. Department of Surgery, Sahlgrenska University Hospital/Ostra, Gothenburg, Sweden mortality after groin hernia surgery. Ann Surg. 2007;245(4):656–60.
4. Sanchez-Manuel FJ, Lozano-García J, Seco-Gil JL. Antibiotic prophylaxis for hernia repair. Cochrane Database Syst Rev. 2007;18(3):CD003769.
5. Simons M, Aufenacker T, Bay-Nielson M, et al. European guidelines on the treatment of inguinal hernia in adult patients. Hernia. 2009;13(4):343–403.
6. Angelini GD, Butchart EG, Armistead SH, Breckenridge IM. Comparative study of leg wound skin closure in coronary artery bypass graft operations. Thorax. 1984;39:942–5.
7. Gilbert AI, Felton LL. Infection in inguinal hernia repair considering biomaterials and antibiotics. Surg Gynecol Obstet. 1993;177:126–30.
8. Devlin HB, Gillen PHA, Waxman BP, Macnay RA. Short stay surgery for inguinal hernia: experience of the Shouldice operation 1970–1982. Br J Surg. 1986;73:123–4.
9. Glassow F. Is post-operative wound infection following simple inguinal herniorrhaphy a predisposing cause of recurrent hernia? Can Med Assoc J. 1964;91:870–1.
10. Howes EL. Effects of suture material on the tensile strength of wound repair. Ann Surg. 1933;98:153–5.
11. Howes EL. The strength of wounds sutured with catgut and silk. Surg Gynecol Obstet. 1933;57:309.
12. Douglas DM. The healing of aponeurotic incisions. Br J Surg. 1952;40:79–82.
13. Douglas DM, Forrester JC, Ogilvie RR. Physical characteristics of collagen in the later stages of wound healing. Br J Surg. 1969;56:219–22.
14. Mason ML, Allen HS. The rate of healing of tendons: an experimental study of tensile strength. Ann Surg. 1941;113:424.
15. LeBlanc KA, Bellanger DE, Rhynes KV, Baker DS, Stout R. Tissue attachment strength of prosthetic meshes used in ventral and incisional hernia repair: a study in the New Zealand white rabbit adhesion model. Surg Endosc. 2002;16(11):1542–6.

16. Ellis H, Gajraj H, George CD. Incisional hernias, when do they occur? Br J Surg. 1983;70:290–321.
17. Hamlin JA, Kahn AM. Herniography in symptomatic patients following inguinal hernia repair. West J Med. 1995;162:28–31.
18. Van Winkle W, Hastings JC, Barker E, Hines D, Nichols W. Effect of suture materials on healing wounds. Surg Gynecol Obstet. 1975;140:7–12.
19. Rath AM, Chevrel JP. The healing of laparotomies: review of the literature. Part 1. Hernia. 1998;2:145–9.
20. Klinge U, Prescher A, Klosterhalfen B, Schumpelick V. Origin and pathophysiology of abdominal wall defects. Chirurg. 1997;68: 293–303.
21. Hunt TK, Goodson WH III. Wound Healing. In: Way LW, editor. Current surgical diagnosis and treatment, 9th ed. Norwalk: Appleton and Lange; 1991. p. 95–108.
22. Forrest I. Current concepts in soft connective tissue wound healing. Br J Surg. 1983;70:133–40.
23. Sandblom P. The tensile strength of healing wounds: an experimental study. Acta Chir Scand Suppl. 1944;891–1088 +.
24. Schilling JA. Advances in knowledge related to wounding, repair and healing: 1885–1984. Ann Surg. 1985;201:268–77.
25. Aird I. Companion in surgical studies. 2nd ed. Edinburgh: Churchill Livingstone; 1957.
26. Artandi C. A revolution in sutures. Surg Gynecol Obstet. 1980; 150:235–6.
27. Sanchez-Montes I, Deysine M. Spigelian hernias. Arch Surg. 1998;133:670–2.
28. Van Winkle WJR, Hastings JC. Considerations in the choice of suture materials for various tissues. Surg Gynecol Obstet. 1972;135:113–26.
29. Moynihan BGA. The ritual of a surgical operation. Br J Surg. 1920;8:27–35.
30. Andrew DR, Williamson KM. Meckel's diverticulum—rare complications and review of the literature. J R Army Med Corps. 1994;140:143–5.
31. Tagart REB. The suturing of abdominal incisions. A comparison of monofilament nylon and catgut. Br J Surg. 1967;54:952–7.
32. Lerwick E. Studies of the efficacy and safety of polydioxanone monofilament absorbable suture. Surg Gynecol Obstet. 1983;156: 51–5.
33. Ray IA, Doddi N, Regula D, Williams JA, Melveger A. Polydioxanone (PDS) a novel monofilament synthetic absorbable suture. Surg Gynecol Obstet. 1981;153:497–507.
34. Irvin TT, Koffman CG, Duthie HL. Layer closure of laparotomy wounds with absorbable and non-absorbable suture materials. Br J Surg. 1976;63:793–6.
35. Halsted WS. The radical cure of hernia. Bull Johns Hopkins Hosp. 1889;1:12–3.
36. Leaper DJ. Laparotomy closure. Br J Hosp Med. 1985;33:317–22.
37. Whipple AO. The use of silk in the repair of clean wounds. Ann Surg. 1933;98:662–71.
38. Mayer AD, Ausobsky JR, Evans M, Pollock AV. Compression suture of the abdominal wall: a controlled trial in 302 major laparotomies. Br J Surg. 1981;68:632–4.
39. Herman RE. Abdominal wound closure using a new polypropylene monofilament suture. Surg Gynecol Obstet. 1974;138:84–6.
40. Herrman NIB. Tensile strength and knot security of surgical suture materials. Am Surg. 1971;37:209–17.
41. Jones DJ. Braided versus monofilament sutures in inguinal hernia. Br J Surg. 1986;73:414.
42. Jenkins TPN. Incisional hernia repair: a mechanical approach. Br J Surg. 1980;67:335–6.
43. Israelsson LA, Jonsson T. Overweight and healing of midline incisions: the importance of suture technique. Eur J Surg. 1997;163: 175–86.
44. Israelsson LA. The surgeon as a risk factor for complications of midline incisions. Eur J Surg. 1998;164:353–9.
45. Hodgson NCF, Malthaner RA, Ostbye T. The search for an ideal method of abdominal fascial closure: a meta-analysis. Ann Surg. 2000;231:436–42.
46. Muysoms F, Miserez M, Berrevoet G, et al. Classification of primary and incisional abdominal wall hernias. Hernia. 2009;13(4):407–14.
47. Paterson-Brown S, Dudley HAF. Knotting in continuous mass closure of the abdomen. Br J Surg. 1986;73:676–80.
48. Pelosa OA, Wilkinson LH. The chain stitch knot. Surg Gynecol Obstet. 1974;139:599–600.
49. Trimbos JB. Factors relating to the volume of surgical knots. Int J Gynecol Obstet. 1989;30:355–9.
50. Eaton AC. A controlled trial to evaluate and compare sutureless skin closure technique (op-site skin closure) with conventional skin suturing and clipping in surgery. Br J Surg. 1980;67:857–60.
51. Pearse HE. Strangulated hernia reduced en masse. Surg Gynecol Obstet. 1931;53:822–8.
52. Taube M, Porter RJ, Lord PH. A combination of subcuticular suture and sterile micropore tape compared with conventional interrupted sutures for skin closure. Ann R Coll Surg Engl. 1983;65:164–6.
53. Pickford IR, Brennan SS, Evans M, Pollock AV. Two methods of skin closure in abdominal operations: a controlled clinical trial. Br J Surg. 1983;70:226–8.
54. Ramshaw BJ, Escartia P, Schwab J, et al. Comparison of laparoscopic and open ventral herniorrhaphy. Am Surg. 1999;65:827–32.
55. Larson GM, Harrower HW. Plastic mesh repair of incisional hernia. Am J Surg. 1978;135:559–63.
56. Larson GM, Vandertoll DJ. Approaches to repair of ventral hernia and full thickness loss of the abdominal wall. Surg Clin North Am. 1984;64:335–50.
57. Usher FC. The repair of incisional and inguinal hernias. Surg Gynecol Obstet. 1970;131:525–30.
58. Usher FC. New technique for repairing incisional hernias with Marlex mesh. Am J Surg. 1979;138:740–1.

Prostheses and Products for Hernioplasty

Karl A. LeBlanc

Introduction

The use of prosthetic biomaterials in the repair of hernias of the abdominal wall is now very commonplace throughout the world. In the USA and Europe over 90% of all inguinal and ventral hernias are repaired with a prosthetic material or device. In other parts of the world, this is not the case. Limitations on the use of these products include a natural reluctance to place a foreign material into a primary hernia or the cost of these products. This is changing rapidly, however, as illustrated by the experience in the approach to inguinal hernia repair in the Department of Surgery in the Hospital Bludenz in Bludenz, Austria, where the Bassini and Shouldice repairs were used in 39% of the cases in 1993. By 1996, these two repairs were done in only 18% of patients because there was a marked increase in the use of prosthetic products to repair inguinal hernias [1]. This expansion is commonplace all over the world.

Incisional hernias will develop in approximately 13% of laparotomy incisions. The risk of herniation is increased by fivefold if a postoperative wound infection occurs. Other factors that predispose to the development of a fascial defect include smoking, obesity, poor nutritional status, steroid usage, etc. While some of these may be avoided, those patients that are found to have such a hernia can present difficult management problems due to the high potential for recurrence. Without the use of a prosthetic material, the recurrence rate is as high as 51% [2]. The use of a synthetic material will reduce this rate to 10–24% [3].

The laparoscopic repair of incisional and ventral hernias was first performed in 1991 and introduced in 1993 using the Soft Tissue Patch made by W.L. Gore and Associates (Elkhart, DE, USA) [4]. The recurrence rate that has been reported in recent literature varies from 0 to 11% but averages approximately 5.5%. The "ideal" prosthetic product has yet to be found. Many of the current materials have been developed to meet the requirements of this procedure but many of these, of course, have found a place in the open repair as well. In fact, modifications of these prostheses have occurred to the extent that many of the "laparoscopic" products can now be used interchangeably as "open" products and vice versa. This chapter will identify these goals and the properties of the various biomaterials that are on the market today. The rational for the choice of a material in the open and laparoscopic repairs of hernias of the abdominal wall will be developed.

There are several hundred different products that can be used in the repair of inguinal, ventral, incisional, and other hernias of the abdominal wall. In many of the products listed below, there is a paucity of published literature that verifies the claims that are made by the manufacturers. While this is the situation at the time of the production of this textbook, the reader is advised to reference the available journals to identify the uses and results of these materials. Much of the information discussed was obtained from the manufacturer directly.

Indications for Use of Prosthetic Materials

Surgeons recognize that the main purpose in the use of these materials will be the repair of a fascial defect in the abdominal wall. The main indications of use of the materials are listed in Table 7.1.

Musculofascial tissue strength can be lost in a variety of ways. The most common, of course, would be due to the external etiology of the weakness that develops after a laparotomy or other abdominal incision that is larger than that of the 5 mm laparoscopic trocar (although even this small incision can rarely develop a hernia). Another example would be the loss of tissue with trauma such as gunshot wounds. The increase of intra-abdominal pressure that results from significant weight gain will result in an internal source of weakening of the abdominal wall musculature. Poor nutritional

K.A. LeBlanc (✉)
Surgeons Group of Baton Rouge/Our Lady of the Lake Physician
Group, Baton Rouge, Louisiana, USA
e-mail: Karl.LeBlanc@ololrmc.com

A.N. Kingsnorth and K.A. LeBlanc (eds.), *Management of Abdominal Hernias*,
DOI 10.1007/978-1-84882-877-3_7, © Springer Science+Business Media London 2013

Table 7.1 Indications for prostheses

Replacement of lost musculofascial tissue caused by:
Trauma
External
Internal
Infection
Reinforcement of native tissue weakness
Aging (laxity of tissues)
Neurological deficit (denervation)

Table 7.2 Natural prosthetic products

Autogenous dermal grafts	Whole skin grafts
Dermal collagen homografts	Porcine dermal collagen
Autogenous fascial heterografts	Lyophilized aortic homografts
Preserved dural homografts	Bovine pericardium

Table 7.3 Nonmetallic synthetic products "ideal surgical" material are listed in Table 7.4

Fortisan fabric (cellulose)	Polytetrafluoroethylene
Polyvinyl sponge	Polypropylene mesh/gelatin film
Polyvinyl cloth	Polyester-reinforced silicon sheeting
Nylon mesh	Silastic
Carbon fiber	Polyester (as a solid sheet)
Silicon-velvet composite	Carbon fiber

Table 7.4 Ideal surgical clinical characteristics of synthetic products

Permanent Repair of the Abdominal Wall (i.e., no recurrences)
Ingrowth characteristics that result in a normal pattern of tissue repair and healing
Does not alter the compliance of the abdominal wall musculature
Lack of adhesion predisposition
Cuts easily and without fraying
Inexpensive
Lack of long-term complications such as pain or fistualization
From Cumberland [10] and Scales [11]

or protein malnutrition is also a source of such problems. Other predisposing factors such as emphysema or the chronic bronchitis of individuals that smoke tobacco products results in a constant increase in intra-abdominal pressure because of a frequent cough. Life-threatening infections such as fasciitis and gangrene will produce large areas of necrosis and resultant tissue loss. More frequently, the development of a postoperative wound infection will increase the risk of herniation by as much a five times. In fact, almost 30% of patients that develop a postoperative incisional wound infection will eventually develop an incisional hernia [5].

The effects of aging and the declining ability of the elderly patients to repair the native tissues will lead to the loss of fascial integrity. This is commonly seen with the direct inguinal hernia. It also occurs with the enlargement of the linea alba that is referred to as diastasis recti. These latter defects can enlarge and occasionally become symptomatic, requiring repair. The disruption of collagen that is seen by the effects of smoking will have a similar effect (i.e., metastatic emphysema).

The most common defect that results from a denervation phenomenon follows the flank incision that is utilized in a nephrectomy, lumbar sympathectomy, or an anterior approach to the lumbar interbody fusion for degenerative disc disease. In these entities, there is usually not the defined fascial edge that is seen with the more common anterior abdominal wall defects. This is due to the broad surface of the denervated musculature that has intact fascia but lacks the reinforcement of healthy muscle tissue.

Prosthetic Materials: History

The use of materials for the repairs of hernias can be found in antiquity. It is believed that Heliodorus used the cellulose from a cotton or flax plant to effect scarification in the inguinal area to treat herniation in A.D. 25. The use of silver as a synthetic prosthesis was reported in 1900 [6]. Metallic biomaterials have also included the use of tantalum gauze mesh and stainless steel mesh. None of these materials gained wide acceptance because of the complications that were associ-

ated with their usage. These included lack of pliability, seroma development, wound infection, fatigue fractures, herniation through the fracture sites, abnormal scarification, adhesions, loss of structural integrity, and allergic reactions. Reoperation in these patients was particularly challenging.

Natural prostheses were considered as myofascial replacement shortly after the use of silver filigree [7]. Other materials that have been used are listed in Table 7.2.

These materials were used with good results in some cases but scarcity and cost limited their widespread adoption. Additionally, there were concerns of viral transmission as one case of Creutzfeld-Jacobs disease developed in a patient that had the use of a dural homograft. The development of other synthetic biomaterials that were closer to the ideal prosthesis hastened the demise of the use of these products in the past. As we now have seen over the last several years, some of these products have seen resurgence. Updated methods of processing these products have allowed for improved safety and efficacy resulting in an expansion of their use.

A series of nonmetallic synthetic prosthetic biomaterials were used as well (Table 7.3). As with the metal materials, there were significant disadvantages with these products also. These included infections, sinus tract formation, alteration of the product in vivo, and lack of incorporation into the native tissues. The use of the carbon fiber in humans has never been attempted because of concerns of potential carcinogenicity (although it functioned fairly well in the experimental model). With some of these materials, newer hernia repair products have used these materials again because of more modern manufacturing capabilities.

The synthetic prosthetic materials can be divided into the absorbable and nonabsorbable products. There has been a recent introduction of non-synthetic biomaterials designed for usage in the repair of hernias, commonly referred to as the "biologics". These are based upon the use of porcine, bovine or cadaveric tissues to produce a collagen matrix. All of these products are not truly absorbable as they are intended to provide a scaffold for the native fibroblasts to incorporate natural collagen to repair a fascial defect. It is the goal of these devices to repair the hernia defect with the tissues of the patient as these will be degraded and replaced over time.

The synthetic nonabsorbable materials are of many types, sizes, and shapes. The use of these products is commonplace in the repair of inguinal hernias. The current use of the prosthesis in the tension-free concept of a repair of the incisional hernias has gained widespread acceptance within the last several years. With the exception of the very smallest of hernias, every laparoscopic approach employs a prosthesis. There is a growing trend to use a synthetic or, more commonly, biologic material to repair even the diaphragmatic hernias associated with gastroesophageal reflux disease.

The materials that are presented below are given in an arbitrary arrangement and with an accurate information that could be obtained. An effort was made, however, to stratify these products in a classification that grouped similar products together. I have attempted to identify all of the currently available products that are used in most parts of the world at the time of publication. Some of these materials have either no published clinical data or very scanty information as to the clinical performance characteristics. Therefore, it is certain, that some products and/or details have been overlooked despite my efforts to present all that I could identify. Due to the very large variation in the sizes of the products, little comment regarding the sizes of these products will be given. The reader is referred to the respective manufacturer for these details. Additionally, if a product or photo of a product is not shown, it is likely due to lack of assistance from a manufacturer in the provision of that information. It should also be noted that not all of these products are available in all countries. Manufacturers have limited the release of many of them to only selected areas of the world or have not obtained the necessary governmental approvals for clinical distribution at the time of this writing. Finally, it is certain that all of the available products are not included in this compilation. Many companies are quite small or have limited production. Therefore, if any of these that are not included it was not because of an intended omission but rather a lack of available information.

Absorbable Prosthetic Biomaterials

The general purpose of these is the temporary replacement of absent tissue (Table 7.5). The strength of these materials and the lack of permanency make some of them unsuitable for the permanent repair of any hernia.

Bio-A, TephaFLEX, and TIGR meshes represent a different type of mesh product. These products represent a new generation of materials that might fill a gap in the products that are available today. The clinical performance characteristics of these are somewhere between the biologic and synthetic materials. The exact fit for the repair of tissue defects has yet to be defined at this time. The *Bio-A* (Fig. 7.1) product is supplied in flat sheet. It is made of trimethylene carbonate and polyglycolic acid. It will maintain approximately 70% of its tensile strength for 21 days. Its use is multifaceted but it is touted for use instead of a biologic product. It serves as a scaffold to allow for fibroblastic infiltration and replacement by the patient's native collagen.

Safil Mesh (Fig. 7.2) is a polyglycolic acid material that will retain 50% of its strength for 20 days. It is not to be

Table 7.5 Absorbable products

Dexon, US Surgical Corp./Davis & Geck, Norwalk, CT, USA
Safil Mesh, B. Braun Surgical, Germany
TIGR mesh, Novus Scientific Pte Ltd., Singapore
TephaFLEX Mesh, Tepha, Inc, Lexington, MA, USA
Vicryl (knitted) mesh, Ethicon, Inc., Somerville, NJ, USA
Vicryl (woven) mesh, Ethicon, Inc., Somerville, NJ, USA

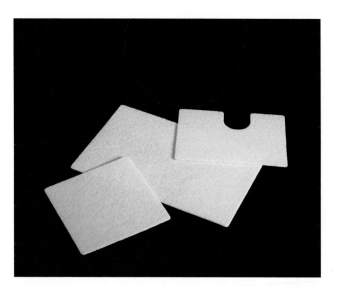

Fig. 7.1 Bio-A (flat sheets and hiatal hernia patch)

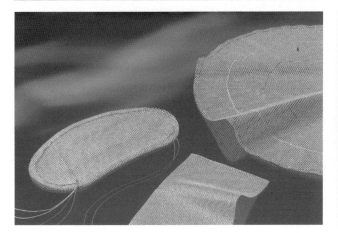

Fig. 7.2 Safil Mesh

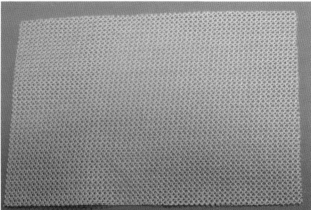

Fig. 7.4 TIGR Matrix Surgical Mesh

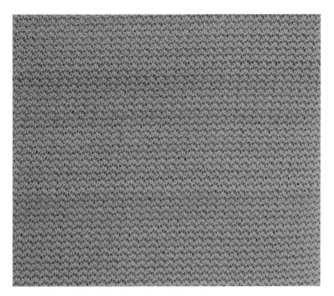

Fig. 7.3 TephaFLEX

considered a permanent repair for tissue. It is said to be used to strengthen the closure of the abdominal and chest walls. The above photo also shows the bags into which this material is also shaped for use in splenic preservation.

TephaFLEX (Fig. 7.3) is composed of poly-4-hydroxybu-tyrate (P4HB). It is degraded by hydrolysis and hydrolytic enzymatic processes. The absorption of the material is minimal until about 26 weeks postimplantation and is essentially complete in about 52 weeks.

TIGR Matrix Surgical Mesh (Fig. 7.4) is knitted from two different synthetic resorbable fibers, polyglycolic acid and polylactic acid (PLA). The Matrix is warp-knitted in a proprietary way, allowing it to gradually increase its relative degradation over time. The strength of the Matrix is comparable to conventional mesh implants for the initial 6–9 months following implantation. The first fiber (polyglycolic acid) appears to lose its functional capabilities in 2 weeks

while the second fiber (PLA) maintains its strength for approximately 9 months.

The *Vicryl* and *Dexon* meshes are primarily PLA (Fig. 7.5). They can be affixed onto the fascia directly with sutures but are not of sufficient strength to formally repair a defect. Most frequently these are used to provide a buttress of support for the temporary closure of an infected incisional wound of the abdomen or in the patient with intra-abdominal sepsis or abdominal compartment syndrome. They have also been used in the treatment of complex or very large hernias that will be repaired in a staged fashion. In that instance, this product will be placed as a bridge and the patient will be returned to the operating room within a few days to perform the definitive procedure.

Biologic Products

As noted earlier, these products do not represent a new concept in hernia repair. They are marked improvement of the materials developed earlier in the last century. They are based upon a harvested collagen matrix that is manufactured into sheets of tissue-engineered materials that can be used to repair defects in the abdominal wall. The concept of these materials is that the biologic material will allow the migration of the patient's own fibroblasts onto them so that collagen will be deposited to form a "neo-fascia." Studies have shown that the extracellular matrix scaffolds from these materials show rapid degradation that is associated with remodeling to a tissue with strength that exceeds that of the native tissues [8]. For the most part, these are used in open techniques but there is some usage in laparoscopic methods especially in the repair of hiatal hernias.

There are similarities of all of the biologic products. They are all harvested from an organism that was alive. The type of source will dictate the size of the material and in most cases, the thickness of the product. The thickness will be variable in

Fig. 7.5 Vicryl mesh, knitted (*left*) and woven (*right*)

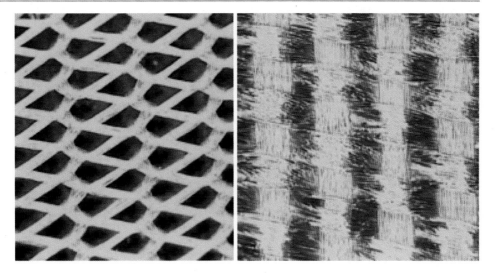

nearly all of them. Some manufacturers have found creative techniques to increase the size of the materials available. All of the products are processed to eliminate all cellular and nuclear material as well as any prions. Following this, a few undergo another process to cross-link the collagen at the molecular level (these are noted when discussed below). The final stage is the sterilization of the prosthesis. It is beyond the scope of this chapter to cover all of these in detail. However, it should be considered, when using any of these materials, that the processing plays a large part into the characteristics and the clinical behavior of them postimplantation.

In general, the biologic products were introduced for use in contaminated fields such as a synthetic mesh infection. While they can be used in this manner, it is recommended that the wound should not possess gross pus as the collagenases of some bacteria and inflammatory cells can degrade these products. These products are finding a place in the repair of very complex noninfected hernias as well. One concern will be that if the patient possesses a collagen deficiency disorder, the remodeling of these products will not occur properly, leading to a predictable failure of the repair. It has also been learned over the last few years that these products perform best if they have direct contact with some type of vascularized tissue. Intuitively, if the expectation of these biologic scaffolds becomes infiltrated by fibroblasts and subsequent collagen deposition, blood supply will deliver these cells more rapidly. Consequently, a higher failure rate will be noted if a biologic prosthesis is used as a "bridge" between fascial edges.

Cadaveric Products

The human cadaveric products have a long history (Table 7.6). These products are similar in that they are not available in exceedingly large sizes. There is significant variability in the amount of stretch that each of these will undergo either at the

Table 7.6 Cadaveric biologic prostheses

Alloderm, LifeCell Inc., Branchburg, NJ, USA (Fig. 7.6)
AlloMax, Davol, Inc., Warwick, RI, USA (Fig. 7.7)
DermaMatrix, Synthes CMF, West Chester, PA, USA
Flex HD, Ethicon, Inc., Somerville, NJ, USA (Fig. 7.8)

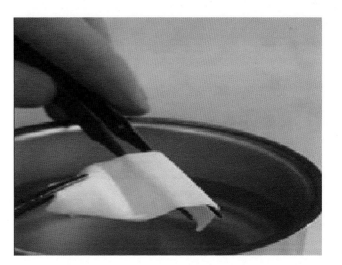

Fig. 7.6 AlloDerm

time of implantation and subsequent to the procedure. This stretch varies from product to product and should be accounted for at the time of implantation. These products are not cross-linked and require rehydration. These are also commonly used in the repair of hiatal hernias.

Bovine Products

The bovine products are from dermis, pericardium, or tendon (Table 7.7). Only the *SurgiMend* (Fig. 7.9) is fetal (dermal) tissue. There is a very unique product, *Easy Prosthesis (PPM/collagen)*, which is a combination of collagen from bovine

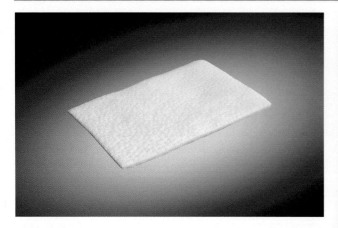

Fig. 7.7 AlloMax

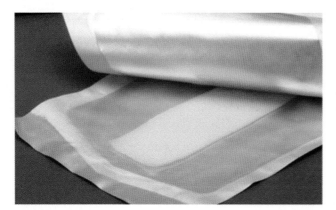

Fig. 7.8 FlexHD

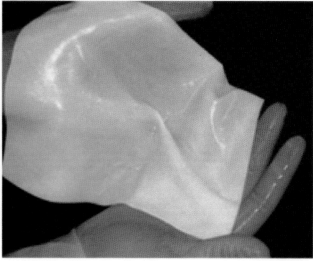

Fig. 7.9 SurgiMend

Fig. 7.10 Tutopatch

Table 7.7 Bovine biologic prostheses

Easy Prosthesis (PPM/Collagen), TransEasy Medical Tech.Co. Ltd., Beijing, China

SurgiMend, TEI Biosciences, Boston, MA, USA

Tutopatch, RTI Biologics, Alachua, FL, USA

Tutomesh, RTI Biologics, Alachua, FL, USA

Veritas, Synovis Surgical Innovations, St. Paul, MN, USA

tendon with polypropylene (PP) (see Fig. 7.116). It is discussed in the section titled "Prostheses for Incisional and Ventral Hernioplasty with an Absorbable Component." Because of the source of all of these products, there will be limitations on the size ranges available.

These are flat sheets. *Tutopatch* (Fig. 7.10) and *Tutomesh* (Fig. 7.11) are of the same source (pericardium) and processing. However, Tutomesh is perforated (unlike the other three products). The use of all of these bovine products has generally been limited to the incisional hernia repair. However there has been increasing application in the repair of hiatal hernias and occasionally in inguinal hernias. *Veritas* is pericardium also.

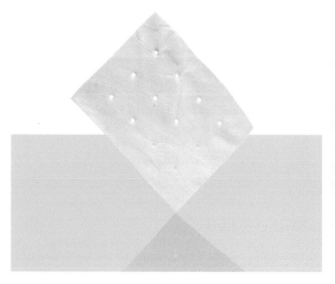

Fig. 7.11 Tutomesh

Table 7.8 Porcine biologic prostheses

CollaMend FM, Davol, Inc., Warwick, RI, USA

Fortagen, Organogenesis, Inc., Canton, MA

Permacol, Covidien, Inc., Mansfield, MA, USA

Strattice, LifeCell Inc., Branchburg, NJ, USA

Surgisis, Cook Surgical, Inc., Bloomington, IN

XenMatrix, Davol, Inc., Warwick, RI, USA

XCM Biologic Tissue Matrix, Synthes CMF, West Chester, PA, USA

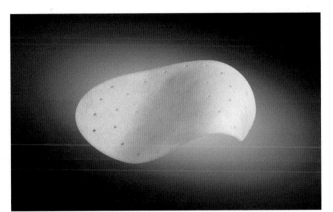

Fig. 7.12 CollaMend FM

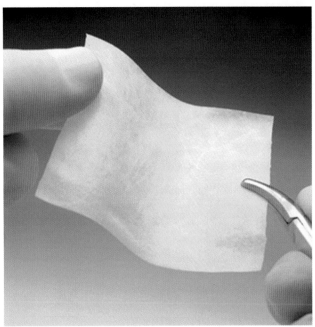

Fig. 7.13 FortaGen

Porcine Products

A number of these materials are available (Table 7.8). Depending on the manufacturer, they are in different sizes and shapes and construction. Some are laminated, some are cross-linked, some are perforated, some require rehydration, and others do not. These are specific to the product and it is recommended that the user follow the instructions for use that is provided with each product.

CollaMend FM (Fig. 7.12) is a cross-linked product derived from porcine dermis. All cross-linked products are bonded at the molecular level with one of the several different chemicals. The level of cross-linking will vary with the product and will impact the longevity of the matrix within the body. Generally, the cross-linked products will remain longer in the intact state and, as such, tend to behave more like a synthetic material than an absorbable one. However, all are eventually resorbed. This product requires rehydration and is fenestrated.

FortaGen (Fig. 7.13) is based upon porcine small intestinal submucosa as is the Surgisis below. The FortaGen material is a three or five-layer construct with a low level of cross-linkage that allows cellular infiltration and remodeling. *Permacol* (Fig. 7.14) is a dermal collagen-based product that is cross-linked and does not require rehydration. It, too, will be present for a prolonged period of time due to the cross-linkage of the collagen fibers. *BioDesign Surgisis Hernia Grafts* (Figs. 7.15, 7.16, and 7.17) are three products that are designed for the repair of specific hernias, ventral, inguinal, and hiatal. They all

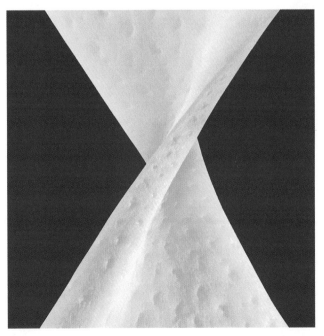

Fig. 7.14 Permacol

are developed from porcine small intestinal submucosa. These are laminated, sewn together, and fenestrated. It is one of the older products in the biologic market.

Strattice is available in two thicknesses, firm and pliable. It is made from dermis. One of the more recent additions to the biologic market is *XenMatrix* (Fig. 7.18). However, it has really been available for several years but has only recently been brought to an expanded market. It is dermal based and is not cross-linked. It does not require rehydration or

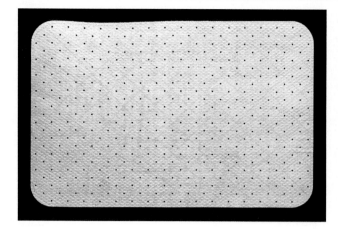

Fig. 7.15 Biodesign Surgisis Hernia Graft

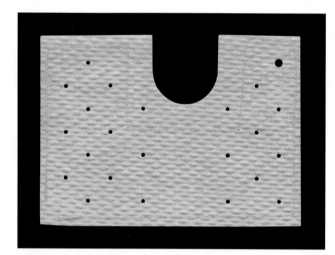

Fig. 7.16 Biodesign Surgisis Hiatal Hernia Graft

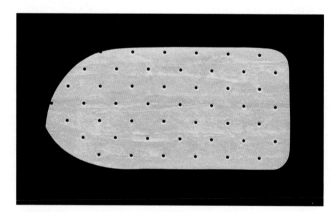

Fig. 7.17 Biodesign Surgisis Inguinal Hernia Graft

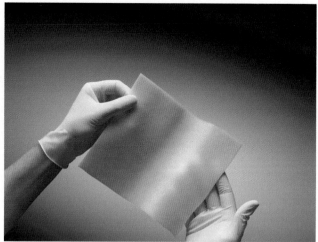

Fig. 7.18 XenMatrix

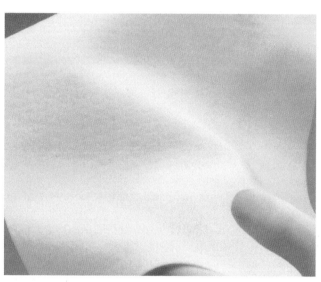

Fig. 7.19 XCM Biologic Tissue Matrix

Flat Prosthetic Biomaterials

The currently available products in use today are polypropylene (PP), polyester (POL), polytetrafluoroethylene (PTFE), expanded PTFE (ePTFE), or condensed PTFE (cPTFE). All are available in a variety of sizes and can be cut to conform to the dimensions that are necessary. There are currently so many products on the market today that it is quite difficult to become well versed in all of these materials. In fact, the similarities of these biomaterials may result in many of them to be considered a "commodity" type of a product, whereupon only the pricing of the material will influence the use of it. The most prominent and commonly used are PP materials (Table 7.9). These, typically, can be used either in the open or laparoscopic applications. Because of the complexities of

refrigeration. As with many of the biological materials, it can vary in thickness. *XCM Biologic Tissue Matrix* (Fig. 7.19) is also a non-cross-linked porcine dermal product and does not require rehydration.

Table 7.9 Flat polypropylene products

Basic mesh, Di.pro Medical Devices, Torino, Italy

Basic Evolution mesh, Di.pro Medical Devices, Torino, Italy

Bard mesh, Davol, Inc., Warwick, RI, USA

Bard Soft mesh, Davol, Inc., Warwick, RI, USA

Biomesh P1, Cousin Biotech, Wervicq-Sud, France

Biomesh P8, Cousin Biotech, Wervicq-Sud, France

Biomesh P9, Cousin Biotech, Wervicq-Sud, France

Combi Mesh Pro, Angiologica, S. Martino Sicc., Italy

DynaMesh PP-Standard t, FEG Textiltechnik mbH, Aachen, Germany

DynaMesh PP- Light, FEG Textiltechnik mbH, Aachen, Germany

Easy Prosthesis, TransEasy Medical Tech.Co. Ltd., Beijing, China

Easy Prosthesis Lightweight, TransEasy Medical Tech.Co. Ltd., Beijing, China

Hertra 0, HerniaMesh, S.R.L., Torino, Italy

Hermesh 3,4,5,6,7,8, HerniaMesh, S.R.L., Torino, Italy

HydroCoat Mesh, Promethean Surgical Devices, East Hartford, CT, USA

Lapartex, Di.pro Medical Devices, Torino, Italy

Optilene, B. Braun Melsungen AG, Melsungen, Germany

Optilene LP, B. Braun Melsungen AG, Melsungen, Germany

Optilene Mesh Elastic, B. Braun Melsungen AG, Melsungen, Germany

Parietene, Covidien plc, Dublin, Ireland

Parietene LIGHT, Covidien plc, Dublin, Ireland

Premilene, B. Braun Melsungen AG, Melsungen, Germany

Prolene, Ethicon Inc., Somerville, NJ, USA

Prolene Soft Mesh, Ethicon Inc., Somerville, NJ, USA

Prolite, Atrium Medical Corporation, Hudson, NH, USA

Repol Angimesh 0,1,8,9, Angiologica, S. Martino Sicc., Italy

Restorelle, Mpathy Medical Devices, Raynham, MA

Surgimesh 1,2, XLight, Aspide Medical, St. Etienne, France

SurgimeshWN, Aspide Medical, St. Etienne, France

Surgipro Monofilamented, Covidien plc, Dublin, Ireland

Surgipro Multifilamented, Covidien plc, Dublin, Ireland

Surgipro Open Weave, Covidien plc, Dublin, Ireland

TiMESH, GfE Medizintechnik, Nuremburg, Germany

Trelex, Meadox Medical Corporation, Oakland, NJ, USA

VitaMESH—Proxy Biomedical Limited, Galway, Ireland

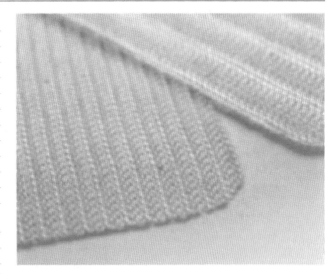

Fig. 7.20 Basic mesh

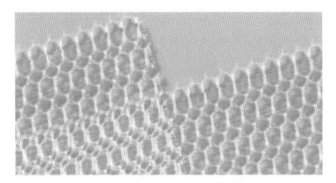

Fig. 7.21 Basic Evolution mesh

pore sizes and the multitude of differing weights and shapes of the PPM within each of these materials, this chapter could not expound upon all of them. The reader is referred to the manufacturer for further information in the exact densities, weights, and pore sizes of these products.

Basic mesh (Fig. 7.20) is a lightweight mesh. Di.pro has developed an ultra-lightweight version that is called Basic Evolution mesh (Fig. 7.21). Although most market penetration is in Europe, there are sites across the globe that have availability of this material. *Bard Mesh* (Fig. 7.22) is probably the oldest flat sheet of heavy weight polypropylene in existence, having been brought to market in the early 1960s. It is still in use today and like many of these prostheses, a lightweight version have been developed, the *Bard Soft Mesh* (Fig. 7.23). *Biomesh P1, P3, and P9* (Figs. 7.24, 7.25, and 7.26) products are differentiated from each other on the basis

of the weight of the material. *Combi Mesh Pro* (Fig. 7.27) is a combination product that is also designed for incisional and ventral hernia repair. It is made of a thin layer of PPM bonded on one side with a thin polyurethane sheet. A colored thread that can be seen in the photo is added to facilitate the identification of the polyurethane layer. It can be easily pulled out after insertion of the product. While this product is designed for the laparoscopic repair, the manufacturer describes its use in the open technique.

DynaMesh (Fig. 7.28) comes in two weights; the standard is twice the weight of the lightweight product. *Easy Prosthesis* (Fig. 7.29) is available as *PPM* (medium weight) and *PMM*, which is lighter in weight and thinner than PPM. The *Easy Prosthesis Lightweight* (Fig. 7.30) is the lightest product of these. The *Hertra 0* mesh is designed for open repair of inguinal hernias, not laparoscopic, especially for the Trabucco repair. The *Hermesh 3–8* can be used either open or laparoscopic (Fig. 7.31). The graduated weights of these vary from the heaviest (3) to the lightest (8). *HydroCoat Mesh* is a new product that only recently received governmental approval

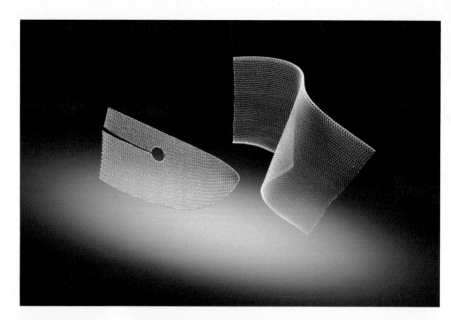

Fig. 7.22 Bard Mesh

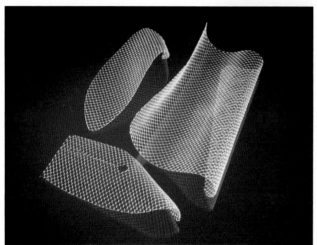

Fig. 7.23 Bard Soft Mesh

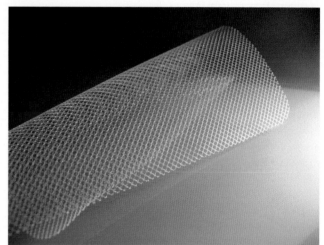

Fig. 7.25 Biomesh P3

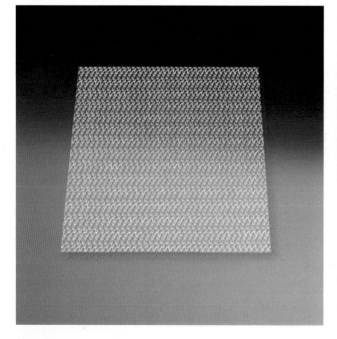

Fig. 7.24 Biomesh P1

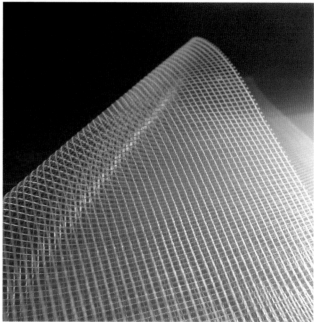

Fig. 7.26 Biomesh P9

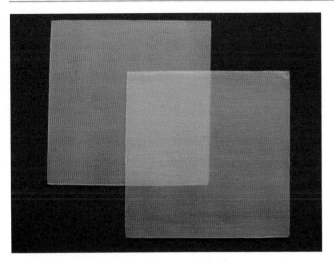

Fig. 7.27 Combi Mesh Pro

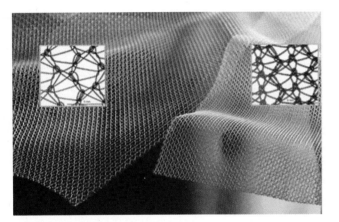

Fig. 7.28 DynaMesh: Light and Standard

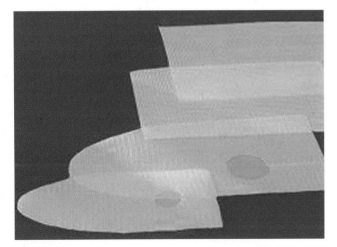

Fig. 7.29 Easy Prosthesis

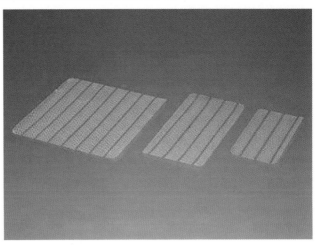

Fig. 7.30 Easy Prosthesis: Lightweight

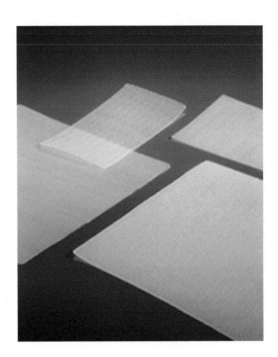

Fig. 7.31 Hermesh variety

for clinical use. It is manufactured with PP that is coated with polyurethane. It is available with different configurations in differing thicknesses and differing microporous structures. It is unknown at this time if this can be placed in the intrap-

eritoneal space. *Lapartex* (Fig. 7.32) is a heavier product than some of the other materials.

The *Optilene* products vary from the heaviest by that name to the lighter *LP* and the *Elastic*, the latter is very light and has larger pores than the other materials (Figs. 7.33, 7.34, and 7.35). Unlike some of the other prostheses, the blue lines in the Optilene do not signify an absorbable component. *Parietene and Parietene LIGHT* products are flat sheet products. *Premilene* (Fig. 7.36) is the heaviest weight product in the Braun flat mesh product line. *Prolene* (Fig. 7.37) is also a heavier weight mesh material and it is one of the older products available. Its lighter weight companion product, *Prolene Soft Mesh* (Fig. 7.38) has larger pores than the original mesh and blue lines to help differentiate it. *Prolite* (Fig. 7.39) was

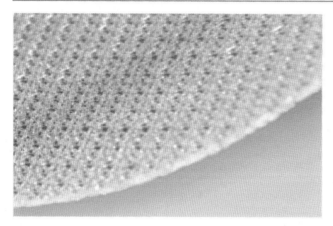

Fig. 7.32 Lapartex

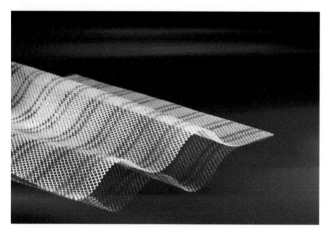

Fig. 7.33 Optilene

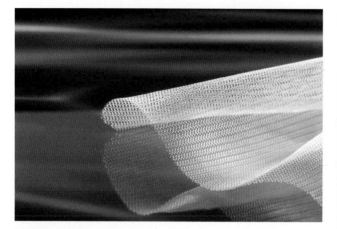

Fig. 7.34 Optilene LP

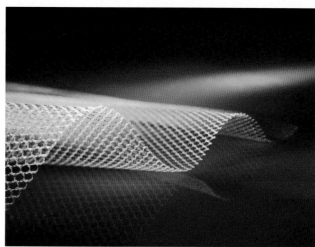

Fig. 7.35 Optilene Elastic

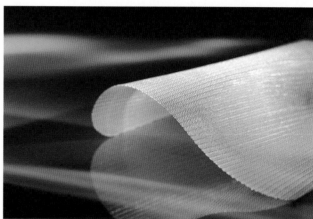

Fig. 7.36 Premilene

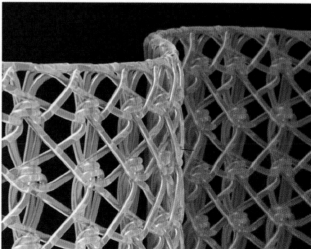

Fig. 7.37 Prolene

one of the earliest meshes that were introduced as a lighter weight material. The more recent *Prolite Ultra* (Fig. 7.40) possesses even less weight of mesh than the older one.

Restorelle is available but has little history in the hernia repair market as it has only recently received governmental

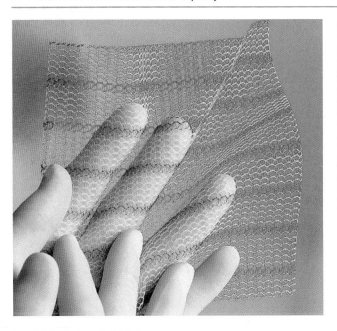

Fig. 7.38 Prolene Soft Mesh

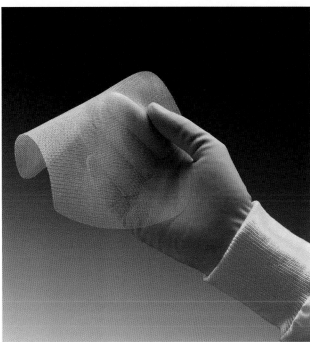

Fig. 7.40 Prolite Ultra

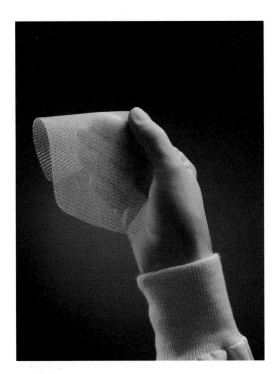

Fig. 7.39 Prolite

approval. *Repol Angimesh 0, 1, 8,* and *9* (Fig. 7.41) are all similar and differentiated in the weights and weaves from each other. The 0 is the lightest and 9 is the heaviest. *SurgiMesh 1, 2,* and *XLight* are PP products similar to the other PP products. *SurgiMesh WN* (Figs. 7.42 and 7.43), however, is a nonwoven microfiber PP product that is extremely lightweight and has a differing microstructure

than the other materials listed in this section. *Surgipro* was originally introduced as a multifilamented mesh (Fig. 7.44). Because of the demand for a monofilamented product (Fig. 7.45), the second-generation product was released. The multifilament material is noticeably softer than the monofilamented one. There is now an open weave product called the *Surgipro Open Weave* (Fig. 7.46).

TiMESH (Fig. 7.47) is similar to the lightweight materials but differs from all of them in that there is a bonded layer of titanium on the fibers of the PP using nanotechnology (Fig. 7.48). This is supposed to allow ingrowth in a flexible manner while inhibiting the development of a scar plate. *Trelex* mesh is an older product that is heavier weight material. *VitaMESH* is of a single lightweight material promoted for laparoscopic inguinal repair.

The differences in the appearance of the prosthetics are easily seen in these photos. The size of the pores of these materials as well as the thickness of the product will have a significant impact on the stiffness. These factors affect the degree of scarring within the tissues. Additionally, the pore sizes vary greatly from each of these products. Since the last edition of this textbook, the lighter weight products have significantly impacted the prosthetic repair of hernias. The current thought is that, for the most part, there is less pain and a scar plate with these lightweight, larger pore meshes. In some cases, these may have become "too thin" and there are a few anecdotal reports of mesh fracture and hernia recurrence. Generally, these meshes are well accepted in the inguinal arena but one should be sure of the strength of these products in the ventral and incisional hernia repair.

Fig. 7.41 Repol 0, 1, 8, 9

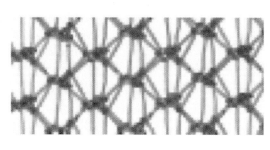

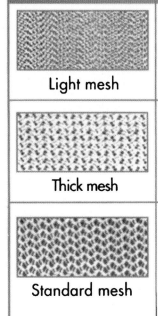

Light mesh

Thick mesh

Standard mesh

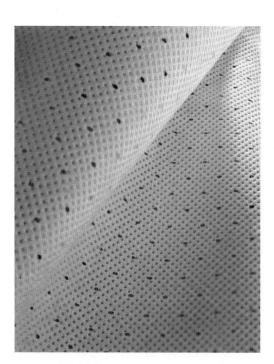

Fig. 7.42 SurgiMesh WN

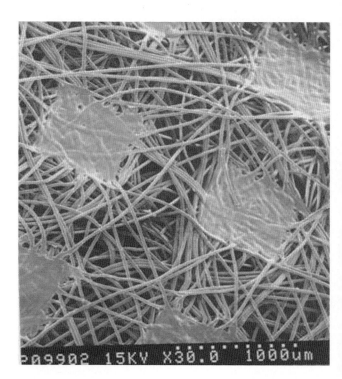

Fig. 7.43 SurgiMesh WN (scanning electron microscopic view)

The polyester biomaterials have seen more acceptance in Europe than in the USA in the past (Table 7.10). Currently, because of the development of newer products, these are used more frequently across the world than in prior times. Like the PP materials, these flat sheets listed can be used in inguinal and ventral hernia repair and can be placed either via an open approach or a laparoscopic technique. The majority of the polyester products that are currently available are produced in various configurations and most have some type of coating. Consequently, these are listed elsewhere in this chapter.

These flat sheets are the *Mersilene* (Fig. 7.49) mesh that has been available for many years and Angimesh R2 (Fig. 7.50). The *Parietex Flat Sheet Mesh* is available in two- or three-dimensional weaves, while the *Parietex Lightweight* (Fig. 7.51) product is a monofilament product.

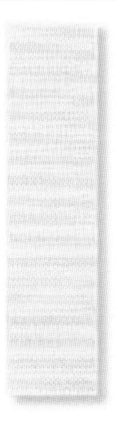

Fig. 7.44 Surgipro, multifilamented

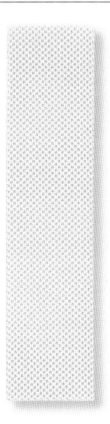

Fig. 7.46 Surgipro Open Weave

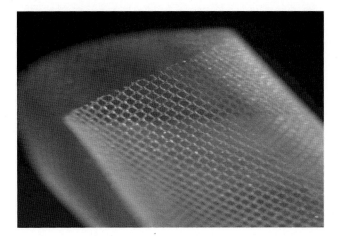

Fig. 7.47 TiMESH

Expanded PTFE prostheses (Table 7.11) have also been available in a flat sheet configuration for many years. In fact, the earliest products used in the intraperitoneal space for incisional hernia repair were of ePTFE. Because of their structure, they are solid and white unless an antimicrobial agent has been added.

The current DualMesh products are very similar in construction (Fig. 7.52). These represent the second generation

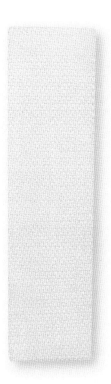

Fig. 7.45 Surgipro, monofilamented

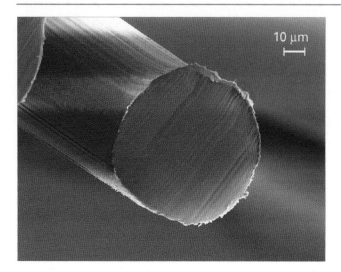

Fig. 7.48 TiMESH (scanning electron microscopic view)

Table 7.10 Flat polyester products

Angimesh R2, Angiologica, S. Martino Sicc., Italy

Mersilene, Ethicon Inc., Somerville, NJ, USA

Parietex Flat Sheet Mesh, Covidien plc, Dublin, Ireland

Parietex Lightweight Mesh, Covidien plc, Dublin, Ireland

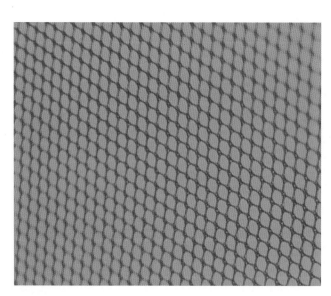

Fig. 7.49 Mersilene

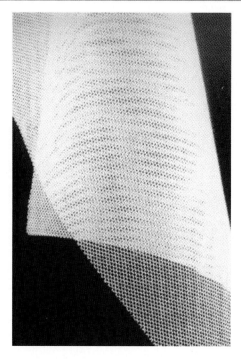

Fig. 7.50 Angimesh R2

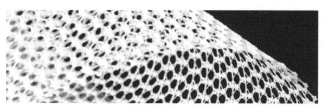

Fig. 7.51 Parietex Lightweight

Table 7.11 ePTFE products

DualMesh, W. L. Gore and Associates, Elkhart, DE, USA

DualMesh Plus, W. L. Gore and Associates, Elkhart, DE, USA

DualMesh Plus with Holes, W. L. Gore and Associates, Elkhart, DE, USA

Dulex, Davol, Inc.,Warwick, RI, USA

MycroMesh, W. L. Gore and Associates, Elkhart, DE, USA

MycroMesh Plus, W. L. Gore and Associates, Elkhart, DE, USA

Soft Tissue Patch, W. L. Gore and Associates, Elkhart, DE, USA

of this prosthetic material. These all have two distinctly different surfaces. One side is very smooth and has interstices of 3 μm while the other has the appearance of corduroy with an approximate "ridge to ridge" distance of 1500 μm. This prosthesis is designed for use in the intraperitoneal space. The smooth side must therefore be placed facing the viscera as this minimizes the potential for adhesion formation. The rough surface is applied to the abdominal wall so that maximum parietal tissue penetration will occur. *DualMesh* is

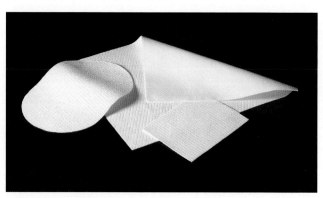

Fig. 7.52 DualMesh

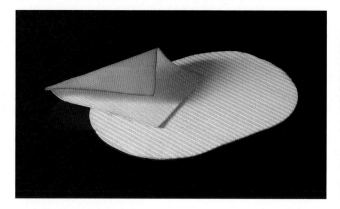

Fig. 7.53 DualMesh PLUS

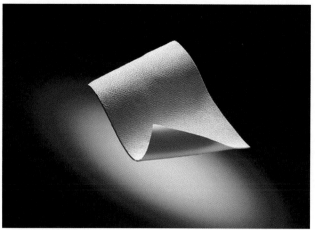

Fig. 7.55 Dulex

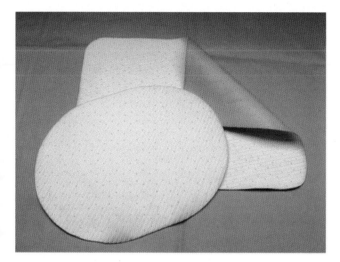

Fig. 7.54 DualMesh PLUS with Holes

available in one thickness, 1 mm. It is available with or without the impregnation of silver and chlorhexidine as *DualMesh PLUS* (Fig. 7.53). The 2-mm product is only available as DualMesh Plus with the antimicrobial agents within it. These two chemicals are antimicrobial agents that are added to decrease the risk of infection and, because of the silver, impart a brown color to the "PLUS" products. At this time, these products are the only materials impregnated with any type of any antimicrobial or bactericidal agents. *DualMesh PLUS with Holes* (Fig. 7.54) is of the same construction as that of the DualMesh. The penetration of the holes requires that this product is of 1.5 mm in thickness. The concept of the addition of these perforations is that there may be greater penetration of the fibroblasts and other cells across the material. Additionally, seroma formation might be diminished.

Dulex (Fig. 7.55) is manufactured of laminated ePTFE. One surface of the material is studded with numerous outcroppings as seen on the scanning electron microscopic view that are approximately 400 μm apart. This gives the product the gross appearance of sandpaper. The intent of this surface

is to provide for greater fibroblastic attachment and subsequent greater collagen deposition on this parietal surface. When used in the intraperitoneal fashion, the smooth surface should contact the intestine.

MycroMesh (Fig. 7.56) is also a dual-sided perforated prosthetic with one surface of 3 μm and the other of 17–22 μm. The latter surface is textured. This material is perforated for reasons that are similar to that of the DualMesh Plus with holes. It is only 1 mm thick, however. *Mycromesh PLUS* (Fig. 7.57) is impregnated with the antimicrobials silver and chlorhexidine. It is not designed for intraperitoneal usage.

The earliest implant of these ePTFE products was the *Soft Tissue Patch* (Fig. 7.58). The variety of available configurations of this product has increased over the last several years. Its use, however, has waned because of the development of the other products that are listed in Table 7.12. Like the MycroMesh, it should not contact any viscera when applied.

Miscellaneous Flat Products

There are newer products that are PTFE-based (Table 7.12). The newest available one is that of INFINIT mesh (Fig. 7.59). This is pure PTFE that has been manufactured into a large pore mesh prosthetic material, which is very supple. This is not recommended for intraperitoneal use. The two other prostheses are made of condensed PTFE (cPTFE) and are designed for use in contact with the intestine. The MotifMesh (Fig. 7.60) and Omyra (Fig. 7.61) are similar in appearance. MotifMESH Tissue Engineering Biomaterial (Fig. 7.62) is based upon cPTFE technology but little is known of its properties or indications. It is sold as a product "that can be used to create a controlled extracellular matrix (ECM) through guided tissue regeneration".

Fig. 7.56 MycroMesh

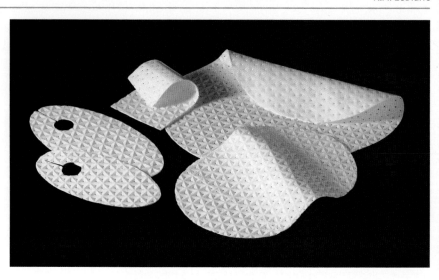

Table 7.12 Plug type prosthetic devices and manufacturer

INFINIT mesh, W. L. Gore & Associates, Elkhart, DE, USA

MotifMESH, Proxy Biomedical Ltd, Galway, Ireland

MotifMESH Tissue Engineering Biomaterial, Proxy Biomedical Ltd, Galway, Ireland

Omyra, B. Braun Melsungen AG, Melsungen, Germany

REVIVE, Biomerix Corporation of Fremont, CA, USA

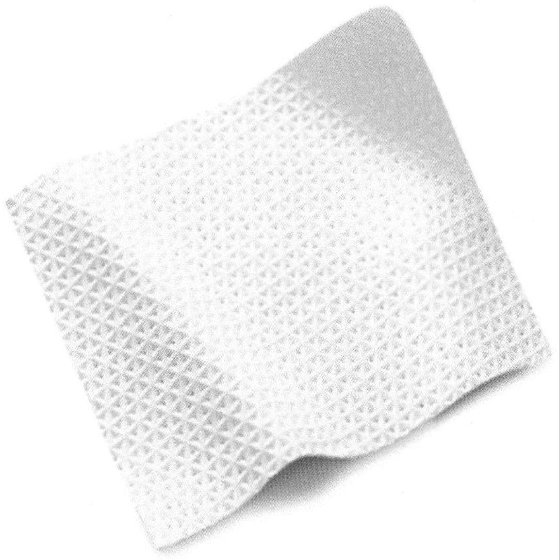

Fig. 7.57 MycroMesh PLUS

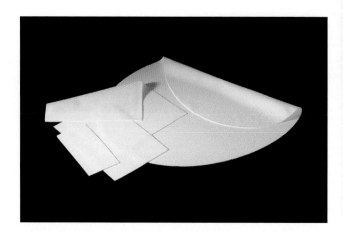

Fig. 7.58 Soft Tissue Patch

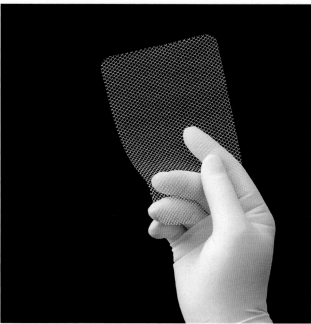

Fig. 7.59 INFINIT

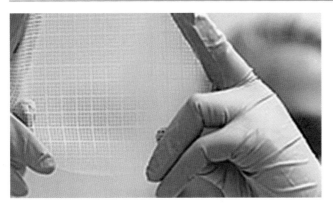

Fig. 7.60 MotifMESH

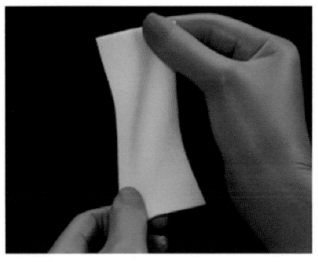

Fig. 7.63 REVIVE

Table 7.13 Flat mesh devices

Angimesh Pre 5,8,9, Angiologica, S. Martino Sicc., Italy
Angimesh Pre 5D, 8D, 9D, Angiologica, S. Martino Sicc., Italy
Bard Mesh, Davol, Inc., Warwick, RI, USA
Bard Soft Mesh, Davol, Inc., Warwick, RI, USA
Biomesh A2, Cousin Biotech, Wervicq-Sud, France
EaseGrip, Covidien plc, Dublin, Ireland
Easy Prosthesis, TransEasy Medical Tech.Co. Ltd., Beijing, China
Folded mesh A5 A5-XCO, A9-XCO, Angiologica S. Martino Sicc., Italy
HydroCoat Mesh, Promethean Surgical Devices, East Hartford, CT, USA
MycroMesh, W. L. Gore & Associates, Elkhart, DE, USA
Optilene mesh, B. Braun, Melsungen AG, Melsungen, Germany
P3, Di.pro Medical Devices, Torino, Italy
P3 Evolution, Di.pro Medical Devices, Torino, Italy
SurgimeshPET, Aspide Medical, St. Etienne, France
SurgiMesh WN, Aspide Medical, St. Etienne, France
T4 Pre-shaped Mesh with Hertra onlay mesh, HerniaMesh, S.R.L., Torino, Italy
T5 Pre-shaped Mesh with Hertra onlay mesh, HerniaMesh, S.R.L., Torino, Italy
TiPATCH, GfE Medizintechnik GmbH, Nuremburg, Germany

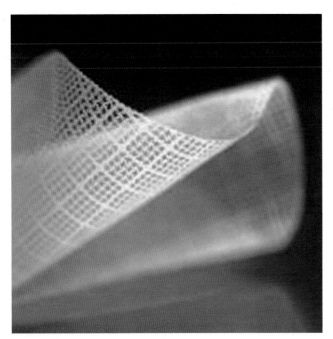

Fig. 7.61 Omyra

An interesting product that is different from all of the other products listed above is the *REVIVE* mesh (Fig. 7.63). It is made of their proprietary Biomerix Biomaterial that is a cross-linked and reticulated polycarbonate polyurethane-urea. It is a three-dimensional, open-cell, macroporous structure. There is no clinical data at the time of this writing as it has just received governmental approval for clinical use.

Flat Mesh Devices for Inguinal Hernioplasty

There are several modifications of the shape of the synthetic meshes described above. For the most part, the ones listed in Table 7.13 are merely the same permanent material that is

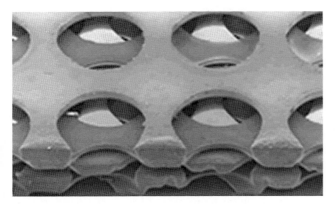

Fig. 7.62 MotifMESH Tissue Engineering Biomaterial

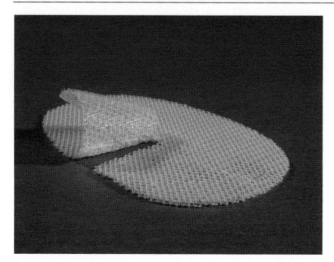

Fig. 7.64 EaseGrip

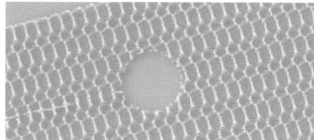

Fig. 7.66 P3 Evolution

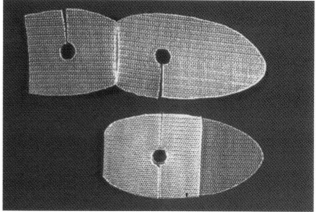

Fig. 7.67 Folded Mesh

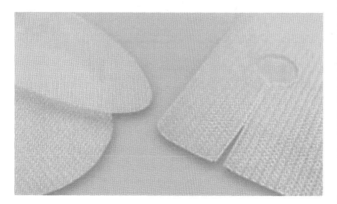

Fig. 7.65 P3

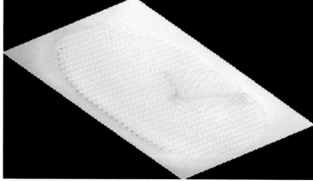

Fig. 7.68 SurgiMesh PET (open)

either pre-shaped with rounded edges and/or have a slit and/ or keyhole to be used for open inguinal hernia repair. Some of these keyholes will be located on the long axis of the mesh to be placed while others will be placed on the short axis of the mesh. If there is a significant modification, it is noted below.

EaseGrip (Fig. 7.64) is composed of the three-dimensional POL of Parietex (see above) and is manufactured with a left and a right mesh. It is elliptical in shape with a colored marker on the median edge of the prosthesis to indicate the location of the suture that is placed at the pubic tubercle for fixation. There is a self-gripping flap that is designed to overlap the slit that is precut into the biomaterial, which allows for the exit of the cord structures through the mesh. This flap is placed in the inferior position of the inguinal floor. The manufacturer recommends that the external oblique fascia be closed below the cord structures so that there is no direct contact with the polyester fabric.

The *P3* (Fig. 7.65) is manufactured in light, medium, and heavy weight PPM with products for the male and

female patient. The "male" product is supplied with a slit and keyhole for the cord structures to pass while the "female" product has no slit or hole. Only the "male" mesh is provided in the heavy weight mesh. The *P3 Evolution* (Fig. 7.66) version is similar but ultra-lightweight. The *Folded Mesh* (Fig. 7.67) has two connected pieces of PPM. The larger piece is placed onto the floor of the inguinal canal and the smaller piece overlaps the larger to cover the internal inguinal ring. *SurgiMesh PET* (Fig. 7.68) is a

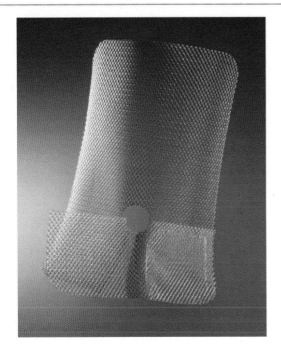

Fig. 7.69 TiPATCH

Table 7.14 Combination products

Adhesix, Cousin Biotech, Wervicq-Sud, France
Easy Prosthesis II, TransEasy Medical Tech.Co. Ltd., Beijing, China
Parietene ProGrip, Covidien plc, Dublin, Ireland
Parietex ProGrip, Covidien plc, Dublin, Ireland
Vypro, Ethicon, Inc., Somerville, NJ, USA
Vypro II, Ethicon, Inc., Somerville, NJ, USA
Ultrapro, Ethicon, Inc., Somerville, NJ, USA

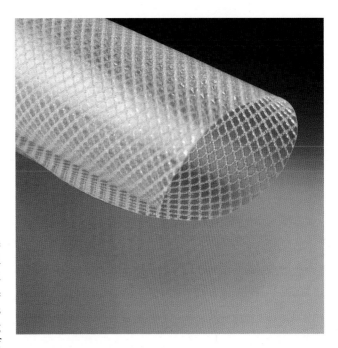

Fig. 7.70 Adhesix

three-dimensional POL product that has a hole to allow the passage of the cord during open repair and a flap designed to cover the slit in the product. *SurgiMesh WN* (Figs. 7.42 and 7.43) is available in two different thicknesses. The *TiPATCH* (Fig. 7.69) is made of the same material as TiMESH (Figs. 7.47 and 7.48) but this has two overlapping pieces of the mesh to cover behind the cord structures of the inguinal hernia repair.

Combination Flat Synthetic Prosthetics for Hernioplasty

This grouping of these products is made because there is a permanent portion of these materials and an absorbable component to the product. These prostheses are not meant to contact any viscera. (Table 7.14)

Adhesix (Fig. 7.70), *Parietene ProGrip*, and *Parietex ProGrip* (Fig. 7.71) all have self-attaching portions of the prosthesis so that once placed onto the tissue surface, they will fixate themselves. These "gripping portions" are absorbable. The permanent portions of Adhesix and Parietene ProGrip are made of PP while the Parietex ProGrip is POL. Adhesix has a coating on one side that is made of polyvinylpyrrolidone and polyethylene glycol. This coating turns into an adhesive gel when it comes into contact with both heat and humidity. Both of the ProGrip products contain grippers, which are prominent in Fig. 7.71, made of PLA. These all can be used either open or laparoscopically. Because

of the gel coating rather than grippers on the Adhesix, it is easier to reposition, if necessary.

Easy Prosthesis II (Fig. 7.72) is a partially absorbable product. It is a combination of PP and poly(glycolide-cocaprolactone) [PGCL] monofilaments. The PGCL portion will be completely absorbed within 90–120 days. The materials, *Vypro* and *Vypro II* (Fig. 7.73) are actually a combination of PP and the absorbable polymer polydioxanone (PDO). The combination of these materials results in a very pliable and malleable material. Once the PDO has been absorbed, the PP that remains has very large interstices into which the fibroblasts and collagen are deposited. The aim of these products is the improvement in the abdominal wall compliance that is more normal in function because of the very lightweight PP that remains. *Ultrapro* (Fig. 7.74) mesh is a similar concept and is manufactured from approximately equal parts of the absorbable poliglecaprone-25 monofilament fiber and the nonabsorbable lightweight PP. A portion of the PP is dyed. The absorbable portion is essentially absorbed by 84 days.

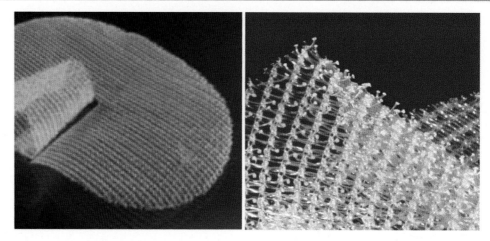

Fig. 7.71 Parietex ProGrip (Close-up of the grippers on the right)

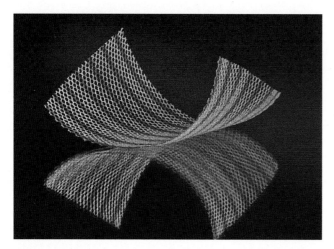

Fig. 7.72 Easy Prosthesis II

Preformed Prosthetic Devices for Open Hernioplasty

There has been a significant amount of interest in the repair of inguinal and femoral hernias utilizing one of the many preformed prosthetic devices in the last several years. The manufacturers of these prostheses have developed several ingenious products for this use. All are of a polypropylene biomaterial with the exception of the Parietex Plug (Table 7.15). There is currently an increasing interest by a few surgeons in the application of some of these for the repair of other hernias of the abdominal wall such as umbilical and ventral hernias.

The first commercially successful device was that of the PerFix Plug and patch. The repair of inguinal hernias with this product simply involves the insertion of the plug through the fascial defect into the extraperitoneal plane, which is then secured to the edges of the fascia. Additionally, they also employ the use of an overlay of an additional piece of mesh to complete the repair. There are structural differences with these products that alter the concept of each one. Some surgeons also modify these plugs prior to insertion to more completely protect the preperitoneal space.

There are several "self-forming" plugs. These are flat, round, and without a hole rather than being pre-shaped, as one would expect a true plug-like product. The *Basic plug* is one of these (Fig. 7.75). The makers of such devices believe that this is a "one-size fits all" concept in that they can be utilized in any size of a fascial defect. Other products that correspond to this design are the *Self-Forming Plug* (Fig. 7.76) and the *SurgiMesh EasyPlug Standard* (Fig. 7.77) and the *Parietex Plug*. The Self-Forming Plug differs from the other two single layer products in that it is made of three circular flat meshes constructed of Atrium mesh. These are bonded together with a tab on one surface to allow for the grasping of the product by forceps during insertion. This is still soft and pliable so that it assumes the shape of the defect rather than forcing itself into the defect. It is available in different sizes.

The *Easy Prosthesis Plug* (Fig. 7.78) is a traditionally designed plug with petals within it. These can be modified, if needed, depending upon the choice of the surgeon. The *4D Dome* (Fig. 7.79) is different from all of the other plug type devices. It is a single layer of PP but it is shaped into a rounded, rather than a pointed, shape. The insertion and fixation is the same as the more traditional plugs.

The *PerFix Plug* (Fig. 7.80) is available in four different sizes. This is the most mature of these commercial products. Because of the trend to lighter weight PP in the repair of hernias, it is also available in the *PerFix Light Plug* (Fig. 7.81). These allow for modification of the plug in that the surgeon can remove the inner petals at the time of implantation. Some

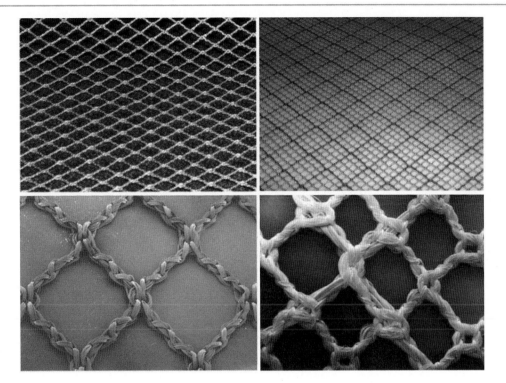

Fig. 7.73 Vypro (left) and Vypro II (*right*)

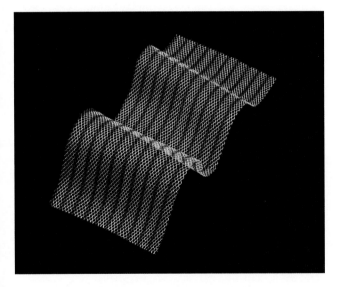

Fig. 7.74 Ultrapro

Table 7.15 Plug type products

Basic plug, Angiologica, S. Martino Sicc, Italy
Easy Prosthesis Plug, TransEasy Medical Tech.Co. Ltd., Beijing, China
4D Dome, Cousin Biotech, Wervicq-Sud, France
Parietex Plug, Covidien plc, Dublin, Ireland
PerFix Plug, Davol Inc., Warwick, RI, USA
Perfix Light Plug, Davol Inc., Warwick, RI, USA
Premilene Mesh Plug, B. Braun Melsungen AG, Melsungen, Germany
Proloop Plug, Atrium Medical Corporation, Hudson, NH, USA
Repol Plug Cap, Angiologica, S. Martino Sicc., Italy
Repol Plug Flower, Angiologica, S. Martino Sicc., Italy
Self-Forming Plug, Atrium Medical Inc., Hudson, NH,
SurgiMesh EasyPlug Standard, Aspide Medical, St. Etienne, France
SurgiMesh WN EasyPlug, Aspide Medical, St. Etienne, France
SurgiMesh WN EasyPlug "No Touch", Aspide Medical, St. Etienne, France
T2 Plug, HerniaMesh, S.R.L., Torino, Italy
T3 Plug, HerniaMesh, S.R.L., Torino, Italy
TEC Evolution plug—Di.pro Medical Devices, Torino, Italy
TiLENE plug, GfE Medizintechnik, Nuremburg, Germany WEB
TP plug, Di.pro Medical Devices, Torino, Italy
TiPLUG—GfE Medizintechnik, Nuremburg, Germany WEB
Ultrapro Plug, Ethicon Inc., Somerville, NJ, USA

surgeons have reported good results with completely opening the petals in the preperitoneal space [9]. Other products that are also fluted but do not allow any modification are the *Premilene Mesh Plug* (Fig. 7.82) and the *Repol Flower* (Fig. 7.83). The *Proloop Plug* (Fig. 7.84) is a pointed type of plug but it lacks any internal structure so it, too, cannot be modified. As shown in the photo, this product is quite different in appearance in the other plug devices. Although pre-

formed into a cylindrical shape, it is very supple and conforms to the defect into which it is inserted.

The *Repol Plug Cap* represents a concept that combines a small piece of a flat PPM and a cone-shaped plug (Fig. 7.85).

Similar products are the T2 and T3 *Plugs.* These devices are also significantly different from all of the other plugs. The *T2 Plug* (Fig. 7.86) has a circular piece of flat mesh that has a rounded plug portion affixed to it whereas the *T3 Plug* (Fig. 7.87) has a rectangular piece of mesh affixed to it. There are differing sizes that are chosen based upon the size of the defect. With any of these three devices, one can insert the plug component into the preperitoneal space and use the flat portion to sew to the fascial edges as a small onlay or underlay.

The *SurgiMesh WN EasyPlug* (Fig. 7.88) differs in several ways. It is of the non-knitted PP and also has two strips to allow for easier fixation. The *SurgiMesh WN EasyPlug* "No Touch" (Fig. 7.89) device is a preformed plug with variable geometry and is adjustable to the size of the defect. An applicator is supplied to make this a "no touch" implantation. As purse-string suture is part of the device to help in sizing of the plug.

The *TEC Evolution* plug (Fig. 7.90) is made in the conical shape and is fluted, as are most plugs, but of an ultra-lightweight PP material. There is a second design of the TEC Evolution plug (Fig. 7.91) that has lightweight petals and a medium weight base. The *TiLene Plug* (Fig. 7.92) is of the TiMesh product that has been previously described. It is a flat product that will conform to the hernia defect as it is inserted. The outer layers of the petals are medium weight PP and the inner petals are a lighter weight PP. The *TP* plug is a rounded mesh with or without an eccentric hole and with or without a slit to that hole. The TiPLUG (Fig. 7.93) is also made of TiMESH. It has a flap through which the cord structures are to be placed. As such, it differs from all of the other plugs listed. The *Ultrapro Plug* (Fig. 7.94) is made from the previously described Ultrapro mesh. The absorbable and nonabsorbable portions are connected by the absorbable poliglecaprone-25 fibers.

Extraperitoneal Prosthetic Devices for Open Inguinal Hernioplasty

The posterior repair of open inguinal hernias is based upon the approach into the preperitoneal space. The use of a preformed prosthetic device in this space represents an emulation of the Stoppa repair and the giant prosthetic repair of the visceral sac of Wantz. The products that have been manufactured

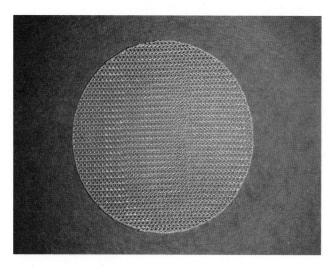

Fig. 7.75 Basic Plug

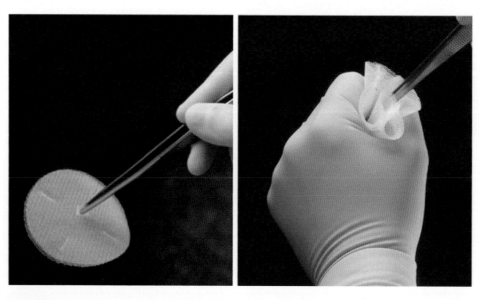

Fig. 7.76 Self-forming Plug

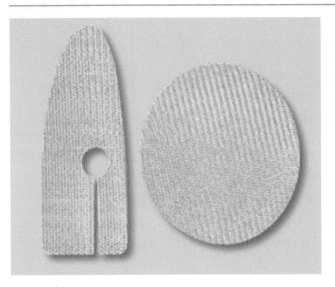

Fig. 7.77 SurgiMesh EasyPlug Standard

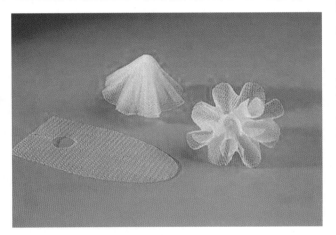

Fig. 7.78 Easy Prosthesis Plug

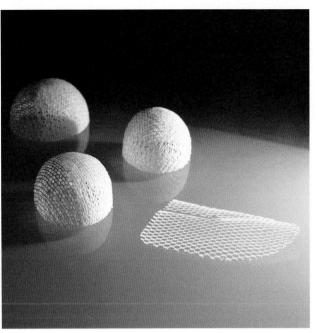

Fig. 7.79 4D Dome

for this concept are not "giant" prostheses, however (Table 7.16).

Easy Prosthesis (self-forming) hernia repair patch (Fig. 7.95) has two bonded PP layers. One will lie in the preperitoneal space and the other as an onlay in the inguinal hernia repair. The *Easy Prosthesis (preperitoneal)* hernia repair patch (Fig. 7.96) also has an underlay portion but instead of the flat sheet of PP, there are petals that can be stitched to the fascial edges of the hernia itself. This is similar to the plug and patch repair as the product is supplied with an onlay patch to place underneath the external oblique.

The *Kugel Patch* (Fig. 7.97) consists of two oblong circular flat meshes of Bard mesh. One of these has a slit to allow the insertion of a finger to aid in the positioning of the product. Near the edge of the device is a polyester ring that maintains the shape of the device after insertion into the preperitoneal space. There are several sizes of this product as well as those that are in a circular configuration. The *Modified Kugel Patch* (Fig. 7.98) adds a strap of PP to assist in the positioning of the product. In addition, this strap can be sewn to the edges of the fascial defect in the inguinal floor. This device also comes with an onlay piece of PP to be placed onto the internal oblique aponeurosis. The *Polysoft Patch* (Fig. 7.99) is similar to the Kugel patch in that it is designed for placement exclusively in the preperitoneal space. Its shape is very similar to the laparoscopic 3D Max (see Fig. 7.109). It currently is available only in Europe.

The *Prolene Hernia System* (Fig. 7.100) is similar to the Easy Prosthesis (Fig. 7.95) in that it is designed to place mesh in the extraperitoneal plane and onto the inguinal floor as a traditional tension-free repair. The difference between the two products is that the older PHS has a connector piece that attaches the rounded underlay portion and the elliptical portion. There are three size of the PHS, medium, large, and extended. The choice of the size will depend upon the size and type of defect as well as the size of the patient and location of the hernia. These have also been used for umbilical and ventral hernias. The *Ultrapro Hernia System* (Fig. 7.101) is a combination product that is made from Ultrapro flat mesh that has the identical shape as the PHS that has incorporated poliglecaprone-25. The latter product is wound with the PP fibers and is placed as a film to ease the use of the device. This absorbable component of the Ultrapro will leave behind a very lightweight PPM to repair the hernia.

Fig. 7.80 PerFix Plug

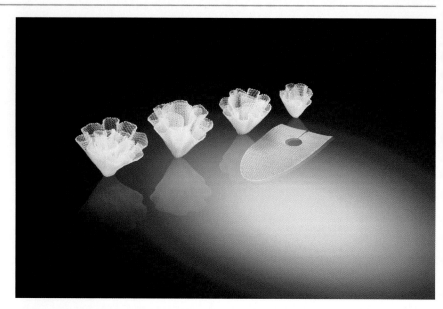

Fig. 7.81 PerFix Light Plug

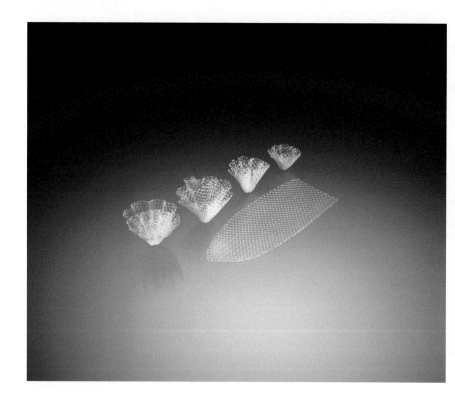

The *Prolene 3D Patch* (Fig. 7.102) is a three-dimensional device, which possesses two different portions of this product. The diamond-shaped portion is inserted into the preperitoneal space. A single pull of the suture causes the diamond to flatten out underneath the tranversalis fascia. The overlay portion is then secured as in the tension-free repairs. It is available in two sizes of the diamond portion and with or without a pre-shaped overlay.

Pre-shaped Products for Laparoscopic Inguinal Hernioplasty

The history of laparoscopic repair of inguinal hernias involved flat meshes of one type or another. This continues to be the most frequently used prosthetic product for this operation (Tables 7.10, 7.11, and 7.12). There are, however, a number of devices that have been constructed for this

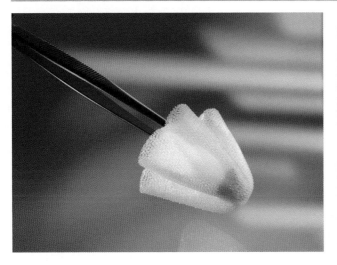

Fig. 7.82 Premilene Mesh Plug

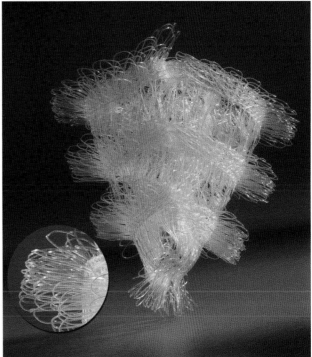

Fig. 7.84 Proloop Plug

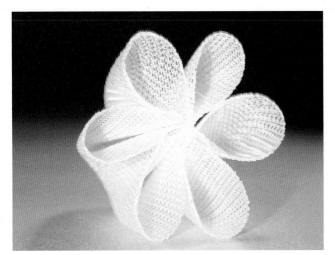

Fig. 7.83 Repol Flower

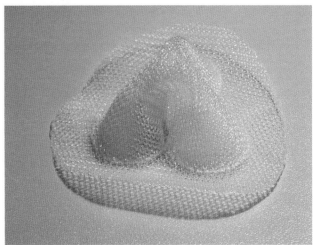

Fig. 7.85 Repol Plug Cap

procedure (Table 7.17). These all attempt to ease the placement of the prosthetic over the myopectineal orifice or serve to conform to the anatomic surfaces at that site of the repair. These can be placed with either the transabdominal preperitoneal (TAPP) or totally extraperitoneal (TEP) approaches. A few are manufactured to make fixation with any type of fastener unnecessary.

The *C-LAP* (Fig. 7.103) lightweight PP prosthesis is designed for laparoscopic inguinal hernia repair. It is a PP product with slits, curves, and shapes to conform to the inguinal floor. These are labeled as male with direct and indirect designs or female in a single design. *Parietex Anatomical Mesh* (Fig. 7.104) is of the same three-dimensional weave of POL as the other Parietex products on the lower portion of the product which is softer and designed to lie on the vessels. The portion that is placed on the posterior aspect of the inguinal floor is a more rigid two-dimensional weave to aid in

handling. It is generally used with the application of some type of fixation but some surgeons do not see the need to add these fasteners. It has a left and right design. The *Folding Mesh with Suture* (Fig. 7.105) is shaped as a flat polyester mesh with rounded edges. To aid in the insertion and deployment of this mesh in the preperitoneal space during the laparoscopic repair, there is a suture that is woven through the material. This suture is placed such that when it is pulled tight the mesh will be drawn into a small somewhat cylindrical shape. It is then placed into the preperitoneal space

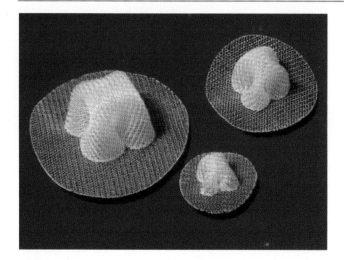

Fig. 7.86 T2 Plug

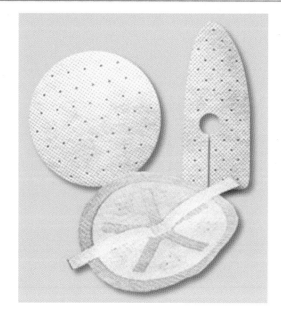

Fig. 7.88 SurgiMesh WN EasyPlug

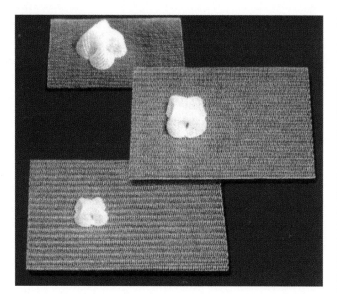

Fig. 7.87 T3 Plug

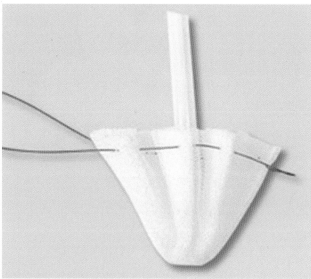

Fig. 7.89 SurgiMesh WN EasyPlug "No Touch"

whereupon the suture is cut, allowing the mesh to resume its original shape. It can then be positioned appropriately. This device is also available with a slit if one desires to place the cord structures within the slit.

Rebound HRD (Fig. 7.106) is a rather unique concept in hernia repair. This device is designed to maintain the shape of the product after introduction into the preperitoneal space by the incorporation of a self-expanding nitinol alloy frame at the perimeter of the mesh. There is an introducing tube that is also shown in the figure. The mesh itself is also unusual in that it is a macroporous cPTFE, which is tied to the frame with a polyethylene-braided suture. This prosthesis can also be used with an open approach. Because of the presence of this nitinol, this is the only prosthesis that can be visualized on radiologic studies postoperatively.

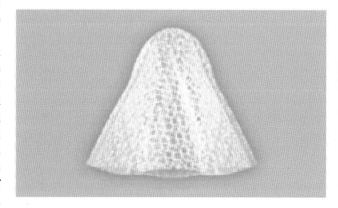

Fig. 7.90 TEC Evolution

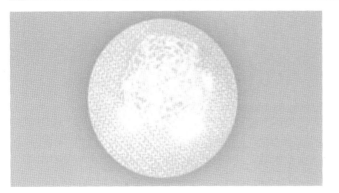

Fig. 7.91   TEC Evolution (second design)

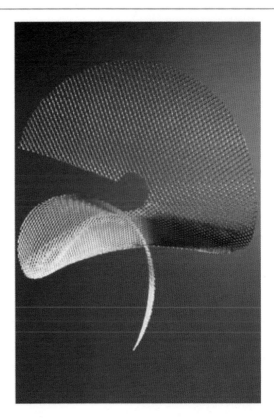

Fig. 7.93   TiPLUG

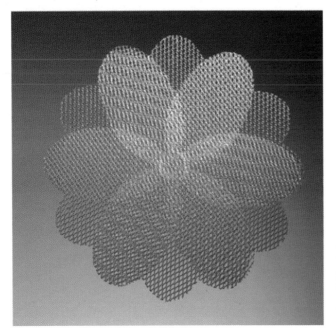

Fig. 7.92   TiLENE Plug

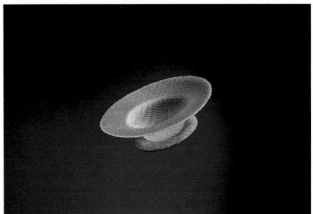

Fig. 7.94   Ultrapro Plug

SurgiMesh WN (Figs. 7.42 and 7.43) has the same structure as that of most of the SurgiMesh products listed in the prior tables. There are two laparoscopic products. One is a single flat square sheet with a rounded portion cutout on one corner. This is to be placed at Cooper's ligament. The other product has a keyhole and a flap to allow the product to be placed onto the posterior wall of the inguinal canal with the cord structures placed in the keyhole. The flap then covers the slit and keyhole to seal this defect in the mesh. *SurgiMesh PET* (Fig. 7.107) is a POL product that is available in an anatomical shape requiring limited fixation. The two-dimensional structure (not the three-dimensional) is designed for laparoscopic use. *SurgiMesh XD* (Fig. 7.108) is of two different types of PP. It is of a shape to allow placement in the inguinal floor laparoscopically. As shown in the photo, the majority of the product is perforated and composed of non-

woven, non-knitted PP. The smooth portions of the prosthesis are of knitted PP. The vertical portion is to align with the spermatic cord and the horizontal portion is to align with Cooper's ligament.

The *3D Max* and *3D Max Light* (Fig. 7.109) products are similar in shape and sizes (medium, large, and extra large). They differ in the weight of the PP within each product. The former is of the heavy weight Bard mesh and the latter is of the lighter Bard Soft Mesh. Both have an "M" and an arrow on the medial aspect of the product to indicate the positioning

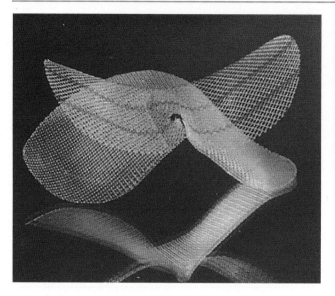

Fig. 7.95 Easy Prosthesis Self-forming Hernia Repair Patch

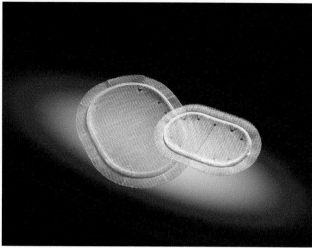

Fig. 7.97 Kugel Patch

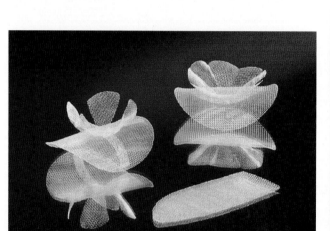

Fig. 7.96 Easy Prosthesis Preperitoneal Hernia Repair Patch

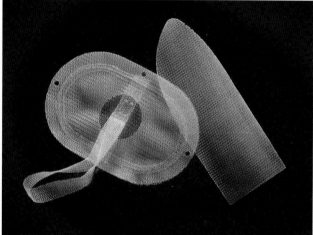

Fig. 7.98 Modified Kugel Patch

Table 7.16 Flat devices and their manufacturer

Easy Prosthesis (Self-forming), TransEasy Medical Tech.Co. Ltd., Beijing, China

Easy Prosthesis (Preperitoneal), TransEasy Medical Tech.Co. Ltd., Beijing, China

Kugel Patch, Davol Inc., Warwick, RI, USA

Modified Kugel Patch, Davol Inc., Warwick, RI, USA

Polysoft Patch, Davol Inc., Warwick, RI, USA

Prolene Hernia System, Ethicon Inc., Somerville, NJ, USA

Prolene 3D Patch, Ethicon Inc., Somerville, NJ, USA

Ultrapro Hernia System, Ethicon Inc., Somerville, NJ, USA

of the prosthesis. These are curved to conform to the shape of the pelvis. Because of this curved shape, there is a right and left product. There is also an indentation on the inferior aspect of the product to indicate the location of the iliac

vessels. *Visilex* (Fig. 7.110) is flat Bard mesh that has a stiffer border designed to ease the manipulation of the product in the preperitoneal space.

Prostheses for Incisional and Ventral Hernioplasty with an Absorbable Component

The original impetus behind the development of these products was the popularity of the laparoscopic methodology. In general, however, all of these prosthetic devices can or have been used in both open and laparoscopic incisional hernioplasties. All of these have the common purpose to repair the hernia and prevent the development of adhesions with the attendant complications associated with this result of the healing processes. These are generally referred to as "tissue-separating" meshes as they create an

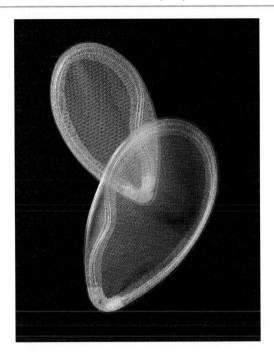

Fig. 7.99 PolySoft Patch

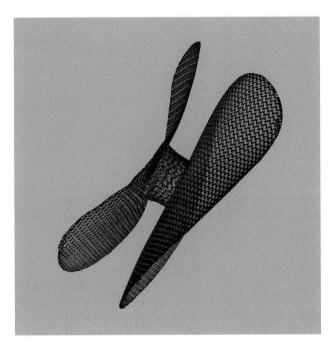

Fig. 7.100 Prolene Hernia System (PHS)

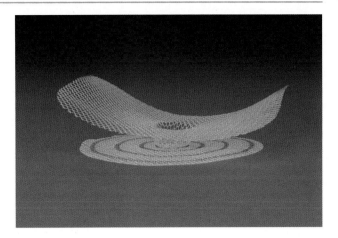

Fig. 7.101 Ultrapro Hernia System (UHS)

absorbable barrier between the permanent product and the viscera (Table 7.18).

The resorption of that nonpermanent substance leaves a permanent layer of mesh that will incorporate into the tissues of the patient. The controversial part of this idea is the fact that the problems that are related to the development of adhesions following the implantation of a synthetic biomaterial do not become manifest for many years postimplantation. Therefore, the late effects of these products will necessitate many years of follow-up to validate these claims. At the present time, however, these meshes do seem to live up to their expectations.

Adhesix is the same product that was listed in Table 7.14. It is touted that this can be used in the preperitoneal position, the retrorectus space, or as an onlay but it is not designed for use in contact with the viscera. Consequently if differs for all of the other products listed in Table 7.18 below. *Biomerix Composite Surgical Mesh* is composite of three products, the Biomerix Biomaterial, REVIVE, described in the "Miscellaneous Flat Mesh section," PP, and a resorbable lactide-caprolactone film (Fig. 7.63).

CA.B.S.' Air SR (Fig. 7.111) has a permanent component of 25% lightweight PP and 75% resorbable poly-L-lactic acid (PLLA). It differs from all of the other products in that it has two permanent sutures with needles that are attached and it is also accompanied by a balloon dissection device as it the CA.B.S.' Air described below (see Fig. 7.123). This device is designed for use in umbilical hernia repair. The entire product is inserted; the balloon is used to dissect the tissues and is then removed, leaving behind the prosthesis with the attached sutures to fixate it.

C-QUR (Fig. 7.112) is made of a lightweight PP onto which Omega-3 Fatty Acid (O3FA) has been into and onto the product. These fatty acids are in a cross-linked gel that covers both sides of the material and impart a characteristic dark yellow color. O3FA will absorb over a period of 3–6 months. *C-QUR EDGE* (Fig. 7.113) adds a reinforced edge to the product to enhance fixation stability and ease of use. *C-QUR Lite* (Fig. 7.114) is like the C-QUR but contains a thinner layer of the O3FA such that the coating will last only about 30 days. *C-QUR OVT* is a single-layer product like the C-QUR but adds as second layer of the product that is cut into flaps to ease its fixation in open hernia repair. The *C-QUR V-Patch* (Fig. 7.115) is designed for umbilical hernia

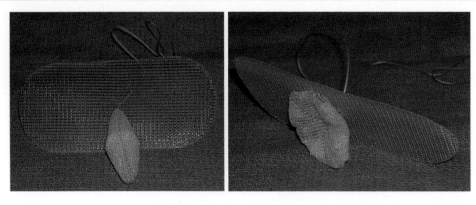

Fig. 7.102 Prolene 3D Patch, pre-deployment (*left*), and post-deployment (*right*)

Table 7.17 Pre-shaped products for laparoscopic inguinal hernia repair

CLAP, Di.pro Medical Devices, Torino, Italy
Parietex Anatomical Mesh, Covidien plc, Dublin, Ireland
Parietex Folding Mesh with Suture, Covidien plc, Dublin, Ireland
Rebound HRD, Minnesota Medical Development, Plymouth, MN, USA
SurgiMesh WN, Aspide Medical, St. Etienne, France
SurgiMeshPET, Aspide Medical, St. Etienne, France
SurgiMesh XD, Aspide Medical, St. Etienne, France
3D Max, Davol, Inc., Warwick, RI, USA
3D Max Light, Davol, Inc., Warwick, RI, USA
Visilex, Davol, Inc., Warwick, RI, USA

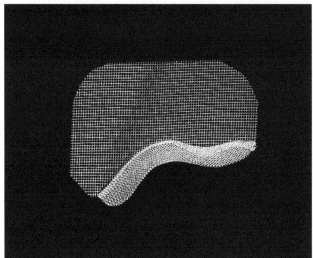

Fig. 7.104 Parietex Anatomical Mesh

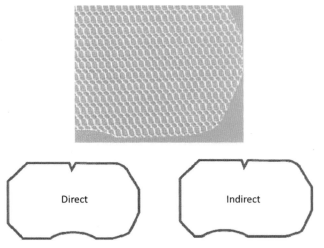

Fig. 7.103 C-LAP

repair but one could see its use for smaller incisional hernias as well. There is an O3FA reinforcement washer that stiffens the product to ease insertion. The fixation straps are secured to the edge of the defect and the excess is removed.

Easy Prosthesis (PPM/Collagen) (Fig. 7.116) is a very unique concept at this time. Bovine tendon is configured and bonded to PP. At the time of this writing there are no other combination biologic/synthetic meshes available, although several are in research stages. This collagen layer becomes a continuous gel within 1 h of implantation. It is said to minimize visceral attachment and, as such, can be used intraperitoneally. Little is known of the clinical results of this product. It is available in several sizes and shapes and can be used for parastomal and hiatal hernia repairs as well, as shown in the photo.

Parietene Composite is a little known PP described earlier that is coated with the hydrophilic collagen and other substances that are used in the better-known Parietex Composite discussed below. *Parietex Composite* (Fig. 7.117) is the same POL biomaterial that is described earlier in this chapter. It has an incorporated hydrophilic layer of a mixture of oxidized Type I atelocollagen, polyethylene glycol, and glycerol, which is absorbable. It is also available as the *Parietex Composite Skirted Mesh* (Fig. 7.118). The skirt is a second layer placed over the larger mesh itself to allow for easier

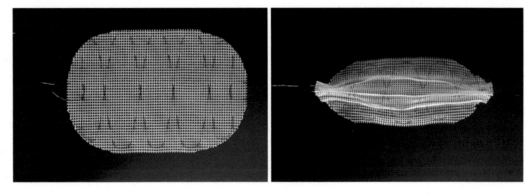

Fig. 7.105 Folding Mesh with Suture, unfolded (*left*) and folded (*right*)

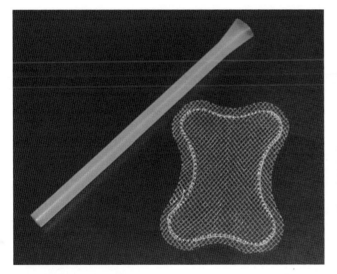

Fig. 7.106 Rebound HRD

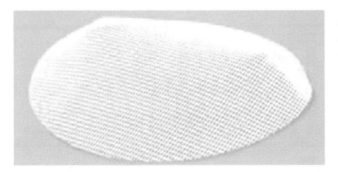

Fig. 7.107 SurgiMesh PET (laparoscopic)

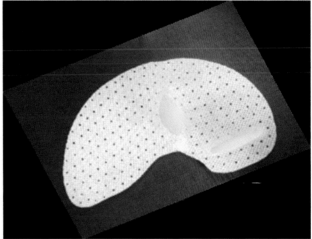

Fig. 7.108 SurgiMesh XD

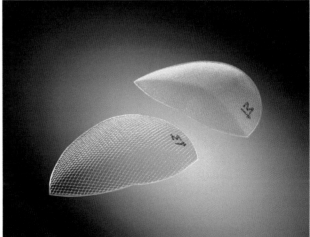

Fig. 7.109 3D Max, light (*left*), and regular (*right*)

placement of the fixation devices that can be used to fix the product to the anterior abdominal wall in the open technique. *Parietene ProGrip* and *Parietex ProGrip* (Fig. 7.71) also differ in that: the former is of PP and the latter is of POL. Both have the PLA grippers (described earlier in this chapter) so that they do not need fixation.

PHYSIOMESH Flexible Composite Mesh (Fig. 7.119) is made of macroporous PP laminated between two undyed polyglecaprone-25 films, which are absorbable. Another PDO film bonds these three layers together. For orientation

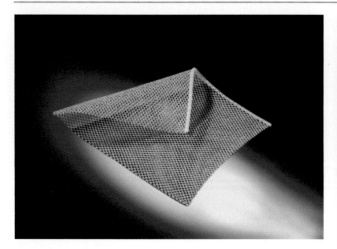

Fig. 7.110 Visilex

Table 7.18 Prostheses with an absorbable component

Adhesix, Cousin Biotech, Wervicq-Sud, France
Biomerix Composite Surgical Mesh, Biomerix Corporation, Fremont, CA
CA.B.S. 'Air SR, Cousin Biotech, Wervicq-Sud, France
C-QUR, Atrium Medical Corp., Hudson, NH, USA
C-QUR EDGE, Atrium Medical Corp., Hudson, NH, USA
C-QUR Lite, Atrium Medical Corp., Hudson, NH, USA
C-QUR OVT Mesh, Atrium Medical Corp., Hudson, NH, USA
C-QUR V-Patch, Atrium Medical Corp., Hudson, NH, USA
Easy Prosthesis (PPM/Collagen), TransEasy Medical Tech.Co. Ltd., Beijing, China
Parietene Composite (PPC), Covidien plc, Dublin, Ireland
Parietex Composite (PCO), Covidien plc, Dublin, Ireland
Parietex Composite (PCO) Skirted Mesh, Covidien plc, Dublin, Ireland
Parietene ProGrip, Covidien plc, Dublin, Ireland
Parietex ProGrip, Covidien plc, Dublin, Ireland
PHYSIOMESH, Ethicon, Inc., Somerville, NJ, USA
Proceed, Ethicon, Inc., Somerville, NJ, USA
PVP, Ethicon, Inc., Somerville, NJ, USA
SepraMesh IP, Davol, Inc., Warwick, RI, USA
Ventralex ST, Davol, Inc., Warwick, RI, USA
Ventrio ST, Davol, Inc., Warwick, RI, USA

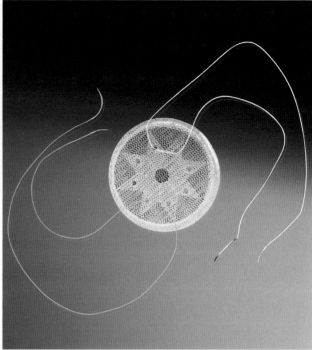

Fig. 7.111 CA.B.S' Air SR

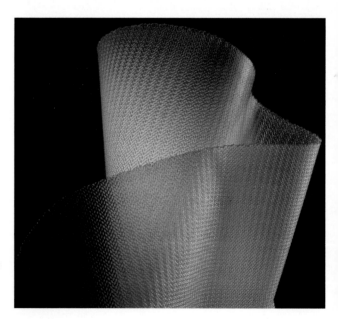

Fig. 7.112 C-QUR

purposes a dyed PDO film marker of the is added. *Proceed* (Fig. 7.120) is composed of an oxidized regenerated cellulose (ORC) fabric and Prolene Soft Mesh which is encapsulated by a PDO polymer that holds this together. The fabric acts as a barrier to separate the PP from the tissue. The ORC is absorbed within 4 weeks. An issue with this product is the fact that the instructions for use state "Proceed Mesh has an ORC component that should not be used in the presence of uncontrolled and/or active bleeding as fibrinous exudates may increase the chance of adhesion formation." The *PVP* or *Proceed Ventral Patch* (Fig. 7.121) has an ORC layer that is placed toward the intestine to protect it from the PPM product above it. In this product, there is an additional layer of

PDO polymer and a positioning ring to provide memory. Vicryl mesh (polyglactin 910) is placed on top of the PDO and is encapsulated with a PDO film. The sutures that are seen in the photo are of polyester.

SepraMesh (Fig. 7.122) is a single layer of polypropylene is covered by barrier that is a combination of carboxymethylcellulose and hyaluronic acid. It is bound together with

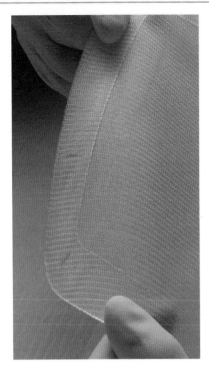

Fig. 7.113 C-QUR EDGE

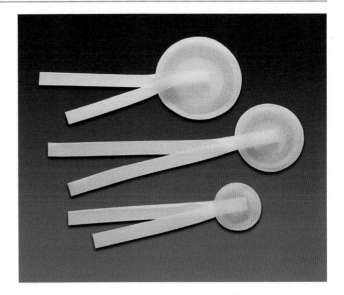

Fig. 7.115 C-QUR V-Patch

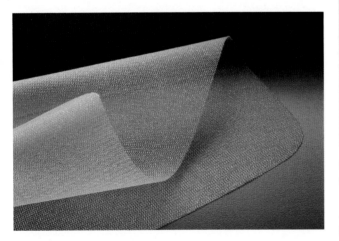

Fig. 7.114 C-QUR Lite

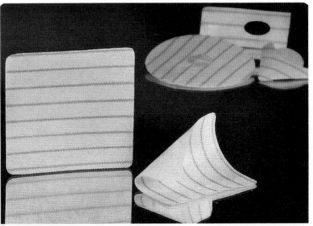

Fig. 7.116 Easy Prosthesis (polypropylene/collagen composite surgical mesh)

polyglycolic acid fibers and a hydrogel. This is the only product in this section that requires brief immersion into saline solution prior to its use to activate the gel. This hydrogel swells following implantation to cover the fixation devices that are used. This portion of the product is stated to last approximately 4 weeks, at which point, it has been resorbed. The "Sepra" technology has been extended to the Ventralex (see Fig. 7.135) and Ventrio (see Fig. 7.136) products. The ePTFE surface has been replaced with the tissue-separating hydrogel that is used on the SepraMesh prosthesis. These products are called *Ventralex ST* and *Ventrio ST*.

Combination Permanent Materials for Incisional and Ventral Hernioplasty

There has been an incredible increase in the number of permanent products available for the open and/or laparoscopic repair of incisional and ventral hernias since the last edition of this textbook (Table 7.19). All of those listed below are a combination of a single product that is manufactured in two different forms or, more commonly, a combination of two different products. The method of fixation of these products differs from each manufacturer. There are some that have been described earlier in this chapter that are single products and are not described again here (Table 7.11). What is consistent in all of the prostheses is the creation of some type of a barrier to adhesion formation while allowing for

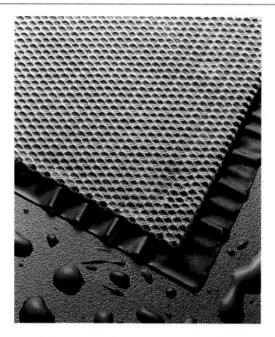

Fig. 7.117 Parietex Composite

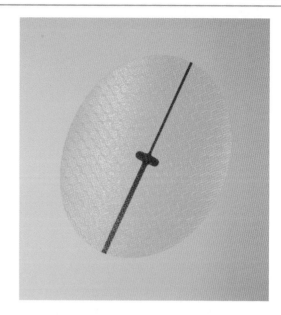

Fig. 7.119 PHYSIOMESH

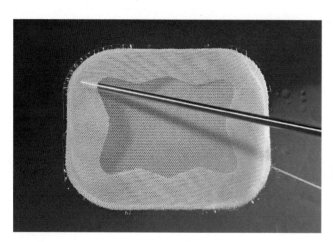

Fig. 7.118 Parietex Composite Skirted Mesh

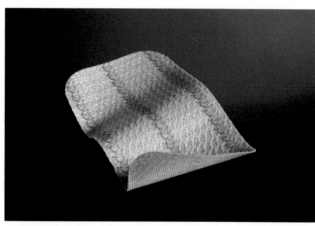

Fig. 7.120 Proceed

ingrowth on the parietal side of these meshes to repair a hernia effectively.

The *CA.B.S.* '*Air* (Fig. 7.123) is similar to the *CA.B.S.*' *Air SR* (Fig. 7.111) device described above. They both are constructed of two materials and inserted with the aid of a balloon dissection device that is removed (Fig. 7.124). The SR device is semi-resorbable while the CA.B.S.' Air is totally made of permanent material. These materials are PP on the parietal surface and ePTFE on the visceral surface. It is available in three sizes and with two or four sutures. They are both marketed for umbilical hernia repair but undoubtedly other hernias will lend themselves to these devices.

ClearMesh Composite (CMC) is a pure PP mesh (Fig. 7.125). There is a textured side that is composed of a

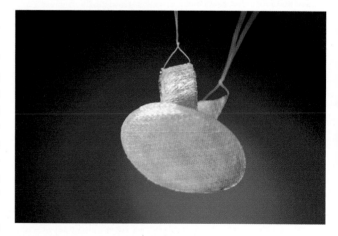

Fig. 7.121 Proceed Ventral Patch (PVP)

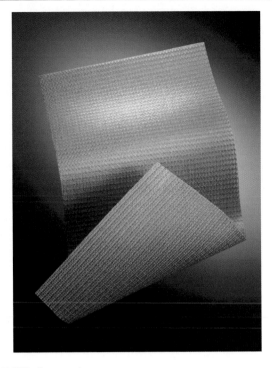

Fig. 7.122 Sepramesh

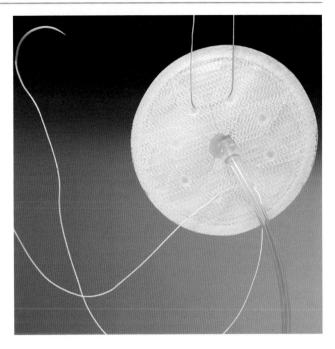

Fig. 7.123 CA.B.S. 'Air

Table 7.19 Ventral hernia products entirely of permanent material

CA.B.S 'Air, Cousin Biotech, Wervicq-Sud, France
ClearMesh Composite (CMC), Di.pro Medical Devices, Torino, Italy
Combi Mesh, Angiologica, S. Martino Sicc., Italy
Composix E/X Mesh, Davol, Inc., Warwick, RI, USA
Composix Kugel (CK) Patch, Davol, Inc., Warwick, RI, USA
Composix L/P Mesh, Davol, Inc., Warwick, RI, USA
DynaMesh IPOM, FEG Textiltechnik mbH, Aachen, Germany
IntraMesh T1, Cousin Biotech, Wervicq-Sud, France
IntraMesh W3, Cousin Biotech, Wervicq-Sud, France
Intramesh PROT1, Cousin Biotech, Wervicq
Omyra Mesh, B. Braun Melsungen AG, Melsungen, Germany
MotifMESH, Proxy Biomedical Ltd., Galway, Ireland
Rebound HRD V, Minnesota Medical Development, Plymouth, MN, USA
Relimesh, HerniaMesh, Torino, Italy
SurgiMesh XB, Aspide Medical, St. Etienne, France
SurgiMesh TintraP, Aspide Medical, St. Etienne, France
TiMesh, GfE Medizintechnik, Nuremburg, Germany
Ventralex (ST), Davol, Inc., Warwick, RI, USA
Ventrio (ST) Hernia Patch, Davol, Inc., Warwick, RI, USA

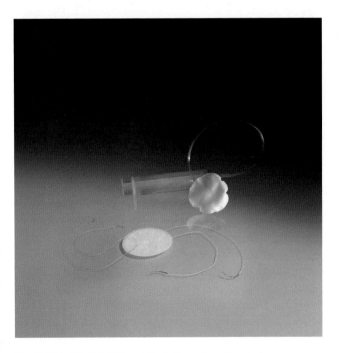

Fig. 7.124 CA.B.S. 'Air and the balloon dissection device

single filament macroporous weave and a nonadhesive side that is composed of a nonporous smooth PP film. It is for use in the intraperitoneal space. The 2P is elliptical in shape and the 2P-C is round. *Combi Mesh* is virtually identical to the Combi Mesh Pro described in the inguinal hernia section (Fig. 7.27). The only difference is that these are larger sizes. This product is designed for placement into the intraperitoneal position with the polyurethane layer facing the viscera.

Composix E/X Mesh (Fig. 7.126) is flat Bard mesh on one side and ePTFE on the other side. The edge of the perimeter of the elliptically shaped product is sealed to prevent contact of viscera to the PP. It is a low profile mesh that is best suited for laparoscopic repairs. *Composix Kugel (CK) Patch* (Fig. 7.127) is a self-expanding product that has Bard mesh on one side and ePTFE on the other as does the E/X and L/P

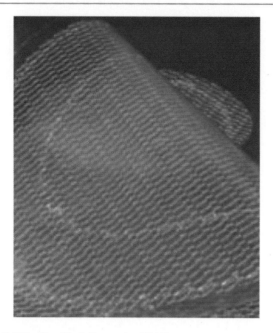

Fig. 7.125 ClearMesh Composite (CMC)

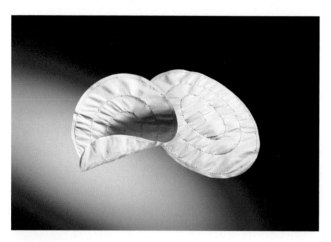

Fig. 7.126 Composix E/X

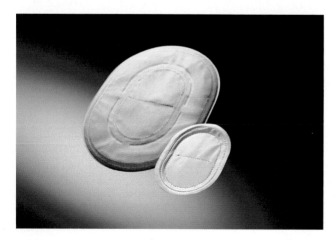

Fig. 7.127 Composix Kugel (CK) Patch

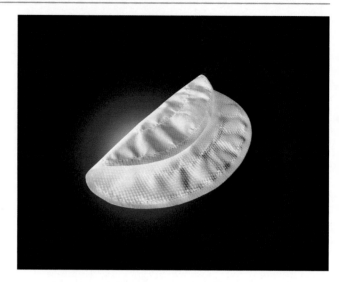

Fig. 7.128 Composix L/P

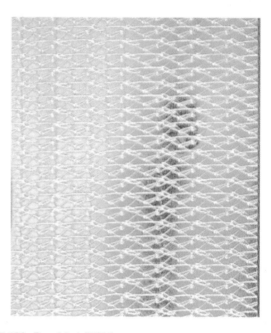

Fig. 7.129 DynaMesh IPOM

products. There is an additional POL ring that causes it to assume its shape after introduction into the abdominal cavity to facilitate fixation. This ring is of a smaller diameter with an improved weld than the earlier version of the product. *Composix L/P* (Fig. 7.128) is very similar to the Composix E/X except that the former uses the lighter Bard Soft Mesh rather than the Bard mesh. It is specifically designed for laparoscopic usage and can be used with an optional introduction tool. The two mesh layers are sutured together with ePTFE suture for all three of these prosthetic devices.

DynaMesh IPOM (Fig. 7.129) is a similar PP weave as the DynaMesh described above but it is slightly lighter than the latter product. This version is intertwined with polyvi-

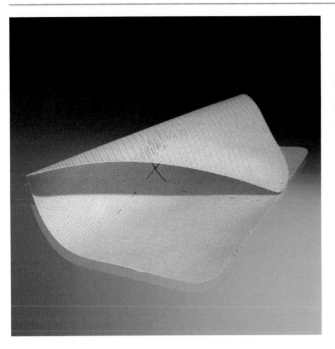

Fig. 7.130 IntraMesh T1

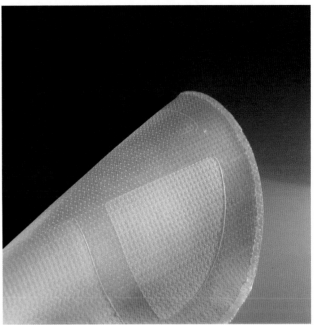

Fig. 7.132 IntraMesh PROT1

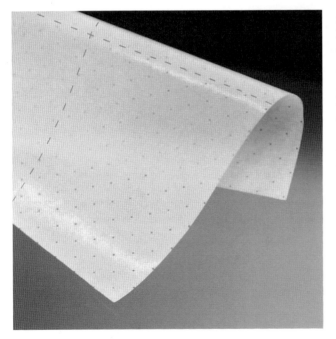

Fig. 7.131 IntraMesh W3

nylidene fluoride (PVDF), which is also a monofilament. Because of this PVDF tissue-separating component it can be placed onto the viscera. *IntraMesh T1* (Fig. 7.130) is similar to the Composix product line in that it is composed of one layer of PP and a second layer of ePTFE. There are lines on the product to delineate the midportions of each side to ease positioning for the laparoscopic approach. *IntraMesh W3* (Fig. 7.131), like the other IntraMesh products, is designed

for intraperitoneal usage. This mesh is also marked but is POL based. There is one layer of nonwoven polyethylene terephthalate with microperforations for parietal attachment and a visceral surface with dimethyl siloxane. *IntraMesh PROT1* (Fig. 7.132) is a combination of the other two IntraMesh prostheses. It is round with two layers of PP and ePTFE. In addition, as can be seen in the photo, there is another layer of dimethyl siloxane designed to strengthen the fixation points. Cousin Biotech also sells a "mesh roller" which is a device to aid in the rolling of these materials to ease insertion via a trocar.

MotifMESH (Fig. 7.60) *and Omyra Mesh* (Fig. 7.61) were discussed the "Miscellaneous Flat Mesh Section" (Table 7.13). Omyra Mesh is said to be a bacterial resistant anti-adhesive mesh. Unlike the W. L. Gore & Associates products, there is no antimicrobial or antibacterial substance added to the product. It is made of lightweight cPTFE.

Rebound HRD V is of the same concept as the Rebound HRD described above. It has a nitinol ring around the perimeter of the oval shape. The mesh product in this version is cPTFE. It is designed for use in the intraperitoneal space. *Relimesh* (Fig. 7.133) is another product that incorporates the PP on one surface and ePTFE on the other to allow placement against the viscera. It is a lighter weight product compared to other HerniaMesh products. Because of this, it can be rolled for insertion via a trocar.

SurgiMesh XB (Fig. 7.134) has a nonwoven, non-knitted structure as does the SurgiMesh WN described earlier. It has an additional layer of silicone to allow contact with the viscera and is microperforated. *SurgiMesh TintraP* is a

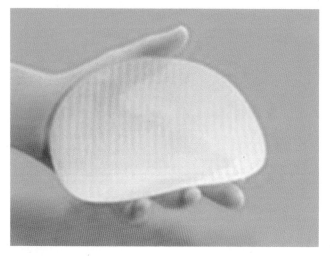

Fig. 7.133 Relimesh

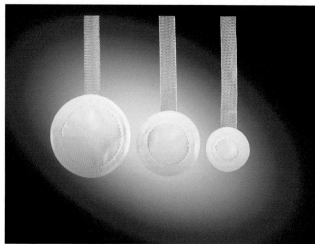

Fig. 7.135 Ventralex

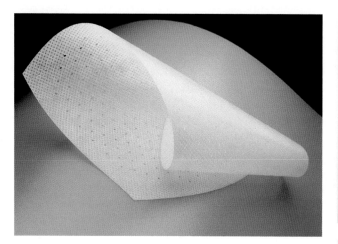

Fig. 7.134 SurgiMesh XB

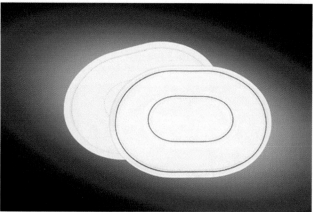

Fig. 7.136 Ventrio Hernia Patch

similar product but is round and to be used with smaller hernias such as trocar and umbilical hernias. TintraP is made to include strips to fix the product to the edge of the fascia. Additionally, the prosthesis is supplied "pre-loaded" over an introducer that aids in deployment of the device in the preperitoneal space. *TiMesh* (Figs. 7.47 and 7.48) is the same material that has been described in several locations within this chapter. The titanized PPM can be used in the intraperitoneal location (per the manufacturer).

Ventralex (Fig. 7.135) is a self-expanding PP device (because of the outer ring of POL) that is fixed with ePTFE on one side to allow placement adjacent to viscera. It is round but smaller than the larger products such as the Composix products described above. It is intended for use in the smaller defects of the abdominal wall such as trocar or umbilical hernias. There is a pocket to allow for a digit to be inserted for placement. Two long straps are attached and are to be used for fixation to the fascia. They are very long as this product can be inserted through a laparoscopic trocar to aid in the prevention

of trocar hernias. The *Ventrio Hernia Patch* (Fig. 7.136) comprises two layers of mesh product. PP that is stitched to an ePTFE layer as the tissue-separating component. Within the PP surface there are "tubes" (similar to the Composix Kugel mesh) that house the absorbable PDO monofilament rings to give the mesh rigidity to aid in positioning and fixation. The purple PDO ring is absorbed within 6–8 months. A second-generation product is due to be released in which the anterior PP will be constructed of a lighter weight PP. There are other minor differences that will not be noted by the surgeon.

Stomal Hernia Prevention and Repair Products

The development of a hernia, wherever a stoma is created, has been the challenge in the life of all patients with some type of an ostomy. Traditionally, relocation or primary closure was used to repair these hernias. It is now recognized that this is fraught with failure in most cases. Consequently,

Table 7.20 Stomal prostheses

Colostomy Mesh, HerniaMesh, Torino, Italy

CK Parastomal Patch, Davol, Inc., Warwick, RI, USA

DynaMesh-IPST, FEG Textiltechnik mbH, Aachen, Germany

Easy Prosthesis (PPM/Collagen), TransEasy Medical Tech.Co. Ltd., Beijing, China

Parietex Composite (PCO) Parastomal Mesh, Covidien plc, Dublin, Ireland

Stomaltex, Di.pro Medical Devices, Torino, Italy

2P-ST, Di.pro Medical Devices, Torino, Italy

TiLENE Guard, GfE Medizintechnik, Nuremburg, Germany

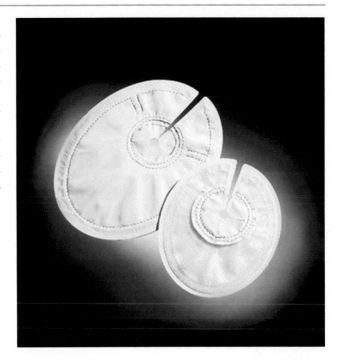

Fig. 7.138 CK Parastomal Patch

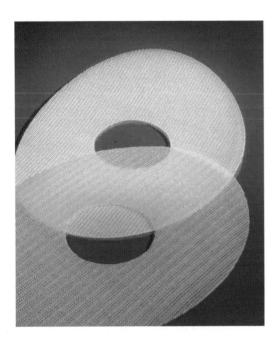

Fig. 7.137 Colostomy Mesh

the use of a prosthetic material has become nearly standard to repair these hernias. In fact, recent trends indicate that the use of a mesh of some type when the stoma is created may be the preferred option. Prevention has become the new effort in mesh construction (Table 7.20). As with many of the other products in this chapter, these can generally be used with the open or laparoscopic technique.

Colostomy Mesh (Fig. 7.137) is a single layer PP product. It has a 5-cm hole in the center of the material through which the intestine can be placed during stomal creation. Of course, the mesh can be cut if this product is used to repair a parastomal hernia. It is available in a "rigid" and a "semi-rigid" construction. The *CK Parastomal Patch* (Fig. 7.138) is to be used to repair an existing parastomal hernia. Like the other CK products, it has a POL memory recoil ring and is made of PP and ePTFE. It has a precut slit and a circular opening to allow passage of the intestine. The ePTFE around the collar is reinforced to inhibit stretching of the opening. Additionally,

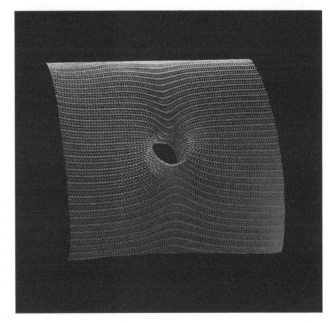

Fig. 7.139 DynaMesh-IPST

there are flaps of ePTFE that will lie on the intestine at the completion of the implantation.

DynaMesh-IPST (Fig. 7.139), like its parent material, is made of both PVDF and PP. It is pre-shaped and three-dimensional. *Easy Prosthesis (PPM/Collagen)* (Fig. 7.116) was previously discussed in the section titled "Prostheses for Incisional and Ventral Hernioplasty with an Absorbable

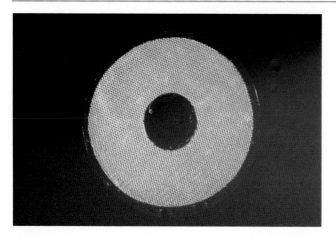

Fig. 7.140 Parietex Composite Parastomal Mesh with hole

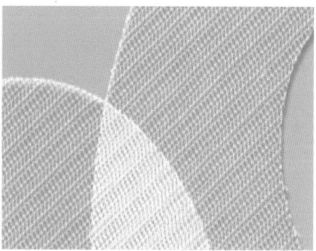

Fig. 7.142 Stomaltex

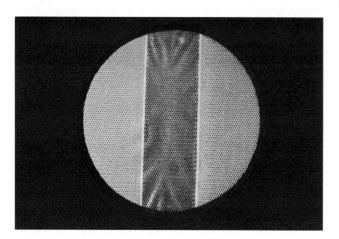

Fig. 7.141 Parietex Composite Parastomal Mesh without hole

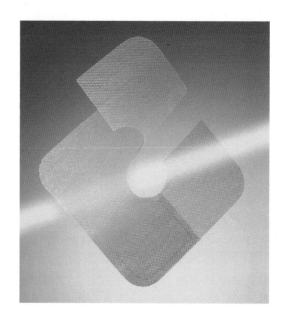

Fig. 7.143 TiLENE Guard

Component." As seen in the figure, there is a shape that is similar to many of these products designed for stomal hernia prevention and repair. *Parietex Composite Parastomal Mesh* is of the same material as that described previously. This is supplied in two sizes and is available with a hole (Fig. 7.140) or without a hole and only a central band (Fig. 7.141). The opening of the hole can either be 3.5 or 5.0 cm.

Stomaltex (Fig. 7.142) is a macroporous heavyweight PP product similar to their Basic flat mesh (Fig. 7.20) described in the earlier section on flat PPM meshes. It does not include any tissue-separating material. The *2P-ST* prosthesis is of the "protected" CMC material as their flat sheets for intraperitoneal usage. It is supplied with a central hole that is either 3 or 5 cm in diameter. *TiLENE Guard* (Fig. 7.143) is of titanized PP (Fig. 7.48). It is supplied with a flap, which is closed after the intestine is placed through the central hole. It is supplied in the light and dual-weight (light and medium) meshes. There is a set, which contains TiLENE mesh that is to be applied as a "sandwich" technique to repair or prevent herniation through the stoma location.

Hiatal Hernia Repair Products

The use of permanent meshes to repair hiatal hernias has been commonplace for many years. The introduction of the biologic products has resulted in a decline in the application of the permanent products at this position. The real concern is of erosion of the product into the esophagus or infection with a permanent prosthesis. While the application of flat meshes such as unprotected PP or POL has been used, these products were designed to mitigate against these concerns (Table 7.21).

CruraSoft Patch (Fig. 7.144) is made of two products. One surface is of PTFE mesh designed to encourage tissue penetration and ingrowth. The other is ePTFE, which will

Table 7.21 Permanent hiatal hernia repair products

CruraSoft, Davol, Inc., Warwick, RI, USA

Easy Prosthesis (PPM/Collagen), TransEasy Medical Tech.Co. Ltd., Beijing, China

Parietex Composite (PCO) Hiatal Mesh, Covidien plc, Dublin, Ireland

TiSURE, GfE Medizintechnik, Nuremburg, Germany

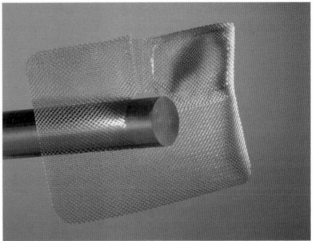

Fig. 7.146 TiSURE

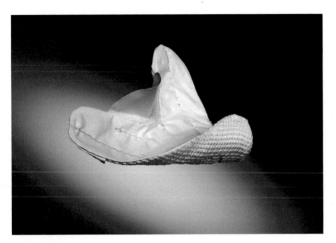

Fig. 7.144 CruraSoft

Parietex Composite Hiatal Mesh (Fig. 7.145) is made of the same material as the parent PCO product. It possesses a U-shaped defect that is slightly off-center that is to be positioned below the esophagus. The legs of the product will lie on the crura. It is available in two sizes also.

TiSURE (Fig. 7.146) is a rectangular mesh that has a central hole and a flap made from TiMESH (Fig. 7.47). It differs from the other products listed in that it possesses that flap which mandates complete encirclement of the esophagus. It can be fixed with either fibrin glue or sutures. It is not recommended to use metal fixation devices on this product because of the risk of complications from these devices.

Fixation Devices

Fixation devices became prevalent early in the development of the laparoscopic repair of hernias. The earlier versions were 10 or 12 mm devices, some of which are still available today. More commonly the 5 mm versions have become the most popular. Most recently, recognition of the requirement of these devices on a temporary basis has led to the introduction of absorbable platforms. Currently, there is a variety of these devices that one may choose to fixate the meshes placed in hernia repair, whether inguinal or ventral and via an open or laparoscopic technique (Table 7.22). Surgeon preference and the mesh chosen will dictate the decision. One should consider the total length of these fasteners, as the depth of penetration will be dependent upon the thickness of the mesh used to repair the hernia. For example, a 5 mm fastener will provide no more of tissue penetration than 4 mm when used with 1 mm prosthesis.

The *AbsorbaTack* (Fig. 7.147) is a 5 mm fixation device which provides an absorbable synthetic polyester copolymer screw-like fastener derived from lactic and glycolic acid.

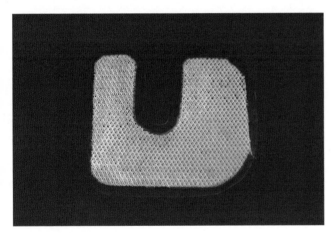

Fig. 7.145 Parietex Composite Hiatal Mesh

have visceral contact to diminish adhesions. There is an additional flap of ePTFE to cradle the esophagus and decrease the risk of adhesion and erosion into it. This prosthesis can be placed either over an open hiatus or re-approximated crura. The latter approach will represent a tension-free repair. It is available in two sizes and can be either sutured or stapled in place. *Easy Prosthesis (PPM/Collagen)* (Fig. 7.116) was previously discussed in the section titled "Prostheses for Incisional and Ventral Hernioplasty with an Absorbable Component." As seen in the figure, there is a shape that is similar to the CruraSoft above, which is designed for use in repair of the hiatal crura.

It measures 5.1 mm in length. It is offered in both a 10 or 20 tack configuration. The tacks are significantly absorbed within 3–5 months with complete absorption within 1 year. The *Amid Hernia Stapler* (Fig. 7.148) is designed to fixate the onlay mesh in a Lichtenstein hernia repair of the groin but will likely find applications for other type of hernias. It contains 17 titanium "box" type staples. Its contents can also be used to close the skin at the completion of the procedure.

The *Endo Universal Stapler* (Fig. 7.149) is to be used via a 10 or 12 mm trocar. It delivers a "box-type" staple of titanium and can be rotated 360° and has 65% of articulation. It can be used in four different positions. The *MultiFire Hernia Stapler* (Fig. 7.150) is introduced through a 12 mm trocar. It has "box-shaped" staples that will fixate the prosthesis into which it is fired. The *MultiFire VersaTack Stapler* (Fig. 7.151) is designed for open usage. It, too, can be rotated 360°. These three staplers can be used with interchangeable disposable loading units that contain either the 4.0 or 4.8 mm staples and delivering ten staples. These staples are usually acceptable for use with MRI and NMR up to three Tesla.

The *PermaSorb* (Fig. 7.152) device delivers a poly (D,L)—lactide (PDLLA) fastener that has two barbs on the end of it. They are delivered over an introducer needle. This product is available in either a 5 or 12 shot shaft; the latter being longer is best suited for laparoscopic procedures while the former is

for open methods. These fasteners are fully absorbed at 16 months. *PermaFix* and *SorbaFix* (Fig. 7.153) deliver the same size (6.7 mm) screw-type fasteners by an identical delivery mechanism with a pilot tip and mandrel. Both of these fasteners are available in either 15 or 30 devices delivered via a 5 mm product. Sorbafix is made of the same material as the PermaSorb ad is purple, while the Permafix is made of grey molded permanent polymer, making it nonabsorbable.

The *ProTack* (Fig. 7.154) was one of the earlier products that delivered a fastener by a 5 mm device. It delivers a permanent titanium helical fastener. It is available with 30 tacks. These are the easiest fixation products to visualize on a plain radiologic study. They are 3.9 mm in total length.

The *SECURESTRAP* (Fig. 7.155) is a new 5 mm laparoscopic device for hernia repair. It is a multi-fire, single-use device pre-loaded with 25 absorbable straps. The straps are composed of a blend of PDO and L(-)-lactide and glycolide dyed with D&C Violet No. 2. This product does not screw into the tissues and has two legs similar to the staplers. The ends of these straps are barbed to aid in fixation. The width between the points is 3.5 mm. The length of the entire device is 6.7 mm but the distance from the inner portion of the strap to the point of fixation of the strap is 4.9 mm (i.e., the "grip").

The *Stat Tack* (Fig. 7.156) and Tacker (Fig. 7.157) devices deliver helical titanium tacks virtually identical to the ProTack (Fig. 7.154). The former device is shorter and designed for open hernia repair, delivering only 15 tacks. The Tacker is longer as it is designed for laparoscopic techniques and delivers 30 tacks in the single-use device. There is an available multiuse handle of the Tacker that can be attached to an available tube of 20 tacks. This is a unique concept for fixation products. The multiuse product has a shorter tube than the single-use product.

Mesh Delivery Devices

At the time of this writing, there are a few devices that have been developed to ease the insertion of the meshes used in laparoscopic repair of hernias, mainly the incisional and

Table 7.22 Fixation devices for hernia repair

AbsorbaTack, Covidien plc, Dublin, Ireland
Amid Stapler, SafeStitch Medical Inc., Miami, FL, USA
Endo Universal Stapler, Covidien plc, Dublin, Ireland
Multifire Endo Hernia Stapler, Covidien plc, Dublin, Ireland
Multifire VersaTack Stapler, Covidien plc, Dublin, Ireland
PermaFix, Davol, Inc., Warwick, RI, USA
PermaSorb, Davol, Inc., Warwick, RI, USA
ProTack, Covidien plc, Dublin, Ireland
SecureStrap, Ethicon Inc., Somerville, NJ, USA
SorbaFix, Davol, Inc., Warwick, RI, USA
Stat Tack, Covidien plc, Dublin, Ireland
Tacker, Covidien plc, Dublin, Ireland

Fig. 7.147 AbsorbaTack

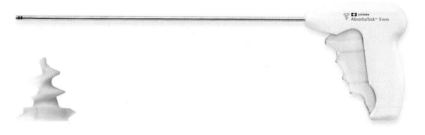

ventral locations. These include the *Mesh GPS* device by Surgical Structure Ltd. (Moshav Herev Le'Et, Israel), the *PrecisionPass Laparoscopic Delivery Device* (Davol, Inc., Warwick, RI, USA), and the *PatchAssist* (Polytouch Medical Ltd., Tel Aviv, Israel). Davol, Inc. recently purchased the Mesh GPS product and may change the name to Echo. This is not certain at this time, however.

The *Mesh GPS* device comprises three components, an inflatable spreading balloon, an adaptor, and an inflation unit/pump. These combine to assist spreading and deploying the mesh used to repair the hernias. The *PrecisionPass* device assists in the rolling of a mesh into a tubular shape for intro-

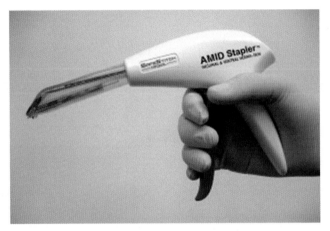

Fig. 7.148 Amid Hernia Stapler

duction via a laparoscopic trocar (Fig. 7.158). The *PatchAssist* (Fig. 7.159) fixes the mesh to itself allowing it to be rolled into a tube and introduced. Upon introduction, the device is opened, deploying the mesh and holding the mesh onto the abdominal wall to ease positioning and fixation.

Conclusion

The use of a prosthetic material for all hernia repairs is the norm rather than an isolated event. The purpose of this chapter is to identify and differentiate the products that can be used in hernioplasties. It is as complete as we could make this at this time. Undoubtedly by the time of the printing of this textbook, others will have become available. The surgeon should choose carefully.

I believe that the ideal material has not yet been developed. There are, however, many that have been described above that do function quite well for the surgeon and the patient. Perhaps in the future, the use of genetic engineering will produce a product that is based from the protein of the patient and will allow the patient to incorporate a "natural" and "native" product into the tissues without fear of infection or adhesions. A permanent solution to the quest of the perfect biomaterial may be the result.

Acknowledgment I want to thank the following for the valuable inclusive photos that were supplied for inclusion in this chapter: Atrium Medical Inc., Davol, Inc., Ethicon Inc., W.L. Gore & Associates.

Fig. 7.149 Endo Universal Stapler

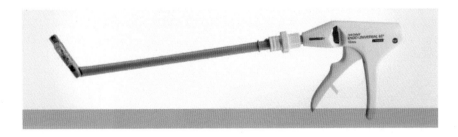

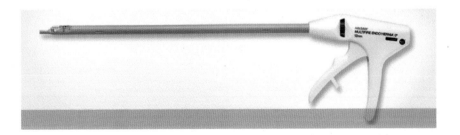

Fig. 7.150 Multifire Hernia Stapler

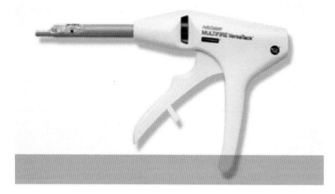

Fig. 7.151 MultiFire VersaTack Stapler

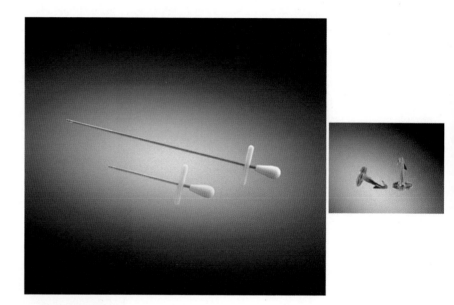

Fig. 7.152 PermaSorb

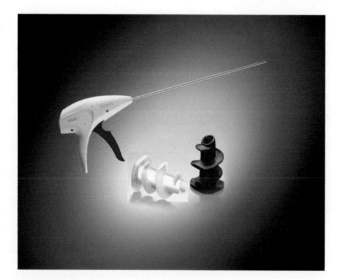

Fig. 7.153 SorbaFix device with SorbaFix (*purple*) and PermaFix (*grey*) fasteners

Fig. 7.154 ProTack

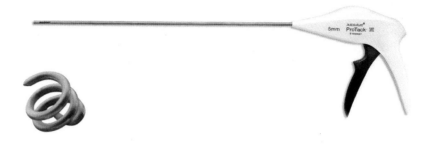

Fig. 7.155 SECURE*STRAP* and the Strap
fastener

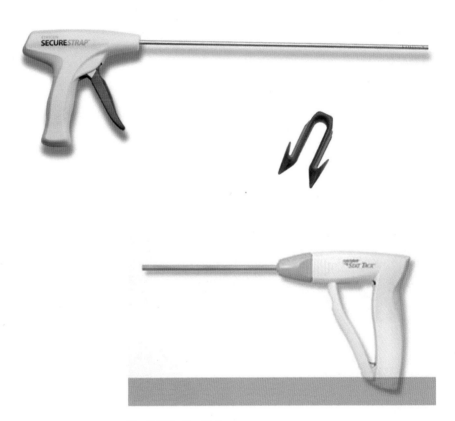

Fig. 7.156 Stat Tack

Fig. 7.157 Tacker

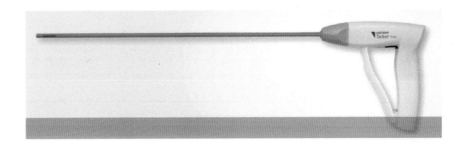

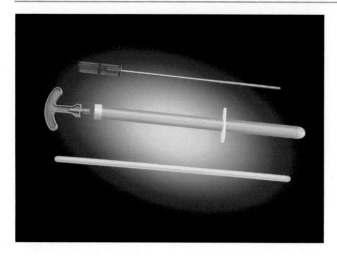

Fig. 7.158 PrecisionPass Laparoscopic Delivery Device

Fig. 7.159 PatchAssist

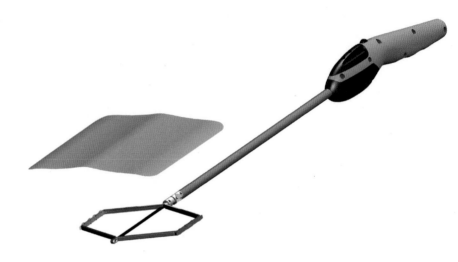

References

1. Scheyer M, Arnold S, Zimmermann G. Minimally invasive operation techniques for inguinal hernia: spectrum of indications in Austria. Hernia. 2001;5:73–9.
2. Hesselink VJ, Luijendijk RW, de Wilt JHW, Heide R. An evaluation of risk factors in incisional hernia recurrence. Surg Gynecol Obstet. 1993;176:228–34.
3. Luijendijk RW, Hop WCJ, van den Tol P, et al. A comparison of suture repair with mesh repair for incisional hernia. N Engl J Med. 2000;343(6):393–8.
4. LeBlanc KA, Booth WV. Laparoscopic repair of incisional abdominal hernias using expanded polytetrafluoroethylene: preliminary findings. Surg Laparosc Endosc. 1993;3:39–41.
5. Bucknall TE, Cox PJ, Ellis H. Burst abdomen and incisional hernia: a prospective study of 1129 major laparotomies. Br Med J. 1982;284:931–3.
6. Goepel R. Uber die verschliersung von bruchpforten durch einleilung gerflochtener fertiger silberdrahtnetze. Verh Deutsch Ges Pathol. 1900;29:4.
7. Kirschner M. Die praktischen Ergebnisse der freien Fascien-Tranaplantation. Arch Klin Chir. 1910;92:888–912.
8. Badylak S, Kokini K, Tullius B, Whitson B. Strength over time of a resorbable bioscaffold for body wall repair in a dog model. J Surg Res. 2001;99:282–7.
9. Millikan K. Doolas. "A Long-Term Evaluation of the Modified Mesh-Plug Hernioplasty in Over 2,000 Patients". Hernia. 2008;12(3):257–60.
10. Cumberland O. Ueber die Verschliessung von Bauchwunden und Brustpforten durch Bersenkte Siberdragrnetze. Zentralbl Chir. 1900;27:257.
11. Scales JT. Discussion on metals and synthetic materials in relation to soft tissues: tissue reactions to synthetic materials. Proc R Soc Med. 1953;46:647.

Bruce Ramshaw and Sheila Grant

History of Mesh

The search for a material to be used to strengthen a hernia repair was initiated in the late 1800s. Marcy experimented with a variety of animal tendons including whale, ox, and deer. In 1887, he used kangaroo tendon as suture material; however, there were problems identified with marked tissue reaction. In the early 1900s a variety of metallic materials such as silver, tantalum, and stainless steel were tried without lasting success. In 1935, with the discovery of synthetic plastics by Carothers, the foundation for the modern materials used for hernia mesh was laid.

In 1958, Francis Usher introduced the modern hernia repair by using a polypropylene mesh design [1]. Until that time, simple tissue re-approximation method was standard practice for hernia repair, which left the sutured area under tension and at high risk for hernia recurrence. The role of mesh in hernia repair is to provide a tension-free bridge between the fascial defects or to be a buttress for approximated defects. Since the introduction of synthetic mesh material as a repair patch for hernias, the recurrence rate has dropped. A Danish study demonstrated that the recurrence rate dropped by at least half with the introduction of mesh inguinal hernia repairs. In the arena of incisional hernia repair, several randomized control studies have also shown the benefit of mesh [2]. Hernia recurrence with a sutured tissue repair, which just re-approximated the edges of the hernia, resulted in a 63% recurrence rate, as opposed to a 32% recurrence rate using a synthetic mesh [3]. The principles of wide coverage with adequate overlap and good fixation of the mesh to the fascia have led to even more successful repairs [4].

One early thought was that a heavy mesh was necessary in order to prevent rupture and re-herniation. The fact that the heavyweight polypropylene induced a large fibrotic, inflammatory response was considered beneficial. The theory was that more scaring would lead to a stronger abdominal wall and less recurrence. In recent years, this theory has been challenged. There are now concerns that a thick scar plate formation may lead to changes in the abdominal wall compliance, changes in mesh properties, and thus higher chance of patient pain and recurrence.

For over 40 years, polypropylene (Marlex, monofilament polypropylene, and Prolene, dual-filament polypropylene) had been the predominant mesh used for hernia repair. But due to adverse clinical effects possibly resulting from heavyweight polypropylene and from the expanding mesh market in dollars (now approximately $1 billion per year), the number and variety of synthetic mesh materials available for hernia repair have increased significantly in the more recent past.

Alternatives to polypropylene mesh have been introduced over the years. For example, expanded polytetrafluoroethylene (ePTFE) was first marketed in the 1970s. Additionally, multifilament polyester mesh, popular in France, was introduced in the United States in the early 1990s, but did not find widespread use until recently. Absorbable synthetic meshes, such as macroporous Vicryl mesh, have also been used in some clinical settings. Newer degradable hernia meshes are being investigated and are currently marketed under trade names of BioA (W.L. Gore & Associates) and TIGR mesh (Novus Scientific). These mesh materials are typically composed of a degradable polymer (such as polylactic acid/polyglycolic acid) that resorbs over time and is eventually, in theory, replaced with collagen. It is believed that in most patients these resorbable meshes will last less than a one-year period, ideally inducing healing that will result in strength necessary to prevent a recurrence. While in vivo animal models have shown success, the medical community has been somewhat reluctant to use resorbable mesh due to the concern of hernia recurrence.

While heavyweight polypropylene has demonstrated some adverse effects, it is still being utilized either in its

B. Ramshaw (✉)
Department of General Surgery, Transformative Care Institute,
Daytona Beach, FL, USA
e-mail: herniateam@yahoo.com

S. Grant
University of Missouri, Columbia, MO, USA

A.N. Kingsnorth and K.A. LeBlanc (eds.), *Management of Abdominal Hernias*,
DOI 10.1007/978-1-84882-877-3_8, © Springer Science+Business Media London 2013

heavyweight form or in modified forms. For example, medium and lightweight polypropylene meshes are available and first came to market in 1998 (marketed as Vypro). It was thought that less amounts of foreign material would elicit a less-enhanced foreign body response. Coated polypropylene or polyester meshes were also introduced to minimize fibrotic tissue/scar tissue formation, particularly to prevent adhesions and ingrowth to the viscera. Today, there are many different types of coatings consisting of collagen, titanium, hyaluronic acid, omega-3 fatty acid, and other degradable polymers. Some of these coatings are applied to individual mesh fibers (i.e., titanium in TiMesh), and some are microporous coatings applied on the visceral side of macroporous mesh to prevent adhesions and ingrowth. Despite all the "new" types of hernia mesh being approved by the FDA, most of the available mesh materials continue to be composed of the basic polypropylene, PTFE, or polyester materials, with or without the various coatings.

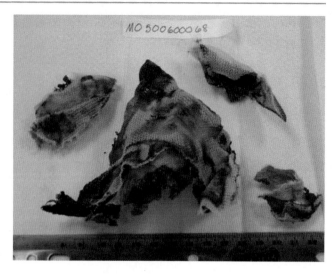

Fig. 8.1 An example of explanted heavyweight polypropylene mesh after cleaning

Synthetic Mesh Design

1. Polypropylene: Polypropylene is synthesized via addition reaction from the monomer propylene. With its methyl side groups off of the carbon backbone, polypropylene is hydrophobic, and it is usually resistant to many chemical solvents, bases, and acids. Since polypropylene is classified as a thermoplastic polymer, it can be remelted and reformed.

   For hernia meshes, semicrystalline polypropylene fibers are extruded and then are woven into particular monofilament or multifilament mesh designs. Recently, microporous, nonwoven mesh design of polypropylene fibers are also reaching the market. Unfortunately, polypropylene mesh has been shown to oxidize and degrade in vivo. Oxidation occurs when the C–H bonds are compromised, creating a free radical that will bind with oxygen. Chain scission and/or cross-linking may occur, and this "embrittlement" may change the physicochemical properties of the polypropylene. For example, polypropylene mesh may become stiff and/or can shrink, which can result in pain or recurrence of the hernia in some patients (Fig. 8.1).

   The dense, small-pore-size heavyweight polypropylene mesh is defined as having greater than 90 g/m² area of material and pore size <3–5 mm. Clinical data has shown that the heavyweight polypropylene induces an intense foreign body response with thick scar plate formation. While this may enhance the strength of the repair, problems such as mesh extrusion, wound sepsis, erosion into intra-abdominal organs, refractory seromas, and bowel fistulas have been known to occur with heavyweight polypropylene. To try to minimize these responses, lighter-weight polypropylene meshes and coated meshes have been introduced. Newer mid- and lightweight meshes are less dense and have an increased pore size compared with the heavyweight mesh. Not only is there less foreign body material but these meshes with the larger pore sizes have been shown to promote better tissue response. Studies have confirmed that increasing the pore size and decreasing the density of polypropylene can mitigate some of the foreign body response [5, 6]. Alternatively, there are many polypropylene meshes on the market that have been coated with degradable or nondegradable coatings in order to reduce the severity of the inflammatory response and lead to less fibrosis and contraction of the mesh [7]. As mentioned earlier, titanium-coated polypropylene mesh marketed as TiMesh (Biomet, Inc.) has been utilized to try to mask the body's response to the polypropylene. A recent FDA-approved mesh using a proprietary synthetic polyurethane-hydrogel coating (marketed by STS) has shown good in vivo results. Natural coatings, such as omega-3 fatty acid-coated polypropylene mesh, marketed as C-Qur (Atrium), have also been produced with the intent to improve healing. While coatings may reduce the initial onslaught of the inflammatory response, stability may be important for long-term success. Clinical evidence has shown that some of the coatings are unstable over time and disintegrate, thus potentially leaving the underlying polypropylene susceptible to degradation.

2. Polyethylene Terephthalate: Polyethylene terephthalate (PET) is a member of the polyester family, and hence it is commonly referred to as "polyester mesh" in the medical market (Fig. 8.2). Unlike polypropylene, PET is synthesized via a condensation reaction, where the starting monomer (bis-β-hydroxyterephthalate) can be synthesized either by an esterification reaction (water as a

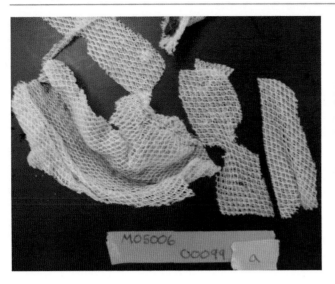

Fig. 8.2 An example of explanted polyester mesh after cleaning

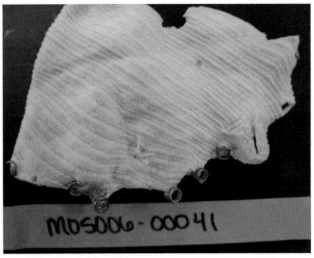

Fig. 8.3 An example of explanted ePTFE mesh after cleaning

by-product) or by a transesterification reaction (methanol as a by-product). Like polypropylene, PET is also a thermoplastic polymer so it can be remelted and reformed, but it is less hydrophobic than polypropylene. PET can be extruded into synthetic fibers wherein it can be woven into particular mesh designs. Additionally, PET can exist as an amorphous (transparent) or as a semicrystalline material, depending on its processing and thermal history.

Polyester's known mechanism of degradation includes hydrolytic, thermal, and thermal oxidation. However, hydrolysis is the degradation mechanism of concern with implanted PET meshes. When PET degrades, several physicochemical changes can occur which include discoloration, chain scissions resulting in reduced molecular weight, formation of acetaldehyde, and formation of cross-links. Additionally, because of its open macroporous design, a significant inflammatory reaction with gross tissue ingrowth into the interstices of the mesh is produced, resulting in a variable degree of scar formation. To alleviate some of the inflammatory response and ingrowth potential when placed in contact with the viscera, PET mesh can be coated. For example, Parietex composite mesh (Covidien) has been coated with collagen in order to avoid ingrowth of abdominal viscera and to potentially prevent adhesions.

3. Polytetrafluoroethylene: Another commonly utilized mesh material is polytetrafluoroethylene (PTFE), which is a fluorocarbon-based polymer. PTFE is usually synthesized via a free radical polymerization of tetrafluoroethylene. This reaction creates a carbon backbone chain containing two fluorine atoms per carbon atom. PTFE is highly crystalline, extremely hydrophobic, and one of the most chemically inert polymers on the market. This inertness or stability of PTFE is the result of the high strength of the fluorine–carbon bond. Expanded PTFE (ePTFE) is commonly produced and utilized as hernia mesh. ePTFE is produced when a sheet of PTFE is heated and then stretched, creating micropores. Because of its many desirable properties, PTFE and ePTFE are utilized in many applications besides hernia mesh, including arterial grafts, catheters, sutures, and in reconstructive surgery.

DualMesh® is an expanded PTFE hernia mesh marketed by W.L. Gore and Associates. DualMesh® has a two-surface design with one side possessing a closed smooth surface structure (prevent adhesions) while the other side is "rough" or corduroy (microporous) to allow tissue ingrowth (Fig. 8.3). There is another product, Dulex (Davol, Inc.), which is also an all-PTFE hernia mesh with a smooth and a rough side. While PTFE is one of the most chemically inert materials, the microporous structure results in poor integration and/or poor recapitulation of host tissue (i.e., scar tissue formation). This can cause mesh contraction and shrinkage, resulting in the possibility of recurrence.

Another product has been introduced that allows better tissue integration is a monofilament PTFE mesh with an open macroporous design (INFINIT® by W.L. Gore and Associates). Another macroporous PTFE mesh on the market is MotifMESH™ (Proxy Biomedical). The former product is not designed for intraperitoneal whereas the latter is marketed for intraperitoneal usage.

4. Hernia Mesh for specific operations

There have been hernia meshes that are designed for particular hernia operations. For example, a variety of meshes have been designed for intra-abdominal placement, particularly for the laparoscopic ventral hernia repair and other minimally invasive abdominal wall reconstruction operations. The main goal of these meshes is to prevent the ingrowth of bowel and other abdominal organs when they are potentially in contact with mesh. In an attempt to pre-

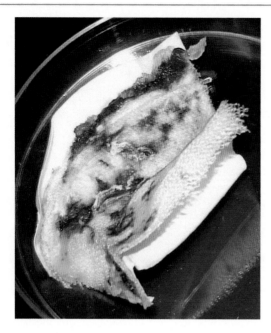

Fig. 8.4 An example of an explanted composite mesh (heavyweight polypropylene/PTFE) after cleaning

vent adhesions, a solid permanent (PTFE) or absorbable (many types) barrier is used on a variety of polypropylene and polyester meshes. These mesh combinations would be considered "composite" meshes (Fig. 8.4). There are also PTFE meshes which each has a rough (toward the abdominal wall) and a smooth (toward the viscera) side. For synthetic meshes placed in the abdominal cavity or with the potential to be exposed to abdominal viscera, one surface is designed to prevent ingrowth into the mesh, which can lead to erosion and complications such as bowel obstruction and fistula formation. The other side of these meshes is intended to promote in growth into the abdominal wall. This side of these meshes is either "rough" PTFE, heavy- or lighter-weight polypropylene or polyester. For any macroporous mesh without a barrier, there is potential for dense adhesions and ingrowth, which can lead to obstruction, fistula formation, and an increase in complications at any future abdominal operation.

5. Design parameters

Despite recent advances, all of these meshes incite a foreign body response and undergo some type of reaction in the body (chemically and/or biologically). In order to improve mesh response, the design of the synthetic material could be better optimized while still achieving its primary goal of mechanical support to prevent hernia recurrence. Material parameters can be considered when optimizing the mesh for the appropriate tissue response, such as weight, weave design, and pore size. Unfortunately, there is little evidence that the designs of the current synthetic mesh materials are optimized to elicit favorable clinical results, such as a favorable tissue integration

response. For example, an important criterion is that the mesh must have the necessary tensile strength to withstand the maximum intra-abdominal forces, which is estimated to be approximately 170 mmHg during coughing [8]. To achieve the needed strength, heavyweight meshes with small pores were initially designed. While these meshes possessed very high tensile strength and burst pressures, they were potentially over engineered for most people. Additionally, the resulting scar plate formation was rigid, due to the small pores size forming granuloma bridging. From these clinical findings, mid- and lightweight mesh with larger pores (>1 mm) and smaller filaments were designed that still could withstand the intra-abdominal pressures but also would have less material per square meter, which would reduce the foreign body response and avoid granuloma bridging [9]. While most of the lightweight meshes do improve the foreign body response, clinical evidence still indicates granulomas and scar tissue forming around the fibers, and hence reformation/formation of normal host tissue usually does not occur, i.e., lower ratio of type I/III collagen occurs. Additionally, some of the newer, lighter-weight mesh with larger, open pore design may suffer from premature failure due to mesh displacement or rupture, highlighting the need for additional research [10].

A design parameter that is often overlooked is the weave. The design of the weave will dictate the overall mechanical properties, pore size, and also the foreign body response. While there are numerous weave designs for hernia mesh that display hexagonal pores, square pores, triangulated pores, etc., there is little scientific evidence in predicting which design would elicit better clinical results. Additionally, the isotropic or anisotropic properties of the mesh are determined by the weave design. Isotropic mesh designs display equal mechanical properties in any direction of applied stress, while anisotropic mesh displays different mechanical properties depending upon the direction of applied stress. Anisotropic mesh design results in a mesh that is stronger in one direction than in the other so that it may be possible to initiate different complexities of the foreign body response. In addition, when stress is applied to mesh (such as coughing and jumping), the mesh can change shape dramatically depending upon the weave, which can lead to enhanced inflammatory and foreign body response. Modeling of weave designs in conjunction with the biomechanics of the abdominal wall could possibly lead to better mesh designs.

Adverse Events from Synthetic Mesh

Because many hernia mesh materials are brought to the market with an FDA 510K application process, no clinical studies are typically required prior to use in patients. We are now learning about some of the problems that all meshes can cause in some patients. A biomaterial is defined as a "nonviable material used in a medical device, intended to interact with biological systems" [11]. However, biocompatibility is defined as "the ability of a material to perform *with an appropriate host response* in a specific application" [11]. While the FDA has approved synthetic mesh materials for use, most of these materials do not elicit an appropriate biocompatibility response. As stated earlier, the response is usually a fibrotic, foreign body response that results in unwanted collagen I/III ratios, which can contribute to mesh contraction, pain, and/or recurrence of the hernia in some patients. Most synthetic meshes are not inert, biologically and/or chemically.

The explanting of mesh, primarily in patients who have had mesh-related complications, has allowed the opportunity to study what truly happens to these materials during their tenure in vivo. Coda's group in Turin, Italy, examined not only explanted mesh but pristine mesh exposed to agents such as water, saline, blood, formalin, and bleach. This group looked at change in pore size of the mesh but also included some intriguing electron micrographs of the mesh surface, which demonstrated flaking and fissuring of the surface [12]. Our group has taken this further and has applied scanning electron microscopy (SEM) as well as materials analysis to demonstrate that the mesh is indeed not inert in vivo [13–15].

Polypropylene, polyester, and PTFE will initiate a biological and/or chemical response. Hydrolysis and oxidation occurs due to the natural wound healing response and the foreign body reaction, which produces very powerful oxidants, such as hydrogen peroxide and hypochloric acid. This ionic environment constantly bathes the mesh, exposes it to attack by the inflammatory cells, which can lead to breakdown of the mesh structure in some areas of the mesh in some patients. The variability of this reaction in different patients and even differences in the different parts of a single mesh in one patient illustrate the complexity of this problem.

According to the FDA Center for Devices and Radiological Health (CDRH), more adverse events occur with polymeric mesh than any other general surgery device. The number of deaths related to surgical polymeric mesh has significantly increased, from 2 reported deaths in 2000 to 40 in 2008. Additionally, there were over ten times more injuries reported in 2008 than were reported in 2000. It should be noted that this type of reporting is relatively uncontrolled and therefore unscientific. For example, it is not uncommon that lawyers enter data related to a patient that presumably is involved in a lawsuit against the medical provider and/or the hernia mesh company.

Problems with these mesh materials have resulted in class I and class II recalls. For example, the Davol Composix

Kugel Mesh was recalled in 2007 due to the memory recoil ring potentially breaking and leading to bowel perforation and/or chronic enteric fistula. Ethicon initiated a voluntary recall of PROCEED™ in 2006; the recall was due to the polypropylene surgical mesh delaminating during certain hernia repairs. These mesh products accounted for approximately 75% of the medical device reports (MDRs) during the time period of the recalls.

The Safe Medical Devices Act of 1990 (finalized in the December 11, 1995 *Federal Register*) requires user facilities (those using the medical devices) to report device-related deaths to the FDA and/or the manufacturer. Serious injuries are required to be reported to the manufacturer, who then reports to the FDA. However, current regulations do not enforce what physically happens to the device. The FDA encourages return of the device to the manufacturer, but there is no specific legislation on evaluation of returned devices [16]. It is not known how manufacturers are studying hernia mesh that has been returned to them.

There is a second reporting mechanism the FDA maintains to improve post-market surveillance of medical devices. Unlike MDR (medical device report) reporting, this is a voluntary program, known as MedWatch [17]. This web-based form allows consumers and health-care professionals the opportunity to directly report adverse events to the FDA. CDRH is also studying methods to improve mandatory reporting and post-market surveillance; the Medical Product Safety Network (MedSun) is a pilot program that was begun in 2002 which has enrolled approximately 350 hospitals and nursing homes into a secure, internet-based reporting system for both mandatory and voluntary reporting on adverse events with devices [18]. The most recent Summary of MedSun Reports describing adverse events with surgical mesh products for hernia repair only lists 29 reports from 30 products in 30 patients. Since most of these reports are voluntary, it is likely these numbers significantly under represent the actual numbers of occurring complications. Only twenty hospitals contributed to these reports which were collected between February 2007 and April 2009 [19]. The most common adverse event related to hernia mesh was the need for additional surgical procedures. Mesh was removed in a majority of these patients, but there is no mention of how or if the materials themselves were subjected to study. Despite the dramatic improvement in recurrence rates using mesh technology, there are still significant attendant complications that patients suffer.

Contraction and Migration

In a variety of animal studies, heavyweight polypropylene meshes have been shown to have more contraction compared to lightweight polypropylene and polyester. In reoperations for recurrent hernias, mesh contraction and/or migration are often found to be the cause of the recurrence. It is becoming recognized that mesh shrinkage, especially heavyweight small-pore mesh, can result in up to a 66% reduction in the surface area [20]. A difference can be seen between different types of mesh materials. A swine study demonstrated that polypropylene mesh placed in a supra-fascial position shrank from a surface area of 100 cm^2 to an average of 67 cm^2, while an identically sized polyester mesh shrank to an average of 87 cm^2 [21]. However, coating the mesh with omega-3 fatty acids (C-Qur Atrium) has shown to reduce contraction. In a 120-day in vivo study performed using 41 New Zealand white rabbits, seven different mesh materials, Atrium C-Qur, Mesh ProLite Ultra, Composix, Parietex, Proceed, Sepramesh, and DualMesh, were sewn to the intact peritoneum. After 120 days, the C-Qur mesh contracted less (3.3±2.1) than all meshes, significantly less ($p < 0.05$) than DualMesh (39.0±6.0) or Proceed (29.7±12.5), which had the largest contractions [22].

Another study recently compared a multifilament polyester mesh (Parietex™ Composite) coated with an absorbable layer of collagen on the visceral side to a monofilament polypropylene mesh (DynaMesh IPOM) covered with anti-adhesive polyvinylidene fluoride (PVDF) on the visceral side. The meshes were implanted intra-abdominally in sheep for up to 19 months, and mesh shrinkage was evaluated. The results showed a significant difference between the two meshes with respect to shrinkage at all time points (3, 6, 9, 19 months) with the PET demonstrating a shrinkage rate of 41% at 3 months as compared to 20% for the DynaMesh [23].

Another recent study was performed to investigate the relationship between shrinkage and fixation method. Parietene composite meshes were fixed either with transfascial sutures or metal spiral tacks for intraperitoneal fixation. The study concluded that while the transfascial sutures were associated with more pain within the first six postoperative weeks, after 6 months, there was less mesh shrinkage as compared to the metal spiral tacks [24]. These results concurred with another study which suggested that mesh contraction could be minimized by suture fixation and running fixation suture, which may provide a more balanced tension around the mesh, which seemed to decrease contraction rate [25].

Mesh Ingrowth and Adhesions

All macroporous synthetic meshes, if they are placed in the abdominal cavity, have the potential to allow ingrowth of bowel and other abdominal organs. This can lead to dense adhesions making future abdominal operations more difficult, and it could cause fistula formation, obstruction, and/or chronic pain. Although it would be ideal for a mesh to prevent adhesions, the prevention of ingrowth into the mesh is the key characteristic for a mesh designed to be placed in the abdominal cavity.

A study by Pierce et al. [22] investigated in vivo adhesion formation in seven different mesh materials, using New Zealand white rabbits. It was discovered that the polypropylene mesh, Proceed, exhibited both the highest-grade adhesions and the largest surface area covered by adhesions, but it was only significant when compared to either DualMesh (1.4% coverage) or Sepramesh (1.0% coverage). No other significant differences between the meshes were noted.

Newer mesh designs have been incorporated and examined for adhesion formations when utilized in an intraperitoneal position. A recent study assessed histology and adhesion formation on four different synthetic meshes (woven polypropylene, nonwoven polypropylene, ePTFE, and compressed PTFE). The four types of synthetic materials were implanted into 12 pigs to compare histology and adhesion formation after 90 days. They discovered that the best performance was that of nonwoven polypropylene, which incorporated extremely well intraperitoneally and displayed few adhesions, while both ePTFE and cPTFE also performed well with few adhesions, but cPTFE did have adhesions at raised edges if the mesh was not secured well around its circumference [26].

Mesh Infection

All synthetic meshes are at risk for infection. One of the factors leading to an increased risk for infection is an open incision for a ventral hernia repair. Sometimes a mesh, particularly a lightweight macroporous mesh, can be salvaged using drainage and antibiotics or appropriate wound care if the mesh is exposed. Often, however, the mesh (particularly if it is a microporous mesh) must be removed to completely clear an infection.

Rare Mesh Complications

There are rare but significant reactions to synthetic meshes. Some patients report systemic, flu-like symptoms after placement of a synthetic mesh. The body will continue to interact with the mesh, and this could lead to degradation and potentially to mechanical failure. We have also seen rare chronic seromas with PTFE material. The pseudo-peritoneum can actively secrete inflammatory fluid, and the patient presents with increasing abdominal pressure and abdominal girth. We have had some success with laparoscopic internal drainage of these seromas to attempt to salvage the mesh, but sometimes the mesh must be removed to prevent recurrence of the seroma.

Biologic Mesh

In the past decade, a new class of hernia mesh has evolved based on experience with allografts and autografts from other surgical applications, particularly orthopedic surgery. Both human- and animal-derived tissues have been used as abdominal wall hernia mesh, but there are many questions yet to be answered about the best applications for these products.

Biologic mesh initially was used in contaminated and other types of operations when a surgeon was not comfortable using a permanent synthetic mesh, usually due to the potential for mesh infection. In surgeons' early experience, the biologic mesh was often sewn to the edges of the fascial defect or used to bridge a hernia defect, often resulting in failure (true recurrence or mesh eventration) within the first year. Due to this experience, most surgeons now recommend not bridging a gap when at all possible when using a biologic mesh.

In general, biologic meshes have been able to be used in contaminated environments and in patients and procedures at high risk for infection. However, there is very limited experience and clinical data to demonstrate where these products have value for the patient and the health-care system. If the biologic mesh can be used to assist in the closure of the complex abdominal wall reconstruction and the costs of care can be reduced from reduced complications, then the costs for these products may be justified. Due to the complexity of these patients and clinical situations, we will need to use methods of analysis that are designed for complex situations and are designed to determine true value, for the patient and for our health-care system.

New Model to Evaluate Clinical Outcomes

In an effort to evaluate and improve clinical outcomes related to hernia disease, we have started a new patient-centered, team approach for care. Using principles of clinical quality improvement and systems science, all patients will be cared for utilizing defined, dynamic clinical pathways. The mesh choice, often determined by the patient in a shared decision process, will be one of many variables measured. Quality, satisfaction, and financial outcomes will also be defined and measured. With this "systems" approach and using the knowledge gained from analyzing the explanted hernia meshes, we hope to continuously modify the clinical pathways to achieve improved outcomes. One way to improve clinical outcomes may be to determine better mesh selection based on specific patient characteristics and/or clinical situations. This new understanding of the biology of prosthetics changes our understanding about the potential of achieving the "ideal mesh." The complexity of our patients requires us to learn what mesh is best for which patient, with the reality that different mesh products, designs, weaves, etc. will be better (or worse) for different patients.

Conclusion

While the use of synthetic mesh has reduced recurrence rates, there is an opportunity to design improved mesh prosthetics through an increased knowledge of the biology of prosthetics. The ideal mesh (for each individual patient) would be able to incorporate itself with strength and a minimum inflammatory reaction into the musculofascial component of the abdominal wall allowing for true recapitulation of host tissue. Choosing from the currently available mesh has to be a decision based on the individual patient needs, surgeon preference, and hospital materials contracts, but it is foreseeable in the near future that optimal mesh designs for specific patients and patient groups will occur within a patient-centered, clinical quality improvement model.

References

1. Read RC. The contributions of Usher and others to the elimination of tension from groin herniorrhaphy. Hernia. 2005;9:208–11.
2. Kehlet H, Bay-Nielsen M. Denmark. In: Schumpelick V, Nyhus LM, editors. Meshes: benefits and risks. New York: Springer; 2004. p. 15.
3. Burger JWA, Luijendijk RW, Hop WCJ, Halm JA, Verdaasdonk EGG, Jeekel J. Long-term follow-up of a randomized control trial of suture versus mesh repair of incisional hernia. Ann Surg. 2004;240(4):578–85.
4. Heniford BT, Park A, Ramshaw BJ, Voeller G. Laparoscopic repair of ventral hernias nine years experience with 850 consecutive hernias. Ann Surg. 2003;238(3):391–400.
5. Conze J, Rosch R, Klinge U, Weiss C, Anuroy M, Titkowa S, et al. Polypropylene in the intra-abdominal position: influence of pore size and surface area. Hernia. 2004;8(4):365–72.
6. Klosterhalfen B, Junge K, Klinge U. The lightweight and large porous mesh concept for hernia repair. Expert Rev Med Devices. 2005;2(1):1–15.
7. Scheidback H, Tamme C, Tannapfel A, Lippert H, Kockerling F. In vivo studies comparing the biocompatibility of various polypropylene meshes and their handling properties during endoscopic total extraperitoneal (TEP) patchplasty: an experimental study in pigs. Surg Endosc. 2004;18(2):211–20.
8. Cobb WS, Burns JM, Kercher KW, Matthews BD, James Norton H, Todd Heniford B. Normal intraabdominal pressure in healthy adults. J Surg Res. 2005;129:231–5.
9. Brown CN, Finch JG. Which mesh for hernia repair? Ann R Coll Surg Engl. 2010;92:272–8.
10. Gemma Pascual G, Rodrıguez M, Gomez-Giln V, Garcıa-Honduvilla N, Bujan J, Bello JM. Early tissue incorporation and collagen deposition in lightweight polypropylene meshes: bioassay in an experimental model of ventral hernia. Surgery. 2008;144(3):427–35.
11. Ratner BD, Hoffman AS, Schoen FJ, Lemons JE, editors. Biomaterials science: an introduction to materials in medicine. 2nd ed. London: Elsevier Academic Press; 2004.

12. Coda A, Bendavid R, Botto-Micca F, Bossotti M, Bona A. Structural alterations of prosthetic meshes in humans. Hernia. 2003;7:29–34.

13. Cozad M, Ramshaw BR, Grant DN, Bachman SL, Grant DA, Grant SA. Materials characterization of explanted polypropylene, polyethylene terephthalate, and expanded polytetrafluoroethylene composites: spectral and thermal analysis. J Biomed Mater Res B. 2010;49B:455–62.

14. Costello CR, Bachman SL, Ramshaw BR, Grant SA. Materials characterization of explanted heavyweight polypropylene hernia meshes. J Biomed Mater Res B Appl Biomater. 2007;83B: 44–9.

15. Costello CR, Bachman SL, Grant SA, Cleveland DS, Loy TS, Ramshaw BR. Characterization of heavyweight and lightweight polypropylene prosthetic mesh explants from a single patient. Surg Innov. 2007;14(3):168–76.

16. Lowe NS, W.L. Medical device reporting for user facilities. Center for Devices and Radiological Health 1996.

17. Medwatch. 2012. http://www.fda.gov/safety/medwatch/default.htm. Accessed 3 Feb 2012.

18. MedSun A. 2012. http://www.fda.gov/MedicalDevices/Safety/MedSunMedicalProductSafetyNetwork/default.htm. Accessed 3 Feb 2012.

19. FDA/CDRH. Medical Product Safety Network Newsletter #36 2009.

20. Klinge U, Klosterhalfen B, Muller M, Ottinger AP, Schumpelick V. Shrinking of polypropylene mesh in vivo: an experimental study in dogs. Eur J Surg. 1998;164:965–9.

21. Gonzalez R, et al. Relationship between tissue ingrowth and mesh contraction. World J Surg. 2005;29(8):1038–43.

22. Pierce RA, Perrone JM, Nimeri A, Sexton JA, Walcutt J, Frisella MM, et al. 120-day comparative analysis of adhesion grade and quantity, mesh contraction, and tissue response to a novel omega-3 fatty acid bioabsorbable barrier macroporous mesh after intraperitoneal placement. Surg Innov. 2009;16:46–54.

23. Zinther NB, Wara P, Friis-Andersen H. Shrinkage of intraperitoneal onlay mesh in sheep: coated polyester mesh versus covered polypropylene mesh. Hernia. 2010;14(6):611–5.

24. Beldi G, Wagner M, Bruegger LE, Kurmann A, Candinas D. Mesh shrinkage and pain in laparoscopic ventral hernia repair: a randomized clinical trial comparing suture versus tack mesh fixation. Surg Endosc. 2010;25(3):749–55.

25. Sekmen U, Gurleyik G, Kayadibi H, Saglam A. The role of suture fixation on mesh contraction after abdominal hernia repair. J Invest Surg. 2009;22:117–21.

26. Raptis DA, Vichova B, Breza J, Skipworth J, Barker S. A comparison of woven versus nonwoven polypropylene (PP) and expanded versus condensed polytetrafluoroethylene (PTFE) on their intraperitoneal incorporation and adhesion formation. J Surg Res. 2011;169(1):1–6.

Anesthesia

Pär Nordin

Anesthesia for Groin Hernia Surgery

It is not all surgical procedures granted to have three choices of anesthesia as the open groin hernia operation. The optimal anesthetic method has to meet several demands. It has to be simple and as safe as possible with low postoperative morbidity. It must be able to offer the patient a painless operation, guarantee a fast recovery without postoperative side effects, and has to be cost-effective. Finally, it is essential to remember that for an operation to be successful the patient should be pleased with it.

Background

Groin hernia surgery is one of the most frequent operations performed in general surgery. Outcome evaluation has usually focused on recurrence rates and technical issues, but more recently there has also been a focus on chronic post-herniorrhaphy pain [1]. However, the increasing demand by health care providers for more efficient and cost-effective surgery has resulted in modifications of care to encourage more widespread adoption of day case, outpatient surgery [2]. In this context, the choice of anesthetic method for groin hernia repair plays a significant role regarding costs, morbidity, early pain relief, and recovery. For the important question as to method of anesthesia, there is still no consensus about the best choice.

The choice of anesthesia is still controversial and available data reflect a large variation in anesthetic practice. Only rarely nowadays is the patient totally unfit to undergo a suitably judged general or regional anesthetic. Local anesthesia for hernia repair does have particular advantages—organizational and economic as well as clinical.

P. Nordin (✉)
Department of Surgery, Östersund Hospital,
Östersund, Sweden
e-mail: par.nordin@jll.se

Local anesthesia is used almost exclusively in several either private hernia centers or public hospitals with a special interest in hernia surgery [3–6]. Large amounts of epidemiologic data, reflecting general surgical practice from Scotland [7], Denmark [8], and Sweden [9], have shown that general anesthesia is the preferred method, for hernia repair in 60–70% of cases, regional anesthesia in 10–20%, and local infiltration anesthesia in about 10%. The type of anesthesia employed may depend on the preferences and skills of the surgical team rather than the feasibility of a technique in a given patient, intra- and postoperative pain control, facilitation of early recovery and monitoring requirements, postoperative morbidity, and costs.

Anesthetic Techniques

Ideally inguinal hernia repair should be performed using a simple and safe anesthetic technique that is acceptable for the patient and easily mastered in general surgical practice. The technique should carry a low morbidity risk and also be cost-effective. Postoperative side effects and prolonged hospital stay after groin hernia surgery are often related to the effects of anesthesia.

Preemptive Analgesia

The concept of preemptive analgesia has long been debated. This concept envisages that effective postoperative pain relief benefits the patient by providing comfort in the period after surgery as well as modifying the autonomic and somatic reflexes to pain which delay recovery [10]. The theory is therefore that effective treatment of acute pain facilitates early rehabilitation and recovery and those preemptive analgesic nerve blocks may prevent central sensitization and secondary hyper-analgesia after tissue damage. In a double-blind randomized trial however, utilizing a field block with bupivacaine as preemptive analgesia for inguinal herniorrhaphy, there were

A.N. Kingsnorth and K.A. LeBlanc (eds.), *Management of Abdominal Hernias*,
DOI 10.1007/978-1-84882-877-3_9, © Springer Science+Business Media London 2013

no differences in pain scores or analgesics consumptions up to 7 days after surgery when comparing patients who receive the block either at induction but before surgery, or after surgery but before the end of anesthesia [11].

A further concept in optimal management of postoperative pain relief is that of balanced analgesia [12]. This concept takes the advantage of multimodal additive and synergistic effects of a combination of analgesic drugs including nonsteroidal anti-inflammatory agents given preoperatively, incisional local anesthesia, and postoperative oral analgesics. Acting at different points on pain pathways, this approach allows low doses of individual drugs to be used thus decreasing the risk of side effects and maximizing the analgesic effect [13].

General Anesthesia

General anesthesia (GA) can provide the surgeon with optimal operating conditions in terms of patient immobility and muscular relaxation. It allows the surgeon to perform the procedure considered necessary and may have particular advantages in incarceration or suspected intestine strangulation.

Techniques

Modern GA with short-acting agents and combined with local infiltration anesthesia is safe and fully compatible with day-case surgery [14]. Inhalation anesthesia, intravenous drugs, or a combination of both may be used. In most patients optimal GA for groin hernia repair will include propofol induction supplemented with sevofluran or desfluran inhalation for maintenance. An alternative is the total intravenous variant utilizing propofol and short-acting opioids such as remifentanil, which in most cases leads to a fast recovery.

There are disadvantages in introducing opioids such as fentanyl or alfentanyl into the anesthetic sequence because of the incidence of nausea and vomiting, apnea, occasional awareness, and muscle rigidity. Benzodiazepines have proved useful for sedation; however, recovery from intravenous midazolam is not as rapid as recovery from intravenous propofol, which may be used during general anesthesia.

The disadvantages of GA are risk for airway complications, respiratory function, cardiovascular instability, nausea, vomiting, and urinary complications. Furthermore, recovery from central hypnotic effects may be prolonged and as a consequence the method is not always suitable for day-case surgery. GA also incurs added costs since it requires specialized anesthesia staff and equipment as well as post-anesthetic care facility.

Finally, the administration of a general anesthetic should not be underestimated; irrespective of technique there is incidence of side effects that may persist for up to 24 h, such as drowsiness, headache, cognitive effects, muscle pain, nausea, and vomiting.

The advantages of early ambulation to prevent thromboembolism are negated by the speed of recovery, and hence early ambulation can be achieved with modern general anesthesia.

Regional Anesthesia

Regional anesthetic techniques (RA) for groin hernia repair can be provided by either subarachnoid (spinal), epidural techniques or, more uncommon, paravertebral techniques [15].

It provides good analgesia intraoperatively and can allow the patient to be awake during the procedure if this is desired. It is quite easy to perform in the great majority of patients and avoids many of the airways, respiratory and gastrointestinal complications that may occur with GA. It also has advantages of less postoperative nausea and vomiting, the immediate postoperative period is pain-free, and minimal drug and equipment costs.

The regional anesthetic techniques do have disadvantages, however, and is burdened with a higher (albeit low) risk of inadequate anesthesia. The bilateral motor and sympathetic block may induce a prolonged postoperative recovery due to postoperative urination difficulties. Spinal anesthesia regularly results in urine retention which results in prolonged postoperative recovery [16–20]. It also carries the risk of cardiovascular instability due to high sympathetic blockade. Other disadvantages are post-spinal headache and, very rarely, neurological damage due to direct neural trauma, infection, or vascular complications. The frequency of post-spinal headache (due to dural puncture) is highly dependent on the age of the patients and type of needle use [21–23]. RA requires anesthesia staff during the operation as well as in the post-anesthetic care.

Techniques

In recent years improvements of the regional anesthetic techniques have been made with use of more short-acting local anesthetic agents and small-gauge pencil point needles. Also the use of additional spinal opioids combined with a reduction in the amount of spinal doses may reduce the postoperative side effects [21, 24]. Paravertebral block (PVB) has been used for unilateral procedures such as breast- and chest wall surgery but also inguinal hernia repair.

The most common regional technique for hernia surgery is spinal anesthesia with short-acting agents, although some hernia centers use short-acting epidural anesthesia but without providing specific intraoperative and postoperative data [25]. Because of the sparse data for epidural analgesia this technique is not discussed or recommended until further data are available. More recently, the use of a paravertebral nerve block has been investigated [15, 26], but this technique only provides analgesia equivalent to a conventional intraoperative peripheral nerve block. Two randomized trial found advantages with PVB, compared to conventional spinal anesthesia [27, 28]. In these trials all patients received intravenous infusion with propofol during surgery.

Local Anesthesia

The open treatment of primary reducible inguinal hernias in adults is nearly always possible under local anesthesia (LA) [4, 6, 29] and can be provided by a local infiltration technique [30] or by a specific blockade of the ilioinguinal and iliohypogastric nerves or a combination of the two methods (see below) [31]. The administration is technically quite easy, but it requires training. LA is only successful if the surgeon handles the tissues gently, has patience, and is fully conversant with the anesthetic technique [30, 32]. Among reported advantages are simplicity, safety, extended postoperative analgesia, early mobilization without post-anesthesia side effects, and low cost. The method is ideally suited for day-case surgery as the anesthetic agents used have no significant central effect and motor block is minimal.

The clinical advantages include the prolonged analgesia provided when long-acting local anesthetic solution is employed, enhanced definition of tissue planes afforded by the hydrodynamic dissection by the local anesthetic distending the tissues, and lastly the patient co-operation possible in testing and identifying anatomic defects. The technique is more demanding for the operator: he or she must be more precise and less traumatic to tissue than in the unconscious patient. Above all, when surgery is completed the subject may be asked to cough or strain so that any deficiencies in technique are immediately observed. The patient is saved the anxiety of GA and the hangover effect of recovery. The time taken to infiltrate the local anesthesia sufficiently to gain satisfactory analgesia has been similar to general in comparative studies [14, 18].

The infrequent use of LA may partly be the patient's wish to sleep because of fear of pain during surgery, but also explained by traditions in anesthesia practice, preferences, and skills of the surgical team. Many surgeons have probably also been reluctant to learn the technique as they may find the operation easier to perform with RA or GA.

Some patients may prove unsuitable for LA, notably very young patients, anxious patients, morbid obesity, and patients with suspected incarceration or strangulation. Whether scrotal hernias and obese patients are suitable depends entirely upon the surgeon's familiarity with the technique [32]. LA is rarely appropriate during laparoscopic repair of groin hernias [33].

History

The use of local anesthesia for the repair of groin hernia has a rather exciting history. Cocaine was isolated as a pure alkaloid from the leaves of the coca plant, Erythroxylum coca, by Niemann in 1860. It was then exploited by the Austrian Karl Koller in 1884 when he instilled it into the eye of a rabbit. This latter discovery is attributed by some to Sigmund Freud, who had been experimenting with cocaine but who deserted his experiments, and the reporting of them, for his fiancée [34]. Freud later wrote:

> In the autumn of 1886 I began to practice medicine in Vienna and married a girl who had waited more than four years for me in a distant town. Now I realize it was my fiancée's fault I did not become famous at that time. In 1884 I was profoundly interested in the little known alkaloid of coca, which Merck obtained for me to study its physiological properties. During this work, the occasion presented itself of going to see my fiancée, whom I had not seen for two years. I hurriedly finished my work with cocaine, confining myself in my report to remarking it would soon be put to new use. At the same time I suggested to my friend Konigstein, the ophthalmologist that he should experiment with cocaine in some eye cases. When I came back from holiday, I found it was not to him but to another friend, Karl Koller that I had spoken about cocaine. Koller had completed the research on the eyes of animals and demonstrated the results to the ophthalmological congress in Heidelberg. Quite rightly, the discovery of local anesthesia by cocaine, of such importance in minor surgery, was thereafter attributed to Koller. But I bear my wife no grudge for what I lost!

William Stuart Halsted, in 1885, demonstrated that cocaine could block impulses through nerves and in the process became a lifelong cocaine addict himself. He underwent sanatorium treatment for his addiction before his translation to the chair of surgery at Johns Hopkins. He apparently was never truly cured of this addiction, for he continued to require daily cocaine until his death in 1922. Halsted's resident, Harvey Cushing [35], pursued the development of local anesthesia for groin hernia repair and in 1900 published the original authoritative paper on the nervous anatomy of the inguinal region and his experiences of local anesthesia in the repair of these hernias.

More recently, Glassow and Bendavid have recorded the experience from the Shouldice clinic in Toronto with a history of over 50 years and more than 250,000 repairs, almost exclusively done in LA [5, 36]. Kark, Callesen, Barwell, Amid, and others have described similar results using local anesthesia [4, 6, 37, 38], and Kingsnorth et al. [39] described an increase in use of local anesthesia from 78 to 91% of cases in a specialized hernia service.

The choice of anesthesia is still controversial and available data reflect a large variation in anesthetic practice. LA is preferred at most centers with a special interest in hernia repair, whereas in general surgical practice, however, LA is only used in 5–8% of the patients [7–9].

Local Anesthetic Agents

Several safe and effective anesthetic agents currently are available. In the 1970s lignocaine (lidocaine) was the drug of choice but since 1980 it has been superseded by more long-acting agents as bupivacaine, levobupivacaine, and ropivacaine. However, some surgeons use a combination of agents in order to achieve the advantages of rapid onset of action and longer duration of anesthesia. Adrenaline can be used with both drugs to protract their duration of activity. Bupivacaine is available in concentrations of 0.25%, 0.50%, and 0.75%. Its onset of action is approximately 20 min and the half-life is 2–3 h.

The maximum safe dose of lignocaine is 3 mg/kg body weight and with adrenaline 7 mg/kg. For bupivacaine the maximum dose is 2 mg/kg body weight and 4 mg/kg with adrenaline.

Bupivacaine is more potent and longer acting than lignocaine and maintains the analgesic block for 8–10 h, which is a major advantage in day-case surgery [40]. The safety margin in the recommended maximum safe dose is wide, as illustrated by serial postoperative plasma concentrations following doses approaching the maximum recommended for lignocaine or bupivacaine. For instance, administering lignocaine with adrenaline to the maximum dose of 7 mg/kg, peak lignocaine concentration ranged from 0.23 to 0.9 mg/L, the toxicity threshold being 5 mg/L [41]. The administration of 20 mL of 0.5% plain bupivacaine resulted in peak venous plasma concentrations of 0.07–1.14 m/L, the cardiovascular toxicity occurring at plasma concentrations greater than 4 mg/L [42].

Barwell, reports 2,066 patients with inguinal hernias operated on under local anesthetic, uses 0.5% lignocaine without adrenaline. He has had no cases of anesthetic toxicity and perhaps the worst complication is "the occasional hematoma at the site of injection for the field block" [43]. Glassow, reporting the experience of the Shouldice clinic in Toronto, recommends 150 mL of 2% procaine without adrenaline [44], whereas Wantz recommends a mixture of lignocaine and bupivacaine with adrenaline [45].

Newer local anesthetic agents with improved safety and anesthetic equivalence have been tested in inguinal hernia surgery. In a study testing the efficacy of ropivacaine, 32 patients operated under general anesthesia were randomized to receive subcutaneous infiltration with 40 mL of ropivacaine or bupivacaine [46]. There was no difference in pain or analgesic requirements after surgery. Bay-Nielsen et al. found neither differences in intra- or postoperative pain when comparing levobupivacaine with

bupivacaine [47]. In a double-blind study comparing the efficacy of levobupivacaine with bupivacaine in elective inguinal herniorrhaphy in 66 patients, Kingsnorth et al. concluded that levobupivacaine exerted similar analgesic effects in the early postoperative period compared with bupivacaine, the theoretical advantage of levobupivacaine being its increased safety margin regarding cardiotoxicity and neurotoxicity [48]. Maybe, due to the cardiotoxicity of bupivacaine, ropivacaine or levobupivacaine should be preferred in cases with extensive need of infiltration (more than 40 mL).

Prolongation of the duration of LA by the addition of agents designed to prolong absorption from the local tissues, mainly dextran, has been explored by several investigators. For the present, additional agents are of no proven advantage and therefore it is recommended that local anesthetic agents are used plain or with adrenaline [49].

Wantz claims that the burning pain caused by the administration of LA can be eliminated by neutralizing the agent [50]. The addition of 1 mL of 8.4% sodium bicarbonate solution to 9 mL of plain local anesthesia brings the pH to a comfortable 7.5, which also enhances the anesthesia and reduces the quantity required. The pH of local anesthetic with adrenaline is 4, and therefore 2.5 mL of the sodium bicarbonate solution is required for neutralization.

Local Anesthetic Techniques

LA can be achieved by a variety of techniques. The most common is local infiltration technique [30] or by a specific blockade of the ilioinguinal and iliohypogastric nerves (see below) or a combination of the two methods [31]. Both are preferably performed by the operating surgeon. The administration is technically quite easy, but it requires training.

The use of LA does not necessarily require an anesthesia staff during post-anesthetic care [6], but in the operating theater a nurse anesthetist should be available if supplementary sedation or analgesia is needed or anesthesia monitored care is used. An anesthetist should be available if the need arises, for instance in case of conversion from LA to GA, or when unexpected complications are met. The equipment needed for LA performance is insignificant.

The recommended local anesthetic agent is a 50:50 mixture of bupivacaine and lignocaine with the possibility to addition of adrenaline 1:200,000. The benefits of this mixture are the rapid onset of action of the lignocaine solution and the prolonged duration of the bupivacaine.

Care must be taken to avoid direct intravascular injection during the infiltration, which is a very rare event since the only major vein in the region is the femoral vein, which should be far from the wandering tip of the infiltrator's needle.

Because oxygen desaturation is common in procedures carried out under sedation [51] oxygen supplementation and measurement of arterial oxygen saturation by a pulse oximeter should be mandatory. Oxygen saturation and clinical monitoring should be supplemented by devices that continuously display the heart rate, pulse volume, or arterial pressure and electrocardiogram [52]. The patient must be able to respond to commands throughout the procedure: if they are unable to do so the seditionist has become an anesthetist. The same standards should be applied to sedative techniques (and RA), when there is depression of consciousness or cardiovascular or respiratory complications.

A small dose of intravenous midazolam (2–4 mg) reduces anxiety and makes the patient more relaxed and co-operative. However, recovery from intravenous midazolam is not as rapid as recovery from intravenous propofol. Anecdotal evidence suggests that administration of propofol reduces local anesthetic requirements [51]. In some centers propofol is used in nearly every case to make the procedure easier.

Local anesthesia should achieve the following main steps:

1. Ensure skin anesthesia in the line of incision.
2. Block the nerve supply to the aponeurotic layers, which must be dissected and manipulated.
3. Ensure anesthesia of the parietal peritoneum of the hernia and especially of the neck of the sac, which is very sensitive.

Anatomy of the Groin Area

Knowledge of the fundamental physiology and neuroanatomy of pain in the abdominal wall is essential if adequate local analgesia is to be obtained. Free nerve endings are distributed throughout the skin; stretch and pain receptors occur in each of the aponeurotic layers and in the parietal peritoneum. The skin and subcutaneous tissue are sensitive to all noxious stimuli. Pin-prick, pressure, and chemical stimuli (e.g., hypertonic solutions) cause pain in these tissues. The parietal peritoneum is also sensitive to pin-prick, stretching, and chemical stimuli. In contrast, the visceral peritoneum and hollow organs are insensitive to touch, to clamp, to knife, and to cautery, but the visceral arteries to these organs are sensitive. There is no pain when viscera are handled under local anesthesia, until a clamp is placed on the vascular pedicle.

The inguinal area is mainly supplied by three nerves which all come from the lumbar plexus. The iliohypogastric nerve (L1) runs between the transverses and internal oblique muscles and supplies the skin above the inguinal ligament. The ilioinguinal nerve (L1) runs parallel to but below the iliohypogastric nerve and on top of the cord through the external ring and gives supply to the adjacent skin and to the scrotum. The genitofemoral nerve (L1 and L2) via its genital

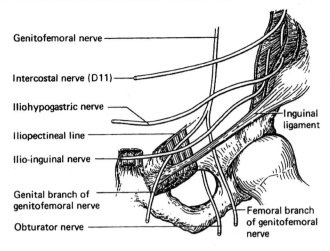

Fig. 9.1 Sensory nerve supply of the inguinal, femoral, and obturator regions

branch supplies the cord structures and anterior scrotum and via its femoral branch the skin and subcutaneous tissue in the femoral triangle. All the nerves of the anterior abdominal wall communicate with each other and thus their cutaneous distribution overlaps (Fig. 9.1). Autonomic nerve fibers accompany the cord to the testis.

Inguinal Block Technique

Inguinal and femoral hernias lie in the borderland between the regular anatomy of the abdominal wall and the complex anatomy of the lower limb. However, the same technical sequence ensures adequate regional anesthesia:

1. An injection is made between the internal oblique and transversus muscles about 1 cm superior to the anterior superior spine in an endeavor to block the ilioinguinal and iliohypogastric nerves. To do this the needle is pushed in vertically; the "give" as the needle penetrates the aponeurosis of the external oblique allows easy estimate of the depth of the injection. Twenty milliliters of local anesthetic is injected at this site (Fig. 9.2).
2. A local weal is raised in the line of the incision. This weal starts 2 cm above and medial to the anterior superior iliac spine. Long spinal needles may be used to deliver this 20 mL infiltration (Fig. 9.3).
3. The medial end of the oblique subcutaneous weal is now "topped up" with 2 mL of local solution, taking care to carry the injection down to the pubic tubercle and the origin of the rectus muscle from the pubis.
4. The final 20 mL syringe of local anesthetic mixture is infiltrated along the direction of the spermatic cord and through the skin, subcutaneous fat, and external oblique aponeurosis (the "give" is felt as the needle penetrates adjacent peritoneal sac, beginning at the deep ring. To achieve this the tip of the infiltration needle is inserted

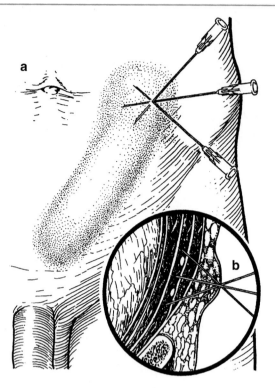

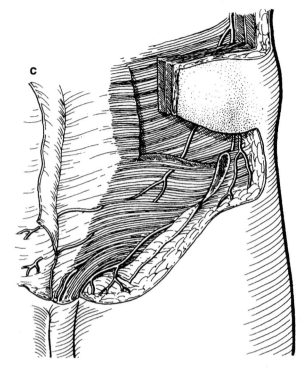

Fig. 9.2 (**a**, **b**) At the upper end of the previous weal, at a point approximately 1 cm above and medial to the anterior superior iliac spine, some 3 mL of the anesthetic solution is injected deep to the aponeurosis of the external oblique. The needle is pushed in until the external oblique aponeurosis is felt as a firm resistant structure. (**c**) The needle is pushed through the aponeurosis and the anesthetic solution distributed to block the ilioinguinal and iliohypogastric nerves which run between the external and internal oblique muscles at this point

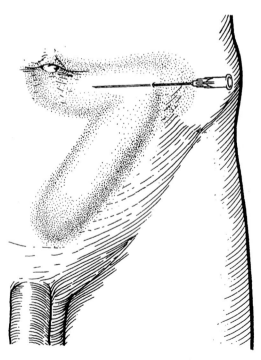

Fig. 9.3 Local anesthesia for an inguinal hernioplasty: using a long spinal needle a weal of local anesthetic solution is made in the line of the groin incision

into the aponeurosis), the syringe aspirated to ensure that the skin at the surface marking of the deep ring, traversed pampiniform plexus has not been penetrated, and the content of the syringe is then gently injected obliquely along the direction of the spermatic cord towards and including the pubic tubercle. This solution will anesthetize the deeper structures including the sac and the genital branch of the genitofemoral nerve (Fig. 9.4).

5. This anesthetic block can conveniently be applied by the surgeon or anesthetist under strict aseptic conditions but before scrubbing up and gowning. In the 5 or 10 min between application of the block, scrubbing, gowning, and preparing the skin and draping the patient, the infiltration will have become completely effective.

6. Patients should be informed that the slightest discomfort will be supplemented with additional local anesthetic solution. This event is the patient's greatest anxiety and the nature of previous anesthetic experience is the prime determinant of any anxiety preoperatively [53].

Local Infiltration Technique

This method is based on preventing pain by infiltration before the incision and, as always when LA is applied, the use of a

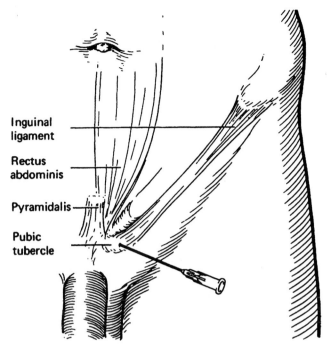

Fig. 9.4 The medial end of the oblique groin (incision) weal is topped up down to the pubic tubercle and origin of the rectus

Labels on figure:
- Inguinal ligament
- Rectus abdominis
- Pyramidalis
- Pubic tubercle

7. Now the cord can be released and infiltrated around its proximal section.
8. *Hernia sac infiltration*: This is the final step of the infiltration. A few milliliters is placed around the neck of the hernia sac.

Laparoscopic Hernia Repair

Hernia surgery requiring intraabdominal manipulation is rarely advisable under local anesthetic and the technique is rarely appropriate during laparoscopic repair of inguinal hernias [33]. However, there are some who are attempting to pursue laparoscopic hernia repair under local anesthetic approaches combined with sedation. It is technically much more difficult to perform and requires extensive experience. In general surgical practice GA should be the preferable choice if laparoscopic repair is to be adopted.

Complications of Local Anesthetics

The possible major complications are allergic reactions, CNS toxicity, cardiac arrhythmias, and cardiovascular collapse due to inadvertent intravascular injection of the local anesthetic. However, all is rare with the local infiltration technique and has never described in large hernia series (Callesen, Amid, Kark, Bendavid). A possible minor complication is a transient femoral nerve blockade, due to a deep injection or spread between fascia planes [54]. Apart from this, the technique is considered extremely safe. Patients undergoing local anesthesia should be questioned about previous side effects from local anesthetics.

Complications of local anesthetics are systemic and local:

Systemic:
(a) Excitation of the nervous system, nervousness, nausea, and convulsions—these are very rare; Increased patient excitability and garrulousness, a rising pulse rate, and an increasing blood pressure are the early signs of CNS intoxication.
(b) Depression of the cardiovascular system with hypotension and arrhythmias.
(c) Hypersensitivity reactions are very rare with lignocaine and bupivacaine.

Local:
(a) Ecchymoses and bruising
(b) Local ischemia and tissue necrosis if too much adrenaline is injected at one site
(c) These local complications can compromise wound healing

gentle and atraumatic surgical technique. Forty milliliters of the 50:50 mixture of a short- and a long-acting agent is usually sufficient for a unilateral hernia operation. It is a simple step-by-step infiltration procedure well described by Amid et al. [30] and contains no field blocks at all, only local infiltration. The method should contain the following steps:

1. *Subdermal infiltration*: 10 mL along the line of the incision.
2. *Deep subcutaneous infiltration*: 10 mL deep into the adipose tissue by vertical insertions 2 cm apart. It's often possible to feel the external aponeurosis with the top of the needle.
3. These first steps should be performed 5 or 10 min before the start of the operation (before scrubbing, gowning, and preparing the skin and draping the patient). Then the infiltration will have become completely effective.
4. *Subfascial infiltration*: 10 mL immediately underneath the aponeurosis through a window created in the adipose tissue at the lateral corner of the incision.
5. While the rest of the subcutaneous tissue is incised, the injection floods the enclosed inguinal canal and anesthetizes all three major nerves in the inguinal region. This injection also separates the external oblique aponeurosis from the underlying ilioinguinal nerve when the aponeurosis is incised.
6. *Pubic tubercle infiltration*: A few milliliters is infiltrated as early as possible in the soft tissue over the tubercle, which is a sensitive area.

Local Anesthesia for Other Small Abdominal Wall Hernias

The same concept of local anesthesia—a combination of regional block and field infiltration—can be employed for small incisional, umbilical, and epigastric hernias. Important points are to adequately infiltrate the subcutaneous layer, especially cranial to the proposed incision, and then to adequately anesthetize the intercostal nerves, which run deep to the internal, oblique/rectus sheath aponeurosis to within 2 cm of the midline.

The intercostal nerves run from their intercostal space forwards between the internal oblique and transversus muscles to the lateral margin of the rectus sheath. They enter the sheath on its posterior aspect, supply the rectus muscle, pierce the anterior sheath, and then ramify in the subcutaneous tissue and supply the adjacent skin. Each of these nerves gives a lateral cutaneous branch, which pierces the flat muscles and becomes subcutaneous in the midaxillary line. Once subcutaneous, this lateral cutaneous branch gives anterior and posterior branches to supply the skin and subcutaneous tissue.

The anterior portions of the six lower intercostal nerves are continued forward from their respective spaces onto the anterior abdominal wall, and are accompanied by the last thoracic (subcostal) nerve.

For local anesthesia nerve block to be successful, the intercostal nerve must be blocked before the lateral cutaneous branch is given off. The site of election for the local anesthetic injection is in the posterior axillary line. If the intercostal nerve is blocked too far anteriorly, the anterior division of the lateral cutaneous branch will remain sensitive (Fig. 9.5).

It should be remembered that the intercostal nerve is tucked under the lower border of the rib in its posterior third and in the center of the intercostal space more anteriorly (Fig. 9.6).

When the hernia is exposed, it is important to infiltrate the neck of the hernial sac (parietal peritoneum) to ensure adequate anesthesia while the sac is dissected, incised, emptied, and closed (if this is the done rather than mere reduction into the preperitoneal space).

Hernia surgery requiring extensive dissection, major intraabdominal manipulation, fluid shifts, or blood transfusion is rarely advisable under local anesthetic and the technique is rarely appropriate during laparoscopic repair of inguinal hernias [33].

Postoperative Outcome of the Anesthetic Techniques

Postoperative Pain

Effective postoperative pain relief benefits the patient by providing comfort in the period after surgery as well as modifying

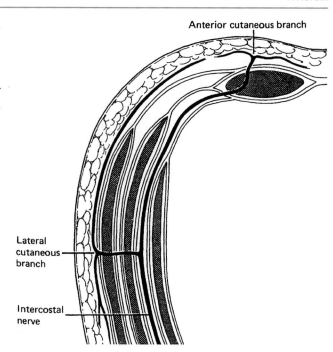

Fig. 9.5 Transverse section through the abdominal wall. The lateral cutaneous branch of an intercostal nerve gives an anterior and posterior division; the anterior division must be blocked for effective abdominal wall anesthesia

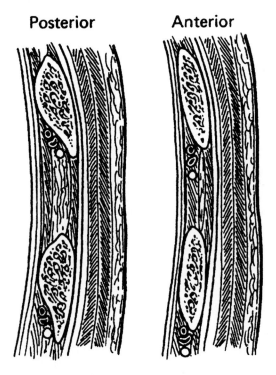

Fig. 9.6 The relative positions of the ribs and the intercostal nerves vary. Posterior to the midaxillary line the intercostal nerves and vessels are tucked under the rib next above, anteriorly they lie midway between the ribs in the mid-intercostal space

the autonomic and somatic reflexes to pain which delay recovery. Treatment of pain facilitates early rehabilitation and recovery [10]. Maximum pain is found on postoperative day 1 and often significant problems are present until the end of the first week [55].

Early postoperative pain is reduced when the operation is performed under LA with the use of a long-acting local anesthetic (bupivacaine, levobupivacaine, ropivacaine) that lasts 4–6 h. This is longer than that for RA or GA, as documented in large, randomized trials comparing the three anesthetic techniques [14, 18]. In earlier reports regarding postoperative pain one study found no difference [56] between anesthetic methods, and five studies observed less pain with LA [6, 57–60]. An exception is the randomized controlled trial of Teasdale et al. [61], where patients with LA required more postoperative analgesics than those in the GA group. Perhaps their use of a short-action agent may be held responsible.

For patients undergoing inguinal hernia repair under GA [62] the benefits of instillation of a long-acting local anesthetic agent into the wound are so well documented that omission of this step should be considered suboptimal care [63, 64]. Patients given GA do not differ in pain scores or analgesic consumption whether given inguinal field block before the surgical incision or after wound closure [65, 66].

Several NSAID drugs have been proven effective after hernia surgery in controlled studies [67–69]. The combination of nonsteroidal anti-inflammatory drugs and local anesthesia acting at different points on pain pathways can maximize analgesic effects and minimize side effects of opioids. A suppository of 100 mg diclofenac sodium administered 1 h before surgery has now become an established part of balanced analgesia regimens in many areas. However, this drug should be used with caution in patients with previous gastrointestinal ulceration, asthma, renal failure, heart failure, or bleeding diatheses.

Regular oral paracetamol for up to 1 week should be recommended to supplement local anesthetic wound blockade and preoperative diclofenac. Opioids are frequently necessary and used routinely in some areas of the world.

Early Complications

The reported risk of urinary retention is usually around 3% [17]. Spinal anesthesia regularly results in urine retention which results in prolonged postoperative recovery [16–20].

In large epidemiologic and consecutive series and several randomized clinical studies, the lowest risk of urinary retention has been obtained with local infiltration anesthesia amounting to 0–1% [4, 6, 17–20] and without an increase in local surgical complications.

The risk of hematoma, infection, and other complications in relation to the anesthetic technique has not been accurately

elucidated but is probably inconsiderable owing to the otherwise low morbidity rate associated with elective groin hernia repair.

Recovery

Postoperative side effects after groin hernia surgery such as nausea and vomiting, time to first meal, and daily activities are often related to anesthesia. Of 13 randomized studies comparing LA with GA and/or RA [14, 18, 20, 58–61, 70–76], 12 bear witness of faster discharge and faster short-term recovery with local. This held true for length of postoperative hospital stay as well as for number of unplanned overnight admissions. The main reason was greater postoperative pain, requiring opioid analgesics after RA and GA, and the large numbers of patients, especially in the RA group, with pronounced micturition difficulties necessitating catheterization. One study did not reveal any difference [76], but interpretation was hindered because of the use of large doses of sedatives and intraoperative and early postoperative potent, long-acting opioids, which often leads to unnecessary nausea, sedation, and discomfort. The few data available from other reports concerning postoperative recovery also reported advantages for LA [6, 56].

Recurrence

Although complication rates are low and hernia recurrence rates lower in many reported series using LA, it is difficult to suggest that the anesthetic has a direct effect on the recurrence rate, which is governed so much by surgical and technical factors. The long-term outcome of hernia repair is generally assumed not to be affected by method of anesthesia used. However, the evidence on which this assumption is based is far from convincing. The few studies on the topic have rendered conflicting results [29, 77–80]. Moreover, information from most randomized trials is limited since follow-up periods are relatively short.

In a register study from Sweden where 59,823 hernia repairs were recorded [81] LA was found to be associated with a somewhat higher reoperation rate in primary hernia repair. No similar association was found after operations for recurrence. In a study on the effect of smoking, Sorensen et al. [82] accidentally found LA to carry a higher risk of recurrence than GA and RA combined. In contrast, no such connection was found in a prospective nationwide register study in Denmark, with data from more than 50,000 patients [29]. Kingsnorth et al. [79] found that the surgeon's personal experience was the factor that most strongly influenced recurrence.

This leads us to stress the importance of proper training before adopting the local anesthetic technique, which is quite easy to learn, but only successful if the surgeon handles the tissues gently and has patience. Since skill and experience seem to be of such great importance in LA, substandard results are likely to occur if surgeons use the technique without appropriate training. In conclusion, a potentially increased risk of a recurrent hernia should not be an argument against LA.

Patient Satisfaction

Most reviews and case series as well as randomized trials indicate that LA has the edge on its rivals GA and RA. But for an operation to be entirely successful the patients should be satisfied with all aspects of management and is hardly likely to be so if they consider themselves to have been exposed to more pain than was absolutely necessary. Data from randomized studies comparing the three anesthetic techniques have shown similar patient satisfaction. The total satisfaction rate of patients operated under LA varies between 80 and 96% [4, 6, 14, 56, 57, 61, 83–85]. The main reason for dissatisfaction with local seemed to be intraoperative pain and discomfort [6, 85]. A great majority of patients from all three groups was satisfied or very satisfied with their anesthesia and the proportion of patients who would prefer the same kind of anesthesia in the future was similar among the three groups [14, 20, 72, 84, 85].

However, in a dedicated ambulatory unit undertaking inguinal hernia repair under unmonitored local anesthesia, 1,000 patients were sent a questionnaire after the surgical intervention [6]. The questionnaire was returned by 940 patients of whom 124 expressed dissatisfaction with the local anesthesia, the day-case setup, or both. The primary reason for complaint by the patients was intraoperative pain (7.8%). This is a relatively high rate of dissatisfaction and suggests that the local anesthetic care pathway still has room for improvement in the intraoperative phase.

Patient preference in the choice of anesthetic cannot be discounted and LA is only successful if the surgeon handles the tissues gently, has patience, and is fully conversant with the technique [32]. When these conditions are fulfilled surgeons should be able to offer the patient painless surgery, which no doubt is crucial for patient acceptance. Insufficient local infiltration technique may be accompanied by the risk of insufficient analgesia and unacceptable anxiety, emphasizing the need for optional supplementary sedation or analgesia [6]. Halsted and Cushing noted over a 100 years ago that pain during surgery under LA depends entirely upon the surgeon's familiarity with the technique an experience that is presumably still valid today [35]. However, the learning curve required to provide effective local anesthesia is short.

Costs

Ideally inguinal hernia repair should be performed using a simple and safe technique that is acceptable for the patient and easily mastered by the surgeon. The technique should carry a low morbidity risk and also be cost-effective. The latter aspect, cost-effectiveness, has so far attracted only slight attention, but scrutiny to ensure that limited healthcare resources are used rationally is of the utmost importance.

Cost comparisons for the anesthetic alternatives have given similar results. LA provides cost advantage over both RA and GA, regarding both total intraoperative as well as postoperative costs [14, 86–89]. Of three randomized controlled trials [14, 76, 89] two found local to be cheaper than both GA and RA [14, 89], while one observed no major difference between LA and GA [76]. The probable explanation is that in the latter trial (O'Dwyer) all operations were performed on an in-patient basis with a mean hospital stay of 3 days. In day-case surgery, prolonged hospital stay after groin hernia surgery is often due to the effects of anesthesia. It follows that for cost saving purposes the avoidance of such side effects is of crucial importance. Shorter total theater time, earlier discharge, and to some extent, anesthetic equipment requirements were the main factors for the great difference in total costs.

Conclusions

Either general, regional, or local anesthesia is suitable for open groin hernia repair. The available scientific data support the use of local anesthesia. A great majority of randomized studies comparing the anesthetic techniques bear witness to advantage for local anesthetic such as less postoperative pain, less anesthesia-related complaints, less micturition difficulties, faster discharge, faster short-term recovery, and fewer costs. This knowledge has not been translated into general practice. There seems to be a discrepancy between existing scientific data and clinical practice. This may be due, in part, to patient preferences to undergo GA rather than either RA or LA.

The development of new short-acting intravenous general anesthetics (propofol, remifentanil) may be a valid alternative to local infiltration anesthesia alone, as the former can be combined with intraoperative local infiltration anesthesia for early postoperative pain relief.

Regional anesthesia especially when using high dose and/or long-acting agents seems to have no documented benefits in open inguinal hernia repair and increases the risk of urinary retention, prolonged recovery, and delayed discharge.

References

1. Aasvang E, Kehlet H. Surgical management of chronic pain after inguinal hernia repair. Br J Surg. 2005;92:795–801.

2. Kingsnorth A, LeBlanc K. Hernias: inguinal, incisional. Lancet. 2003;362:1561–71.

3. Amid PK, Shulman AG, Lichtenstein IL. Open tension-free repair of inguinal hernias: the Lichenstein technique. Eur J Surg. 1996;162:447–53.

4. Kark AE, Kurzer MN, Belsham PA. Three thousand one hundred seventy-five primary inguinal hernia repairs: advantage of ambulatory open mesh repair in local anaesthesia. J Am Coll Surg. 1998;186:447–55.

5. Bendavid R. Symposium on the management of inguinal hernias. 4. The Shouldice technique: a canon in hernia repair. Can J Surg. 1997;40:199–207.

6. Callesen T, Bech K, Kehlet H. One thousand consecutive inguinal hernia repairs under unmonitored local anaesthesia. Anesth Analg. 2001;93:1373–6.

7. Hair A, Duffy K, Mclean J, et al. Groin hernia repair in Scotland. Br J Surg. 2000;87:1722–6.

8. Bay-Nielsen M, Kehlet H, Strand L, et al. Quality assessment of 26,304 herniorrhaphies in Denmark; a nationwide questionnaire study. Lancet. 2001;358:1124–8.

9. Nilsson E, Haapaniemi S. Assessing the quality of hernia repair. In: Fitzgibbons Jr R, Greenburg AG, editors. Nyhus and condon: hernia. Philadelphia: Lippincott Williams & Wilkins; 2000.

10. Wheatley RG, Samaan AK. Postoperative pain relief. Br J Surg. 1995;82:292–5.

11. Gill P, Kiami S. Pre-emptive analgesia with local anaesthetic for herniorrhaphy. Anaesthesia. 2001;56:414–7.

12. Kehlet H. Balanced analgesia: a prerequisite for optimal recovery. Br J Surg. 1998;85:3–4.

13. Callesen T, Kehlet H. Post-herniorrhaphy pain. Anesthesiology. 1997;87:1219–30.

14. Song D, Greilich NB, White PF, Watcha MF, Tongier WK. Recovery profiles and costs of anesthesia for outpatient unilateral inguinal herniorrhaphy. Anesth Analg. 2000;91:876–81.

15. Klein SM, Pietrobon R, Nielsen KC, et al. Paravertebral somatic nerve block compared with peripheral nerve blocks for outpatient inguinal herniorrhaphy. Reg Anesth Pain Med. 2002;27:476–80.

16. Finley Jr RK, Miller SF, Jones LM. Elimination of urinary retention following inguinal herniorrhaphy. Am Surg. 1991;57:486–8.

17. Jensen P, Mikkelsen T, Kehlet H. Postherniorrhaphy urinary retention—effect of local, regional, and general anesthesia: a review. Reg Anesth Pain Med. 2002;27:612–7.

18. Nordin P, Zetterstrom H, Gunnarsson U, Nilsson E. Local, regional, or general anaesthesia in groin hernia repair: multicentre randomised trial. Lancet. 2003;362:853–8.

19. Ryan Jr JA, Adye BA, Jolly PC, Mulroy MF. Outpatient inguinal herniorrhaphy with both regional and local anesthesia. Am J Surg. 1984;148:313–6.

20. Sultana A, Jagdish S, Pai D, Rajendiran KM. Inguinal herniorrhaphy under local anaesthesia and spinal anaesthesia—a comparative study. J Indian Med Assoc. 1999;97:169–70, 175.

21. Salinas FV, Liu SS. Spinal anaesthetics and adjuncts in the ambulatory setting. Best Pract Res Clin Anaesthesiol. 2001;16:195–210.

22. Halpern S, Preston R. Postdural puncture headache and spinal needle design. metaanalyses. Anesthesiology. 1994;81:1376–83.

23. Kehlet H, Dahl JB. Spinal anaesthesia for inguinal hernia repair? Acta Anaesthesiol Scand. 2003;47:1–2.

24. Gupta A, Axelsson K, Thörn SE, Matthiessen P, Larsson LG, Holmström B, et al. Low-dose bupivacaine plus fentanyl for spinal anesthesia during ambulatory inguinal herniorrhaphy: a comparison between 6 mg and 7,5 mg of bupivacaine. Acta Anaesthesiol Scand. 2003;47:13–9.

25. Robbins AW, Rutkow IM. Mesh plug repair and groin hernia surgery. Surg Clin North Am. 1998;78:1007–23.

26. Weltz CR, Klein SM, Arbo JE, et al. Paravertebral block anesthesia for inguinal hernia repair. World J Surg. 2003;27:425–9.

27. Bhattacharya P, Mandal MC, Mukhopadhyay S, Das S, Pal PP, Basu SR. Unilateral paravertebral block: an alternative to conventional spinal anaesthesia for inguinal hernia repair. Acta Anaesthesiol Scand. 2010;54(2):246–51.

28. Akcaboy EY, Akcaboy ZN, Gogus N. Ambulatory inguinal herniorrhaphy: paravertebral block versus spinal anesthesia. Minerva Anestesiol. 2009;75(12):684–91.

29. Kehlet H, Bay NM. Anaesthetic practice for groin hernia repair—a nation-wide study in Denmark 1998–2003. Acta Anaesthesiol Scand. 2005;49:143–6.

30. Amid PK, Shulman AG, Lichtenstein IL. Local anesthesia for inguinal hernia repair step-by-step procedure. Ann Surg. 1994;220:735–7.

31. Heidemann Andersen F, Nielsen K, Kehlet H. Combined ileoinguinal blockade and infiltration anaesthesia for inguinal hemiorrhaphy. Br J Anaesth. 2005;94:520–3.

32. Ponka JL. Hernias of the abdominal wall. Philadelphia: WB Saunders; 1980.

33. Edelman DS, Misiakos EP, Moses K. Extraperitoneal laparoscopic hernia repair with local anaesthesia. Surg Endosc. 2001;15:976–80.

34. Margotta R. An illustrated history of medicine. In: Lewis L, editor. English translation. Middlesex: Hamlyn; 1968.

35. Cushing H. The employment of local anaesthetics in the radical cure of certain cases of hernia with a note on the nervous anatomy of the inguinal region. Ann Surg. 1900;31:1.

36. Glassow F. Inguinal hernia repair using local anaesthesia. Ann R Coll Surg Engl. 1984;66:382–7.

37. Barwell NJ. Results of conventional inguinal hernia surgery in England. In: Buchler MW, Farthmann EH, editors. Progress in surgery, vol. 21. Basel and London: Karger; 1996. p. 100–4.

38. Amid PK, Lichtenstein IL. Long-term result and current status of the Lichtenstein open tension-free hernioplasty. Hernia. 2003;2:89–94.

39. Kingsnorth AN, Porter C, Bennett DH. The benefits of a hernia service in a public hospital. Hernia. 2000;4:1–5.

40. Armstrong DN, Kingsnorth AN. Local anaesthesia in inguinal herniorrhaphy: influence of dextran and saline solutions on duration of action of bupivacaine. Ann R Coll Surg Engl. 1986;68:207–8.

41. Karatassas A, Morris RG, Walsh D, Hung P, Slavotinek AH. Evaluation of the safety of inguinal hernia repair in the elderly using lignocaine infiltration anaesthesia. Aust N Z J Surg. 1993;63:266–9.

42. Kastrissios H, Triggs EJ, Sinclair F, Moran P, Smithers M. Plasma concentrations of bupivacaine after wound infiltration of a 0.5% solution after inguinal herniorrhaphy; a preliminary study. Eur J Clin Pharmacol. 1993;44:555–7.

43. Barwell NJ. Recurrence and early activity after groin hernia repair. Lancet. 1981;2:985.

44. Glassow F. Short stay surgery (Shouldice technique) for repair of inguinal hernia. Ann R Coll Surg Engl. 1976;58:133–9.

45. Glassow F. Ambulatory hernia repair (a discussion with M. Ravitch and G. Wantz). Contemp Surg. 1984;24:107–30.

46. Erichsen CJ, Vibits H, Dahl JB, Kehlet H. Wound infiltration with ropivacaine and bupivacaine for pain after inguinal herniotomy. Acta Anesthesiol Scand. 1995;39:67–70.

47. Bay-Nielsen M, Klarskov B, Bech K, et al. Levobubivacaine vs bupivacaine as infiltration anaesthesia in inguinal herniorrhaphy. Br J Anaesth. 1999;82:280–2.

48. Kingsnorth AN, Porter CA, Cummings GC, Bennett DH. A randomized, double-blind study to compare the efficacy of levobupivacaine with bupivacaine in elective inguinal herniorrhaphy. Eur J Surg. 2002;168:391–6.

49. Kingsnorth AN, Wijesinha SS, Grixti CJ. Evaluation of dextran with local anaesthesia for short stay inguinal herniorrhaphy. Ann R Coll Surg Engl. 1979;61:456–8.

50. Wantz GE. Atlas of hernia surgery. New York: Raven Press; 1991.

51. Charlton JE. Monitoring and supplemental oxygen during endoscopy. Br Med J. 1995;310:886–7.

52. Association of Anaesthetists of Great Britain and Ireland. Recommendations for standards of monitoring during anaesthesia and recovery, revised edn. London: AAGBI; 1994.

53. MacKenzie JW. Daycase anaesthesia and anxiety: a study of anxiety profiles amongst patients attending a day bed unit. Anaesthesia. 1989;44:437–40.

54. Skinner PP, Raftery AT, Rosario DJ. Transient femoral nerve palsy complicating preoperative ilioinguinal nerve blockade for inguinal herniorrhaphy. Br J Surg. 1994;81:897.

55. Callesen T, Bech K, Nielsen R, et al. Pain after groin hernia repair. Br J Surg. 1998;85:1412–4.

56. Young DV. Comparison of local, spinal, and general anesthesia for inguinal herniorrhaphy. Am J Surg. 1987;153:560–3.

57. Peiper C, Tons C, Schippers E, et al. Local versus general anaesthesia for Shouldice repair of the inguinal hernia. World J Surg. 1994;18:912–5.

58. Knapp RW, Mullen JT. Clinical evaluation of the use of local anaesthesia for the repair of inguinal hernia. Am Surg. 1976;42:908–10.

59. Godfrey PJ, Greenan J, Ranasinghe DD, et al. Ventilatory capacity after three methods of anaesthesia for inguinal hernia repair: a randomized controlled trial. Br J Surg. 1981;68:587–9.

60. Alsarrage SAM, Godbole CSM. A randomised controlled trial to compare local with general anaesthesia for inguinal hernia repair. J Kuwait Med Assoc. 1990;24:31–4.

61. Teasdale C, McCrum A, Williams NB, et al. A randomised controlled trial to compare local with general anaesthesia for short-stay inguinal hernia repair. Ann R Coll Surg Engl. 1982;64:238–42.

62. Spittal MJ, Hunter SJ. A comparison of bupivacaine instillation and inguinal field block for control of pain after herniorrhaphy. Ann R Coll Surg Engl. 1992;74:85–8.

63. Dierking GW, Ostergaard E, Ostergard HT, Dahl JB. The effects of wound infiltration with bupivacaine versus saline on postoperative pain and opioid requirements after herniorrhaphy. Acta Anaesthesiol Scand. 1994;38:289–92.

64. Tverskoy M, Cozacov C, Ayache M, Bradley Jr EL, Kissin I. Postoperative pain after inguinal herniorrhaphy with different types of anesthesia. Anesth Analg. 1990;70:29–35.

65. Dierking GW, Dahl JB, Kanstrup J, Dahl A, Kehlet H. Effect of pre- vs postoperative inguinal field block on postoperative pain after hernoirrhaphy. Br J Anaesth. 1992;68:344–8.

66. Møiniche S, Kehlet H, Dahl JB. A qualitative and quantitative systematic review of pre-emptive analgesia for postoperative pain relief: the role of timing of analgesia. Anesthesiology. 2002;96:725–41.

67. Iles JD. Relief of postoperative pain by ibuprofen: a report of two studies. Can J Surg. 1980;23:288–90.

68. Dueholm S, Forrest M, Hjortsö E, et al. Pain relief following herniotomy: a double-blind randomized comparison between naproxen and placebo. Acta Anaesthesiol Scand. 1989;33:391–4.

69. Mentes O, Bagci M. Postoperative pain management after inguinal hernia repair: lornoxicam versus tramadol. Hernia. 2009;13(4):427–30.

70. Kingsnorth AN, Bowley DMG, Porter C. A prospective study of 1000 hernias: results of the Plymouth Hernia Service. Ann R Coll Surg Engl. 2003;85:18–22.

71. Özgün H, Kurt MN, Kurt I, et al. Comparison of local, spinal and general anaesthesia for inguinal hemiorrhaphy. Eur J Surg. 2002;168:455–9.

72. Behnia R, Hashemi F, Stryker SJ, Ujiki GT, Poticha SM. A comparison of general versus local anesthesia during inguinal herniorrhaphy. Surg Gynecol Obstet. 1992;174:277–80.

73. Friemert B, et al. [A prospective randomized study on inguinal hernia repair according to the Shouldice technique. Benefits of local anesthesia]. Chirurg. 2000;71:52–7.

74. Gonullu NN, Cubukcu A, Alponat A. Comparison of local and general anesthesia in tension-free (Lichtenstein) hernioplasty: a prospective randomized trial. Hernia. 2002;6:29–32.

75. Gultekin FA, et al. A prospective comparison of local and spinal anesthesia for inguinal hernia repair. Hernia. 2007;11:153–6.

76. O'Dwyer PJ, et al. Local or general anesthesia for open hernia repair: a randomized trial. Ann Surg. 2003;237:574–9.

77. Schmitz R, Shah S, Treckmann J, Schneider K. [Extraperitoneal, "tension free" inguinal hernia repair with local anesthesia—a contribution to effectiveness and economy]. Langenbecks Arch Chir Suppl Kongressbd. 1997;114:1135–8.

78. van Veen RN, et al. Spinal or local anesthesia in lichtenstein hernia repair: a randomized controlled trial. Ann Surg. 2008;247:428–33.

79. Kingsnorth AN, Britton BJ, Morris PJ. Recurrent inguinal hernia after local anaesthetic repair. Br J Surg. 1981;68:273–5.

80. Morris GE, Jarrett PEM. Recurrence rates following local anaesthetic day case inguinal hernia repair by junior surgeons in a district general hospital. Ann R Coll Surg Engl. 1987;69:97–9.

81. Nordin P, Haapaniemi S, van Der Linden W, et al. Choice of anesthesia and risk of reoperation for recurrence in groin hernia repair. Ann Surg. 2004;240:187–92.

82. Sorensen LT, Friis E, Jørgensen T, et al. Smoking is a risk factor for recurrence of groin hernia. World J Surg. 2002;26:397–400.

83. Flanagan L, Bascom JU. Repair of the groin hernia. Outpatient approach with local anesthesia. Surg Clin North Am. 1984;64:257–67.

84. Nordin P, Hernell H, Unosson M, et al. Type of anaesthesia and patient acceptance in groin hernia repair: a multicentre randomised trial. Hernia. 2004;8:220–5.

85. Aasbø V, Thuen A, Ræder J. Improved long-lasting postoperative analgesia, recovery function and patient satisfaction after inguinal hernia repair with inguinal field block compared with general anesthesia. Acta Anaesthesiol Scand. 2002;46:647–78.

86. Bay-Nielsen M, Knudsen MS, Christensen JK, Kehlet H. [Cost analysis of inguinal hernia surgery in Denmark]. Ugeskr Laeger. 1999;161:5317–21.

87. Callesen T, Bech K, Kehlet H. The feasibility, safety and cost of infiltration anaesthesia for hernia repair. Hvidovre Hospital Hernia Group. Anaesthesia. 1998;53:31–5.

88. Kendell J, Wildsmith JA, Gray IG. Costing anaesthetic practice. An economic comparison of regional and general anaesthesia for varicose vein and inguinal hernia surgery. Anaesthesia. 2000;55:1106–13.

89. Nordin P, Zetterstrom H, Carlsson P, Nilsson E. Cost-effectiveness analysis of local, regional and general anaesthesia for inguinal hernia repair using data from a randomized clinical trial. Br J Surg. 2007;94:500–5.

Complications of Hernia in General

10

Morten Bay-Nielsen

Except for episodes of acute obstruction and strangulation, complications per se of having a hernia are rare. As a consequence, the description of general complications is based on single cases or case series, often from publications otherwise considered historical. While the age of the publications by itself may not be a problem, the applicability to the present patient population and current medical knowledge and technology may in some instances be questionable. Presently, only a few well-designed trials and population-based studies exist, on which to describe current complications of hernia in general.

Incarceration, Obstruction, and Strangulation

Incarceration is the state of an external hernia, which cannot be reduced into the abdomen (the term "irreducible" is sometimes used as a synonym for incarceration). Incarceration is important because it implies an increased risk of obstruction and strangulation. Incarceration is caused by (a) a tight hernial sac neck; (b) adhesions between the hernial contents and the sac lining—these adhesions are sometimes a manifestation of previous ischemia and inflammation; (c) development of pathology in the incarcerated viscus, e.g., a carcinoma or diverticulitis in incarcerated colon; (d) impaction of feces in an incarcerated colon.

Incarceration is an important finding. It should urge the surgeon to undertake operation sooner rather than later. If reduction of a hernia is performed, it should be gentle; forcible reduction of an incarcerated hernia may precipitate reductio-en-masse (see below).

If bowel with a compromised blood supply is reduced, stricturing and adhesions between gut loops will follow. This will lead to intestinal obstruction some weeks or months later [1, 2]. The best policy is to operate on incarcerated hernias and check the viability of the gut at operation.

Incarceration in an inguinal hernia is the commonest cause of acute intestinal obstruction in infants and children in the UK. In adults, postoperative adhesions account for 40% of cases of obstruction, external hernias for 30%, and malignancy for 25% of cases. In tropical Africa, strangulated external hernia is the commonest cause of intestinal obstruction in all age groups [3]. In West Africa, strangulated inguinal hernia is the commonest cause of obstruction, with indirect inguinal hernia accounting for 85% and direct hernias 15% of these cases. In the African experience, Richter's hernias are more common with direct than with indirect sacs [4].

Patients presenting with symptoms of intestinal obstruction should have all potential hernial sites carefully examined. The sites of obstruction are inguinal, femoral, umbilical, incisional, Spigelian, and obturator and perineal hernial orifices in that order.

A partial enterocele (Richter's hernia) is a particularly treacherous variety of hernia, especially in infancy (see below). Partial enterocele is a potentially lethal and easily overlooked complication of trocar site hernia following laparoscopy [5, 6].

Strangulated External Hernia in General

Strangulation is the major life-threatening complication of abdominal hernias. In strangulation the blood supply to the hernial contents is compromised. At first there is angulation and distortion of the neck of the sac; this leads to lymphatic and venous engorgement. The herniated contents become edematous. Capillary vascular permeability develops. The arterial supply is occluded by the developing edema, and now the scene is set for ischemic changes in the bowel wall.

The gut mucosal defences are breached, and intestinal bacteria multiply and penetrate through to infect the hernial sac contents. Necrobiosis and gangrene complete an irreversible

M. Bay-Nielsen (✉)
Department of Gastroenterology, Surgical Section,
Hvidovre University Hospital, Hvidovre, Denmark
e-mail: morten.bay-nielsen@regionh.dk

and lethal cycle unless surgery or preternatural fistula formation saves the patient. Hypovolemia and septic shock predicate vigorous resuscitation if surgery is to be successful [7].

The average annual incidence of strangulated external hernia in the UK is 13/100,000 population [8], with a higher prevalence in the winter months (October to March) [9].

Strangulation in Groin Hernias

During the period 1991–1992, 210 deaths occurring following inguinal hernia repair and 120 deaths following femoral hernia repair were investigated by the UK National Confidential Enquiry Into Perioperative Deaths [10]. This enquiry is concerned with the quality of delivery of surgery, anesthesia, and perioperative care. Expert advisers compare the records of patients who have died with index cases. In this group of 330 patients many were elderly (45 were aged 80–89 years) and significantly infirm unfit; 24 were ASA grade III and 21 ASA grade IV. Postoperative mortality was attributed to preexisting cardiorespiratory problems in the majority of cases. In a nationwide study in Denmark of 158 patients dying after acute groin hernia repair, Kjaergaard et al. also found that these patients were old (median age 83 years) and fragile (>80% with significant comorbidity), with frequent delay in diagnosis and subsequent treatment [11]. Clearly this group of patients requires high-quality care by an experienced surgeon and anesthetist with skills equivalent to that of the ASA grade of the patient. Postoperative care should necessarily take place in a high-dependency unit or intensive therapy unit; this may necessitate transfer of selected patients to appropriate hospitals and facilities. Sensible decisions must be made in consultation with relatives of extremely elderly, frail, or moribund patients to adopt a humane approach, which may rule out interventional surgery.

Forty percent of patients with femoral hernia are admitted as emergency cases with strangulation or incarceration, whereas only 3% of patients with direct inguinal hernias present with strangulation [12]. This clearly has implications for the prioritization on waiting lists when these types of hernia present electively to outpatient clinics. A groin hernia is at its greatest risk of strangulation within 3 months of its onset [13]. For inguinal hernia at 3 months after presentation, the cumulative probability of strangulation is 2.8%, rising to 4.5% after 2 years. For femoral hernia the risk is much higher, with a 22% probability of strangulation at 3 months after presentation rising to 45% at 21 months.

Right-sided hernias strangulate more frequently than left-sided hernias; this is possibly related to mesenteric anatomy (Fig. 10.1).

In both the UK and the USA the annual death rate due to inguinal and femoral hernia has decreased in the last two to three decades [14, 15]. In the UK, deaths for inguinal and

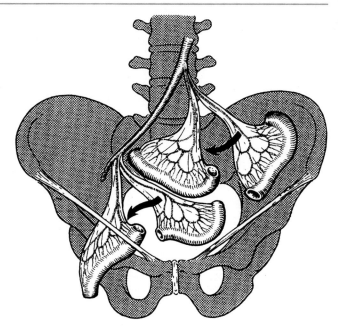

Fig. 10.1 The mesenteric anatomy determines that right-sided inguinal, femoral, and obturator hernias strangulate more frequently than left-sided ones

femoral hernia declined from 22 to 55% respectively from 1975 to 1990. The annual deaths in the USA per 100,000 population for patients with hernia and intestinal obstruction decreased from 5.1 in 1968 to 3.0 in 1988. For inguinal hernia with obstruction, 88% of patients underwent surgery with a mortality rate of 0.05%. These figures could be interpreted as showing that elective groin hernia surgery has reduced overall mortality rates. In support of this contention is the fact that strangulation rates are lower in the USA than in the UK, which could be a consequence of the three times higher rate of elective hernia surgery in the USA. Even so, the available statistics show that rates of elective hernia surgery in the USA per 100,000 population fell from 358 to 220 between 1975 and 1990 [14], although this may be an artifact of the data collection systems rather than a real decline [16].

In a randomized trial, evaluating an expectative approach to minimally symptomatic inguinal hernias, Fitzgibbons et al. in the group of patients randomized to watchful waiting found a risk of an acute hernia episode of 1.8 in 1,000 patient years [17]. In another trial, O'Dwyer and colleagues, randomizing patients with painless inguinal hernias to observation or operation, found two acute episodes in 80 patients randomized to observation [18]. In both studies, a large percentage of patients randomized to nonoperative care were eventually operated due to symptoms.

Neuhauser, who studied a population in Columbia where elective herniorrhaphy was virtually unobtainable, found an annual rate of strangulation of 0.29% for inguinal hernias [19].

The risk of an acute groin hernia episode is of particular relevance, when discussing indication for operation of painless or minimally symptomatic hernias. A sensible approach in groin hernias would be, in accordance with the guidelines from the European Hernia Society [20] to advise a male patient, that the risk of an acute operation, with an easily reducible ("disappears when lying down") inguinal hernia with little or no symptoms, is low and that the indication for operation in this instance is not absolute, but also inform, that usually the hernia after some time will cause symptoms, eventually leading to an operation.

In contrast, female patients with a groin hernia, due to the high frequency of femoral hernias and a relatively high risk of acute hernia episodes, should usually be recommended an operation [12, 13].

Strangulation in Ventral Hernias

Only very few population-based studies exist regarding ventral hernias. In a nationwide study, 661 acute operations for a ventral hernia were found in a population of approximately five male inhabitants over a 2-year period, of which 69% were periumbilical, 22% incisional, 3% parastomal, and 2% in trocar sites, giving a incidence of 6.6 acute hernia operations per 100,000 inhabitants/year [21]. Discussion of indication for surgery in incisional hernias should probably be based more on evaluation of symptoms and risk of postoperative complications, than on risk of acute hernia episodes [22].

Strangulation in Other Hernias

Obturator hernias are very prone to strangulation; however, their elective repair is rarely feasible, and a high index of suspicion particularly in elderly, emaciated female patients with symptoms of intestinal obstruction is required. Clinical suspicion (Romberg-Howship sign: pain on medial side of thigh when extending or abducting leg, positive in 15–25% of patients) combined with preoperative CT scan can in some instances diagnose an obturator hernia preoperatively, and although surgery can be successful, this group of patients has a high mortality risk [23–26]. Recently, the magnetic resonance imaging of these patients has identified these hernias readily [27].

Management of Strangulation

Diagnosis is based on symptoms and signs supplemented by diagnostic imaging when indicated. Pain over the hernia site is invariable, and obstruction with strangulation of intestine will cause colicky abdominal pain, distension, vomiting, and constipation. Physical examination may reveal degrees of dehydration with or without CNS depression, especially in the elderly if uremia is present, together with abdominal signs of intestinal obstruction. Femoral hernias can be easily missed, especially in the obese female, and a thorough examination should be performed in order to make the correct diagnosis. Frequently, however, physical examination alone is insufficiently accurate to confirm the presence of a strangulating femoral hernia vs. lymphadenopathy vs. a lymph node abscess. In these instances, one may elect to perform radiographic studies such as an ultrasound or a CT scan on an urgent or emergent basis.

Preoperative laboratory investigations should include full blood count to assess leukocytosis as an indicator of intestinal infarction and hematocrit to assess hydration. Blood biochemistry may reveal features suggestive of dehydration, such as electrolyte imbalance or raised creatinine and urea. A period of resuscitation is essential to bring these laboratory parameters in line for safe anesthesia. In the elderly a chest radiograph and electrocardiograph will complete the preoperative workup and may indicate the need for additional preoperative monitoring, such as venous pressure monitoring or atrial wedge pressure. Treatment begins with nasogastric suction, bladder catheterization, and intravenous fluid replacement. Broad spectrum antibiotics to cover both Gram-negative and Gram-positive organisms should be instituted. The period of resuscitation must be finely judged: the merits of optimizing the patient's state of hydration, electrolyte balance, and cardiopulmonary status must be balanced against the systemic toxic complications of unresected, infarcted bowel.

The choice of anesthetic is dependent upon the general fitness of the patient, patient preference, and the skills of the surgeon or anesthetist. Nevertheless, a bowel resection and anastomoses is always more safely performed through a peritoneal route; this operation should be carried out under general anesthesia. Alternatives include regional anesthesia (epidural or spinal) and, rarely, local anesthetic. Inflamed skin and tissues overlying strangulated hernial sacs have a low pH, and local anesthetic solutions may be ineffective. This should be borne in mind when selecting local anesthesia.

The choice of incision will depend on the type hernia if the diagnosis is confident. When the diagnosis is in doubt, a half Pfannenstiel incision 2 cm above the pubic ramus, extending laterally, will give an adequate approach to all types of femoral or inguinal hernia. The fundus of the hernia sac can then be approached and exposed and an incision made to expose the contents of the sac. This will allow determination of the viability of its contents. Nonviability will necessitate conversion of the transverse incision into a laparotomy incision followed by release of the constricting hernia ring, reduction of the contents of the sac, resection, and reanastomosis. Precautions should be taken to avoid contamination of the general peritoneal cavity by gangrenous bowel or intestinal contents. In the majority of cases, once the constriction of the hernia ring has been released, circulation to the intestine is reestablished and viability returns. Intestine that is initially dusky, aperistaltic, or dull in hue may pink up with a short period of warming with damp packs once the constriction band is released. If viability is doubtful, resection should be performed. A small Richter's hernia resulting in ischemia of a limited area of the intestinal circumference may be adequately treated by over sewing with a serosal suture, taking care not to reduce the bowel lumen circumference.

A viable alternative to this approach for the laparoscopic surgeon is the use of a diagnostic laparoscopy with an easy inspection of the inguinofemoral area. If a Richter's hernia, as noted above, is found, then this too can be over sewn laparoscopically. Conversion to either an open inguinal approach or a laparotomy could still be performed if needed.

Intestinal resection in children with strangulated hernias is rarely required. Resection rates are highest for femoral or recurrent inguinal hernias and lowest for inguinal hernias. Other organs, such as bladder or omentum, should be resected, as the need requires. After peritoneal lavage and formal closure of the laparotomy incision, specific repair of the groin hernia defect should be performed. In this situation prosthetic mesh should not be used in an operative field that has been contaminated and in which there is a relatively high risk of wound infection. The hernia repair should follow the general principles for elective hernia repair. It should be kept in mind, that in this group of predominantly frail and elderly patients with a very high postoperative mortality risk, the primary objective of the operation is to stop the vicious cycle of strangulation, and only secondary to repair the hernia defect.

Reductio-en-Masse

Mass reduction of a hernia is nowadays a great rarity in Western nations, where elective operation is the treatment of choice and where incarcerated or strangulated hernias are subjected to early open operation. Mass reduction is, therefore, not a complication with which surgeons are well acquainted, and for this reason the diagnosis may be overlooked. Pearse, in 1931, calculated that it occurred in 0.3% of strangulated hernias treated by taxis (gentle external reduction of the hernial contents) [28].

Reductio-en-masse (mass reduction) refers to reduction of the external herniation with continued incarceration or strangulation of the internally prolapsed hernial contents. The most commonly reported instances followed reduction of inguinal, more frequently indirect than direct, and femoral hernias. However, examples of reductio-en-masse of obturator and other rare hernias have been reported [29].

Barker and Smiddy reviewed the topic in 1970 and added considerably to our understanding of the condition. More importantly, they were able to describe additional clinical signs to enable more accurate diagnosis [30].

Reductio-en-masse is not a single anatomical entity. There are at least three varieties encountered [28]:

1. The sac still containing its strangulated contents can be forced away from the parietal muscles and come to lie in the abdominal cavity [28]. For this to occur, the neck of the sac must be small, fibrosed, and unyielding and, once irreducibility has occurred, must grip the contents preventing their reduction. The neck of the sac must also be surrounded by a weak internal ring to which it is not adherent (Fig. 10.2a). Enthusiastic manipulation by the patient or his attendants can then force the sac and its contents from their moorings and reduce them intact inside the abdominal wall. Reduction of the hernia in these circumstances causes traction on the spermatic cord with retraction of the testis. In these circumstances the reduced mass may still be palpable in the iliac fossa, the testis will be retracted on the same side, and gentle traction on the testis and spermatic cord will elicit pain—"Smiddy's sign" (Fig. 10.2b) [30].

2. The sac may separate but the constriction ring at the neck remains intact, so that although the external hernia reduces into the extraperitoneal plane, the obstruction/strangulation remains. This is the most commonly reported type, accounting for 92.8% of recorded cases [28].

3. The contents could be reduced from an external sac into a preperitoneal communicating sac if one were present. Moynihan described apparent mass reduction of an incarcerated inguinal hernia into an associated preperitoneal sac, the obstruction at the neck of the sac where it joined the main peritoneal cavity remaining unaltered. This complication can only occur in bilocular sacs. Bilocular sacs are rare, except in patients who have worn a truss for many years and developed adhesions of the superficial inguinal ring. Hence, Moynihan's type of reductio-en-masse is also very rare nowadays [31].

In all cases of reductio-en-masse, although the external hernial mass has gone, palpation of its egress site will demonstrate the empty ring. Usually there is adjacent tenderness around the egress ring and careful gentle palpation of the nearby abdomen will reveal the globular obstructed viscera in it. More importantly, the symptoms of obstruction will persist. Central colicky abdominal pain, increasing distension, vomiting, constipation, and hypovolemia should alert the clinician. Abdominal radiographs will point up the stigmata of intestinal obstruction, dilated loops, and fluid levels.

Operation through an extraperitoneal approach to the groin will allow simultaneous hernia repair if the hernia is inguinal, femoral, or obturator in type. The use of preoperative CT scanning may obviate the need for the extraperitoneal approach in this manner. Certainly the use of diagnostic

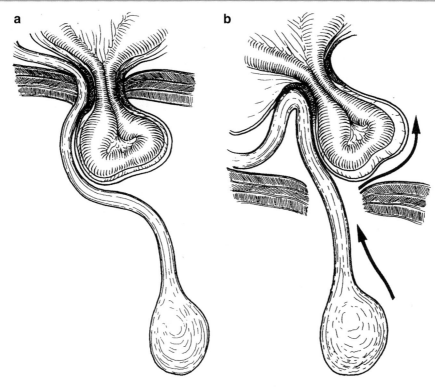

Fig. 10.2 Reductio-en-masse. (**a**) An incarcerated inguinal hernia with a tight unyielding neck which is not attached securely to the parieties at the deep ring can be forcefully reduced into the abdomen. (**b**) The bowel remains incarcerated; the sac and its contents are "reduced" into the abdomen where they remain as a tender mass in the inguinal region. The spermatic cord is dragged in by its attachment to the neck of the sac at the deep ring and consequently the testicle is retracted. Attempts to reposition the testicle (traction on the cord) will elicit pain (Smiddy's sign)

laparoscopy may provide excellent visualization of the reduced bowel, and additionally, the surgeon could then proceed with a laparoscopic hernia repair.

Maydl's Hernia and Afferent Loop Strangulation

In 1895, Maydl [32] described the hernie-en-W or double-loop hernia, in which segments of bowel proximal and distal to an infolded loop become incarcerated within a hernial sac but without loss of viability. However, the infolded or intra-abdominal loop may become infarcted by strangulation even in the presence of viable loops incarcerated in the hernial sac. When more than one loop is gangrenous, it is always the intra-abdominal loops rather than the intrahernial loops that are involved. Isolated gangrene of an intrahernial loop without gangrene of the intra-abdominal loop has not been reported (Fig. 10.3).

Maydl's hernia is most common in men and on the right side. Both small bowel and large bowel are found in these hernias; Maydl originally described the strangulated appendix vermiformis in a hernial sac (see below). On the left side the sigmoid colon and transverse colon have been described in the hernia [33]. One patient in whom all the loops were large bowel has been reported. This patient needed a right hemicolectomy because the loops of cecum, ascending colon and hepatic flexure were all gangrenous [34].

Maydl's hernia is rare in Western series of strangulated hernias. Frankau reviewed 1,487 strangulated hernia from centers in the British Isles; there were 654 strangulated inguinal hernias, and in four of these a Maydl's hernia was found (0.6%) [35]. In West Africa, where strangulated inguinal hernia is the commonest cause of intestinal obstruction, Maydl's hernia accounts for 2% of all cases [4, 36].

Afferent loop strangulation is a complication in which intra-abdominal strangulation of small intestine occurs proximal to an obstructed inguinal hernia. It is a common complication of right inguinal hernia obstruction in East Africa. The afferent loop is imprisoned behind the cecum, which is obstructed in the inguinal hernial sac. The internal herniation of the loop of ileum passes from medial to lateral, behind the pendulous cecum, which is fixed in the hernial sac. The cecum retains its circulation from the ileocecal vessels, which form the anterior component of the constriction, imprisoning the loop of ileum and infringing its mesenteric marginal blood

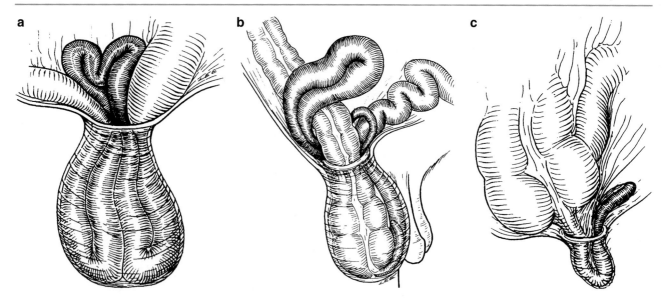

Fig. 10.3 (**a**) Maydl's hernia or W or "double-loop" hernia. The infolded, intra-abdominal loop is strangulated. It is important when operating on a strangulated hernia to inspect in continuity all the loops of gut in the sac so that an infolded loop is not overlooked. (**b**) Afferent loop strangulation. This is a complication of large inguinoscrotal hernias in Africans who have a long pendulous scrotum. The cecum is incarcerated in the hernial sac; a loop of small bowel passes behind the ascending colon and is strangulated to the right of the colon. Formal laparotomy is required. (**c**) A Maydl's hernia of the appendix is a complication of an incarcerated inguinal hernia in an infant

vessels. At operation for strangulation, if the cecum when released is pendulous and free, not sliding, the ileum for at least 1 m proximal should be checked to ensure it has not suffered entrapment and infarction [37] (Fig. 10.3).

Davey draws attention to these variations of strangulated hernia when the sac contains the cecum in Africans. As a precaution the surgeon should always count the loops in the sac and inspect the gut for 1 m proximal and distal. The use of the laparoscope in this type of patient would relieve any doubt about the viability of the bowel if this exists. A diagnosis of strangulated middle or afferent loop Maydl's hernia should be suspected in any patient who presents with a painful but not tender inguinoscrotal swelling, a tender mass in the lower abdomen, and a scaphoid empty upper abdomen [3]. Here again, the diagnostic laparoscopy will assist in the determination of the intestinal strangulation.

In small tight-necked indirect inguinal hernia in infants, a Maydl's hernia of the appendix can occur. Appendectomy at herniotomy is an appropriate surgery [38] (Fig. 10.3). Maydl's hernia can also occur after laparoscopic operations by herniation of small bowel through a trocar site [39].

Strangulation of the Appendix in a Hernial Sac

The appendix is seen frequently, in an inguinal or femoral hernial sac. Strangulation (as opposed to appendicitis) is rare. On clinical and histological grounds, separation of the two diseases should not present difficulties. In strangulation, inflammation is accompanied by venous infarction; it involves all coats of the appendix and is clearly delimited proximally where the constriction is applied [32]. In acute appendicitis, suppuration begins in the mucosa, spreads outward, and is associated with intracavity purulent distension. A strangulated appendix behaves clinically like a Richter's partial enterocele [40].

Richter's Hernia

Partial enterocele, the eponymous Richter's hernia, was not first described by Richter! And the condition has a variety of other names in the English and American literature: nipped hernia and pinched hernia. It was Sir Frederick Treves who gave an excellent overview on the topic and proposed the title Richter's hernia [41].

In the partial enterocele, the antimesenteric circumference of the intestine becomes constricted in the neck of a hernial sac without causing complete intestinal luminal occlusion (Fig. 10.4).

Richter's hernia has recently again come into prominence, this time as a complication of continuous ambulatory peritoneal dialysis (CAPD), used in the treatment of renal failure [42], and as a complication of port site hernias following laparoscopy [6]. There is a significantly greater risk of the development of such a hernia when 10-mm (or larger) trocars are used. This risk can probably be decreased if the surgeon uses a non-cutting trocar or a dilating type of trocar and can be reduced if the surgeon sutures the fascia closed after the completion of the laparoscopic procedure.

According to localization and the mode of herniation and entrapment, the clinical picture and course can vary considerably. Steinke and Zellweger have described four main

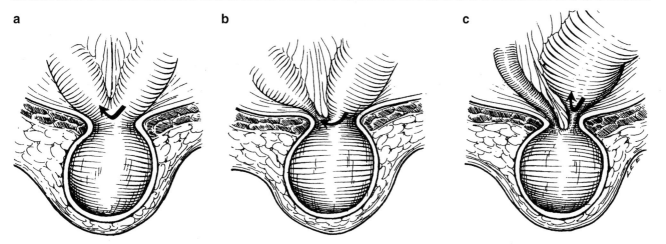

Fig. 10.4 Richter's hernia (partial enterocele). The antimesenteric circumference of the bowel is first held by the rigid neck of the hernial sac, usually a femoral or obturator hernia. The situation is progressive: from (**a**) partial involvement of the bowel circumference without obstruction to (**b**) subacute obstruction to (**c**) complete obstruction and strangulation of the incarcerated bowel

groups: (1) the obstructive group, in which early diagnosis and therapy leads to an excellent prognosis; (2) the danger group, in which symptomatology is vague and subsequent delay in surgery is responsible for a high death rate; (3) the postnecrotic group in which local strangulation and perforation leads to formation of an enterocutaneous fistula (similar to the noble woman described by Fabricius in 1606)—the fistula may close spontaneously ("the miracle cure") or remain chronic; and (4) the "unlucky" perforation group, in which the postnecrotic abscess, as a result of unlucky anatomical constellations, accidentally finds its way into another compartment, resulting either in a large abscess with severe septic/toxic load or in peritonitis; both of these would lead to a high death rate [41].

Richter's hernias occur in infantile indirect inguinal hernias. Colic and distension occur, but absolute constipation for feces and gas is a late phenomenon. Vomiting is also often absent. On physical examination there is tenderness but no palpable lump at the hernial site. Strangulation and gangrene of the bowel wall nipped in the hernial sac sets in rapidly, and perforation of the gut into the sac may occur without immediate catastrophic peritonitis. It is important to recognize the condition at operation—to return the nonviable bowel to the peritoneal cavity is to precipitate disaster.

Littre's Hernia: Hernia of Meckel's Diverticulum

Alexis Littre, in 1700, reported three cases of an incarcerated femoral hernia containing an ileal diverticulum. Littre interpreted the ileal diverticulum as a secondary phenomenon related to the hernial ring and arising from the intestine opposite it.

Meckel's diverticulum is the most common congenital anomaly of the gastrointestinal tract arising as a result of incomplete dissolution of the vitellointestinal duct. Approximately 4% of patients with Meckel's diverticulum develop complications,

Littre's hernia being one of the least common [43]. A Meckel's diverticulum may be a chance finding in an inguinal hernia. It has been described in incarcerated inguinal hernia in infants: in infants the diverticulum frequently becomes adherent to the sac, and as a consequence the hernia becomes irreducible. This can be diagnosed when after taxis of a right inguinal hernia in an infant, part of the hernia remains unreduced [44].

Meckel's diverticulum has also been described in an umbilical hernia. This is not unsurprising when it is recalled that the omphalomesenteric duct is a component of the normal fetal umbilicus [45]. Meckel's diverticulum in femoral hernia is also described; a most unusual variant is the presentation of the diverticulum as a small bowel fistula resulting from strangulation of the diverticulum progressing to a groin abscess which discharged externally with a persistent small bowel fistula [46] (Fig. 10.5).

Hernia of Ovary, Fallopian Tube, and Uterus

The first case of hernia of the ovary was reported by the Greek physician Soranus of Ephesus about AD 97. Watson reports two cases and comments that the uterus may become impregnated while in the hernial sac or the pregnant uterus may enter the sac and become irreducible as the pregnancy proceeds [38].

The tube and ovary may also enter the hernial sac. Ectopic pregnancy in a hernial sac is reported in these circumstances [38].

In contemporary practice, internal genitalia are frequently found in inguinal hernia in baby girls. The frequency with which they occur warrants caution to open and inspect each hernial sac to exclude their presence.

In older females the tube and ovary are sometimes the contents of inguinal, femoral, or obturator hernias, usually as components of sliding sacs. Pathology may complicate these

Fig. 10.5 Meckel's diverticulum in a hernial sac. A Meckel's diverticulum may be the only occupant of the sac (**a**); alternatively, adjacent loop ileum may be in the sac too (**b**). A Meckel's diverticulum may become adherent to the sac (**c**) or form a fistula (**d**)

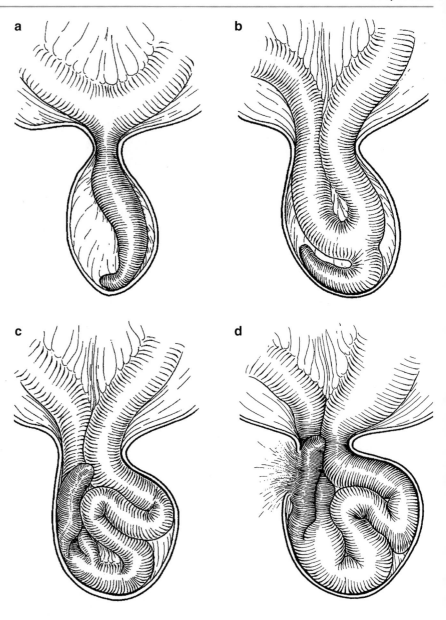

hernial contents, hydrosalpinx being common in irreducible inguinal hernia [47].

A uterus has been described in a male intersex with inguinal hernias. Routine examination of the scrotum for normal testicles should be the drill in all boys with inguinal hernias. If developmental anomalies are then found in the wall of a hernial sac, they can be excised [48].

Urinary Tract Complications

The bladder is a very frequent component of the medial wall of direct inguinal and of femoral hernias (Fig. 10.6). Herniation of the bladder proper is a rare phenomenon; the involvement of a small part of the organ, often a diverticulum, is more frequent and usually associated with hypertrophy of the prostrate [49]. This partial bladder herniation is rarely diagnosed preoperatively, but in cases where there is a strong suspicion, preoperative cystography is indicated [50]. Usually the bladder is easily identified during dissection, but when difficulty is encountered, the obliterated umbilical artery is a useful landmark. If the bladder is near the protrusion of the hernia or part of the hernia, the risk of injury is particularly high during a laparoscopic repair. This situation is even more problematic in the recurrent hernia repair. The inexperienced laparoscopist should not attempt these difficult repairs and should either refer the patient or perform a careful open hernioplasty. The bladder is a very common finding in the medial wall of indirect inguinal hernias in boys (see pp. 116, 121).

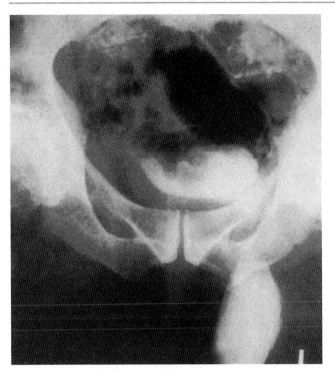

Fig. 10.6 An intravenous urogram demonstrating the left wall of the bladder in a femoral hernia sac in a man with bladder neck obstruction

Testicular Strangulation

The testicular blood supply is compromised when a tight strangulation compresses it in its passage from the abdomen to scrotum. This may occur in three circumstances:

1. In male infants with incarcerated inguinal hernias, the venous drainage becomes obstructed at the rigid external ring. This is a not infrequent complication of infantile incarceration.

2. In giant inguinoscrotal hernia, spontaneous infarction of the testicle has been described [55].

3. In Africans with strangulated indirect inguinal hernia, testicular infarction due to vascular obstruction at the deep ring is reported. At operation the gangrenous testicle should be excised [55].

The site of the vascular damage in these instances, the superficial ring in infancy and the deep ring in adulthood, emphasizes the different anatomy and structure of the inguinal canal in the pre- and postpubertal male. It is important to differentiate the diagnosis from that of testicular torsion. In either event, however, surgery is required.

Spontaneous and Traumatic Rupture

Spontaneous rupture (dehiscence) of hernia is a well recognized though very rare complication. Helwig, in a comprehensive article, reported 47 cases of spontaneous exteriorization of hernial contents; of these, 17 were through incisional hernia, while the remainder were through inguinal, femoral, umbilical, or epigastric hernia or through recurrences of these [56]. Spontaneous rupture of an umbilical hernia with evisceration is a very rare event. The complication is so rare that it should not influence the accepted surgical practice of initial conservative management of infantile umbilical hernia [57].

Four such cases are described in the British literature and one in India. In two cases there was no precipitating cause [58, 59], in one a bout of severe coughing precipitated rupture and evisceration [60] and in another damage to the overlying skin and trauma [61], and in the remaining case umbilical sepsis may have been to blame [62]. All of the children were under 4 months at the time of rupture. Damage to the bowel did not occur in any of the four British cases and complete recovery followed reduction of the bowel and standard umbilical hernioplasty.

A special case of spontaneous rupture of umbilical hernias is in patients with incompensated liver disease and ascites, where several reports exist in the literature. In case of ascites leakage, an aggressive approach to reduce ascites production by TIPS or otherwise, followed by a semi-elective repair, has been advocated [63].

Care will protect the bladder from trauma during surgery. If the bladder is injured, closure with two layers of absorbable polymer suture is required, followed by catheter drainage for a week.

Herniation of the ureter is a rare and often misdiagnosed event, and serious surgical complications are possible. Two types of the uretero-inguinal hernia can be identified: paraperitoneal (more frequent, acquired, always presenting a peritoneal hernia sac, frequently associated with other herniated abdominal structures) and extraperitoneal (very uncommon, congenital, never associated with a true peritoneal sac, always composed only of ureter [51]). The paraperitoneal type usually presents in the lateral wall of giant sliding inguinal hernias. Knowledge, suspicion, and care are all that are needed to avoid damaging the ureter. The ureter should be identified; dissected away, preserving its blood supply; and returned to the abdomen. If the ureter is injured or its vasculature in doubt, a pigtail ureteric catheter for several days is best advised [52]. Preoperative intravenous urogram and micturating cystogram are advisable before operation on giant inguinoscrotal hernias, to exclude ureteric complications or bladder diverticula in the hernial sac [53].

Prolapse of an ileal conduit into an indirect inguinal hernia is described [54]. The patient presented with an ischemic blue stoma and anuria. The ileal loop was twisted around its distal fixed point (the stoma) and prolapsed into the hernial sac.

The majority of spontaneous hernia ruptures are in lower abdominal, inguinal, and incisional hernias. Many develop insidiously and present in emergency departments some time after an apparently painless disruption. Others are associated with episodes of straining or coughing. The dehiscence would appear to be a degenerative process, with the relatively avascular and thin hernial sac, undergoing progressive stretching, becoming increasingly ischemic, and finally giving way. This process is accelerated in some cases by skin ulceration due to tight corsets or to intertrigo and skin infection in pendulous sacs.

Surprisingly, the mortality is low and is only potentially fatal in remote areas where medical assistance is far distant [64]. The main peritoneal cavity is uncontaminated, the tight neck usually preventing reduction of the contents and contamination of the main peritoneal cavity.

Spontaneous rupture leading to fistula and then "cure" was described by Cheselden [65]. A more remarkable example of a spontaneous cure of an incarcerated right inguinal hernia in a 7-week-old Chinese male child whose hernia remained irreducible for 10 days and who then developed a cecal fistula is reported by Stock [66].

Rupture of the intestine in an unreduced hernia in a male subjected to trauma is not excessively rare; deaths from this cause appear in nineteenth-century literature [67]. Except in one case in which the colon was damaged in a sliding hernia, the perforated loop of small intestine is invariably found in the general peritoneal cavity. There is an association between small bowel rupture due to blunt trauma and inguinal hernia. Small bowel perforation is more likely to have occurred if the trauma was sustained when a hernia is "down" or in the presence of a voluminous incarcerated inguinoscrotal hernia [68].

Where the violence is applied directly to the hernia, the explanation is simple—the intestine is damaged locally where it lies unprotected in the hernial sac. Alternatively the force of the blow first opposes the walls of the incoming and outgoing bowel, sealing the loop. Then additional pressure that is applied will raise the loop's intraluminal pressure to the point that traumatic perforation occurs [69]. When blunt trauma is applied to the abdomen, loops of mobile gut slide around to absorb the violence. Fixed gut is most at risk; hence the duodenum and terminal ileum are most frequently damaged. A hernia which is "down" is another fixed point contributing to gut immobility and predisposing to serious injury.

A number of cases have been reported of sudden rupture of an indirect inguinal hernial sac with extravasation, in patients on CAPD [70]. It is recommended that when patients with inguinal hernias require long-term peritoneal dialysis, even when the inguinal hernia is asymptomatic, repair should be carried before CAPD is commenced.

Involvement of Hernial Sac in Disease Process

Nodular Mesothelial Hyperplasia and Mesothelioma

The peritoneum has a great capacity to undergo metaplasia, to form papillary projections, pseudo-acini, squamous nests, and even cartilaginous nodules in response to repeated mechanical trauma [71]. Cirrhotic ascites and collagen vascular disease are associated with marked mesothelial hyperplasia. Nodular mesothelial hyperplasia can develop in hernial sacs, particularly those subject to trauma. A truss can be an initiating factor. Nodular mesothelial hyperplasia has been described in hernial sacs in infants and children and in these cases is associated with repeated episodic incarceration or strangulation. A total of 1,494 inguinal hernia sacs were pathologically evaluated from 1,077 pediatric patients by Partrick et al. [72]. Nodular mesothelial hyperplasia was a rare and incidental finding, not affecting clinical management.

The pathological features are the presence in the sac of cellular nodules up to 1.0 cm in diameter. These nodules are composed of cells with a pale acidophilic cytoplasm derived from the peritoneum. The cells show a moderate to severe pleomorphism; most are round cells when lying free in the intercellular fluid, but they are polygonal when compressed together by neighboring cells to form the characteristic nodules. The nodules may coalesce to form cystic spaces grossly resembling a pseudomyxoma [73].

If injury to the hernial sac is sustained and of sufficient intensity, the mesothelial proliferation can exceed the simple needs of regeneration and acquire pseudomalignant cytologic features. The consummate ability of mesothelial cells to simulate carcinoma should be remembered, and pathologists need to be cautious in interpreting the microscopic features of hernial sacs [73].

Nodular mesothelial hyperplasia is more common in infants and children, and in them it exhibits its most exuberant characteristics. The condition is entirely benign—no radical surgery is required and follow-up data confirms the harmless nature of the lesion. It is important to make the correct diagnosis to avoid pointless and potentially dangerous therapy. Ordonez et al. have suggested that the term nodular mesothelial hyperplasia should be replaced by the term nodular histiocytic hyperplasia because the lesions are primarily reactive histiocytic proliferations and occur in other locations aside from the serosal membrane. If any doubt exists in the diagnosis of these histiocytic proliferations because of mitotic activity or cellular atypia, then staining for keratin or the histiocytic marker CD68 may be appropriate. By this means lesions, which present high mitotic activity, can be differentiated from malignancy [74].

On the other hand, genuine peritoneal mesothelioma has been encountered within a hernial sac [75]. The mesothelioma may be found by chance, or alternatively the patient can present with a mass in the hernial sac wall. While mesothelioma generally arises in the main peritoneal cavity, it can arise from the hernial sac itself or from the cord or the tunica vaginalis. If the mesothelioma arises from the cord structures or from mesothelial remnants in them, in addition to the mass the patients usually also feature a hydrocele.

Malignant mesothelioma has been encountered in hernial sacs in patients with no history of exposure to asbestos, further evidence for a relationship with local trauma and the occurrence of mesothelial hyperplasia. Grove et al. describe three histologically and immunohistochemically well-documented cases of mesothelioma of the tunica vaginalis testis and hernia sac [76]. Analysis and follow-up of these three patients and a review of 30 previously reported cases revealed a varied and often unpredictable clinical course. A classification into high- and low-grade malignant tumors was suggested based on clinical and pathological findings. In the high-grade variety, intraperitoneal deposits appear and intestinal obstruction and other complications then ensue [75].

Solitary fibrous tumor (SFT) is a further tumor of mesenchymal origin, which is classified as a variant of fibroma and has been found arising in abdominal wall hernia sacs [77]. SFT of the peritoneum has also been called fibrous mesothelioma, and the site of origin is felt to be a submesothelial mesenchymal cell. Two primary tumors arising in hernia sacs were reported by Lee and colleagues associated with copious myxoid material mimicking pseudomyxoma peritonei. Wide local surgical excision is the treatment of choice with the degree of resectability being a powerful predictor of outcome.

Carcinoma as a Complication of Hernial Sacs

Malignancy involving inguinal hernial sacs is uncommon but not rare. Suspicion should always haunt the surgeon's mind, particularly when he is confronted with an elderly patient with the recent onset of a groin hernia [78, 79]. If the sac is thickened or ascitic fluid is present in it at operation, it should be subjected to histological evaluation and the ascitic fluid to full cytology. The hernial sac offers a unique opportunity for peritoneal biopsy, which should not be missed. If a suspicious sac is found at hernioplasty, immediate frozen section may elucidate the pathology, while digital palpation through the hernial orifice may give more information. The index of suspicion should be particularly high for male patients of advanced age and especially those who have previously undergone surgery for colorectal carcinoma [80]. Immediate laparotomy is not advised: repair the hernia and subject the patient to early elective operation after bowel preparation and antibiotic prophylaxis.

Lejars [81] classified malignant involvement of inguinal hernial sacs into three varieties: extrasaccular, saccular, and intrasaccular. While this classification has merit, it does not easily fit contemporary concepts of pathology and surgery. A better classification is:
1. Primary carcinoma: (a) extrasaccular and (b) intrasaccular
2. Secondary carcinoma—predominantly intrasaccular: derived, by metastatic spread from lung, breast, stomach, colon, ovary, or any other intraperitoneal viscus

Extrasaccular carcinoma can arise from the bladder or from a diverticulum of the bladder that is sliding into the medial side of a direct hernia. Similarly, a carcinoma may occur in the colon, which is a component of the wall of a sliding hernia. Such a carcinoma may obstruct, and a mistaken diagnosis of a strangulated hernia be made. Careful history taking can avoid this error. In the six examples recorded in the literature, all the hernias were large and scrotal, and all had been present and irreducible for some considerable time before they presented with intestinal obstruction [82]. The carcinoma is usually bulky and locally advanced and may be palpated in the sac, which is not so discreetly tender as the sac containing strangulated small bowel [83]. A liposarcoma of the cord, which invaded the adjacent hernial sac, is reported reminding surgeons that not all malignancy in groin hernias is derived from the peritoneal cavity [79].

Intrasaccular carcinoma is a primary carcinoma arising from an organ which is a permanent denizen of a hernial sac. The most frequent examples are colon or cecal cancers. Malignant tumors arising from an appendix in a hernial sac also occur [84].

Carcinomas in hernial sacs are often locally fixed and advanced when the diagnosis is made. This should not prevent wide local excision being successfully undertaken. Intrasaccular carcinoma can also occur in Spigelian, umbilical, and incisional hernias.

Routine histological examination of hernial sacs is not recommended. Kassan et al. routinely examined 1,020 hernial sacs after surgery; the incidence of unexpected findings, the discovery of an occult tumor, in those specimens, which appeared normal to the surgeon at operation, was 1 in 1,020 (0.098%). The incremental cost per unexpected finding was $49,041, and the only unexpected and abnormal finding in the series was one atypical lipoma [85]. If at operation the hernial sac is seen to be abnormal or if it is thickened, then histology should always be performed. However, there is no positive benefit to be gained by the patient from routine histological examination of an apparently normal sac. However, in some areas of the world (notably the United States), the hernia sac, if it is excised, is sent for pathologic examination for documentation of its removal as a medico-legal issue.

Gynecological Tumors: Endometriosis and Leiomyomas

Endometriomas are not infrequently encountered in incisional hernias related to caesarean section. These can also be seen in inguinal or femoral hernia sacs. The characteristic cyclical pain should enable a preoperative diagnosis. Endometriosis in the hernia sac maybe the only evidence of the disease and may mimic incarceration [86, 87].

Leiomyomas arising from uterine fibroids are also encountered in inguinal, femoral, obturator [88], and umbilical hernial [89] sacs in women.

Acute Inflammation: Peritonitis and Appendicitis as Complications of a Hernial Sac

Intraperitoneal sepsis producing pus and presenting as a painful distended hernial sac is an important differential diagnosis of strangulated hernia; in these circumstances the hernia is behaving as a peritoneal recess in which pus can loculate. Zuckerkandl first described this phenomenon in 1891. His patient was a 55-year-old male with a 6-day history of a painful irreducible right inguinal hernia. At operation the hernial sac contained pus only, and the perforated appendix lays in the peritoneal cavity just above the sac. The appendix was not removed and the patient recovered [90]. Cronin and Ellis reported five patients from Oxford in which a pus-filled hernia misled surgeons into a preoperative diagnosis of strangulated hernia [40]. This complication of pus in a hernial sac most frequently occurs in right inguinal [91], then right femoral [92], then left inguinal, and, least often, in left femoral hernias [93]. The syndrome has been encountered in epigastric and umbilical hernias. Underlying pathologies include acute appendicitis (the most common), perforated peptic ulcer, pneumococcal peritonitis, acute pyosalpinx, acute pancreatitis, and biliary peritonitis [40, 94].

In acute appendicitis the appendix may itself be contained in an external hernial sac. Ryan, in 1937, collected 537 cases. An overall incidence of 0.3% of cases of acute appendicitis was found to occur in a hernial sac [95]. Although the appendix is frequently encountered within an inguinal or femoral hernial sac, it is rarely inflamed. The first reported case of appendicitis in a femoral hernial sac is that of De Garengeot [96]. Doolin described a case in which a tender femoral hernial sac was found to contain pus and the gangrenous tip of the appendix. In this patient there were no abnormal findings in the abdomen above the inguinal ligament [97]. Hernial appendicitis usually occurs in a right inguinal or right femoral hernia [98] and in cases of perforated appendix is often misdiagnosed as a strangulated groin hernia [99, 100]. Claudius Amyand performed the first successful appendectomy in 1736, which was contained in a right inguinal hernia [101].

Amyand, a Huguenot, was a pioneer of smallpox vaccination and surgeon to King George II at St George's Hospital, London—the appendix had given rise to a fistula in the right groin where it had been perforated by a pin and was discharging through an inguinal hernia. Most reported cases of appendicitis are in femoral hernias of postmenopausal women or in inguinal hernias in males of all ages from 6 weeks to 88 years. Appendicitis has been reported in a left inguinal hernia [102], in an umbilical hernia [103], in an obturator hernia, and in incisional hernias [102, 104].

Before the advent of modern radiology, the preoperative diagnosis of acute hernial appendicitis was rarely made [105]. Luchs et al. reported two cases of Amyand's hernia which were clinically thought to be incarcerated inguinal hernias but were correctly prospectively diagnosed as having Amyand's hernia on the basis of preoperative computed tomography (CT) examinations [106]. These cases show the utility of CT of the acute abdomen and pelvis in revealing a previously unsuspected diagnosis and rapidly triaging patients to the appropriate management. Laparoscopy is an alternative diagnostic modality, which can be turned to therapeutic advantage to perform the appendicectomy and repair the hernia [107]. The history usually suggests a strangulated hernia with local peritonitis. The differential diagnosis is a Richter's hernia or strangulated omentum. The pain in both these conditions is classically continuous and penetrating, whereas in early appendicitis, periumbilical colic is a typical feature [108].

Treatment is operation, if possible appendectomy via the hernial sac, with repair of the hernia. In a series of seven cases, four femoral and three inguinal, from Bristol and Exeter (England), the preoperative diagnosis was a strangulated hernia in each instance; appendicitis was not suspected. Appendectomy via the sac and hernia repair was performed in each. All the patients recovered, although wound infection created postoperative problems in three patients. Preoperatively only three patients had right iliac fossa pain, but all had histories lasting longer than 24 h before the diagnosis was reached [104]. Acute appendicitis in a hernial sac must be distinguished from acute strangulation of the appendix in a hernia [109]. In case of appendicitis repaired through a hernia orifice, the use of mesh repair should be avoided.

References

1. Magnus R. Late bowel obstruction due to kinking of the damaged loop following reduction of a strangulated hernia. Br J Surg. 1965;52:121–2.
2. Moore CA. Hypertrophic fibrosis of the gut causing chronic obstruction: a sequel to a strangulated hernia. Br J Surg. 1913;1:361–5.
3. Davey WW. Companion to surgery in the tropics. Edinburgh: Livingstone; 1968.
4. Badoe EA. Acute intestinal obstruction in Korie Bu Teaching Hospital, Accra: 1965–1969. Ghana Med J. 1970;9:283–7.

5. Krug F, Herold A, Wenk H, Bruch HP. Incisional hernias after laparoscopic interventions. Chirurg. 1995;66:419–23.

6. Tonouchi H, Ohmori Y, Kobayashi M, Kusunoki M. Trocar site hernia. Arch Surg. 2004;139:1248–56.

7. Vowles KDJ. Intestinal complications of strangulated hernia. Br J Surg. 1959;47:189–92.

8. Quill DS, Devlin HB, Plant JA, Denham KR, McNay RA, Morris D. Surgical operation rates: a twelve year experience in Stockton on Tees. Ann R Coll Surg Engl. 1983;65:248–53.

9. Andrews NJ. Presentation and outcome of strangulated external hernia in a district general hospital. Br J Surg. 1981;68:329–32.

10. Campling EA, Devlin HB, Hoyle RW, Lunn JN. The report of a national confidential enquiry into perioperative deaths 1991/1992. London: NCEPOD; 1993.

11. Kjaergaard J, Bay-Nielsen M, Kehlet H. Mortality following emergency groin hernia surgery in Denmark. Hernia. 2010;14:351–5.

12. Dahlstrand U, Wollert S, Nordin P, Sandblom G, Gunnarsson U. Emergency femoral hernia repair: a study based on a national register. Ann Surg. 2009;249:672–6.

13. Gallegos NC, Dawson J, Jarvis M, Hobsley M. Risk of strangulation in groin hernias. Br J Surg. 1991;78:1171–3.

14. Milamed DR, Hedley-Whyte J. Contributions of the surgical sciences to a reduction of the mortality rate in the United States for the period 1968 to 1988. Ann Surg. 1994;219:94–102.

15. Williams M, Frankel S, Nanchalal K, Coast J, Donovan J. Hernia repair: epidemiologically based needs assessment. Health care evaluation unit. Briston: University of Bristol Print Services; 1992.

16. Rutkow IM, Robbins AW. Demographic, classificatory, and socioeconomic aspects of hernia repair in the United States. Surg Clin North Am. 1993;73:413–26.

17. Fitzgibbons Jr RJ, Giobbie-Hurder A, Gibbs JO, Dunlop DD, Reda DJ, McCarthy Jr M, et al. Watchful waiting vs repair of inguinal hernia in minimally symptomatic men: a randomized clinical trial. JAMA. 2006;295:285–92.

18. Chung L, Norrie J, O'Dwyer PJ. Long-term follow-up of patients with a painless inguinal hernia from a randomized clinical trial. Br J Surg. 2011;98:596–9.

19. Neuhauser D. Elective inguinal herniorrhaphy versus truss in the elderly. In: Bunker JP, Barnes BA, Mosteller F, editors. Costs, risks and benefits of surgery. New York: Oxford University Press; 1977. p. 223–9.

20. Simons MP, Aufenacker T, Bay-Nielsen M, Bouillot JL, Campanelli G, Conze J, et al. European Hernia Society guidelines on the treatment of inguinal hernia in adult patients. Hernia. 2009;13:343–403.

21. Helgstrand F, Rosenberg J, Bay-Nielsen M, Friis-Andersen H, Wara P, Jorgensen LN, et al. Establishment and initial experiences from the Danish Ventral Hernia Database. Hernia. 2010;14:131–5.

22. Lauscher JC, Rieck S, Loh JC, Grone J, Buhr HJ, Ritz JP. Oligosymptomatic vs. symptomatic incisional hernias-who benefits from open repair? Langenbecks Arch Surg. 2011;396(2):179–85.

23. Yokoyama T, Munakata Y, Ogiwara M, Kamijima T, Kitamura H, Kawasaki S. Preoperative diagnosis of strangulated obturator hernia using ultrasonography. Am J Surg. 1997;174:76–8.

24. Gilliam A, Wai D, Perry EP. Ultrasonic diagnosis of strangulated obturator hernia. Eur J Surg. 2000;166:420–1.

25. Green BT. Strangulated obturator hernia: still deadly. South Med J. 2001;94:81–3.

26. Rodriguez-Hermosa JI, Codina-Cazador A, Maroto-Genover A, Puig-Alcantara J, Sirvent-Calvera JM, Garsot-Savall E, et al. Obturator hernia: clinical analysis of 16 cases and algorithm for its diagnosis and treatment. Hernia. 2008;12:289–97.

27. Toms AP, Dixon AK, Murphy JM, Jamieson NV. Illustrated review of new imaging techniques in the diagnosis of abdominal wall hernias. Br J Surg. 1999;86:1243–9.

28. Pearse HE. Strangulated hernia reduced en masse. Surg Gynecol Obstet. 1931;53:822–8.

29. Levack JH. En masse reduction of strangulated hernia. Br J Surg. 1963;50:582–5.

30. Barker AK, Smiddy FG. Mass reduction of inguinal hernia. Br J Surg. 1970;57:264–6.

31. Moynihan BGA. Retroperitoneal hernia. London: Bailliere; 1899.

32. Maydl C. Über retrograde Incarceration der Tuba ond des Processus Vermiformis in Leisten und Schenkelhernien. Wien Klin Rund. 1895;8:17–35.

33. Ganesaratnam M. Maydl's hernia: report of a series of seven cases and review of the literature. Br J Surg. 1985;72:737–8.

34. Moss CM, Levine R, Messenger N, Dardik I. Sliding colonic Maydl's hernia: report of a case. Dis Colon Rectum. 1976;19:636–8.

35. Frankau C. Strangulated hernia: a review of 1,487 cases. Br J Surg. 1931;19:176–91.

36. Bayley AC. The clinical and operative diagnosis of Maydl's hernia: a report of five cases. Br J Surg. 1970;5:687–90.

37. Philip PJ. Afferent limb internal strangulation in obstructed inguinal hernia. Br J Surg. 1967;54:96–9.

38. Watson LF. Hernia: anatomy, etiology, symptoms, diagnosis, differential diagnosis, prognosis and the operative and injection treatment. 2nd ed. London: Harry Kimpton; 1938.

39. Bender E, Sell H. Small bowel obstruction after laparoscopic cholecystectomy as a result of a Maydl's herniation of the small bowel through a trocar site. Surgery. 1996;119:480.

40. Cronin K, Ellis H. Pus collections in hernial sacs; an unusual complication of general peritonitis. Br J Surg. 1959;46:364–7.

41. Steinke W, Zellweger R. Richter's hernia and Sir Frederick Treves: an original clinical experience, review, and historical overview. Ann Surg. 2000;232:710–8.

42. Engeset J, Youngson GG. Ambulatory peritoneal dialysis and hernial complications. Surg Clin North Am. 1984;64:385–92.

43. Andrew DR, Williamson KM. Meckel's diverticulum-rare complications and review of the literature. J R Army Med Corps. 1994;140:143–5.

44. Baillie RC. Incarceration of a Meckel's inguinal hernia in an infant. Br J Surg. 1959;46:459–61.

45. Castleden WM. Meckel's diverticulum of an umbilical hernia. Br J Surg. 1970;57:932–4.

46. Leslie MD, Slater ND, Smallwood CJ. Small bowel fistula from a Littre's hernia. Br J Surg. 1983;70:244.

47. Van Meurs DPP. Strangulation of the ovary and fallopian tube in an obturator hernia. Br J Surg. 1945;32:539–40.

48. Binns JH, Cross RM. Hernia uteri inguinalis in a male. Br J Surg. 1967;54:571–5.

49. Carrieri P, Nardi S, Basuku GC, Vitali A, Nistri R. The involvement of the urinary tract in inguinal hernias. Ann Ital Chir. 1998;69:795–7.

50. Garcia AA, Perales NJ, Schiefenbusch ME, Marquez JL, Polo HE, Cacha LG. Inguinal bladder hernias: a report of two cases. Actas Urol Esp. 1999;23:625–8.

51. Giglio M, Medica M, Germinale F, Raggio M, Campodonice F, Stubinski R, et al. Scrotal extraperitoneal hernia of the ureter: case report and literature review. Urol Int. 2001;66:166–8.

52. Percival WL. Ureter within a sliding inguinal hernia. Can J Surg. 1983;26:283, 286.

53. Pollack HM, Popky GL, Blumberg ML. Hernias of the ureter—an anatomic-roentgenographic study. Radiology. 1975;117:275–81.

54. Ramayya GR. Volvulus of an ileal conduit in an inguinal hernia. Br J Surg. 1984;71:637.

55. Mabogunje OA, Grundy DJ, Lawrie JH. Orchidectomy in a rural African population. Trans R Soc Trop Med Hyg. 1980;74:749–51.

56. von Helwig H. Uber sogennante Spontonrupturen von Hernien. Schweiz Med Wochenschr. 1958;27:662–6.

57. Maniatis AG, Hunt CM. Therapy for spontaneous umbilical hernia rupture. Am J Gastroenterol. 1995;90:310–2.
58. McLean A. Spontaneous rupture of an umbilical hernia in an infant. Br J Surg. 1950;37:239.
59. Strange SL. Spontaneous rupture of an umbilical hernia in an infant. Postgrad Med J. 1956;32:39.
60. Bain IM, Bishop HM. Spontaneous rupture of an infantile umbilical hernia. Br J Surg. 1995;82:35.
61. Hartley RC. Spontaneous rupture of incisional herniae. Br J Surg. 1962;49:617–8.
62. Chatterjee SK. Spontaneous rupture of umbilical hernia with evisceration of small intestine. J Indian Med Assoc. 1972;59:287.
63. Telem DA, Schiano T, Divino CM. Complicated hernia presentation in patients with advanced cirrhosis and refractory ascites: management and outcome. Surgery. 2010;148:538–43.
64. Ogundiran TO, Ayantunde AA, Akute OO. Spontaneous rupture of incisional hernia—a case report. West Afr J Med. 2001;20:176–8.
65. Cheselden W. The anatomy of the human body. 12th ed. London: Livingston, Dodsley, Cadell, Baldwin and Lowndes; 1784.
66. Stock FE. Faecal fistula and bilateral strangulated hernia in an infant. Br Med J. 1951;1:171.
67. Aird I. The association of inguinal hernia with traumatic perforation of the intestine. Br J Surg. 1935;24:529–33.
68. Masso-Misse P, Hamadiko, Yomi, Mbakop A, Yao GS, Malonga E. A rare complication of inguinal hernia. Evisceration by rupture of the scrotum secondary to blunt trauma of the abdomen. J Chir (Paris). 1994;131:212–3.
69. Reynolds RD. Intestinal perforation from trauma to an inguinal hernia. Arch Fam Med. 1995;4:972–4.
70. Ralph-Edwards A, Maziak D, Deitel M, Thompson DA, Kucey DS, Bayley TA. Sudden rupture of an indirect inguinal hernial sac with extravasation in two patients on continuous ambulatory peritoneal dialysis. Can J Surg. 1994;37:70–2.
71. Ackerman LV. Tumours of the retroperitoneum mesentery and peritoneum. Atlas of tumour pathology. Washington, DC: Armed Forces Institute of Pathology; 1954. p. 134–5.
72. Partrick DA, Bensard DD, Karrer FM, Ruyle SZ. Is routine pathological evaluation of pediatric hernia sacs justified? J Pediatr Surg. 1998;33:1090–2.
73. Rosai J, Dehner LP. Nodular mesothelial hyperplasia in hernia sacs: a benign reactive condition simulating a neoplastic process. Cancer. 1975;35:165–75.
74. Ordonez NG, Ro JY, Ayala AG. Lesions described as nodular mesothelial hyperplasia are primarily composed of histiocytes. Am J Surg Pathol. 1998;22:285–92.
75. Brandt WE. Unusual complications of hernia repairs: large symptomatic granulomas. Am J Surg. 1956;92:640–3.
76. Grove A, Jensen ML, Donna A. Mesotheliomas of the tunica vaginalis testis and hernial sacs. Virchows Arch A Pathol Anat Histopathol. 1989;415:283–92.
77. Lee JR, Hancock SM, Martindale RG. Solitary fibrous tumors arising in abdominal wall hernia sacs. Am Surg. 2001;67:577–81.
78. Ficarra BJ. Hernia: masquerader of surgical disorders. Surg Clin North Am. 1971;51:1401–14.
79. Roslyn JJ, Stabile BE, Rangenath C. Cancer in inguinal and femoral hernias. Am Surg. 1980;46:358–62.
80. Matsumoto G, Ise H, Inoue H, Ogawa H, Suzuki N, Matsuno S. Metastatic colon carcinoma found within an inguinal hernia sac: report of a case. Surg Today. 2000;30:74–7.
81. Lejars F. Neoplasmes herniares et peri-herniares. Gaz Hop Civ Mil. 1889;62:801–11.
82. Lees W. Carcinoma of colon in inguinal hernial sacs. Br J Surg. 1966;53:473–4.
83. Griffiths JC, Toomey WF. Large bowel obstruction due to a herniated carcinoma of sigmoid colon. Br J Surg. 1964;51:715–7.
84. Nayak IN. Malignant mucocele of the appendix in a femoral hernia. Postgrad Med J. 1974;50:246–9.
85. Kasson MA, Munoz E, Laughlin A, Margolis IB, Wise L. Value of routine pathology in herniorrhaphy performed upon adults. Surg Gynecol Obstet. 1986;163:518–22.
86. Quagliarello J, Coppa G, Bigelow B. Isolated endometriosis in an inguinal hernia. Am J Obstet Gynecol. 1985;152:688–9.
87. Yuen JS, Chow PK, Koong HN, Ho JM, Girija R. Unusual sites (thorax and umbilical hernial sac) of endometriosis. J R Coll Surg Edinb. 2001;46:313–5.
88. Lung NG, Kit HK, Collins REC. Leiomyoma of the broad ligament in an obturator hernia presenting as a lump in the groin. J R Soc Med. 1986;79:174–5.
89. Coetzee T, Phillips WR. Torsion of a myomatous uterus incarcerated in an umbilical hernia. Br J Surg. 1960;48:342–4.
90. Zuckerkandl M. Hernia inflammata in Folge Typhilitis des Wormfortsatzes in einem Leistebruche. Wien Klin Wochenschr. 1891;4:305.
91. Bennett C. Appendiceal pus in a hernia sac simulating strangulated inguinal hernia. Br Med J. 1919;2:75.
92. Garland EA. Femoral appendicitis. J Indiana State Med Assoc. 1955;48:1292–6.
93. Watkins RM. Appendix abscess in a femoral hernial sac—case report and review of the literature. Postgrad Med J. 1981;57:306–7.
94. Ekwueme O. Strangulated external hernia associated with generalized peritonitis. Br J Surg. 1973;60:929–33.
95. Ryan WJ. Hernia of the vermiform appendix. Ann Surg. 1937;105:135.
96. De Garengeot RJC. Traite des operations de chirurgie. 2nd ed. Paris: Huart; 1731. p. 369–71.
97. Doolin W. Inflamed appendix in a hernial sac. Br Med J. 1919;2:239.
98. Lestor R, Burke JR. Strangulated femoral hernia containing appendices. J R Coll Surg Edinb. 1979;24:102–3.
99. Logan MT, Nottingham JM. Amyand's hernia: a case report of an incarcerated and perforated appendix within an inguinal hernia and review of the literature. Am Surg. 2001;67:628–9.
100. House MG, Goldin SB, Chen H. Perforated Amyand's hernia. South Med J. 2001;94:496–8.
101. Orr KB. Perforated appendix in an inguinal hernial sac: Amyand's hernia. Med J Aust. 1993;159:762–3.
102. Carey LC. Acute appendicitis occurring in hernias: a report of 10 cases. Surgery. 1967;61:236–8.
103. Doig CM. Appendicitis in umbilical hernial sac. Br Med J. 1970;2:113–4.
104. Thomas WE, Vowles KD, Williamson RC. Appendicitis in external herniae. Ann R Coll Surg Engl. 1982;64:121–2.
105. Gray HT. Lesions of the isolated appendix vermiformis in the hernial sac. Br Med J. 1910;2:1142–5.
106. Luchs JS, Halpern D, Katz DS. Amyand's hernia: prospective CT diagnosis. J Comput Assist Tomogr. 2000;24:884–6.
107. Bamberger PK. Revisiting Amyand's hernia in the laparoscopic era. Surg Endosc. 2001;15:1051.
108. Cope Z. The early diagnosis of the acute abdomen. 4th ed. London: Oxford University Press; 1972.
109. Johnson CD. Appendicitis in external herniae. Ann R Coll Surg Engl. 1982;64:283.

Inguinal Hernias in Children

Aly Shalaby and Joe Curry

History

Hernia management in children dates from Antiquity. Described as a swelling on the surface of the belly in ancient papyri, it was treated with tight bandages by the early physicians of Alexandria. The underlying abnormality [patent processus vaginalis (PPV)] leading to the development of congenital (indirect) inguinal hernia or hydrocele was described by Galen in 176 A.D. as a "small offshoot of the great peritoneal sac in the lower abdomen" [1].

The Roman Celsus (first century A.D.), to whom "the earliest reference to hernia repair in children is attributed" [1], "recommended removal of the hernial sac and the testis through a scrotal incision" (op. cit). The practice of testicle amputation was as an essential part of hernia care until it was rejected by William de Salicet in the twelfth century (1210–1277).

The foundation of herniology was set during the Renaissance (fifteenth to seventeenth centuries). The greatest contributor was Pierre Franco, a Swiss barber-surgeon, who, in 1556, "devised an incision of the fascial constriction using a grooved dissector… that allowed him to divide the ring of the constriction of a strangulated hernia without risking damage to the bowel" [2]. Ligation of the hernial sac at the external inguinal ring was practiced by Stromayr, who distinguished between direct and indirect hernias and allowed removal of the testis in the latter type, and by Purmann (1649–1711) who spared the testicle. Contemporaneously, Paré recommended treatment of inguinal hernias found in children, accurately described for the first time by Pott in 1756 [3].

While Bassini, Halsted, and Shouldice were describing methods of repair and reinforcement of adult hernias,

Turner reported in 1912 that, in the majority of children however, no repair was required in treatment of inguinal hernia and that the only procedure necessary was high ligation of the sac [3].

Soon after the advent of laparoscopy for adult inguinal hernias, laparoscopic repair in children gained popularity. And while Shouldice and Lichtenstein repairs are the most favored "tissue repair" approaches to the treatment of groin hernias [2] in adults, the techniques for children continue to evolve.

Currently, inguinal hernia repair in children is done on an outpatient basis, as first recommended by Herzfield in 1938. Early repair in infancy, pioneered by Ladd and Gross in 1941 [3], has developed due to advances in neonatology and anesthesia.

Embryology and Anatomy

Embryology

The gonads arise from the urogenital ridge around the fifth or sixth week of gestation [4]. A core of mesenchymal cells extending from the epidermal ectoderm (future scrotum) to the caudal pole of the gonad condenses to form a cord-like structure: the "gubernaculum." The inguinal canal forms around this gubernaculum as the muscles of the abdominal wall begin to differentiate.

At the end of the second month of gestation, the caudal part of the ventral abdominal wall is horizontal. As it becomes progressively vertical, the umbilical artery pulls up a peritoneal fold, which forms the medial boundary of a peritoneal fossa. This fossa is called the *saccus vaginalis* or *lateral inguinal fossa*. Its lower end protrudes down the inguinal canal along the gubernaculum, as the *processus vaginalis* (PV) (Fig. 11.1) [4]. Some researchers have suggested that formation of the PV is a result of intra-abdominal pressure, whereas others believe that it is an active process [5].

A. Shalaby • J. Curry (✉)
Department of Neonatal and Paediatric Surgery,
Great Ormond Street Children's Hospital Foundation Trust,
London, United Kingdom
e-mail: alyshalaby@nhs.net; Joe.Curry@gosh.nhs.uk

A.N. Kingsnorth and K.A. LeBlanc (eds.), *Management of Abdominal Hernias*,
DOI 10.1007/978-1-84882-877-3_11, © Springer Science+Business Media London 2013

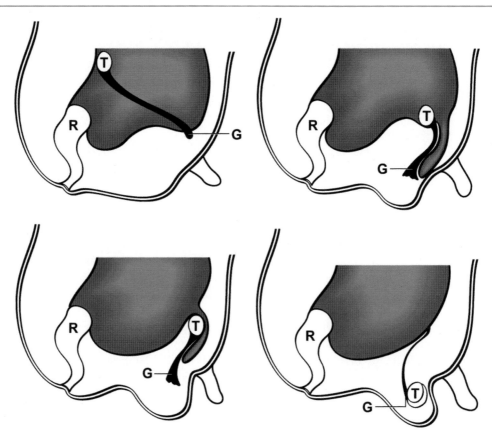

Fig. 11.1 Embryology of the processus vaginalis. *T* testicle, *G* gubernaculum, *R* rectum

In males, the distal end of this processus, into which the testis projects, forms the *tunica vaginalis testis*. The proximal part adjacent to the spermatic cord becomes obliterated, usually leaving a fibrous remnant. The *saccus vaginalis* also appears in females; its prolongation into the inguinal canal (sometimes termed the *canal of Nuck*) normally undergoes complete obliteration.

The mechanisms that govern PV obliteration are currently unknown. Some authors believe that endocrinal factors controlling the final stages of testicular descent such as androgens, peptide neurotransmitter *calcitonin gene-related peptide* (CGRP), and Leydig insulin-like hormone gene (INSL3) may also control subsequent closure of the PV [4, 6]. It is unclear, however, how this is applicable to females as the ovary descends into the pelvis and not the inguinal canal.

Studies have shown that exogenous CGRP in organ culture causes fusion of a patent PV (PPV) by epithelial mesenchymal transformation. Similarly, a hepatocyte growth factor (HGF) was also shown to cause PV fusion as seen in embryonic palatal fusion. Nevertheless, closure of the PV is proving to be a more complex process than previously thought [7].

The exact timing of closure is also uncertain. Studies have suggested that most infants are born with a PPV [5] and that closure is most likely within the first 6 months of life. After that, patency rate falls more gradually and stabilizes around 3–5 years of age. It is also unknown *where* the processus starts its closure: proximal, middle, or distal parts [5].

Anatomy of the Inguinal Canal in Children

The basic anatomy of the inguinal canal is the same in children as in adults. However, there are several differences between the infant and the adult. The inguinal canal is shorter, in relation to body size in infants and children, than in adults. In infants, it is 1–1.5 cm long. The internal and the external rings are nearly superimposed in cases of pubic diastasis (bladder and cloacal exstrophy) or in infants with very large hernias where the external inguinal ring is very stretched. Scarpa's fascia is so well developed that the surgeon may mistake it for the aponeurosis of the external oblique muscle. There may be a layer of fat between the fascia and the aponeurosis. As long as fat is encountered, the external oblique fascia has not been reached.

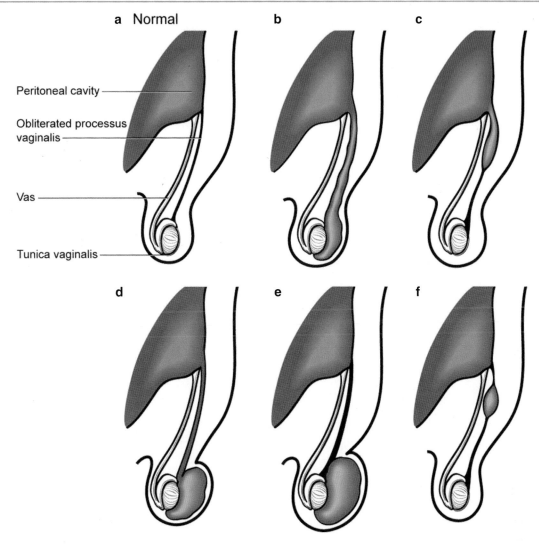

a Normal

Peritoneal cavity

Obliterated processus vaginalis

Vas

Tunica vaginalis

b

c

d

e

f

Fig. 11.2 Inguinoscrotal variations of the processus vaginalis. Normally obliterated (**a**), indirect inguinoscrotal hernia (**b**), inguinal hernia (**c**), communicating hydrocele (**d**), hydrocele of the tunica vaginalis (**e**), hydrocele of the cord (**f**)

Etiology and Clinical Presentation

Etiology

Failure of obliteration of the PV may result in a variety of inguinoscrotal anomalies (Fig. 11.2).

These will include:

- Complete persistence resulting in an *indirect inguinoscrotal hernia* (Fig. 11.2b).
- Distal processus obliteration and proximal hernia patency resulting in an *inguinal hernia* (Fig. 11.2c).
- Complete patency with a narrow opening at the internal ring referred to as a *communicating hydrocele* (Fig. 11.2d).

- Proximal obliteration with distal patency resulting in *hydrocele of the tunica vaginalis* (noncommunicating hydrocele). Its counterparts in girls are called *a hydrocele of the canal of Nuck* (Fig. 11.2e).
- Proximal and distal obliteration with central patency referred to as a *hydrocele of the cord* (Fig. 11.2f).

A PPV is a prerequisite for developing an inguinal hernia, but its patency alone does not mean an *inevitable* hernia. Prematurity is one situation where the normal physiological processes of testicular descent and PV closure are not complete, hence the high incidence of inguinal hernia. A positive family history (see: Clinical Presentation) and other factors (Table 11.1) have also been shown to be associated with inguinal hernia in children. A link between

Table 11.1 Predisposing factors to inguinal hernia in children

| Age (prematurity) |
| Family history |
| Urogenital |
| Undescended testis |
| Pubic diastasis |
| Increased intra-abdominal pressure |
| Repair of exomphalos or gastroschisis |
| Ascites |
| Ventriculoperitoneal shunt |
| Peritoneal dialysis |
| Meconium peritonitis |
| Chronic respiratory disease |
| Cystic fibrosis |
| Connective tissue disorders |
| Congenital hip dislocation |
| Ehlers-Danlos syndrome |
| Hunter-Hurler syndrome |
| Marfan's syndrome |
| Mucopolysaccharidosis |

Table 11.2 Differential diagnosis of a mass in the groin

| Hydrocele |
| Hydrocele of cord (cyst of canal of Nuck) |
| UDT |
| Lymph node |

inguinal hernia and some genetic diseases (viz., connective tissue disorders) is documented [8].

Clinical Presentation

Incidence

The percentage of children with inguinal hernia has been reported to be around 5% [1]. This incidence rises in premature infants, and reported ranges have been anywhere from 11 [9] to 25% [1].

Boys are more commonly affected than girls, three to ten times more often [1, 5]. Sixty percent of inguinal hernias are right sided. This is attributed to later testicular descent and delayed obliteration of the processus vaginalis on the right [1, 3, 10]. Twenty-five percent of inguinal hernias occur on the left side [3] while the remaining 15% are bilateral at presentation [3]. The incidence of bilateral hernia at presentation increases to between 44 and 55% in preterm and low-birth-weight infants, respectively [9].

In girls as in boys, the observation of right-sided inguinal hernias being more common than left-sided ones cannot be explained by the same mechanism of testicular descent, and the cause remains obscure. An inguinal hernia in a girl should not be taken at face value, and the surgeon should always have a suspicion of complete androgen insensitivity syndrome (CAIS) [11] and take the appropriate measures for preoperative and intraoperative investigations.

There is a positive family history in 11.5% of patients [12], with an increased incidence in twins, being 10.6% in male twins and 4.1% in female twins [5].

Clinical Features

An inguinal hernia typically presents with a history of an intermittent swelling in the groin, scrotum, or labia. As with many childhood conditions, the caregiver usually is the first to observe it. Parents might notice it during bathing or when the child is crying; a pediatrician may find it on routine examination.

The first presentation of an inguinal hernia may be an acute one. The swelling is then tense and tender, and the child may have symptoms of bowel obstruction. This specific entity will be discussed in detail in the section on incarcerated hernia below.

Examination

The diagnosis for many children with inguinal hernia is based on a reliable history of an intermittent swelling in the region of the external inguinal ring. Parents will reliably point to this area when prompted. It is also vital, as in adults, that a child presenting with intestinal obstruction should have a thorough examination of the hernial orifices.

Physical examination will often be unremarkable, but some physical signs can be observed to support the diagnosis. To examine for inguinal hernia, the child or infant is placed supine and undressed on an examining table in a warm room. After inspection of the groin for any visible mass or asymmetry, the testis should be localized in the scrotum to account for both testes and to sort out true inguinal swellings from retractile or undescended testes. If a mass is still not apparent, patency of the PV may be determined by the "silk scarf" *sign*. This is performed by laying two fingers over the spermatic cord slightly above the level of the pubic tubercle. The fingers are lightly rolled over the cord from side to side. A positive sign is when the fingers "slide" as the two surfaces of the PPV roll against each other indicating patency. It should be compared with the "normal" non-presenting side, but this remains a somewhat subjective sign.

Differential Diagnosis

There are only a few diagnoses that can present in the infant or child that may mimic an inguinal hernia. It is important to consider these in the differential diagnosis (Table 11.2).

Fig. 11.3 Ultrasound scan of inguinal canal with herniated bowel loop in a child

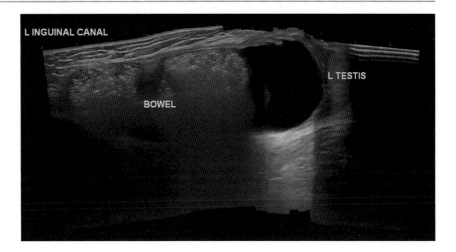

While the underlying cause for an inguinal hernia and hydrocele is the same, differentiating the two is important because it affects subsequent management (see congenital hydrocele below). Transillumination is a pathognomonic physical sign for a hydrocele. A hydrocele usually masks the testis and the latter is thus difficult to palpate. In contrast, the testis is usually palpable with a hernia. A large hydrocele in an infant may be difficult to distinguish from an incarcerated hernia.

An undescended or retractile testis may have been noted, or on examination, failure of localization of the testis in the scrotum would point to that diagnosis. The hemi-scrotum on the side in question may be underdeveloped.

The presence of an inguinal lymph node is a discrete swelling, noncompressible, nonreducible, and usually anatomically distant from the external ring. Palpable inguinal lymphadenopathy is not common, and a local source of infection might be sought, or the examiner should proceed to palpate the other lymph nodes to detect generalized lymphadenopathy.

Investigations

A good clinical history alone is usually sufficient for a pediatric surgeon to operate. Historically, investigations have not been necessary in the management of children with inguinal hernia. Investigations are employed in the rare cases where diagnostic doubt exists, in the assessment of the contralateral side or where there is suspicion of hernia recurrence.

Herniography was performed but has now been abandoned because less invasive examinations are available.

Ultrasound has gained popularity over the past decade. It has the advantage of being rapid, noninvasive, and complication-free. Studies reported by Chen et al. [13]. and Erez et al. [14]. Concluded that ultrasound is a reliable tool and may

even be used for preoperative evaluation of the contralateral groin in cases with unilateral hernias. The upper limit of the normal diameter of the inguinal canal was set to 4 mm. Measurements of 4.9±1.1 mm were associated with a PPV, whereas measurements of 7.2±2.0 mm or greater (Fig. 11.3) were associated with a true hernia. In the hands of an experienced sonographer, ultrasound is equally useful in girls with unilateral or bilateral inguinal hernias, in order to exclude CAIS [11].

Laparoscopy is now used as both an investigative and therapeutic tool. Further discussion is noted below (metachronous hernia).

Management

Treatment in Childhood

After understanding the anatomical causes underlying an inguinal hernia in children, it is clear that such a hernia will not resolve on its own; therefore, surgery is the only recourse. Furthermore, conservative management is never indicated due to the high rate of associated complications [15, 16]. Complications are heralded by incarceration, which may in turn lead to bowel obstruction and/or strangulation. The gonad is at risk of atrophy caused by prolonged compression of the vascular supply by a hernia sac filled with bowel. An incarcerated hernia that cannot be reduced is most at risk of causing intestinal obstruction. Rescorla and Grosfeld reported an incidence of 9% in such cases [17]. Prolonged incarceration could also lead to intestinal resection, estimated at 3–7% of incarcerated hernias [17]. Testicular ischemia is reported by some authors in almost one-third of boys with incarcerated hernia, while other authors suggest that the problem has been much overemphasized [18]. Gonadal infarction secondary to incarceration was found to be more common in infants younger than 3 months [19] compared to similar cases in older age groups [9]. The operation is usually performed shortly after the diagnosis is made. Some reports suggest that the great majority complications can be avoided if repair is done early.

The anesthetic type varies with the patient. Options include general, regional, or local techniques, and the choice depends on several factors, including the patient's age, and the presence of significant comorbidities. The majority of patients receive general anesthesia with endotracheal intubation or laryngeal mask.

Postoperative Care

With the exception of infants who require extended observation, most patients are discharged on the day of surgery. Premature infants at risk of apnea may require prolonged observation or overnight stay based on local protocols [20]. Similarly, an extensive laparoscopic procedure may require hospital admission. Oral intake may be resumed when the effects of anesthesia wear off. The reader is referred to "Good practice in postoperative and procedural pain" [21] for advice on best practice with regard to postoperative pain management. Baths can then be resumed on the third postoperative day. Older children should refrain from bicycle riding, swimming, or other vigorous physical activity for 1 month [3]. However, recent evidence supports the resumption of normal activities as early as the resolution of postoperative pain.

Complications

The most serious intraoperative complication, albeit rare, is injury to the spermatic vessels or vas deferens. Given that most injuries to the vas likely result from crushing or vascular impairment [1, 22], they might go unnoticed intraoperatively. However, if the vas deferens is divided, it should be repaired with interrupted 7/0 or 8/0 monofilament sutures. An experienced practitioner utilizing adequate magnification will make the repair more precise. The potential for vasal and vascular injury should always be included in the process of obtaining informed consent.

Intraoperative hemorrhage is also an unusual complication, unless the floor of the canal is weakened and requires repair. Needle-hole injury to vessels such as the femoral vein can usually be controlled by withdrawal of the suture and direct pressure.

The overall postoperative complication rate after elective inguinal hernia repair is about 2%; this rises to 19% in cases of incarcerated hernia [1, 16, 23]. Therefore, earlier elective repair is preferred. The more common or important complications are described below.

Table 11.3 Etiology of recurrence of pediatric inguinal hernias

Major causes of recurrent inguinal hernia in children [1, 5, 25]
1. Incarceration
2. Missed hernial sac or unrecognized peritoneal tear
3. Broken suture ligature at the neck of the sac
4. Failure to repair a large internal inguinal ring
5. Injury to the floor of the inguinal canal, resulting in a direct inguinal hernia
6. Severe wound infection
7. Increased intra-abdominal pressure
8. Connective tissue disorders
9. Conditions with pubic diastasis

The wound infection rate at most major pediatric centers is low (1–2%) [3]. An increased incidence of infection would be expected in incarcerated hernias.

A postoperative hydrocele may be attributed to incomplete excision of the distal sac and may be avoided by partial resection of the latter. The postoperative hydrocele often resolves spontaneously, rarely requiring aspiration. Even more rarely, long-term persistence of the hydrocele may require a formal hydrocelectomy [24].

The iatrogenic undescended testis or "trapped testicle" is a possible sequel to inguinal hernia repair. It may be attributed to improper replacement of the testicle in the scrotum at the end of the hernia repair, or because it subsequently retracted. Orchidopexy is necessary. It has a low reported incidence of 0.2%, but some authors suggest it might be underreported [5].

A recurrent inguinal hernia is a relatively uncommon complication in children (Table 11.3). The rate following repair on an uncomplicated inguinal hernia is up to 0.8% [1, 5, 35] rising to ~15% in premature infants [5] and up to 20% if the hernia was incarcerated [1, 26]. Of these, 80% is noted within the first postoperative year [25], although there is a suggestion that recurrence rates are underreported due to lack of long-term follow-up in the studies [5].

Interestingly, the surgeon's level of experience was not found to be a factor statistically associable to recurrence [5], although a technical error will certainly contribute to recurrence.

Testicular atrophy after elective inguinal hernia repair is rare and the actual incidence is thus unknown [1, 24]. Atrophy occurs more commonly in incarcerated hernias with an incidence reported to be up to 20% [15]. Intraoperative or early postoperative assessment of the testicle is unhelpful [27]: an intraoperative cyanotic testicle may frequently improve; therefore, an orchidectomy is discouraged unless obvious necrosis is seen [5]; similarly, testicular atrophy may not declare itself till after puberty [27].

Postoperative infertility is uncommon but documented intraoperative vasal injuries are quoted at 0.13% [28], while postoperative examination of excised hernial sacs puts it at

0.23% [29]. As the hernial sac is not routinely sent for histopathological examination and as the vas may also be damaged by crushing, stretch, or mere grasping [1], the true incidence of vasal injury is probably underreported. Subfertility [30], obstructive azoospermia [31], and subsequent circulating spermatic autoagglutinating antibodies [32, 33] have been associated with inguinal hernia repair in childhood. However, unless the injury is bilateral, the ultimate effect on fertility may not be evident.

The quoted mortality rate of elective inguinal hernia is 0.1% [34], and this rises up to 3.0% with incarcerated inguinal hernias [34]. Mortality is also associated with coexisting risk factors such as cardiac disease, prematurity [24], or in the rare neglected case from misdiagnosis [35]. Other identified risk factors include an age younger than 6 months and lack of surgical and/or anesthetic pediatric experience [36].

Histology

The pediatric hernia sac has a lining of simple mesothelium over connective tissue including fibrous, fatty, and muscular components. Abundant adipose tissue may lead to the surgeon's diagnosis of a lipoma. In girls the round ligament may also be normally found [22].

The value of routine histopathological examination of the pediatric hernia sac remains a matter of debate and varies according to hospital policy. Financial considerations aside, there may be merit in not sending adult specimens, but in children it might be warranted because sacs can reflect occult disease or malformations [22]. In that respect, pathologists are stronger proponents than surgeons for keeping the sac [22]. However, the rarity of finding occult disease in hernia sacs is the main argument used in cost-benefit studies against their routine histopathological examination [22, 28].

Special Issues in Management of Hernias in Children

Incarcerated Hernia

Incarceration (Fig. 11.4) may be the first presentation of an inguinal hernia or develops as some children are awaiting a scheduled operation. The incidence of incarceration ranges from 9 to 31%, and the majority of cases occur in children under 1 year of age [1, 3, 9, 18, 25]. Incarceration occurs most commonly in the first 6 months of life and is relatively rare after the age of 5 years. An incidence of up to 31% has been reported in the first 3 months of life [1, 3, 9, 18, 25], down to 24% at 6 months [1], and 15% in children up to 18 years of age [3]. Premature infants have a relatively lower

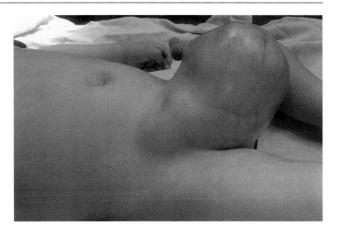

Fig. 11.4   Incarcerated inguinal hernia

Table 11.4   Rate of incarceration in relation to age

Author	Age	No. of patients	No. of incarcerated (%)
De Boer (1957)	0–17 year	2,100	380 (18.1)
Rowe and Clatworthy (1970)	0–16 year	2.764	351 (12.7)
Puri et al. (1984)	<1 year	511	158 (31.0)
Rescrola and Grosfeld (1984)	<2 month	100	31 (31.0)

From Grosfeld [9], with permission

rate of incarceration rate of 13–18%, possibly due to a stretched inguinal canal [1]. Grosfeld (1989) reported a 2–5 times higher rate of incarceration in younger infants than in older children, after comparing four studies on the topic (Table 11.4).

The incarcerated hernia is a clearly defined, tense mass in the inguinal region that may extend into the scrotum. It is tender and does not spontaneously reduce. Occasionally, it will transilluminate and must then be distinguished from a tense hydrocele of the cord. Ultrasound may help to make this distinction. Intestinal obstruction will manifest with vomiting and abdominal distension. With the onset of ischemia due to strangulation, the pain intensifies and there is increasing pyrexia and evidence of intestinal obstruction intensifies: the vomiting becomes bilious and/or there may be blood in the stools. The overlying skin and the testis may be swollen and tender. Abdominal X-ray will show evidence of intestinal obstruction, and gas may be seen within the incarcerated bowel loops in the scrotum.

It is often possible to safely reduce an incarcerated inguinal hernia in infants and convert an emergency problem that requires an immediate operation, to a condition requiring a semi-elective procedure. The success rate in reducing infant hernias is over 70% [1, 3, 9, 18, 25]. Hence, the initial management of incarcerated inguinal hernia without strangulation should be nonoperative [25]. The three basic requirements are a stable environment, adequate resuscitation, and analgesia. The latter is achieved with morphine. The dose is 0.1 mg/kg given intravenously to infants or 0.2 mg/kg as an oral preparation for children over 6 months of age. The dose should be reduced 0.025 mg/kg for the premature infant. Midazolam 0.1 mg/kg may be added for the older child. The respiration and pulse must be monitored. After allowing adequate time for the infant to settle, spontaneous reduction may occur; if not, gentle bimanual compression is usually successful in reduction. Ipsilateral hip flexion with external rotation aids in the ability to achieve reduction. The pressure should be gentle and sustained: a gurgling sensation will indicate emptying of the bowel and subsequent reduction. An elective repair can then be scheduled in 24–48 h [1, 18, 25]. This time allows some resolution of the edema, minimizing the difficulty of the dissection and decreasing the risk of complications.

Failure to reduce the hernia is an indication for an immediate operation. The operative approach is that for the elective procedure, but the external inguinal ring must be opened to allow reduction of the contents of the hernia. Further operative management is determined by the viability of the intestine. If the incarcerated intestine is viable, it is reduced into the abdominal cavity and a high ligation of the sac is performed. If, on the other hand, the intestine is no longer viable, it should be resected, either through the sac or through a separate entry into the peritoneal cavity via the same skin incision. An incarcerated hernia in an infant is technically more difficult and has a higher complication rate since the hernial sac is typically edematous and fragile. The testicular vessels and the vas deferens are particularly susceptible to injury because of the edema and often-difficult dissection. These procedures are safest in the hands of experienced surgeons.

The complication rate in patients with incarcerated hernia has been reported to range from 11 to 31% [18]. Reducible incarcerated hernias have a complication rate of 4.5%, compared to 33% for those that were irreducible and required an emergency operation [9]. Rescorla and Grosfeld (1984) [9] noted a slightly higher complication rate in very low-birth-weight infants younger than 2 months of age at the time of their operation.

Incarcerated Ovary

The management of an asymptomatic irreducible ovary is unclear. In a survey of the variability of technique in inguinal hernia management and repair, Levitt et al. (2002) found that management of an incarcerated non-tender ovary still varied from repair at the first available elective time (50%), repair that week (28%), or repair that day as an emergency (10%) [37]. The herniated ovary and fallopian tube are at a risk of vascular compromise either due to incarceration or, more

likely, torsion. The reported incidence of strangulated irreducible ovaries is as high as 32% [5]. It is therefore our opinion that the risk to the ovary is indeed significant and should be managed as an emergency.

Metachronous Hernia

If patients are observed after ipsilateral hernia repair, a metachronous hernia will appear on the contralateral side from 1 to 31% of the time [38]. Exploration of the asymptomatic side was designed to detect a PPV or nonevident clinical hernia. The goals of identifying these two entities are to avoid a second anesthesia, minimize parental and patient inconvenience, avoid the chance of incarceration, and reduce costs. However, there is no current support for contralateral exploration in any child with a unilateral inguinal hernia and a clinically normal, asymptomatic contralateral groin [39, 40]. Furthermore, contralateral exploration is not done in cases of incarceration [9].

In 2007, a systematic review on the risk of developing a metachronous contralateral inguinal hernia (MCIH) acknowledged that "the success of contralateral exploration cannot be measured by how many PPVs are closed, but by how many MCIHs are prevented" [41]. The results of the review stated that the risk of MCIH for all children having open hernia repair is 7.2%. Overall, 14 contralateral explorations would be required to prevent one metachronous hernia. In boys younger than 2 years, the ratio is still high [41].

Laparoscopy has offered the advantage of closing an incidentally found PPV. Interestingly, some cases in which the contralateral side was deemed closed on laparoscopy were noted to develop an inguinal hernia at a subsequent time (authors' experience).

Premature Infants

It is a well-established fact that premature infants have a higher incidence of inguinal hernias and are likely to have a bilateral presentation. It is known that the more premature the infant, the higher the incidence of an inguinal hernia. Premature infants also show an increased risk of postoperative life-threatening apnea after inguinal hernia repair [20, 42]. Unlike older children who may be treated on a day-case basis, monitoring of these high-risk infants for 12–24 h after operation is recommended [20].

The optimal timing of surgical repair in these neonates is controversial [25]. In a small premature infant, the operation is technically more difficult and associated with a higher morbidity. Furthermore, the anesthetic risk is higher in a premature infant. For those already admitted to a neonatal intensive care unit, it has been suggested that they should have their hernia repaired before discharge [1], but this is a simplistic proposal. Many factors such as gestational age, birth weight, actual weight, comorbidities, pulmonary status, and history of incarceration are all factors that should be taken into consideration in order to formulate an individualized approach to determine the optimal time for surgical repair [25]. For infants diagnosed after discharge from the hospital and who are expected to require ventilatory support or experience episodes of apnea and/or bradycardia, elective repair is usually delayed until 44–60 weeks of corrected conceptional age [17].

Congenital Hydrocele

For infants with congenital hydrocele, the processus vaginalis will usually close and the hydrocele resolve during the first year of life. The recommended management of a hydrocele is therefore to avoid surgery during that period, unless a hernia cannot be excluded. After 2 years of age, a hydrocele is unlikely to resolve and should be operated upon. The recommended operation is high ligation of the processus vaginalis, as for inguinal hernia, with drainage of the distal sac. Splitting, everting, or removal of the distal sac is not only unnecessary, but may even cause a postoperative hematoma. Fluid rarely reaccumulates the sac and if it does, it usually resolves spontaneously.

There is no evidence that a hydrocele will become a hernia, although this is theoretically possible. Occasionally, a previously unapparent hydrocele may present in an older child as a scrotal swelling often presenting during a viral illness.

Sliding Hernia

A number of structures could be involved in a sliding hernia in children. In infants, the bladder may be pulled with the hernia sac. Alternatively the cecum or appendix may share a wall with a right-sided hernia sac. In girls, a fallopian tube or mesosalpinx may share a wall with the sac.

Careful inspection of the neck of the hernia sac before transfixion avoids injury to any of these structures. If, on the other hand, there is any doubt of safety, the sac should be opened and inspected from the inside and subsequently closed with a purse-string suture.

Direct Inguinal Hernia

It occurs due to a defect in the transversalis fascia and presents as a bulge medially in the groin. It is rarely encountered in children and often misdiagnosed as an indirect inguinal hernia. As is often the case, a direct hernia may not be obvious while the patient is anesthetized, and they will return with what appears to be a recurrent indirect inguinal hernia. If this is the case, it is repaired using interrupted nonabsorbable sutures between the inguinal ligament and conjoined tendon. Occasionally a mesh repair is required in the older child. Therefore, a direct hernia should be suspected if a typical PPV cannot be found or in "recurrent" cases.

Operative Techniques

The Open Inguinal Approach (Fig. 11.5)

An incision is made in the lowest inguinal crease. Scarpa's fascia is incised and the external oblique fascia along with the external inguinal ring is identified. At this point the spermatic cord may be accessed either at its exit from the external ring or inside the inguinal canal by incising the external oblique. If the latter approach is used, the ilioinguinal nerve should be identified on the inner surface of the external oblique aponeurosis in order to avoid its entrapment in a suture.

The cremasteric fascia is opened to expose the cord structures (Fig. 11.5a). Care is taken not to grasp either the vas deferens or the vessels. Only loose connective tissue may be handled until the hernia sac is identified. At this point, the latter is grasped with a pair of non-toothed forceps and the remaining cord structures pushed away bluntly (Fig. 11.5b). In boys, delivery of the testicle into the wound is usually unnecessary.

Once free from the vas and vessels, the sac can be divided between clamps and the proximal end dissected superiorly to the level of the internal inguinal ring (Fig. 11.5c). This is identified by appearance of the preperitoneal fat. The contents of the sac are reduced and the sac twisted and transfixed (Fig. 11.5d). The distal end of the sac is left open. Further dissection of this distal sac is discouraged.

In boys, the testicle should be confirmed to be in a normal intrascrotal position at the end of the procedure. Unlike adults, the infantile inguinal hernia does not need reinforcement. Exception is made for children with an underlying collagen disease [8] or perhaps a recurrent hernia.

The external oblique (if opened) and Scarpa's fascia are closed with interrupted absorbable sutures. The skin is closed with a subcuticular absorbable suture.

In girls, the absence of vital cord structures makes repair simpler. The surgical approach to the sac is the same. However, it is important to routinely open the sac in girls because as many as 21% [43] have a sliding component, and to exclude CAIS (Fig. 11.6). The proximal sac is dissected to the level of the internal ring, twisted, and ligated. The wound is closed in a standard fashion (described above).

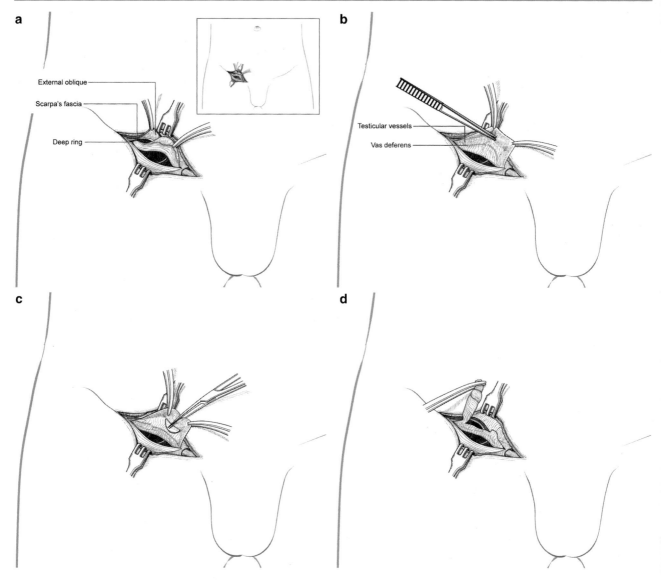

Fig. 11.5 (**a–d**) Open inguinal herniotomy. (**a**)The cremasteric fascia is opened to expose the cord structures. (**b**) The sac is grasped with a pair of non-toothed forceps and the remaining cord structures pushed away bluntly. (**c**) The sac is divided between clamps and the proximal end dissected superiorly to the level of the internal inguinal ring. (**d**) The contents of the sac are reduced and the sac twisted and transfixed

The High Scrotal "Bianchi" Approach

In 1989, Bianchi and Squire [43] hailed the use of their scrotal approach for a palpable undescended testis as an acceptable alternative to the groin incision. A high scrotal crease incision exposes the cord structures. The hernia sac is dissected in the usual manner. Upward traction allows access to the neck of the hernia sac for transfixion. Age may be a limiting factor to this approach. The older the child, the more retraction becomes necessary to reach the neck of the hernia sac. The published literature is not unencouraging [44–46].

Laparoscopic Closure

Laparoscopy was first applied to pediatric inguinal hernias to evaluate the contralateral side for the presence of a PPV [37, 47–49] and can be used to confirm a diagnosis of inguinal hernia [47, 48].

A 0° telescope is inserted via the umbilicus using an open technique. An instrument is inserted in the right and left lower quadrants. Ports are not necessary for these instruments. The internal ring is closed by a purse-string suture that avoids the vas and vessels. Contrary to appearances, this suture does not seem to affect testicular viability [50]. Some

Fig. 11.6 Open inguinal herniotomy in girls

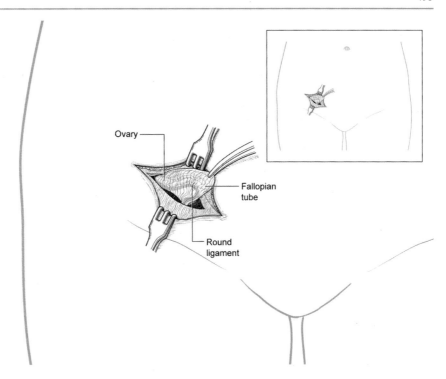

authors incise the peritoneum laterally to reduce mechanical tension, although the benefit of this step has been questioned [47, 48]. Other groups have reported a needlescopic technique, using one or two lateral ports to assist with percutaneous, extraperitoneal ligation of the internal ring [49, 51]. The choice of suture material (absorbable vs. nonabsorbable, monofilament vs. braided) differs according to the surgeon [47, 48]. Proponents of the laparoscopic approach cite a comparable operative time to that of open surgery and a similar complication rate [25, 47].

Improved cosmetic outcome aside, the laparoscopic approach offers the surgeon the ability to easily examine the contralateral groin and to repair any hernia found. Openings no deeper than 2 mm (size of the needle driver shaft) are suggested to be unlikely to cause a hernia and are left open by some authors [48]. Laparoscopy is also advantageous when dealing with sliding components in the hernial sac.

Direct and femoral hernias, which are rare in children, are more readily diagnosed and repaired laparoscopically [47, 48]. Laparoscopy is equally advantageous in cases of recurrent inguinal hernias after open surgery [25], allowing the surgeon to avoid previously operated tissue planes and potentially lowering the risks of injury to the vas and/or vessels. The pneumoperitoneum may widen the internal ring and help in reduction of incarcerated hernias [52], the viability of which can be easily assessed and addressed if needed. In addition, immediate repair could avoid the tissue edema and complications arising from delayed repair after incarceration [52].

Laparoscopic repair, however, remains an intraperitoneal procedure with increased costs, longer operating time (reported by some to range from 25 to 74 min [49]), and a prolonged learning curve. Peritoneal thickening from chronic irritation may hinder the identification of cord structures and put them at risk of entrapment. Nerve entrapment is also a possibility [53]. Finally, the effects of prolonged pneumoperitoneum have not been fully elucidated.

Variations in Laparoscopic Technique

Flip-Flap Closure

A flap of peritoneum is dissected laterally, flipped, and anchored to cover the hernial opening [54]. Initial reports on this technique are unsatisfactory due to intraoperative complications (vas injury, flap avulsion) and high rate of recurrence.

Laparoscopic Inversion Ligation

The hernial sac is inverted into the peritoneal cavity, and the base tied with an endo-loop.

It is only applicable in girls, as the vas and vessels cannot be excluded from the tie (Fig. 11.7). A series of 241 procedures reported only two recurrences [5, 55].

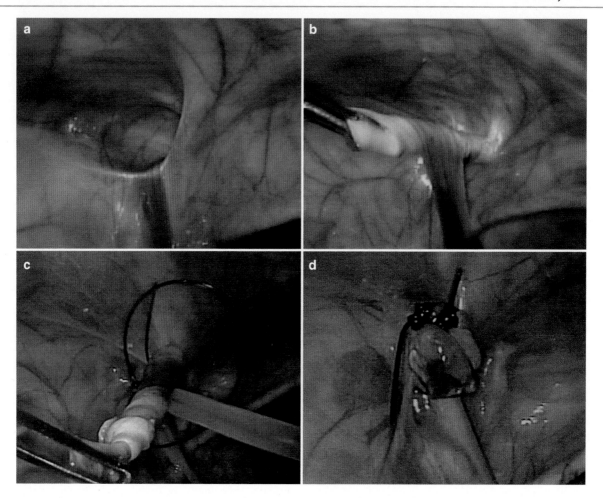

Fig. 11.7 Laparoscopic inversion ligation (LIL). Hernia is identified (**a**), peritoneum inverted (**b**), twisted and double ligated (**c**), and then excised (**d**) (From Lipskar et al. [53], with permission)

The Reverdin* Needle Technique

Reverdin needle (RN) is a surgical needle with an eye that can be opened and closed with a slide. It essentially modifies the delivery of the suture material, creating extracorporeal knot tying (Fig. 11.8). It markedly reduces both operative time and technical difficulty [56].

*Jaques L. Reverdin, Swiss surgeon, 1842–1929

Laparoscopic Percutaneous Extraperitoneal Closure

An Endoneedle [57] devised by the Department of Pediatric Surgery of Saitama Municipal Hospital in Japan is a special instrument that has a wire loop to hold the suture material at

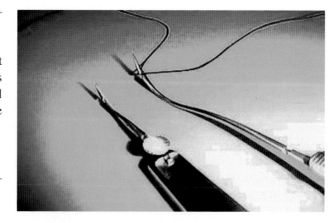

Fig. 11.8 Both components of the Reverdin needle, seen here with mounted suture (From Shalaby et al. [56], with permission)

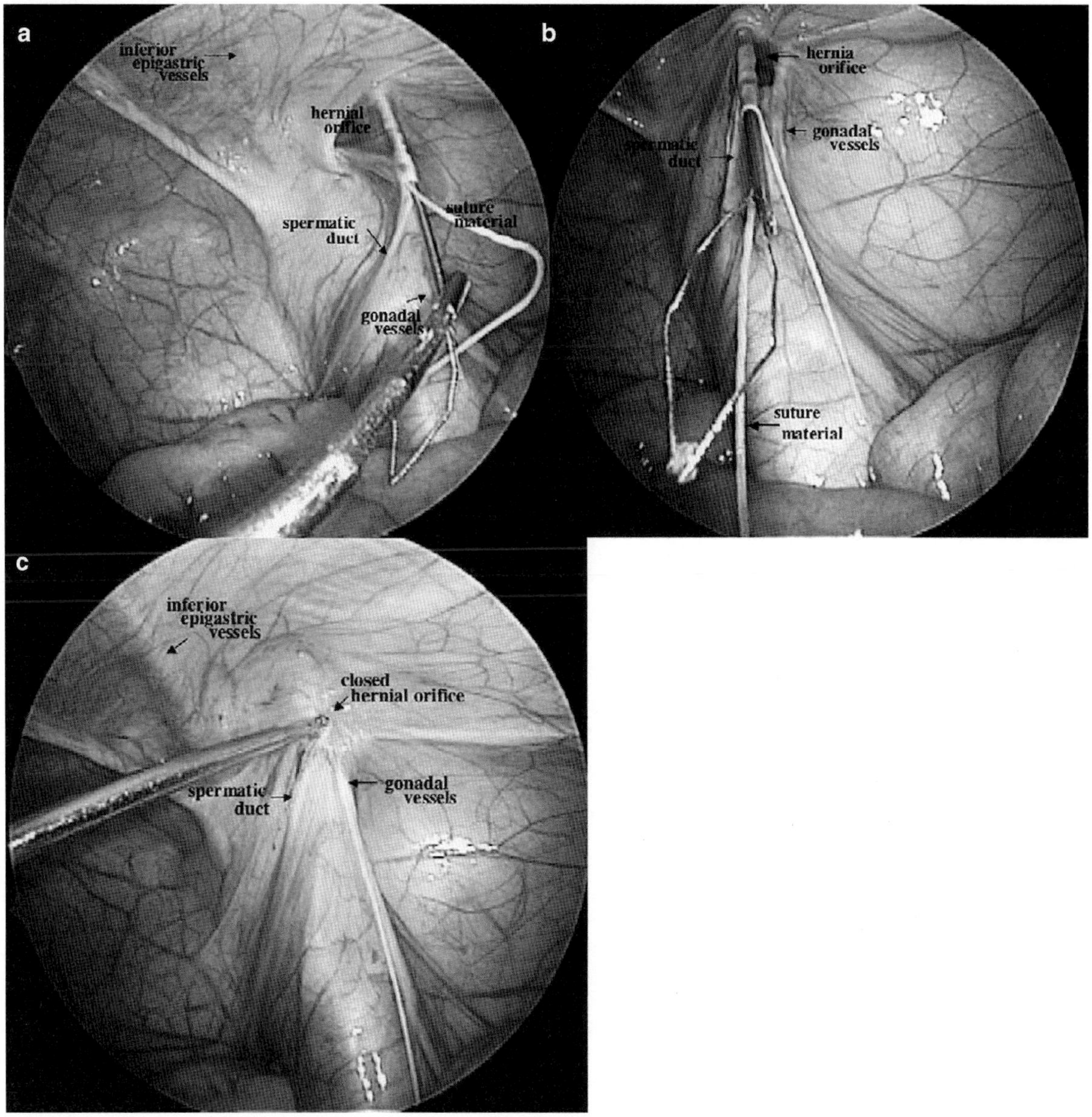

Fig. 11.9 (a–c) Laparoscopic percutaneous extraperitoneal closure (LPEC) of the internal ring (From Takehara et al. [58]; with permission). (a) Half of the purse-string suturing is started extraperitoneally, beginning at the anterior edge and proceeding to the posterior edge on the lateral side of the internal inguinal ring using the LPEC needle. (b) Suturing of the medial side of the internal ring is placed extraperitoneally using the same technique, and the suture material is held in the wire loop inside the LPEC needle. (c) The LPEC needle is then removed from the abdomen together with the suture material. The purse-string is tied extracorporeally

the top and can be used for purse-string suturing around the internal inguinal ring, with extracorporeal knot tying [58] (Fig. 11.9).

complications, the most serious of which was bowel strangulation that required resection anastomosis. Recurrence was in three cases out of 106 children [59].

Percutaneous Internal Ring Suturing

A hollow needle with suture material inside is passed percutaneously under the peritoneum of each half of the internal ring. It allows extracorporeal knot-tying by catching a loop of the suture material and pulling it to the surface. Patkowski et al. (2006) report some intraoperative and postoperative

Subcutaneously Endoscopically Assisted Ligation (Fig. 11.10)

A swaged-on needle is inserted percutaneously and passes extraperitoneally over half of the internal ring. A hollow needle is also inserted percutaneously over the opposite half of the internal ring. Mating of the two allows the suture

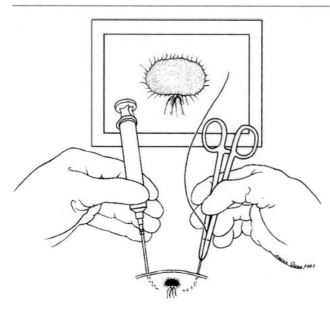

Fig. 11.10 Subcutaneous endoscopically assisted ligation (SEAL) of the internal ring (From Harrison et al. [60], with permission)

material to jump over the vas and vessels and encompass most of the circumference of the internal ring. The swaged-on needle is then backed subcutaneously, completing the circumference; retrieved through its entry point; and tied extracorporeally [60].

Tissue Adhesives

The use of tissue adhesives as an adjunct to closing pediatric inguinal hernias remains at an experimental level. Sealants mentioned in the literature include electrocautery and talc [49] and glue [49, 61]. In a preliminary study on the usefulness of tissue adhesives in repair of inguinal hernias, Kato et al. [2005] reported that only the laparoscopic injection of octylcyanoacrylate (Dermabond®) is effective and scarless. Interestingly it also did not affect fertility [62]. To the best of our knowledge, no sealant or adhesive has yet been approved for use in closure of the hernial sac in humans.

Conclusion

The repair of inguinal hernias in children first requires an accurate affirmation of the diagnosis. Once this is done, a variety of methods exist to repair these hernias. In the majority of cases, no prosthetic material is required, unlike that of the adult population. Long-term consequences, such as infertility, are significant sequelae that may not become apparent until adulthood. Because of this, exacting surgical technique is mandatory.

References

1. Lloyd DA. Inguinal and femoral hernia. In: Ziegler M, Azizkhan R, Weber T, editors. Operative pediatric surgery. 1st ed. New York: McGraw-Hill; 2003. p. 543–54.
2. Lau WY. History of treatment of groin hernia. World J Surg. 2002;26:748–59.
3. Grosfeld JL. Hernias in children. In: Spitz L, Coran AG, editors. Rob & Smith's pediatric surgery. 5th ed. London: Chapman & Hall Medical; 1995. p. 222–7.
4. Collins P. Embryology and development. In: Williams P, Bannister L, Berry M, et al., editors. Gray's anatomy. 38th ed. New York: Churchill-Livingstone; 1995. p. 212–3.
5. Glick PL, Boulanger SC. Inguinal hernias and hydroceles. In: Grosfeld JL, O'Neill Jr JA, Fonkalsrud EW, Coran AG, editors. Pediatric surgery, vol. 2. 6th ed. Philadelphia: Mosby Eslevier; 2006. p. 1172–92.
6. Kolon TF, Patel RP, Huff DS. Cryptorchidism: diagnosis, treatment, and long-term prognosis. Urol Clin North Am. 2004;31:469–80.
7. Ting AYS, Huynh J, Farmer P, Yong EXZ, Hasthorpe S, Fosang A, King S, Deshpande A, Hutson J. The role of hepatocyte growth factor in the humoral regulation of inguinal hernia closure. J Pediatr Surg. 2005;40:1865–8.
8. Barnett C, Langer JC, Hinek A, Bradley TJ, Chitayat D. Looking past the lump: genetic aspects of inguinal hernia in children. J Pediatr Surg. 2009;44(7):1423–31.
9. Grosfeld JL. Current concepts in inguinal hernia in infants and children. World J Surg. 1989;13(5):506–15.
10. Rowe MI, Clatworthy HW. The other side of the pediatric inguinal hernia. Surg Clin North Am. 1971;51(6):1371–6.
11. Deeb A, Hughes IA. Inguinal hernia in female infants: a cue to check the sex chromosomes? BJU Int. 2005;96(3):401–3.
12. Czeizel A, Gardonyi J. A family study of congenital inguinal hernia. Am J Med Genet. 1979;4(3):247–54.
13. Chen KC, Chu CC, Chou TY, Wu CJ. Ultrasonography for inguinal hernias in boys. J Pediatr Surg. 1998;33(12):1784–7.
14. Erez I, Rathause V, Vacian I, Zohar E, Hoppenstein D, Werner M, et al. Preoperative ultrasound and intraoperative findings of inguinal hernias in children: a prospective study of 642 children. J Pediatr Surg. 2002;37(6):865–8.
15. Stylianos S, Jacir NN, Harris BH. Incarceration of inguinal hernia in infants prior to elective repair. J Pediatr Surg. 1993;28(4):582–3.
16. Fette AM, Höllwarth ME. Special aspects of neonatal inguinal hernia and herniotomy. Hernia. 2001;5(2):92–6.
17. Rescorla FJ, Grosfeld JL. Inguinal hernia repair in the perinatal period and early infancy: clinical considerations. J Pediatr Surg. 1984;19(6):832–7.
18. Niedzielski J, Król R, Gawłowska A. Could incarceration of inguinal hernia in children be prevented? Med Sci Monit. 2003;9(1):16–8.
19. Sloman JG, Mylius RE. Testicular infarction in infancy: its association with irreducible inguinal hernia. Med J Aust. 1958;45(8):242–4.
20. Walther-Larsen S, Rasmussen LS. The former preterm infant and risk of post-operative apnoea: recommendations for management. Acta Anaesthesiol Scand. 2006;50(7):888–93.
21. Howard R, Carter B, Curry J, Morton N, Rivett K, Rose M, et al. Good practice in postoperative and procedural pain. Paediatr Anaesth. 2008;18 suppl 1:1–78.
22. Taylor GP. Pathology of the pediatric regio inguinalis: mysteries of the hernia sac exposed. Pediatr Dev Pathol. 2000;3(6):513–24.
23. Phelps S, Agrawal M. Morbidity after neonatal inguinal herniotomy. J Pediatr Surg. 1997;32(3):445–7.

24. Davies BW, Fraser N, Najmaldin AS, Squire BR, Crabbe DC, Stringer MD. A prospective study of neonatal inguinal herniotomy: the problem of the postoperative hydrocele. Pediatr Surg Int. 2003;19(1–2):68–70.
25. Lau ST, Lee YH, Caty MG. Current management of hernias and hydroceles. Semin Pediatr Surg. 2007;16(1):50–7.
26. Steinau G, et al. Recurrent inguinal hernias in infants and children. World J Surg. 1995;19(2):303–6.
27. Walc L, Bass J, Rubin S, et al. Testicular fate after incarcerated hernia repair and/or orchiopexy performed in patients under 6 months of age. J Pediatr Surg. 1995;30:1195–7.
28. Partrick DA, Bensard DD, Karrer FM, et al. Is routine pathological evaluation of pediatric hernia sacs justified? J Pediatr Surg. 1998;33:1090–2.
29. Steigman CK, Sotelo-Avila C, Weber TR. The incidence of spermatic cord structures in inguinal hernia sacs from male children. Am J Surg Pathol. 1999;23:880–5.
30. Matsuda T, Horii Y, Yoshida O. Unilateral obstruction of the vas deferens caused by childhood inguinal herniorrhaphy in male infertility patients. Fertil Steril. 1992;58:609–13.
31. Jequier AM. Obstructive azoospermia: a study of 102 patients. Clin Reprod Fertil. 1985;3:21–36.
32. Friberg J, Fritjofsson A. Inguinal herniorrhaphy and sperm-agglutinating antibodies in infertile men. Arch Androl. 1979;2(4): 317–22.
33. Parkhouse H, Hendry WF. Vasal injuries during childhood and their effect on subsequent fertility. Br J Urol. 1991;67(1):91–5.
34. Jona JZ. Letter: the neglected inguinal hernia. Pediatrics. 1976;58: 294–5.
35. Harper SJ, Bush GH. Deaths in children with inguinal hernia. Br Med J (Clin Res Ed). 1988;296(6616):210.
36. Callum KG, Gray AJG, Hoile RW et al. Extremes of age: the 1999 report of the national confidential enquiry into peri-operative deaths. 1999. Available at: http://www.ncepod.org.uk/1999ea.htm.
37. Levitt MA, Ferraraccio D, Arbesman MC, Brisseau GF, Caty MG, Glick PL. Variability of inguinal hernia surgical technique: a survey of North American pediatric surgeons. J Pediatr Surg. 2002;37(5): 745–51.
38. Miltenburg DM, Nuchtern JG, Jaksic T, et al. Meta-analysis of the risk of metachronous hernia in infants and children. Am J Surg. 1997;174:741–4.
39. Ballantyne A, Jawaheer G, Munro FD. Contralateral groin exploration is not justified in infants with a unilateral inguinal hernia. Br J Surg. 2001;88(5):720–3.
40. Nassiri SJ. Contralateral exploration is not mandatory in unilateral inguinal hernia in children: a prospective 6-year study. Pediatr Surg Int. 2002;18:470–1.
41. Ron O, Eaton S, Pierro A. Systematic review of the risk of developing a metachronous contralateral inguinal hernia in children. Br J Surg. 2007;94(7):804–11.
42. Sale SM. Neonatal apnoea. Best Pract Res Clin Anaesthesiol. 2010;24(3):323–36.
43. Goldstein IR, Potts WJ. Inguinal hernia in female infants and children. Ann Surg. 1958;148(5):819–22.
44. Bianchi A, Squire BR. Transscrotal orchidopexy: orchidopexy revised. Pediatr Surg Int. 1989;5:189–92.
45. Gökçora IH, Yagmurlu A. A longitudinal follow-up using the high trans-scrotal approach for inguinal and scrotal abnormalities in boys. Hernia. 2003;7(4):181–4.
46. Fearne C, Abela M, Aquilina D. Scrotal approach for inguinal hernia and hydrocele repair in boys. Eur J Pediatr Surg. 2002;12(2):116–7.
47. Schier F. Laparoscopic inguinal hernia repair-a prospective personal series of 542 children. J Pediatr Surg. 2006;41(6):1081–4.
48. Schier F, Montupet P, Esposito C. Laparoscopic inguinal herniorrhaphy in children: a three-center experience with 933 repairs. J Pediatr Surg. 2002;37(3):395–7.
49. Ozgediz D, Roayaie K, Lee H, Nobuhara KK, Farmer DL, Bratton B, Harrison MR. Subcutaneous endoscopically assisted ligation (SEAL) of the internal ring for repair of inguinal hernias in children: report of a new technique and early results. Surg Endosc. 2007;21(8):1327–31.
50. Schier F, Turial S, Huckstadt T, et al. Laparoscopic inguinal hernia repair does not impair testicular perfusion. J Pediatr Surg. 2008;43: 131–5.
51. Shalaby R, Desoky A. Needlescopic inguinal hernia repair in children. Pediatr Surg Int. 2002;18:153–6.
52. Kaya M, Huckstedt T, Schier F. Laparoscopic approach to incarcerated inguinal hernia in children. J Pediatr Surg. 2006;41(3):567–9.
53. Lipskar AM, Soffer SZ, Glick RD, Rosen NG, Levitt MA, Hong AR. Laparoscopic inguinal hernia inversion and ligation in female children: a review of 173 consecutive cases at a single institution. J Pediatr Surg. 2011;45:1370–4.
54. Hassan ME, Mustafawi AR. Laparoscopic flip-flap technique versus conventional inguinal hernia repair in children. JSLS. 2007;11(1):90–3.
55. Zallen G, Glick PL. Laparoscopic inversion and ligation inguinal hernia repair in girls. J Laparoendosc Adv Surg Tech A. 2007;17(1):143–5.
56. Shalaby R, Fawy M, Soliman S, Dorgham A. A new simplified technique for needlescopic inguinal herniorrhaphy in children. J Pediatr Surg. 2006;41(4):863–7.
57. Endo M, Ukiyama E. Laparoscopic closure of patent processus vaginalis in girls with inguinal hernia using a specially devised suture needle. Ped Endosurg Innov Tech. 2001;5(2):187–91.
58. Takehara H, Yakabe S, Kameoka K. Laparoscopic percutaneous extraperitoneal closure for inguinal hernia in children: clinical outcome of 972 repairs done in 3 pediatric surgical institutions. J Pediatr Surg. 2006;41(12):1999–2003.
59. Patkowski D, Czernik J, Chrzan R, Jaworski W, Apoznanski W. Percutaneous internal ring suturing: a simple minimally invasive technique for inguinal hernia repair in children. J Laparoendosc Adv Surg Tech A. 2006;16(5):513–7.
60. Harrison MR, Lee H, Albanese CT, Farmer DL. Subcutaneous endoscopically assisted ligation (SEAL) of the internal ring for repair of inguinal hernias in children: a novel technique. J Pediatr Surg. 2005;40:1177–80.
61. Esposito C, Damiano R, Settimi A, De Marco M, Maglio P, Centonze A. Experience with the use of tissue adhesives in pediatric endoscopic surgery. Surg Endosc. 2004;18(2):290–2.
62. Kato Y, Yamataka A, Miyano G, Tei E, Koga H, Lane GJ, Miyano T. Tissue adhesives for repairing inguinal hernia: a preliminary study. J Laparoendosc Adv Surg Tech A. 2005;15(4):424–8.

Anjili Khakar and Simon Clarke

Introduction

Umbilical hernia is a protrusion of intra-abdominal contents through the umbilical ring, within a peritoneal sac, and is one of the most common conditions managed by pediatric surgeons (Fig. 12.1). Debate exists regarding its natural history, expectant management before surgery, and supposed infrequent incarceration rate.

History of Umbilical Hernia Management

Observations regarding the management of pediatric umbilical hernia date back to the first century. Celsus described an operation by "ligature" for umbilical hernia, whereas Soranus (A.D. 98–117) suggested "doubling the cord over, rolling it in wool and laying it gently against the middle of the navel" [1].

In 1884 Erichsen declared that "these small umbilical hernias never strangulated, never caused death, and were rarely seen over the age of ten" [2]. Woods observed that no case of strangulation of an infantile umbilical hernia had ever been recorded, and treatment by strapping may actually delay the disappearance of the hernia or even increase its severity [1].

Surgical closure is now the accepted treatment if spontaneous resolution has not occurred or if complications arise. Recent reports would suggest that incarceration with or without strangulation occur more commonly than was previously thought [3–9].

Umbilical Pathology in Children

Umbilical disorders are common in pediatric surgical practice and usually present with umbilical discharge, pain, or mass.

The majority occur due to abnormal embryologic or physiological processes. Umbilical hernia falls into the spectrum of congenital abdominal wall defects (see Table 12.1)

Formation of the Anterior Abdominal Wall and Its Relation to Umbilical Hernia

During embryonic development the umbilical area is highly complex. After birth however the normal umbilicus is a relatively simple structure. During fetal life anterior abdominal wall development depends on differential growth of embryonic tissues. This occurs by a combination of cranial, caudal, and lateral infolding of the head and tail folds as well as acute ventral flexion beginning in the 4th fetal week. Return of the midgut and a reduction in the relative size of the body stalk also play an important part [10]. The rectus muscles approximate and become closed by the 12th week, except for the umbilical ring. The connective tissue of the umbilical cord originates from the primitive mesoderm, whereas the rectus sheath, the linea alba, and the fascia of the anterior abdominal wall are formed from intraembryonic mesoderm. Fusion of these two types of mesoderm occurs at the embryonic rim which then becomes the umbilical orifice. Proliferation of lateral connective tissue plates is then responsible for closure of the umbilical ring; when this is incomplete, a patent ring is the result [1].

There are also anatomical theories for predisposition to development of umbilical hernia in addition to the embryonic theories (Table 12.2).

Physiology/Natural History of the Umbilicus After Birth

Shortly after birth there is a natural clamping of the blood flow through the umbilical cord, a physiological process triggered by the fall in temperature. Wharton's jelly swells and blood vessels within the cord collapse. After cord ligation,

A. Khakar • S. Clarke (✉)
Department of Pediatric Surgery, Chelsea and Westminster Hospital, London, United Kingdom
e-mail: simon.clarke@chelwest.nhs.uk

A.N. Kingsnorth and K.A. LeBlanc (eds.), *Management of Abdominal Hernias*,
DOI 10.1007/978-1-84882-877-3_12, © Springer Science+Business Media London 2013

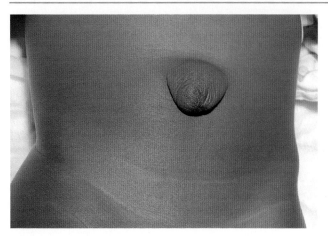

Fig. 12.1 Umbilical hernia

Table 12.1 Congenital umbilical disorders

		Delayed cord separation
Failure of normal physiology		Umbilical granuloma
Congenital	Abdominal wall defects	Hernia of umbilical cord
		Exomphalos/omphalocele (gastroschisis)
		Umbilical hernia
	Others	Dermoid cyst
		Vascular malformation
	Embryological remnants	
	Vitelline duct remnants	Umbilical polyp
		Patent vitellointestinal duct
		Meckel's diverticulum/band/cyst
	Urachal remnants	Umbilical polyp
		Patent urachus
		Urachal sinus/cyst

Table 12.2 Summary of the embryologic and anatomical theories predisposing to development of umbilical hernia

Failure of the recti to approximate in the midline after return of the midgut
Variability in the attachment of the ligamentum teres and median umbilical ligament
Variability in coverage of the umbilical ring by umbilical (Richet's) fascia
Anatomical maturity of the umbilical fascia

the vessels thrombose and the cord dries and sloughs. This leaves a granulating surface that heals by cicatrization and becomes covered by epithelium.

Elastic fibers that reinforce the umbilical ring, together with proliferation of the lateral connective tissue plates, originally from the cord, are responsible. Atrophy and obliteration of the umbilical vessels continue the process with the scar contracting resulting in a retracted umbilicus. Delay in development during the latter stages results in umbilical defects with minor degrees of herniation of the umbilicus observed in many neonates [11].

Table 12.3 Conditions associated with umbilical hernia

Prematurity and low birth weight
Racial variation
Trisomy 21, 13, 18
Beckwith–Wiedemann syndrome
Congenital hypothyroidism
Malnutrition/rickets
Mucopolysaccharidosis type 1

Natural History of Congenital Umbilical Hernias

The expectant approach to management of pediatric umbilical hernias relates to their natural history and asymptomatic nature. Umbilical hernias regress spontaneously in the majority of children. Early reports demonstrated that up to 93% of children resolve automatically in the first year of life [1]. Recent series have established spontaneous closure occurring in most children by the age of 4 years [12–15]. In Africa however some demonstrate resolution continuing up to 14 years of age [16].

If not repaired in childhood, 10% of umbilical hernias will persist to adulthood [17] and have an increased risk of incarceration compared to childhood hernias [18]. Emergency surgery for an incarcerated umbilical hernia in adults has significant morbidity and carries a mortality rate of up to 6% [19].

Some authors have observed that the size of the fascial defect, and even its sharpness, is indicative of its ability to close naturally [12, 20, 21]. Walker demonstrated in a series of 314 children that fascial rings measuring less than 1 cm in diameter tend to close spontaneously, while those larger than 1.5 cm rarely do [21]. A hernia with a thicker, rounded fascial edge is suggested by some as more likely to close than one with a thin, sharper edge [20].

Epidemiology of Umbilical Hernia

As the majority of umbilical hernias resolve naturally, their exact incidence is unknown. A true figure could only be obtained by large population-based studies. Incidence figures in the literature vary, due to differing definitions and methods of patient selection. Incidence is also dependent on factors such as the age and ethnicity of the patient group (Table 12.3).

Age

One author found that 106 (19%) of 583 healthy infants below the age of 6 months attending a welfare clinic had an umbilical hernia. It was also found that in a group of 105 children at nursery school, 10 children (9.5%), all age 2 years, had umbilical hernias. These all resolved by 5 years of age [1].

Prematurity

Umbilical hernias occur in 75–84% of premature (<1,500 g) neonates at birth [22, 23] but only 20% of larger neonates (2,000–2,500 g) [22].

Racial Variation

Umbilical hernias occur in 4–30% of Caucasian infants [1, 12, 13] and are up to ten times more common in persons of African origin [23, 24]. This difference is seen in different parts of the world. In the West Indies, 58.5% of children of African origin have umbilical hernias compared with 1–8% of white, Indian, and Chinese children [17]. Similarly in East Africa, 60% of African origin children have umbilical hernias, compared with 4% of Indian origin [25], and in South Africa 61.8% of children among the Xhosa tribe have umbilical hernias [26].

Meier and colleagues prospectively evaluated the umbilical area of 4,052 Nigerians. "Outies" (umbilical protrusion past the periumbilical skin in an erect subject) were identified in 92% of subjects below the age of 18 years and 49% of those above the age of 18 years. There was no palpable fascial opening in 39% of children with "outies." Umbilical hernias, defined as protrusion of at least 5 mm and a diameter of at least 10 mm, were present in 23% of patients under the age of 18 years [16]. One study from South Africa showed no significant racial disparity in incidence, with umbilical hernias present in 23% of blacks and 19% of white South Africans [12].

An interesting suggestion is the association between umbilical hernia and socioeconomic class. A prospective study of 7,968 Nigerian children seeking admission for private school found only 1.3% had umbilical hernias, a prevalence of 1.8 per 1,000 [27]. This is a much lower frequency than that usually observed in Nigeria [16].

Other factors predisposing to umbilical herniation (Table 12.3) are low birth weight [1, 22, 23], respiratory distress syndrome, and malnutrition [1]. Conditions such as trisomy 21, 13, and 18 [18], Beckwith–Wiedemann syndrome [18], congenital hypothyroidism [18], and mucopolysaccharidosis [18, 28] are also associated with umbilical hernias. However, the majority of umbilical hernias in children occur with no other associated anomaly. There is no gender difference.

Incarceration and Strangulation

Incarceration is the most common complication of umbilical hernia, followed by strangulation of bowel or omentum. Rupture and evisceration of contents is a rare but alarming condition that has a risk of mortality.

Incidence of Incarceration

Historically, obstruction of an umbilical hernia was considered "rare," occurring in approximately 1:1,500 (0.06%) umbilical hernias [12]. In 1975 a large European study of 590 children found 5% of umbilical hernias incarcerated [13]. More recently, several case series and retrospective studies of incarcerated umbilical hernias [3, 5–9] have highlighted that this complication is more common than previously thought. One author reported seven cases in 3 years and suggested a possible increasing trend of this complication [3] (Table 12.4).

There may be geographic, genetic, or socioeconomic factors involved in complication of hernias, though some of the difference in incarceration rates may simply reflect the increased incidence of umbilical hernias in these areas. Retrospective studies from Africa show a relatively high frequency of incarceration and other complications, up to 37.5% for acute incarceration and 54% if those that were recurrently incarcerated were included [5–8]. However, these patients are likely to be a self-selected group with the majority only presenting when symptomatic, as umbilical hernia is considered normal in their society and presentation for cosmesis is rare [16]. In the same continent, a South African study of mainly Caucasian (93%) children observed an incarceration rate of 7% [4], a figure more in line with the 5% from the only comparable European series [13].

Contrary to these findings is a retrospective analysis from Nigeria that only identified two children who had emergency surgery for umbilical hernia in 15 years [16] and a report from Kansas children's hospital where they did not observe any emergency surgery for umbilical hernia over a 15-year period [29]. Clearly there are geographical differences.

Predicting Which Umbilical Hernias will Incarcerate

Conflicting evidence suggest defect size has a role in predicting complications. Lassaletta observed that small defects (<1.5 cm) are at higher risk [13], a finding confirmed by others [3]. Several case series however found the opposite, with their complications arising in defects 1.5 cm or larger [5, 6]. Brown et al. suggest that size has no impact on whether the hernia incarcerates [4].

In the literature, age at presentation of patients with acute incarceration ranged from 14 months to 5 years. Why these age groups are more at risk is not clear, though this may represent a closing defect.

Severe abdominal wall spasm associated with an umbilical hernia incarceration during vigorous swimming has also been described in two children. High intra-abdominal pressures from breathing using the abdominal muscles is suggested as causing umbilical herniation and incarceration under such circumstances [30].

Table 12.4 Table summarizing literature on complicated umbilical hernias

Author	Location of study	Type of study	Time period (years)	Total number children	Age	Incarceration cases/% of total	Comment
Woods [1]	UK	Po		283	Infants only	0	All Caucasian
Lassaletta [13]	Europe			590 / 377 repaired		5% / 3.7% age <1 y / 4.7% age ≥4 y	• 2/3 children of Afro-Caribbean origin • Incarceration most frequent in defects 0.5–1.5 cm
Mawera [8]	Zimbabwe	R	4	38	1 mth–13 y	37.5% / 20% S/RI	• 86% of obstructed group reduced spontaneously • Only 2 needed operative reduction
Vrsansky [9]	France	CS	5	N/A		4	1 strangulated
Papagrigoriadis [20]	UK	CS	20	N/A	22/40/48 mths	3	• Caribbean descent • 2 had mass of undigested material in the incarcerated bowel
Meier [16]	Nigeria	R	15	Unknown	0–18 years (adults also studied)	2	• No denominator
Keshtgar [3]	UK	CS	3	N/A	Median 3 y	7 / 5 acute / 2 recurrent	• 4/5 reduced under G/A or at surgery. 1 with taxis • 1 necrotic omentum • Defects <1.5 cm
Ameh [5]	Nigeria	R	14	47	≤12 y / Median age of: 1) Acute—5 y 2) recurrent—3 y	25 (53%) / 15 A (32%) / 10 RI (21%)	• 1/15 reduced spont • 2/15 had bowel resection • 5 others (11%) had spontaneous evisceration • Complications in hernias ≥1.5 cm
Brown [4]	Cape Town S Africa	Pr	15	389	6 y (average) / Incarcerated—3 y (average)	28 (7%)	• 2 had resection of ischemic omentum • 5 had pica • Only 22 African origin, 6 colored • 5 spontaneously reduced 14 reduced by taxis 9 at surgery • Mean defect size 2.24 cm
Chirdan [6]	Nigeria	CS	8	52	4 y (median) / Median age / Acute—4 y / Recurrent—8.5 y (average)	23 (44%) / 17 A (33%) / 6 RI (11%)	• Acute—defect 2 cm (median). Recurrent 2.5 cm • 1 resection gangrenous bowel and Meckel's • 12/15 reduced by taxis 3/15 at emergency surgery

Fall [7]	Senegal	R	5	Unknown	14 mths	41 (15%)	• 5 necrotic bowel (1 had perforated Meckel's diverticulum) • 5 reduced at anesthetic induction • All operated as emergency
Snyder [29]	USA	R	15	Unknown		0	Statement in review article; Presumed retrospective
Khakhar 2009	UK	R	4	184	20 mths	10 (5%) A 4 (2%) S/RI	Personal series

Po population based, *CS* case series, *R* retrospective, *Pr* prospective, *Y* years, *Mths* months

Pica leading to accumulation of undigested foreign material in bowel, such as chewing gum, sand, or even the presence of ascarids, may predispose to irreducibility of a hernia. They have been observed in incarcerated hernias, and it is presumed that the size of the mass prevents reduction through a narrow neck [4, 20].

Recurrent Incarceration

Recurrent incarceration may be due to intermittent trapping of omentum within a closing hernia and presents as episodes of vomiting with umbilical pain [31]. Studies show this is not uncommon and is reported in a fifth of the patients in African studies [5, 6, 8] and is also described in the United Kingdom [3]. Recurrent incarceration may be significantly underreported as some studies may not have included those patients [4, 13, 15].

Outcome of Incarcerated Umbilical Hernia

Two studies found that 86% of incarcerated umbilical hernias spontaneously reduced, in or just prior to arriving at the hospital [8, 32]. Others showed that only 6–18% of irreducible hernias resolved without intervention with 50–80% being reduced by taxis with sedation or analgesia [4, 6]. Reduction at surgery was necessary in 18–32% of these incarcerated hernias. In contrast to these results, one study from Senegal found that all 41 of their patients were operated on as an emergency, five of which reduced at anesthetic [7].

Strangulation of hernia contents is also reported in up to 13% of incarcerated hernias undergoing bowel resection [4–7, 16] and up to 14% excising omentum only [3, 4]. Postoperative infection is reported to occur in 4–7% of those that had been previously been incarcerated or strangulated [4–7]. There was no mortality in any published study.

Conditions Mimicking Incarcerated Umbilical Hernia

Tender distended umbilical hernias occur in and mirror intra-peritoneal disease, peritonitis, intestinal obstruction, and ascites. Recent reports in the pediatric literature illustrate how other pathology, such as appendicitis [33] or an inflamed Meckel's diverticulum [34], can present as an incarcerated umbilical hernia.

Rupture and Evisceration

Spontaneous rupture is a rare complication of umbilical hernias in children, with only 14 cases in the literature [28, 35, 36].

It is usually bowel that eviscerates [31, 32, 35, 37, 38] but can be omentum alone [26] or more rarely the urinary bladder dome [36]. Factors implicated in spontaneous rupture [35] include local trauma or ulceration of skin [31, 32, 37], umbilical sepsis [38], and prematurity with prolonged positive pressure ventilation [37]. Severe coughing [31] and excessive crying [32, 35] may also contribute. It also appears that those hernias with larger fascial defects ≥1.5 cm are at higher risk [35]. There is one case report of rupture of an umbilical hernia in an infant with Hurler's syndrome (mucopolysaccharidosis type 1), a condition in which umbilical hernias are commonly seen though rarely repaired due to high anesthetic risk and short life expectancy [28]. Spontaneous rupture has also been reported in a previously healthy 8-month-old infant [35].

Clinical Definition of Congenital Umbilical Hernia

A congenital umbilical hernia can be defined clinically as a herniation of intra-abdominal viscera, usually intestine, through the umbilical ring within a peritoneal sac. It is covered by skin and is present from birth. Some authors specify that a true umbilical hernia is a saccular swelling, present and protruding on straining [1, 12, 16]. Others use less strict criteria, with palpability of a gap at the umbilical orifice alone being sufficient [13]. Some studies do not state their definition.

Diagnosing Umbilical Hernia

The diagnosis of umbilical hernia is a clinical one. The usual history is of an umbilical protrusion since birth and a trend of either growth of the size of the hernia or, as in most cases, a reduction. Age at presentation to a surgeon often depends upon the parental or local medical knowledge of the natural history of umbilical hernia.

During a consultation parents will often comment on the size of the hernia and its worsening during crying. A history of recurrent abdominal discomfort and believing the hernia to be responsible is often given, especially as increasing size is associated with crying. The child may repeatedly play with the protruding skin which is also taken as a sign of discomfort.

Clinical examination should focus on the position of the hernia and its differentiation from an epigastric or supraumbilical hernia and embryological remnants such as a residual urachal cyst [39]. An umbilical hernia has at its base a circumscribed central defect, whereas a supraumbilical hernia is often a transverse or irregular defect which is outside the central umbilical area. In addition, the defect in an umbilical hernia is often relatively small in comparison to that of the herniated contents, and the contents reduce without difficulty or discomfort.

Table 12.5 Chelsea and Westminster Hospital Series 2004–2009

185 patients
Median age at surgery—55 months
158 elective (85.4%). Median age—58 months
10 underwent emergency surgery for incarceration (5.4%); Median age 24 months
5 symptomatic hernias/recurrent incarceration (3%) 11 repaired incidentally when other surgery being performed 6%

Table 12.6 Indications for surgery in umbilical hernia

Absolute	Incarceration and/or strangulation
	Spontaneous rupture and evisceration
Relative indications	Hernia causing pain
	Cosmesis
	Large rings—unlikely to close >1.5 cms
	Asymptomatic age 3 years +
Incidental	At time of other surgery?
	At laparoscopic surgery

The diameter and sharpness of the fascial edge of the hernia orifice can be recorded during the examination. A smooth edge and a diameter of less than 1.5 cm are seen by some as predictors of spontaneous closure [12, 20, 21].

Acute incarceration usually presents as an emergency. The clinical picture for incarceration is one of developing tenderness in the umbilical region with a history of umbilical hernia. In our own series of 185 cases over a 10-year period, 10 patients (5%) presented with incarceration, and an additional five patients (3%) reported intermittent abdominal pain associated with a temporary irreducible hernia. The true denominator in our community is of course unknown (Table 12.5).

Consent and Indications for Surgery

Consent

Consent for umbilical hernia repair should focus on the position of the incision, the nature of the repair, the absorbability of the suture used, the dressing immediately following surgery, and the potential complications. Complications occur in 0.5–1% of patients undergoing umbilical hernia repair and include wound infection, hematoma, and recurrence. Excessive skin and hypertrophic scarring should also be mentioned as being possible short-term observations particularly in the proboscoid-type hernia and those of African–Caribbean descent [16, 21, 23, 40].

Indications for Operating on Umbilical Hernia

Indications for surgery include incarceration, recurrent abdominal discomfort associated with herniation, or umbilical port closure following laparoscopy (Table 12.6).

The precise age at which surgery should be carried out in an asymptomatic umbilical hernia is debated. Most pediatric surgeons have a tendency to offer repair for an asymptomatic hernia prior to regular schooling. In our own recent series, the median age at operation for elective patients was 58 months (Table 12.5). For most surgeons cosmetic appearance is not an indication to operate until the natural regression of the defect has occurred. Parental desire is often for

their child not to look different from other children, and teasing from an umbilical bulge is not an infrequent complaint from school-age children. Increasing size as an adult also carries a greater incarceration risk in later life and therefore represents an indication to operate earlier in life.

If there was a desire to avoid surgery at 3–4 years of age, then expectant management could continue. Parents should be made aware of the low risk of incarceration and what to expect if it should occur.

Incidental Closure

Any laparoscopic procedure that results in an umbilical insertion of a Veress needle or open insertion of trocar would, for most pediatric surgeons, result in the closure of an incidental hernia at that time. A recent poll of clinical investigators in a multicenter international randomized controlled trial into pediatric laparoscopic inguinal hernia repair indicated that most would also close an incidental umbilical hernia, regardless of age (S. Clarke. Personal Correspondence). An umbilical procedure that occurs in most laparoscopy converts a natural orifice into an unnatural one, making it unlikely to be subject to the normal forces of closure.

In our own recent series of laparoscopic inguinal hernia repair associated with an umbilical hernia, one umbilical hernia did reoccur [41]. This was presumed to be due to an inadequate umbilical herniotomy at time of umbilical port closure.

Management Options for Umbilical Hernia

Observation

An initial conservative approach is the suggested management for most children presenting at preschool age. Parental reassurance is important, as the size of the herniation can be of considerable concern. Follow-up is not indicated in the majority unless reassurance is difficult to convey. A referral back to a surgeon once the child is of schooling age is typical.

Diagnostic Work-Up

Prenatal diagnosis of congenital umbilical hernia is possible using ultrasound and must be differentiated from persistent omphalomesenteric duct or omphalocele [42]. Postnatally, imaging studies are not usually required for umbilical hernia to be confirmed. An ultrasound may help if there is doubt as to the site of the defect, i.e., paraumbilical or umbilical. However, clinical confusion in children is rare.

Procedural

Preoperative Reduction

Any umbilical hernia incarceration should be considered for reduction following resuscitation. Sedation should always be carried out in a suitable environment that can provide for the resuscitation of children [43]. Reduction after administration of simple analgesia should be attempted first. Discussion with a pediatric anesthetist is advisable if further sedation is thought necessary. Any doubt as to the viability of the herniated contents or failed reduction should result in an examination of the contents and open reduction with repair under general anesthesia.

In the unlikely event of spontaneous rupture with evisceration, the child should be resuscitated, and the eviscerated bowel should be covered with cling film to protect and prevent heat loss. The hernia should then be repaired urgently.

Anesthesia for Umbilical Hernia

General anesthesia is preferred in children. Local anesthesia using 0.25% bupivacaine (0.8 mL/kg) within the fascia or as a pararectal block is recommended. Some evidence also exists for reduced postoperative pain requirement with a preoperative caudal anesthetic [44].

Surgical Options for Umbilical Hernia

Operative technique for umbilical hernia repair was highlighted by Mayo more than a century ago [45]. Over the past few decades, observational studies have continued to describe alterations in technique as well as outcome [12, 14, 15, 46, 47].

The most established accepted technique for strength and closure in an adult is similar to that originally described by Mayo and involves closing of the defect using an overlapping fascial technique. In children, where the defect is usually not large as in adults, the most commonly performed method involves a primary interrupted repair of the defect following control and excision of the sac [15].

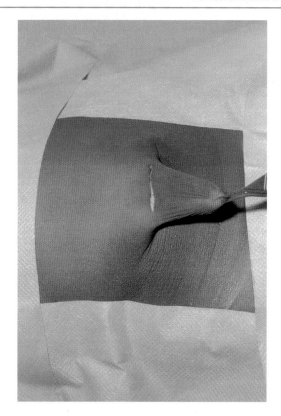

Fig. 12.2 Incision

Position and Prepping of the Patient

The child is placed on his back (supine) on the operating table. A warming device or cotton wool sheets are placed around the child to prevent heat loss during surgery. Antibiotics are not routinely given for umbilical hernia repair. Careful aseptic technique combined with a Betadine or chlorhexidine prep will suffice.

Draping

Drapes are applied so that the umbilical area is exposed throughout the operation.

Incision

Most pediatric surgeons carry out a simple curved sub- or supraumbilical incision, with circumferential dissection of the sac around its base to control it (see Fig. 12.2). The supraumbilical incision is seen by many as preferable, as with growth this is hidden within the superior umbilical fold itself and is not visible to the patient. Hernia reduction has usually occurred following anesthesia, though it is important the operator should confirm reduction of contents before opening the sac.

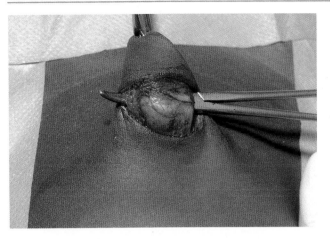

Fig. 12.3 Controlling the sac

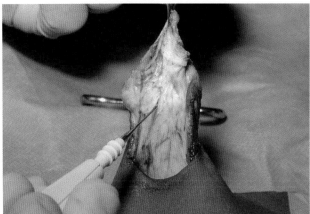

Fig. 12.5 Excising the sac

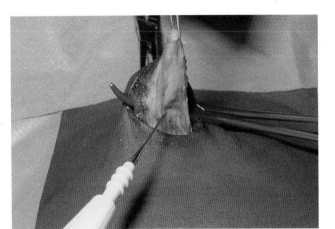

Fig. 12.4 Freeing the sac from the defect

Sac Dissection

A circumferential dissection then begins to isolate the sac (Fig. 12.3). Once controlled, the sac can be incised at its base (Fig. 12.4) and the distal part removed from the overlying skin to avoid a bulky appearance (Fig. 12.5).

An alternative method, or if the sac is particularly large, involves opening the sac immediately following the skin incision. The umbilical ring can be seen from inside the sac. The sac can then be stripped from the umbilical fascia and overlying skin [47–49].

Regardless of technique, removing some of the sac especially in the larger hernias will result in an improved and inverted cosmetic appearance. Care must be taken when stripping the sac off the overlying skin to avoid postoperative skin necrosis and ulceration. It is not customary to excess excise overlying skin in children as this usually resolves with time, and excision may result in a distorted or flattened appearance.

The defect itself, once identified clearly, can be closed with an overlapping fascial technique. A monofilament

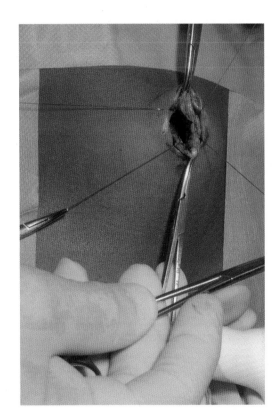

Fig. 12.6 Interrupted sutures to defect

absorbable suture such as PDS (Ethicon) 2-0 or 3-0 will suffice in most children. A monofilament suture runs easily through the thickened umbilical fascia than a braided suture. The peritoneum and muscle are closed as one layer either transversely or in a midline fashion depending on the shape of the umbilical defect. Applying a hemostatic clip to each suture (see Fig. 12.6) and tying after all have been placed allows for a controlled repair as well as superior retraction and avoidance of damage to intraperitoneal viscera (see Fig. 12.7).

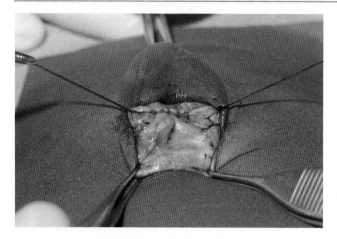

Fig. 12.7 Defect closed with knots buried

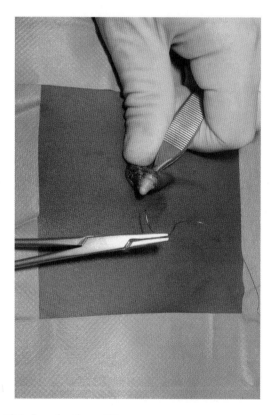

Fig. 12.8 Inverting the umbilicus

One suture is then used to anchor the central subdermal area of the umbilicus to fashion an inverted appearance (see Fig. 12.8). The superficial fascia can then be closed with an interrupted nonabsorbable suture. Finally, the skin can then be closed with either a continuous subcuticular absorbable suture or glue (see Fig. 12.9).

A dressing can be applied which may or may not have a pressure pad to avoid hematoma formation. Some authors doubt the necessity of this step [50].

In larger hernias one can adopt the Mayo technique as used in adults [45], or a patch can be placed if the muscle is weak or the hernia recurrent. This would be unusual in children.

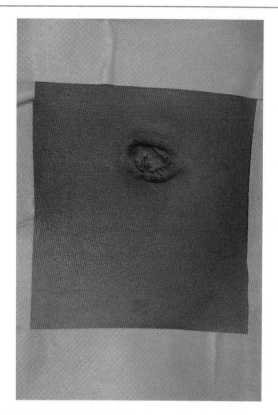

Fig. 12.9 Final appearance

Minimally Invasive Technique for Umbilical Hernia Repair

Minimally invasive techniques have been described for treating umbilical hernia in children. These involve the injection of polymers or using laparoscopy. Feins et al. described twenty-five children with umbilical hernias of 1.5 cm or less, where Deflux, a biodegradable compound of dextranomer microspheres in hyaluronic acid, was injected percutaneously in the border and preperitoneal space in 4 quadrants of the hernia defect occluding the lumen. They reported 21 of the 25 (84%) umbilical hernias as being closed at follow-up. The average age at the time of the procedure was 6 years and 7 months, and the average defect was more than 6.4 mm [51]. Albanese et al. describe a novel technique for the repair of umbilical and epigastric hernia using 3-mm laparoscopy. They repaired 41 umbilical hernias using two 3-mm lateral ports at a mean age of 4.2 years and reported excellent cosmetic and patient satisfaction outcomes [52].

Recommendations Based on Level of Evidence

The surgical method described in this chapter is effective and easily replicated though no level 1 evidence exists for this method of congenital umbilical hernia repair. The Mayo technique is widely used in adults and as such has little to compare it with. Recommendation is therefore based solely on level 2 and level 3 evidence. The lack of need for a pressure dressing is based on one randomized controlled trial in children [50].

Expected Posttreatment Course and Postoperative Care

Children should expect a full and quick recovery following umbilical hernia surgery, provided that no complications occur. A dressing, if used, is usually removed 48–72 h after surgery. Follow-up is not routinely offered in our own unit if the defect is large or at parents' request.

Postoperative Complications and Treatment of Complications

Bleeding

Bruising around the umbilicus is a possibility and often results from the pararectal anesthetic block. Hematoma from the surgical dissection is rare but if large and painful, may require evacuation.

Infection

The incidence of infection in one reported series is 1% and is not influenced by the use or not of a dressing [50]. Infection should be treated with antibiotics and would rarely require abscess drainage.

Cosmetic Concerns

In the author's own series, excess skin has occasionally demanded umbilicoplasty at the patient's request during teenage years. Twelve patients (6.5%) voiced cosmetic concerns, of which four went on to further corrective surgery. Two African–Caribbean patients experienced hypertrophic keloid scarring and were treated conservatively.

Recurrence

In adults the recurrence rate is reported as being between 8 and 20%. Associated risk factors include high body mass index, cirrhosis with ascites, and large defects [53–55].

In children, recurrence is much less common 1–2% [56]. In our own recent series, there were two recurrences (1%). There were no clear indications in either case as both occurred some months after the initial repair, though an incomplete closure at the initial surgery is presumed. Postoperative wound infection, hematoma, or obesity are likely risk factors for recurrence in children.

References

1. Woods GE. Some observations on umbilical hernias in infants. Arch Dis Child. 1953;28:450–62.
2. Erichsen JE. The science and art of surgery, vol. 2. 8th ed. London: Longmans, Green & co. London; 1884. p. 822–3.
3. Keshtgar AS, Griffiths M. Incarceration of umbilical hernia in children: is the trend increasing? Eur J Pediatr Surg. 2003;13(1):40–3.
4. Brown RA, Numanoglu A, Rode HS. Complicated umbilical hernia in childhood. S Afr J Surg. 2006;44(4):136–7.
5. Ameh EA, Chirdan LB, Nmadu PT, Yusufu LM. Complicated umbilical hernias in children. Pediatr Surg Int. 2003;19(4):280–2.
6. Chirdan LB, Uba AF, Kidmas AT. Incarcerated umbilical hernia in children. Eur J Pediatr Surg. 2006;16(1):45–8.
7. Fall I, Sanou A, Ngom G, Dieng M, Sankalé AA, Ndoye M. Strangulated umbilical hernias in children. Pediatr Surg Int. 2006;22(3):233–5.
8. Mawera G, Muguti GI. Umbilical hernia in Bulawayo: some observations from a hospital based study. Cent Afr J Med. 1994;40(11):319–23.
9. Vrsansky P, Bourdelat D. Incarcerated umbilical hernia in children. Pediatr Surg Int. 1997;12(1):61–2.
10. Skandalakis J, Gray SQW, Ricketts R. The anterior abdominal wall. In: Skandalakis JG, editor. Embryology for surgeons. 2nd ed. Baltimore: Williams & Wilkins; 1994. p. 540–93.
11. O'Donnell KA, Glick PL, Caty MG. Pediatric umbilical problems. Pediatr Clin North Am. 1998;45:791–9.
12. Blumberg NA. Infantile umbilical hernia. Surg Gynecol Obstet. 1980;150:187–92.
13. Lassaletta L, Fonkalsrud EW, Tover JA, Dudgeon D, Asch MJ. The management of umbilical hernias in infancy and childhood. J Pediatr. 1975;10:405–9.
14. Cilley RE, Krummel TM. Disorders of the umbilicus. In: O'Neill JA, Rowe MI, Grosfeld JL, editors. Pediatric surgery. 5th ed. St. Louis: Mosby; 1998. p. 1037–41.
15. Spitz L. Operative pediatric surgery. 6th ed. London: Hodder Arnold publication; 2007.
16. Meier DE, OlaOlorun DA, Omodele RA, Nkoi SK, Tarpley JL. Incidence of umbilical hernia in African children: redefinition of "normal" and reevaluation of indications for repair. World J Surg. 2001;25:645–8.
17. Jackson DJ, Mocklen LH. Umbilical hernia: a retrospective study. Calif Med. 1970;113(4):8–11.
18. Garcia VF. Umbilical and other abdominal wall hernias. In: Ashcraft KW, Whitfield Holcomb G, Murphy JP, editors. Pediatric Surgery. Philadelphia: Elsevier Saunders; 2005. p. 670–2.
19. Haller Jr JA, Morgan Jr WW, White JJ, Stumbaugh S. Repair of umbilical hernias in childhood to prevent adult incarceration. Am Surg. 1971;37(4):245–6.
20. Papagrigoriadis S, Browse DJ, Howard ER. Incarceration of umbilical hernia in children: a rare but important complication. Pediatr Surg Int. 1998;14:231–2.
21. Walker SH. The natural history of umbilical hernia. A six-year follow up of 314 Negro children with this defect. Clin Pediatr (Phila). 1967;6(1):29–32.
22. Vohr BR, Rosenfield AG, Oh W. Umbilical hernia in low birth-weight infants (less than 1,500 gm). J Pediatr. 1977;90:807–8.
23. Crump ED. Umbilical hernia. Occurrence of the infantile type in Negro infants and children. J Pediatr. 1952;40:214–23.
24. Evans AG. The comparative incidence of umbilical hernias in coloured and white infants. J Natl Med Assoc. 1941;33:158.
25. Mack NK. The incidence of umbilical hernia in Africans. East Afr Med J. 1945;22:369.
26. James T. Umbilical hernia in Xhosa infants and children. J R Soc Med. 1982;75:537–41.

27. Uba AF, Igun GO, Kidmas AT, Chirdan LB. Prevalence of umbilical hernia in a private school admission-seeking Nigerian children. Niger Postgrad Med J. 2004;11(4):255–7.

28. Hulsebos RG, Zeebregts CJ, de Langen ZJ. Perforation of a congenital umbilical hernia in a patient with Hurler's syndrome. J Pediatr Surg. 2004;39(9):1426–7.

29. Snyder CL. Current management of umbilical abnormalities and related anomalies. Semin Pediatr Surg. 2007;16(1):41–9. Review.

30. Skidmore FD. Umbilical hernia in child swimmers. Br Med J. 1979;2:494.

31. Ahmed A, Ahmed M, Nmadu PT. Spontaneous rupture of infantile umbilical hernia: report of three cases. Ann Trop Paediatr. 1998;18:239–41.

32. Bain IM, Bishop HM. Spontaneous rupture of an infantile umbilical hernia. Br J Surg. 1995;82:35.

33. David OO. Gangrenous retrocolic appendix masquerading as incarcerated umbilical hernia in a 13-month-old boy. J Trop Pediatr. 2009;55(3):202–4. Epub 2008 Nov 26.

34. Komlatsè AN, Komla G, Komla A, Azanledji BM, Abossisso SK, Hubert T. Meckel's diverticulum strangulated in an umbilical hernia. Afr J Paediatr Surg. 2009;6(2):118–9.

35. Durakbasa CU. Spontaneous rupture of an infantile umbilical hernia with intestinal evisceration. Pediatr Surg Int. 2006;22(6):567–9. Epub 2006 Mar 4.

36. Pandey A, Kumar V, Gangopadhyay AN, Upadhyaya VD. Eviscerated urinary bladder via ruptured umbilical hernia: a rare occurrence. Hernia. 2008;12(3):317–9.

37. Weik J, Moores D. An unusual case of umbilical hernia rupture with evisceration. J Pediatr Surg. 2005;40(4):E33–5.

38. Chatterjee SK. Spontaneous rupture of umbilical hernia with evisceration of small intestine. J Indian Med Assoc. 1972;59:287.

39. Carlisle EM, Mezhir JJ, Glynn L, Liu DC, Statter MB. The umbilical mass: a rare neonatal anomaly. Pediatr Surg Int. 2007;23(8):821–4. Epub 2007 Feb 15.

40. Abramson J. Epigastric, umbilical and ventral hernia. In: Cameron JL, editor. Current Surgical Therapy-3. Philadelphia: BC decker; 1989. p. 417.

41. Niyogi A, Tahim AS, Sherwood WJ, De Caluwe D, Madden NP, Abel RM, Haddad MJ, Clarke SA. A comparative study examining open inguinal herniotomy with and without hernioscopy to laparoscopic inguinal hernia repair in a pediatric population. Pediatr Surg Int. 2010;26(4):387–92.

42. Sherer DM, Dar P. Prenatal ultrasonographic diagnosis of congenital umbilical hernia and associated patent omphalomesenteric duct. Gynecol Obstet Invest. 2001;51:61–8.

43. Leroy PL, Gorzeman MP, Sury MR. Procedural sedation and analgesia in children by non-anesthesiologists in an emergency department. Minerva Pediatr. 2009;61(2):193–215.

44. Tobias JD. Postoperative analgesia and intraoperative inhalational anesthetic requirements during umbilical herniorrhaphy in children: post incisional local infiltration versus preincisional caudal epidural block. J Clin Anesth. 1996;8(8):634–8.

45. Mayo WJ. Further experience with the vertical overlapping operation for the radical cure of umbilical hernia. J Am Med Assoc. 1903;41:225–8.

46. Criado FJ. A simplified method of umbilical herniorrhaphy. Surg Gynecol Obstet. 1981;153:904–5.

47. Gilleard O, Gee AS. Paediatric umbilical hernioplasty. Ann R Coll Surg Engl. 2008;90(5):426–7.

48. Ikeda H, Yamamoto H, Fujino J, Kisaki Y, Uchida H, Ishimaru Y, Hasumi T, Hamajima A. Umbilicoplasty for large protruding umbilicus accompanying umbilical hernia: a simple and effective technique. Pediatr Surg Int. 2004;20(2):105–7.

49. Kajikawa A, Ueda K, Suzuki Y, Ohkouchi M. A new umbilicoplasty for children: creating a longitudinal deep umbilical depression. Br J Plast Surg. 2004;57(8):741–8.

50. Merei JM. Umbilical hernia repair in children: is pressure dressing necessary. Pediatr Surg Int. 2006;22(5):446–8. Epub 2006 Apr 25.

51. Feins NR, Dzakovic A, Papadakis K. Minimally invasive closure of pediatric umbilical hernias. J Pediatr Surg. 2008;43(1):127–30.

52. Albanese CT, Rengal S, Bermudez D. A novel laparoscopic technique for the repair of pediatric umbilical and epigastric hernias. J Pediatr Surg. 2006;41(4):859–62.

53. Halm JA, Heisterkamp J, Veen HF, Weidema WF. Long-term follow-up umbilical hernia repair: are there risk factors for recurrence after simple and mesh repair. Hernia. 2005;9(4):334–7.

54. Mark D, Pescovitz MD. Umbilical hernia repair in patients with cirrhosis. Ann Surg. 1984;199(3):325–7.

55. Rodríguez-Hermosa JI, Codina-Cazador A, Ruiz-Feliú B, Roig-García J, Albiol-Quer M, Planellas-Giné P. Incarcerated umbilical hernia in a super-super-obese patient. Obes Surg. 2008;18(7):893–5.

56. Davenport M, Pierro A. Abdominal wall hernias. Oxford handbook of paediatric surgery. Oxford: Oxford University Press; 2009. p. 274.

Diagnosis of a Lump in the Groin in the Adult

Andrew C. de Beaux and Dilip Patel

Swelling and/or pain in the groin are a common presentation for the abdominal surgeon. Nevertheless, diagnosis of a problem in the groin can still, in some cases, be a difficult clinical dilemma. It is fair to say that the diagnosis of an obvious swelling in the groin is usually straight forward, in terms of a hernia being present or not. However, the traditional inguinoscrotal hernia, where the hernial sac passes down into the scrotum, is a relatively uncommon event. Coupled with the increasing body mass index of the population, it is increasingly common for even a large groin hernia not to result in an obvious groin swelling. In some cases, where there is diagnostic doubt, thinking about several key questions may focus the investigation pathway:

Groin symptoms but no swelling: is there a hernia?
Groin swelling, but is it a hernia?
Hernia, but is it causing the symptoms?

Inguinal Hernia: The Adolescent and the Adult

The younger the patient, the more likely the hernia is to be indirect. An indirect hernia is where the hernial sac follows and is closely associated with the spermatic cord. It thus starts at the deep inguinal ring, passing medially and inferiorly down the inguinal canal, where with time it will emerge from the superficial inguinal ring. As the hernia continues to enlarge and follow the spermatic cord into the scrotum, it is then named an inguinoscrotal hernia. In contrast, a direct inguinal hernia exploits a weakness in the transversalis fascia,

in the region of the superficial inguinal ring. The hernial sac in this case is less adherent to the spermatic cord.

The majority of inguinal hernias are diagnosed by the patient when they see or feel a lump in their groin. The taking of a cleansing shower seems to be a common theme to the place of diagnosis, for obvious reasons. Sometimes pain or discomfort draws the patient's attention to the groin, but this is rarely a significant element in the patient's symptoms to begin with. As the hernia enlarges, symptoms in the groin, particularly a dragging sensation, but at times quite marked pain, can be reported. This swelling, discomfort, or pain rapidly settles on lying down but returns as the patient becomes ambulant again. It is not unusual for the patient to report episodes of discomfort in the groin on exercise for months or even a few years prior to the appearance of a swelling in the groin. The natural history of hernia development is very variable, with some patients' hernia remaining small in size for years, while in others, there is rapid progression of a small lump to a large hernia. Symptoms from an inguinal hernia are also very variable, ranging from no symptoms at all apart from the swelling, to pain that significantly interferes with work and recreation of the patient. Patients with a chronic cough, or who have to strain to micturate or defecate, may complain of symptoms while performing these maneuvers. Inguinal hernias in women are more likely to present with pain. It is postulated that the closed inguinal canal in the adult female means that a small indirect hernia in women causes more stretching of the tissues and hence more pain.

As the length of time that the patient has had the hernia increases, the cumulative probability of pain increases to almost 90% at 10 years, and the probability of irreducibility increases from 6.5% at 12 months to 30% at 10 years [1]. Patients who have an asymptomatic hernia may not progress to irreducibility of the hernia as quickly. A recent randomized trial of surgery vs. watchful waiting management of an asymptomatic inguinal hernia reported 23% in the watchful waiting group crossed over to surgery by 4.5 years, with increase in hernia pain being the most common reason offered [2]. Of these 364 men assigned to watchful waiting,

A.C. de Beaux (✉)
Department of General Surgery, Royal Infirmary of Edinburgh, Edinburgh, UK
e-mail: adebeaux@doctors.org.uk

D. Patel
Department of Radiology, Royal Infirmary of Edinburgh, Edinburgh, UK

A.N. Kingsnorth and K.A. LeBlanc (eds.), *Management of Abdominal Hernias*,
DOI 10.1007/978-1-84882-877-3_13, © Springer Science+Business Media London 2013

only 1 had incarceration of the hernia by 2 years and a second by 4 years, a frequency of 1.8/1,000 patient-years.

Inguinal hernias are more common in adult males than in adult females in a ratio of 10:1. However, it must not be forgotten that indirect inguinal hernias in women are as common as femoral hernias in women.

A number of patients will present with bilateral inguinal hernia, although one side is usually significantly larger than the other. Sometimes this can indicate a connective tissue disorder such as Ehlers-Danlos syndrome, although such diseases are rare. Patients with ascites, such as heart or liver failure, are more prone to bilateral hernias, as are patients on continuous ambulatory peritoneal dialysis (CAPD). It is not clear whether the incidence in such groups is higher or whether the fluid in the abdominal cavity results in more symptoms so that such patients present sooner.

Another area that can cause some diagnostic difficulty is recurrent inguinal hernia. Pain tends to be a more prominent feature. The mechanism for this is unclear, although recurrent inguinal hernias often have a tighter neck, perhaps due to fibrosis from the previous mesh or suture repair limiting dilatation of the neck or constriction of the hernial sac contents. However, such patients often give a good history, and the giveaway line is the comment that the symptoms feel similar to when the patient had the hernia previously.

An interesting element to modern hernia practice is the so-called work-related hernia or hernia following a single strenuous event. The patient is aware of sudden pain in the groin while lifting, pulling, or straining at a task. At the same time, or shortly afterward, a swelling in the region of the groin is evident. There has been a debate as to whether this strenuous event causes the hernia or simply brings a pre-existing asymptomatic hernia to the attention of the patient. Current opinion is more of the latter. The strenuous event precipitates identification of the hernia, which would have become evident in a few months to years time anyway, had the strenuous event not taken place. Several studies have reported on this. In one study [3], 129 patients with 145 hernias presenting with an inguinal hernia pursing a negligence claim, only in 9 (7%) did the patient have a "convincing history suggestive" of an associated strenuous event. However, the time from this event to diagnosis of the hernia was up to 4 years. In another study [4], 133 consecutive patients presenting with a hernia (the majority of which were inguinal) were examined. Fourteen (11%) reported a sudden development of the hernia, but on detailed questioning of these patients, there was no good evidence to point to a single strenuous event as the cause. A further similar study [5] reported 108 patients who alleged that their hernia was the result of an accident, clearly a subset of the hernia patient population. While 51% did have an alleged identifiable strenuous event, of the remaining 49%, no hernia was detectable in 23%; there was no single event in 19%; and the hernia

was documented present before the alleged accident in 6%. Nevertheless, work-related hernia has been and continues to be a source of work-related litigation for compensation. The following guidelines have been suggested when considering such a claim [3]:

1. The incident of muscular strain must be reported officially to the patient's line manager.
2. There must be severe groin pain at the time of the strain.
3. A diagnosis of a hernia must be made by a doctor within 30 days and preferably within 3 days.
4. There should be no previous history of a hernia.

While there is little evidence to support the detail of these guidelines, they remain a useful, pragmatic approach to the problem. The compensation level is minimal, as causation is a problem; the strenuous event did not cause the hernia, but simply speeded up the patient being aware that they were developing a hernia anyway.

Femoral Hernia

A femoral hernia accounts for approximately 5–10% of all groin hernias in adult [6]. In an analysis of 379 patients with groin hernia presenting electively at a university department of surgery, 16 patients had a femoral hernia. The correct diagnosis of femoral hernia was made in only three cases by general practitioners and in only six cases by surgical staff of all grades indicating the difficulty in diagnosis.

Most femoral hernias occur in women over 50 years. The incidence of femoral hernias, male to female, is around 1:4. The different pelvic shape and additional preperitoneal fat in women are postulated to increase their risk compared to men. Women with femoral hernias are usually multiparous—multiple pregnancies are said to predispose to femoral herniation. Indeed, femoral hernias are as common in men as nulliparous women.

Forty percent of femoral hernias present as an emergency with an incarcerated or strangulated hernia sac contents. It is a diagnosis that is often missed, with the patient vomiting for several days, often with plain films of the abdomen supporting small bowel dilatation. The patient or the nursing staff (if the patient is confined) then detects the red, painful groin swelling during bathing duties, which prompt calls for a surgeon. It is believed that femoral hernias are more likely to strangulate because of the relatively small neck to the sac, which also makes them less likely to be reduced in the emergency setting [7]. Ischemic bowel appears to be the major risk factor for death in the emergency setting [8], and thus patients, who are fit for surgery, should have femoral hernias repaired in a timely manner, and a watch and wait policy is not recommended. A study reported 111 patients undergoing femoral hernia repair in the Netherlands [9]. In the elective group, 10% of whom had significant comorbidity, there was no mortality and no bowel resection. Of the 33 patients treated as an emergency of which 20% had significant comorbid disease, there were nine bowel resections and three deaths. The remainder of patients with a femoral hernia, who presented electively, complained of a groin lump and/or groin pain. About half of femoral hernias are irreducible at elective presentation.

The accuracy of diagnosis of femoral hernias in the community varies. In a retrospective review [6], letters of referral were traceable in 88% of elective patients with an operative diagnosis of femoral hernia. The correct diagnosis was arrived at by the referring general practitioner in less than 40% of cases, and the diagnostic rate was only improved by 20% in the hands of the surgical staff.

Differential Diagnoses of Groin Bulges

Hydrocele

The presence of a hydrocele in the adult will most commonly be associated with an inguinal hernia. In general, this does not present a diagnostic dilemma. However, there are situations in which either the hernia or the hydrocele is so large that the diagnosis is difficult to ascertain despite all the physical examination maneuvers that are employed. The use of diagnostic ultrasound will easily determine the diagnosis, as the use of transillumination in this circumstance is not always reliable.

Vascular Disease

Arterial—aneurysms of the iliac and femoral vessels: these may be complicated by distal embolization or vascular insufficiency, which will make the diagnosis more straightforward. A recent history of cardiac catheterization or transluminal angioplasty should raise awareness of a possible aneurysm.

Venous—a saphenovarix can be confused with a femoral hernia. Its anatomical site is the same, but its soft feel, fluid thrill, and disappearance when the patient lies down is characteristic. In a thin patient, the swelling may be a blue color. Varicose veins of the leg also support such a diagnosis, although varicose veins and groin hernias are associated through a common etiology of collagen disease.

Inguinal venous dilation secondary to portosystemic shunting can result in a painful inguinal bulge. Again, there is a dramatic change on lying the patient flat. A Doppler ultrasound will confirm this with ease [10].

Lymphadenopathy

Chronic painless lymphadenopathy may occur in lymphoma and a spectrum of infective diseases. Acute painful lymphadenitis can be confused with a strangulated femoral hernia.

A lesion in the watershed area, the lower abdomen, inguinoscrotal area, perineal region, anal canal, or the ipsilateral lower limb will often suggest this. Ultrasonic examination is very helpful to distinguish this pathology.

Tumors

Lipomas are very common tumors. The common "lipoma of the cord," which in reality is an extension of preperitoneal fat, is frequently associated with an indirect or direct inguinal hernia. A study reported on 140 inguinal hernias in 129 patients [11]. A fatty swelling was deemed significant if it was possible to separate it from the fat accompanying the testicular vessels. The fatty swelling was designated as being a lipoma if there was no connection with extraperitoneal fat and was designated as being a preperitoneal protrusion if it was continuous through the deep ring with extraperitoneal fat. Protrusions of extraperitoneal fat were found in 33% of patients and occurred in association with all varieties of hernia. There was a true lipoma of the cord in only one patient. It was concluded that the mechanisms causing the hernia were also responsible for causing protrusion of extraperitoneal fat. Read has commented that occasionally extraperitoneal protrusions of fat may be the only herniation, and therefore inguinal hernia classifications need to include not only fatty hernias but sac-less, fatty protrusions [12]. Indeed, in the laparoscopic approach, it is our impression that a lipoma of the cord may be more common than suggested above. Lipomas can also occur in the subcutaneous fat of the groin and upper thigh. A lipoma is rarely tender; it is soft with lobulated or scalloped edges, is not fixed to the skin, and does not have a cough impulse.

Secondary Tumors

A lymph node enlarged with metastatic tumor usually lies in a more superficial layer than a femoral hernia. Such lymph nodes are more mobile in every direction than a femoral hernia and are often multiple. A metastatic deposit of a tumor arising from the abdominal cavity such as adenocarcinoma can present as a rock-hard immobile mass that can be confused as either a primary incarcerated inguinal hernia or a postoperative fibrotic reaction following inguinal hernia repair.

Genital Anomalies

Ectopic testis in the male—there is no testicle in the scrotum on the same side. Torsion of an ectopic testicle can be confused with a strangulated hernia.

Cyst of the canal of Nuck—these cysts extend toward or into the labia majora. They can be transilluminable.

Obturator Hernia

An obturator hernia, especially in the female, lies in the thigh lateral to the adductor longus muscle. Vaginal examination may sometimes help with the diagnosis. This hernia is nearly always detected as an emergency, with the patient presenting with bowel obstruction with a Richter's-type hernia.

Rarities

A cystic hygroma is a rare swelling; it is loculated and very soft. Usually the fluid can be pressed from one part of it to another.

A psoas abscess is a soft swelling frequently associated with backache. It loses its tension if the patient is laid flat. It is classically lateral to the femoral artery. This will frequently be associated with elevation of the white blood cell count and a fever.

A hydrocele of the femoral canal is a rarity reported from West Africa. In reality it is the end stage of an untreated strangulated femoral epiplocele. The strangulated portion of omentum is slowly reabsorbed, the neck of the femoral sac remains occluded by viable omentum, while the distal sac becomes progressively more and more distended by a protein-rich transudate.

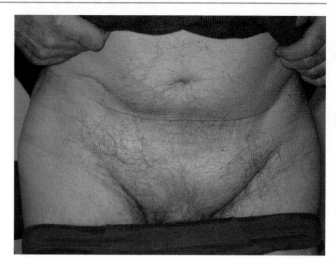

Fig. 13.1 Asymmetrical left groin swelling suggestive of a hernia on that side

Clinical Examination of a Swelling in the Groin

Traditional surgical teaching is that the patients should be undressed and the entire abdomen and lower limbs examined. When the diagnosis of a hernia is suspected from the history, and examination reveals an obvious hernia, then this pursuit of excellence is not necessary and the patient is not expecting such exposure. However, if a hernia is not evident, then such exposure to allow adequate examination is necessary.

In the male, the first step is to observe where the testicles are. Knowledge of testicle position prevents all the confusions of undescended testicles, etc. If there is a significant scrotal swelling, the key question to differentiate between an inguinoscrotal hernia and a scrotal swelling is "can I get above the swelling and palpate a relatively normal cord," which excludes an inguinoscrotal hernia. A lack of a cough impulse is additional support that the scrotal swelling is not a hernia. If the swelling is confined to the scrotum, the next key question is whether a testicle is palpable and if not, a hydrocele is present. If a testicle is palpable, the next question is "is it normal?" If the testicle is diffusely enlarged and painful, then think infection, either bacterial or viral. If eccentrically enlarged, then a tumor is likely. If the swelling is separate from the testicle, but appears to be applied to one side of the testicle, then an epididymocele is likely. If the swelling is separate from the testicle but along the cord, then a spermatocele is likely.

The groin should be examined with the patient standing erect and again with the patient lying flat. Hernias are sometimes only apparent when the patient is standing or when they strain or cough. The majority of moderate and large

hernias, especially in the nonobese, are evident on inspection of the groin in a standing patient with asymmetry evident between the two sides of the groin (Fig. 13.1). This swelling is then gently palpated, the patient asked to cough, and a cough impulse will confirm the presence of a hernia. Sometimes the swelling will visibly increase in size, again consistent with a hernia. In small groin hernias, or in the obese, visual inspection may not show a hernia so obviously. In this case, palpate the groin in both the anatomical positions of an inguinal or femoral hernia, and also over the area where the patient feels pain.

If a cough impulse is not obvious, lie the patient down. Again palpate the groin before and during a cough. As the hernia is likely to have reduced by lying down, the cough impulse is often more prominent when lying down, and indeed the cough thrill of hernial sac contents passing under the examination fingers may be palpated.

As already discussed, the need to differentiate direct from indirect inguinal hernias, and to a lesser degree, inguinal from femoral hernias is largely a hangover from a far from perfect art from the past. The operative approach to groin hernias allows whichever groin hernia is encountered at surgery to be corrected. This is especially true of the laparoscopic approach to groin hernia repair. The key is to be able to make a diagnosis of a hernia and modify the surgical strategy depending on the hernia type found.

Previous surgery may add to the difficulty of hernia diagnosis. Femoral hernias may present as "recurrences" after repair of an inguinal hernia at open surgery. In these circumstances, they are often indistinguishable from inguinal hernias. The diagnostic difficulty is increased by the fact that as a femoral hernia emerges through the cribriform fascia at the fossa ovalis, the fundus comes forward and then turns upward to lie over and anterior to the inguinal ligament. If the external ring and the cord can be palpated, the diagnosis is more easily made. The difficulty is in the female. If the hernia can be reduced, careful palpation of the hernial aperture should enable the examiner to orientate it relative to the inguinal ligament. If the hernia emerges above the inguinal ligament when the patient coughs, the hernia is inguinal: if below the ligament, it is femoral.

Reducing the hernia and then using one finger to hold it reduced while the patient coughs is a useful test, which will enable the inguinal canal or the femoral ring to be identified, almost with certainty. This test become less reliable the fatter the patient becomes, as accurate location of landmarks becomes more difficult. Invagination of the scrotal skin into the inguinal canal, a time-hallowed test, is uncomfortable for the patient and does not provide useful information, except perhaps in small indirect inguinal hernias.

Remember, once you have thought about a lump or swelling in terms of any changes in the skin overlying the lump; the position, size, shape, and consistency of the lump; any fixation to the skin or deep tissues; disappearance of the lump when contracting the muscles in the area; fluctuation or pulsation of the lump; and in the scrotum, transillumination, the diagnosis of the swelling is usually evident. Further investigations may be necessary, not to confirm the type of lump or swelling, but to investigate the cause of the lump, especially if malignancy is expected, but this is out with the remit of this chapter.

Inguinoscrotal Pain

Inguinoscrotal pain may arise in the groin and radiate to the ipsilateral hemiscrotum, thigh, flank, or hypogastrium. Such pain may be neuralgic in type and accentuated by physical exertion. If the cause is a hernia or preperitoneal fat forcing its way out through the deep inguinal ring, it is postulated that these structures are stretched and pain fibers are stimulated. This is thought to cause a local reflex increase of tone in the internal oblique and transversus muscles coupled with neuralgic pain from stretching of the ilioinguinal nerve. The pain due to increase in tone is intermittent, whereas the neuralgic pain leading to hyperalgesia can be constant. This pain can resolve following hernia repair but sometimes can persist following surgery. It is imperative that this fact be made known to the patient preoperatively.

Numerous other conditions can give rise to acute or chronic pain in the inguinoscrotal and neighboring anatomical regions (Table 13.1). These include gynecological and urological pathology and a variety of musculoskeletal syndromes. An important entity increasingly being characterized is the syndrome of Gilmore's groin or the sportsman's hernia (see below). Thus, patients presenting with pain, as opposed to a painless, reducible swelling in the groin, require

Table 13.1 Differential diagnosis of inguinoscrotal pain

Hernia: Direct or indirect inguinal hernia, femoral hernia, lipoma of the cord
Scrotal conditions: Epididymo-orchitis, prostatitis, urinary tract infection, torsion of the testis
Urological conditions: Tumor or stone disease, urethral extravasation
Gynecological conditions: Pelvic inflammatory disease, uterine or ovarian tumor
Musculoskeletal disorders: Adductor tendinitis, adductor avulsion, gracilis syndrome, pubic instability, osteitis pubis, rectus abdominis tendinopathy, iliopsoas injury
Spinal abnormalities
Hip abnormalities
Enthesopathy

a careful history and examination for urological, gynecological, and musculoskeletal disorders.

In many patients presenting with chronic groin pain, a urological disorder is the initial working diagnosis. Chronic prostatitis or seminal vesiculitis is commonly suspected, and many patients may have been treated with multiple courses of antibiotics.

Groin Disruption in Sportsmen/Athletes

This is an interesting area and is often best dealt within a specialist sports injury clinic, with attendant general and orthopedic surgeons, with full support from physiotherapy. The history is variable. Some athletes, such as runners, will tend to describe an insidious onset resulting in a "groin strain" with a persistent, dull, deep ache in the groin. Athletes involved in contact sports may describe sudden tearing sensations giving rise to continuous aching pain in the inguinoscrotal region. The pain is aggravated by physical exertion and may begin to radiate to the thigh, scrotum, or lower abdomen. The classic history in my experience, which requires no investigation but is cured by surgery, is in footballers (soccer players). The history is of running quickly, stretching to cross the ball, and sudden pain is experienced in the groin. Rarely can they continue playing the game but usually need to be substituted. The pain resolves within a few days of rest but returns as soon as they try to sprint again in training. This sequence of rest, pain resolves, train, pain returns can be repeated several times in the hope that the symptom will resolve. A period of rest often settles most of these so-called groin strains, the symptoms returning as soon as training is resumed. Indeed, I often describe what is going on with these sportsmen as akin to a paper cut in the skin—the skin heals but the cut reopens a few days later with more symptoms. Many of these patients experience exacerbations of pain with coughing or straining pointing to an abnormality of the shutter or sphincter mechanism of the inguinal region.

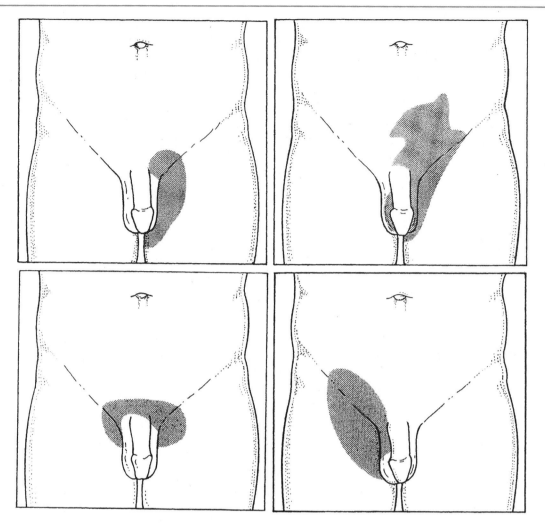

Fig. 13.2 Pain diagrams, each accompanied by the instruction "Please shade the areas where you felt pain prior to your operation"

It is useful to ask patients to shade in pain areas on an anatomical diagram, to identify areas in which the pain occurs and is developing (Fig. 13.2). Sometimes patients will point to an area of spot tenderness with one finger, but a more diffuse area of pain is more typical.

Herniography has been instrumental in identifying the cause of the sportsman's hernia as the syndrome of "broad and deep fossae" [13]. In the UK, Jeremy Gilmore has contributed significantly to the understanding of this problem, and it is still referred to as Gilmore's groin. Gilmore is clear in stating that groin disruption is not a hernia; there is no protrusion of a viscus beyond the normal confines of the abdominal cavity. Groin disruption is a severe musculotendinous injury of the groin. Gilmore described an experience of over 2,000 cases referred [14], 1,400 of which required surgery, 98% were male with the majority football (soccer) players. The severity of the pathology found at operation

varied, but the main features included torn external oblique aponeurosis, torn conjoint tendon, conjoint tendon torn from the pubic tubercle, dehiscence between the conjoint tendon and the inguinal ligament, and no inguinal hernia was evident.

The findings at open operation are said to be characteristic: these include, in addition to the features described by Gilmore, a dilated external ring, absence or attenuation of the transversalis fascia, and a plug of preperitoneal fat at the internal ring. Other explanations are a sheer injury of the common abductor-rectus abdominis anatomical unit [15] and entrapment by the inguinal ligament of the genital branch of the genitofemoral nerve [16]. In acute cases, edema and occasionally evidence of hemorrhage are seen. There is a degree of correlation with the severity of the tear and the patient's symptoms. However, it must be remembered that the detailed anatomy of the inguinal canal is very variable, and an anatomical basis for the sportsman's groin syndrome is elusive.

A period of rest, followed by physiotherapy and rehabilitation, focussing on core stability is indicated for the majority, although in professional football (or other athletes such as hockey) players with the classic description detailed above, early surgery is likely to result in an earlier return to playing. Surgery is indicated in those who fail to respond to conservative treatment. Traditional teaching to a successful operation is said to involve restoration of the normal anatomy by repairing each element. Indeed, Gilmore describes the repair of up to six layers [14]. However, most surgeons would now do this by the insertion of a mesh, either at open or laparoscopic surgery, with similar results [17]. Such surgery results in 9 out of 10 athletes returning to full sporting activity within 3 months, with the symptoms either cured or minimal [18, 19]. A novel technique called the "minimal repair" has recently been described [20].

Clinical Examination of Patients with Groin Pain

Examination will have begun as you observe the patient walking into your office. However, it is useful to ask the patient to walk and observe their gait. Exposure from the abdomen to the toes is necessary while preserving their modesty as best as possible. Palpate the spine. Test for movement of the lumbar spine in forward, backward, and lateral flexion and rotation. Ask the patient to hop on one and then the other foot. Pain elicited over the pubic symphysis while hopping points to instability or osteitis pubis. Perform bilateral femoral nerve stretch tests. Examine the patient standing as described above for a possible hernia in the groin. Then lay the patient flat and perform full active and passive movements of the hip, comparing one side with the other. Sportsmen, especially those with well-developed quadriceps muscles (hockey players) load their hip joint in an abnormal way, and early arthritis can be picked up by subtle reduction in the range of movement on the affected side. Perform bilateral sciatic nerve stretch tests. Palpate carefully the whole of the groin and upper thigh area, although the area of palpation will at times be focussed if the patient reports pain in one spot. Enthesopathy—tennis elbow of the groin (inflammation of the insertion—enthesis—of a ligament or tendon) [21] typically produces point tenderness at the affected site, in particular at the adductor longus insertion, inguinal ligament insertion, rectus abdominis insertion, or along the inguinal ligament at sites where the transversalis and internal oblique muscles insert. Such symptoms may respond to local injection of long-acting local anesthetic and steroid. If no point tenderness is evident, then examine the pectineus muscle, adductor muscles (magnus, brevis, and longus), and gracilis muscle by palpation, passive abduction, and adduction against resistance and hip flexion. The rectus abdominis muscle should be examined by active contraction with both legs elevated and by palpation of its origins. Examine the bony pelvis by palpation of the pubic arches, the crests and tubercles, and the pubic symphysis by compression and direct pressure. Depending on the patient's symptoms, a full neurological examination of the lower limb and affected groin, with particular reference to ilioinguinal or genitofemoral nerve neuralgias, may be appropriate.

In sportsmen's hernia, the clinical findings following a period of rest may be minimal. However, following a period of training or sporting activity, the whole inguinoscrotal region may be tender. While examination is important to rule out other pathology, it is my feeling that the sequence of events in the history are more important in reaching a diagnosis than the examination findings, as there is no single finding or test that easily supports the diagnosis. Palpation of the external ring by invagination of the scrotal skin is an uncomfortable maneuver, but it is typically much more painful on the affected side, which is made worse by coughing, and a more prominent cough impulse may be detected. If the diagnosis is still in doubt, ask the patient to adopt a half sit-up and cough while the margins of the superficial ring and the posterior inguinal wall palpated. An enlarged tender ring and posterior pain as compared to the other side is evidence of inguinal canal disruption [22].

Clinical examination of the scrotum may be necessary if the diagnosis is still not clear or there are symptoms in the scrotum. A small hernia protruding at the deep ring may stimulate the genital branch of the genitofemoral nerve to give scrotal pain in the male or labial pain in the female as its feature. If the patient presents acutely complaining of pain in the groin associated with a lump, the differential examination should look for hernias, torsion of the testicle or testicular appendage, spasm of the cremaster and trauma to the testicle or cord.

Other rare causes of inguinoscrotal pain include abdominal aneurysms, degenerative disease of the lower thoracic and lumbar spines, and degenerative disease of the hip joint. The genital pelvic viscera, prostate, seminal vesicles, and proximal vasa have an autonomic supply from T12 to L2 and from S2 to S4. Referred pain from these organs may radiate via the genital branch of the genitofemoral nerve L1 and posterior scrotal nerves S2 and S3 to the groin and external genitalia.

Investigations in Occult Hernia and Groin Pain

In the majority of cases, a good history and examination is all that is required to establish the likely diagnosis and initiate management. However, there are occasions where help from a radiologist or a laparoscopy may help with the management. The tests will be discussed in turn and then use of such investigations to answer the three questions laid out in the introduction of this chapter summarized.

Herniography

Herniography is still popular with some hernia surgeons, although I have not requested this investigation in 10 years! In those patients referred to me who have had a herniogram demonstrating a symptomatic hernia, I would have been happy to offer hernia surgery on the basis of the history and clinical examination alone. Nevertheless, herniography is used by many surgeons and is a sensitive tool, capable of demonstrating hernias in the groin, especially when clinical examination is negative [23]. One study reported lateral protrusion of the urinary bladder ("bladder ears") into the deep inguinal ring in 9% of 406 patients undergoing intravenous urography and cystograms [24].

Direct herniography was first performed in experimental animals [25] and subsequently performed in children [26]. Herniography with fluoroscopy and peritoneography, performed by puncture of the abdominal wall and injection of nonionic contrast medium, is now the preferred method of investigation [27]. Indications are principally symptoms indicative of a hernia but no palpable lump, obscure groin pain (other diagnoses having been excluded by appropriate investigation), and evaluation of patients who remain symptomatic following primary hernia repair.

Technique is important. The patients must be placed on a tilt table with fluoroscopy, enabling tangential views of the pelvic floor and groin. The bladder should be empty at the time of the examination to avoid inadvertent puncture. A needle puncture is performed using a 22-G spinal needle or occasionally a 21-G Chiba needle at the border of the lateral rectus muscle below the level of the umbilicus on the opposite side to the patient's symptoms. This site of puncture is chosen to minimize the risk of injury to the inferior epigastric vessels. Typically three pops are felt as the needle traverses the anterior rectus sheath, posterior rectus sheath, and transversalis fascia to enter the peritoneal cavity. Correct needle placement within the peritoneal cavity is confirmed by injection of a small volume of nonionic contrast under fluoroscopic guidance, which should freely run away from the needle tip. Approximately 60–80 mL of contrast is then injected with the head of the table elevated 30° to encourage the contrast to pool in the various fossae and hernial orifices. After the contrast has been injected, the patient is turned prone with the head elevated 20°, and PA and oblique views are taken. The patient is then instructed to exercise for 15–20 min, and repeat radiographs are taken with additional views obtained with the patient straining

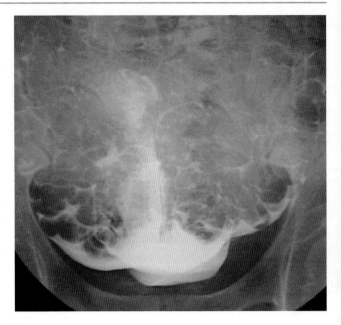

Fig. 13.3 Normal herniogram

and coughing or during any other maneuver, which precipitates the symptoms.

A thorough examination of the entire surgical anatomy of the pelvic and inguinal floor should be performed for exact verification of all potential hernia orifices. Figure 13.3 demonstrates a normal herniogram.

The different types of hernia can be diagnosed from their shape, relation to the pelvic peritoneal folds, and the resulting pelvic fossae. Five pelvic peritoneal folds in the pelvis and groin (lateral umbilical, medial umbilical, and median umbilical) divide the pelvic cavity into five fossae: the supravesical, the left and right medial umbilical, and left and right lateral umbilical fossae. An indirect hernia protrudes lateral to the lateral fold through the lateral (inguinal) fossa. A direct inguinal hernia protrudes lateral to the median fold through the medial (inguinal) fossa whereas a femoral hernia protrudes through the median umbilical fossa in a lateral direction through the femoral canal. Figure 13.4 demonstrates herniograms depicting bilateral indirect hernias in a patient suspected clinically of having a unilateral left-sided hernia.

Herniography can be used in the postoperative evaluation of patients with persistent symptoms in whom clinically detectable hernias are not evident on physical examination. One study [28] performed herniograms in 46 patients with 54 symptomatic sites. Ten recurrent hernias were found, although only two were symptomatic. In addition, 14 hernias were found in the contralateral, asymptomatic groin, and the herniogram was negative in one patient with a clinical hernia. Although herniography can demonstrate a hernia, 22 of the hernias detected in this study had no clinical significance, and the reason for performing the study in the patient with a clinically evident hernia is unclear.

Inguinal and femoral hernias are most easily detected by herniography. Anterior wall defects such as ventral, Spigelian, and obturator hernias are less well demonstrated [29] and are more eloquently demonstrated by CT or MRI.

Complications of herniography occur in around 6% of patients. Fortunately the majority of these are minor, including hematoma of the anterior abdominal wall, adverse reaction to the contrast, and extraperitoneal extravasation of contrast medium. More serious, infrequent complications include bowel perforation, mesenteric hematoma formation, and pelvic peritonitis.

In short, herniography can detect occult hernias and aid in the diagnosis of obscure groin pain, and series of patients

said to benefit from the investigation continue to be reported [30]. It is performed under local anesthesia on an outpatient basis with minimal complications [31]. Visceral perforation is a rare hazard that does not usually require significant intervention [32]. Its use is not widespread, however.

Ultrasonography

Ultrasound examination of the abdominal wall and inguinal region is being used increasingly in the diagnosis of occult hernia and groin pain. This has the advantage of avoiding the use of ionizing radiation, but the quality and accuracy of the study depends on the skill and experience of the sonographer and the body habitus of the patient. The technique is performed using a medium- to high-frequency linear array probe (7–13.5 MHz) depending on the patient's body habitus. The patient is initially examined in the supine position before and during the Valsalva maneuver and with coughing with the transducer placed parallel to the inguinal ligament with the inferior epigastric vessels used as a landmark in an attempt to distinguish between indirect and direct inguinal hernias. Using the same transducer orientation, the femoral canal is then examined to assess for a femoral hernia. Both sides are examined and the procedure should be repeated with the patient in the erect position if the supine examination is negative despite a strong clinical suspicion of an occult hernia.

Although the procedure is operator dependent, in experienced hands, ultrasonography has a reported sensitivity and specificity approaching 100% in determining the nature of groin hernia [33]. When used for the assessment of equivocal groin signs and groin pain, the accuracy of ultrasound is not so good [34]. False interpretation is more likely to occur in cases of femoral hernia. The typical findings and interpretation of a femoral hernia are shown in Fig. 13.5.

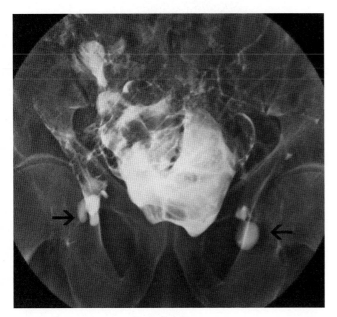

Fig. 13.4 Herniogram demonstrating bilateral indirect inguinal hernias (*arrows*) in a patient suspected clinically of having a unilateral left-sided hernia

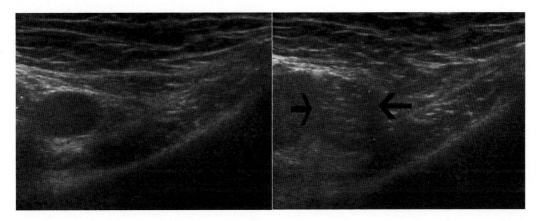

Fig. 13.5 Ultrasound scan demonstrating normal femoral canal at rest (i) with a femoral hernia (outlined by *arrows*) evident during straining (ii)

The antenatal diagnosis of abdominal wall defects is now a successful part of obstetric/pediatric practice. Patients born with significant abdominal wall herniation can be detected prenatally and thus delivered in a unit with the appropriate pediatric surgical expertise.

The use of ultrasound to diagnose hernias in small children is less successful. One study reported ultrasound assessment of the contralateral groin accurately diagnoses a patent processus vaginalis in only 15 of 23 infants, with four false-positive and four false-negative cases [35]. Thus ultrasound alone should be used with caution to plan management of the contralateral groin in infants. An interesting study reported that inguinal hernias could be accurately diagnosed using the parent's digital photographs when the physical examination is not diagnostic [36].

In boys, where there is doubt about the diagnosis, ultrasound is a noninvasive and highly accurate diagnostic tool [37]. Using 4 mm as the upper limit of the normal diameter of the internal ring, occult inguinal hernias can be diagnosed with 98% accuracy.

A small study in 19 patients with clinically diagnosed groin hernias assessed the ability of color Doppler sonography to distinguish between different types of groin hernia in adults [38]. The inferior epigastric artery was used as a landmark to differentiate different types of hernia sac but was only visualized in 55% of cases making this examination an unreliable method for differentiating hernia types.

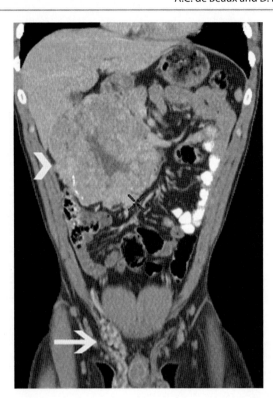

Fig. 13.6 Coronal CT scan demonstrating a right-sided varicocele (*arrow*) as the cause of the patient's right-sided groin discomfort which is secondary to a large retroperitoneal mass pathologically confirmed to represent a neurogenic tumor (*arrowhead*)

Computed Tomography

Cross-sectional imaging by CT scanning can accurately evaluate disorders of the abdominal wall, including hernias. In the elective setting, CT scanning of a lump in the groin is indicated when the lump is not considered on clinical grounds to be a hernia. CT scanning will delineate tumors of the anterior abdominal wall, lymph node masses, and tumors of the abdominal cavity enlarging though hernial orifices. Inflammatory conditions and abscesses within the abdomen and pelvic can also be detected. Sometimes such tumors and other conditions can be the cause of groin pain (Fig. 13.6). Several studies describe the use of CT scanning to differentiate clinically evident hernias of the groin into inguinal or femoral [39, 40] (Fig. 13.7) and between direct and indirect hernias (Fig. 13.8) [41]. The multiplanar high-resolution reconstructions obtained from multidetector CT scans clearly depicts the inferior epigastric vessels to allow differentiation of indirect from direct hernias. The femoral canal can also be directly visualized (using the inguinal ligament, femoral vein, and adductor longus as landmarks), thus allowing the diagnosis of femoral hernias.

To laparoscopic groin surgeons, and I expect to most open groin hernia surgeons also, this is seen as a waste of resource and unnecessary radiation risk to the patient with the usual type of groin hernia.

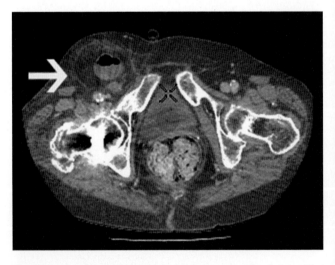

Fig. 13.7 Coronal CT scan demonstrating a strangulated right-sided femoral hernia (*arrow*) containing small bowel lying within the femoral canal presenting as acute small bowel obstruction

The real role of CT scanning is in the assessment of a patient with difficult to diagnosis multiply recurrent herniation or with obstruction of the bowel. Femoral and obturator hernias, with a Richter's-type hernia, can be difficult to detect clinically until infarction and perforation of the bowel has occurred. CT scan eloquently demonstrate these otherwise occult hernias to be the cause of the underlying bowel obstruction (Fig. 13.9). It is also useful to rule out other sources of lower abdominal or groin pathology as the source of pain.

Magnetic Resonance Imaging

MRI of the abdomen and pelvis is also increasing in use for the assessment of groin pain and groin swellings not thought to be a hernia (Fig. 13.10). MRI provides superb soft tissue resolution with multiplanar anatomical depiction and avoids the use of ionizing radiation. It is a useful "screening" tool to detect foci of inflammation that may explain the patient's symptoms, especially in athletes. Osteitic changes particularly in the pubis are detected as areas and low signal intensity

on T1-weighted images of high and homogenous signal intensity on T2-weighted scans [42] (Fig. 13.11). Abnormalities in myotendinous structures are also well documented by this technique as is involvement of the sacroiliac joints [43]. Groin hernias can be detected on MRI, which allows direct visualization of the hernial sac within the inguinal or femoral canal (Fig. 13.12). More rapid sequence times also allow the scan to be performed with a Valsalva technique [44].

Laparoscopy

This investigation has merit as treatment can sometimes be undertaken at the same time. There have always been cases, where the history is suggestive of a hernia (including the

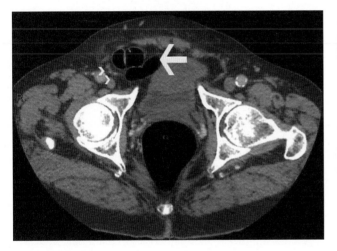

Fig. 13.8 Axial CT scan demonstrating a right-sided direct inguinal hernia (*arrow*), with the neck lying medial to the inferior epigastric vessels (*arrowheads*)

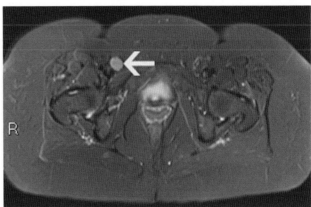

Fig. 13.10 Axial STIR MRI scan demonstrating a right inguinal node in a female patient presenting with a painful right groin mass. Excision biopsy confirmed metastatic squamous cell carcinoma

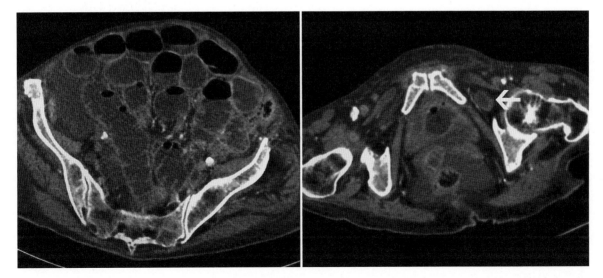

Fig. 13.9 Axial CT scans demonstrating small bowel obstruction (i) secondary to a clinically occult left-sided obturator hernia (ii)

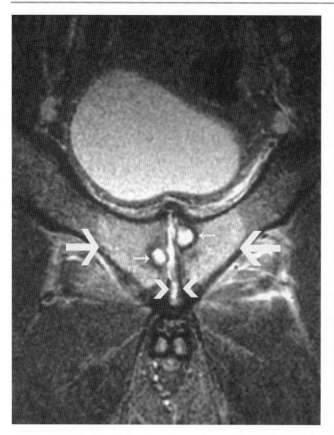

Fig. 13.11 Coronal T2 scan demonstrating osteitis pubis with bone marrow edema in the symphysis pubis (*large arrows*) with associated cystic bone changes (*small arrows*) and high signal change within the fibrocartilaginous disc (*arrowheads*)

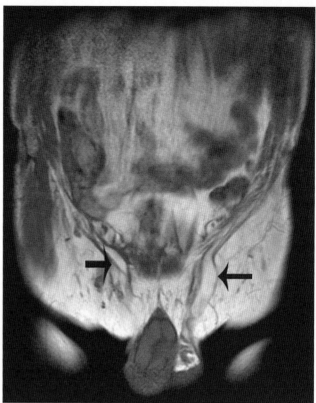

Fig. 13.12 Coronal T1 MRI scan demonstrating bilateral fat containing indirect inguinal hernias

so-called sportsman's hernia), but the clinical findings are equivocal, yet the patient has symptoms that interfere with work or social activities. In such patients, I discuss investigation options, vs. exploring their groin with a laparoscope. While traditional intraperitoneal laparoscopy is within the ability of most general and hernia surgeons, lipomas of the cord, obturator hernias, and small femoral hernias when there is little in the way of hernial sac can be missed by this approach. If a hernia is found by conventional laparoscopy, then the options would be to do a TAPP or convert to a traditional open operation. My preference is to explore the groin with a TEP approach, and I would always mesh the groin following this exploration. I still feel uncomfortable exploring the groin by open surgery, when the diagnosis is not clear, because of the small risk of severe chronic groin pain (in the region of 2–3%), while severe chronic pain following laparoscopic surgery is a very rare event.

Clinical Dilemmas

1. Symptom but no swelling: is there a hernia?

   The investigative options here are to consider an ultrasound scan first, perhaps a herniogram, but my preference

unless significant anesthetic risk or contraindication is to proceed with laparoscopy via a preperitoneal approach, in effect—perform a TEP repair.

2. Swelling, but is it a hernia?

   The investigative options here are to consider an ultrasound scan first, followed by an MRI or CT scan if the ultrasound is equivocal, or further evaluation of deeper aspects of the swelling are necessary.

3. Hernia, but is it causing the symptoms?

   The investigative options here are to consider an MRI scan first. If this is normal or fails to identify an alternate obvious cause for the symptoms, then proceed with laparoscopy (or open exploration) of the groin.

Conclusions

An effort should be made to distinguish inguinal from femoral hernias before surgery to help plan the surgical approach. However, with laparoscopic surgery, this is less important as all the hernial orifices in the groin can be easily exposed during the operation.

Careful identification of the pubic tubercle, the anterior superior iliac spine, and, between them, the inguinal ligament is the prerequisite. Inguinal hernias emerge from the fascia transversalis above this line and femoral hernias below it.

Femoral hernias never pass from the abdomen into the scrotum or labia majora as indirect inguinal hernias do.

The diagnosis of inguinoscrotal pain can be a challenging clinical problem. A diagnosis can often be achieved by taking a detailed history and examination, supported with appropriate radiological investigation.

References

1. Hair A, Paterson C, Wright D, Baxter JN, O'Dwyer PJ. What effect does the duration of an inguinal hernia have on patient symptoms? J Am Coll Surg. 2001;193:125–9.
2. Fitzgibbons RJ, Giobbie-Hunter A, Gibbs JO, et al. Watchful waiting vs repair of inguinal hernia in minimally symptomatic men. JAMA. 2006;295:285–92.
3. Smith GD, Crsoby DL, Lewis PA. Inguinal hernia and a single stressful event. Ann R Coll Surg Engl. 1996;78:367–8.
4. Pathak S, Poston GJ. It is highly unlikely that the development of an abdominal wall hernia can be attributable to a single strenuous event. Ann R Coll Surg Engl. 2006;88:168–71.
5. Schofield PF. Inguinal hernia: medicolegal implications. Ann R Coll Surg Engl. 2000;82:109–10.
6. Hair A, Paterson C, O'Dwyer PJ. Diagnosis of a femoral hernia in the elective setting. J R Coll Surg Edinb. 2001;46:117–8.
7. Harissis HV, Douitsis E, Fatouros M. Incarcerated hernia: to reduce or not to reduce. Hernia. 2009;13:263–6.
8. Derici H, Unalp HR, Bozdaq AD. Factors affecting morbidity and mortality in incarcerated abdominal wall hernia. Hernia. 2007;11:341–6.
9. Kemler MA, Oostvogel HJM. Femoral hernia: is a conservative policy justified? Eur J Surg. 1997;163:187–90.
10. Horn TW, Harris JA, Martindale R, Gadacz T. When a hernia is not a hernia: the evaluation of inguinal hernias in the cirrhotic patient. Am Surg. 2001;67:1093–5.
11. Fawcett AN, Rooney PS. Inguinal canal lipoma. Br J Surg. 1997;84:1169–70.
12. Read RC, White HJ. Lipoma of the spermatic cord, fatty herniation, liposarcoma. Hernia. 2000;4:149–54.
13. Smedberg S, Broome AEA, Gullmo A, Roos H. Herniography in athletes with groin pain. Am J Surg. 1985;149:378–82.
14. Gilmore OJA. Groin disruption in sportsmen. In: Kurzer M, Kark AE, Wantz GE, editors. Surgical management of abdominal wall hernias. London: Martin Dunnitz; 1999. p. 151–7.
15. Syme G, Gibbon W. Groin pain in athletes. Lancet. 1999;353:1444–5.
16. Akita K, Niga S, Yamato Y, Munata T, Sato T. Anatomic basis of chronic pain with special reference to sports hernia. Surg Radiol Anat. 1999;21:1–5.
17. Ingolby JH. Laparoscopic and conventional repair of groin disruption in sportsmen. Br J Surg. 1997;84:213–5.
18. Fon LJ, Spence RAJ. Sportsman's hernia. Br J Surg. 2000;87:545–52.
19. Genitsaris M, Goulimaris I, Sikas N. Laparoscopic repair of groin pain in athletes. Am J Sports Med. 2004;32:1238–42.
20. Muschaweck U, Berger L. Minimal repair technique of sportsmen's groin: an innovative open-suture repair to treat chronic inguinal pain. Hernia. 2010;14:27–33.
21. Ashby EC. Chronic obscure groin pain is commonly caused by enthesopathy: 'tennis elbow' of the groin. Br J Surg. 1994;81:1632–4.
22. Macleod DAD, Gibbon WW. The sportsman's groin. Br J Surg. 1999;86:849–50.
23. Eames NWA, Deans GT, Lawson JT, Irwin ST. Herniography for occult hernia and groin pain. Br J Surg. 1994;81:1529–30.
24. Allen RP, Condon VR. Transitory extraperitoneal hernia of the bladder in infants (bladder ears). Radiology. 1961;77:979–83.
25. Sternhill B, Schwartz S. Effect of hypaque on mouse peritoneum. Radiology. 1960;75:81–4.
26. Ducharme JC, Bertrand R, Chacar R. Is it possible to diagnose inguinal hernia by x-ray? J Can Assoc Radiol. 1967;18:448.
27. Gullmo A. Herniography. World J Surg. 1989;13:560–8.
28. Hamlin JA, Kahn AM. Herniography in symptomatic patients following inguinal hernia repair. West J Med. 1995;162:28–31.
29. Harrison LA, Keesling CA, Martin NL, Lee KR, Wetzel LH. Abdominal wall hernias: review of herniography and correlation with cross-sectional imaging. Radiographics. 1995;15:315–32.
30. Hachem MI, Saunders MP, Rix TE, Anderson HJ. Herniography: a reliable investigation avoiding needless groin exploration—a retrospective study. Hernia. 2009;13:57–60.
31. MacArthur DC, Grieve DC, Thompson JD, Greig JD, Nixon SJ. Herniography for groin pain of uncertain origin. Br J Surg. 1997;84:684–5.
32. Heise CP, Sproat IA, Starling JR. Peritoneography (herniography) for detecting occult inguinal hernia in patients with inguinodynia. Ann Surg. 2002;235:140–4.
33. Djuric-Stefanovic A, Saranovic D, Ivanovic A, et al. The accuracy of ultrasonography in classification of groin hernias according to the criteria of the unified classification system. Hernia. 2008;12:395–400.
34. Depasquale R, Landes C, Doyle G. Audit of ultrasound and decision to operate in groin pain of unknown aetiology with ultrasound technique explained. Clin Radiol. 2009;64:608–14.
35. Lawrenz K, Hollman AS, Carachi R, Cacciagnerra S. Ultrasound assessment of the contralateral groin in infants with unilateral inguinal hernia. Clin Radiol. 1994;49:546–8.
36. Kawaguchi AL, Shaul DB. Inguinal hernias can be accurately diagnosed using the parent's digital photographs when the physical examination is nondiagnostic. J Pediatr Surg. 2009;44:2327–9.
37. Chen KC, Chu CC, Chou TY, Wu CJ. Ultrasound for inguinal hernias in boys. J Pediatr Surg. 1999;34:1890–1.
38. Zhang GQ, Sugiyama M, Hagi H, Urata T, Shimamori N, Atomi Y. Groin hernias in adults; value of colour Doppler sonography in their classification. J Clin Ultrasound. 2001;29:429–34.
39. Cherian PT, Parnell AP. The diagnosis and classification of inguinal and femoral hernia on multisection spiral CT. Clin Radiol. 2008;63:184–92.
40. Kitami M, Takase K, Tsuboi M, et al. Differentiation of femoral and inguinal hernias on the basis of anteroposterior relationship to the inguinal ligament on multidimensional computed tomography. J Comput Assist Tomogr. 2009;33:678–81.
41. Hahn-Pederson J, Lund L, Hansen-Hojhus J, Bojsen-Muller F. Evaluation of direct and indirect inguinal hernia by computed tomography. Br J Surg. 1994;81:569–72.
42. Omar IM, Zoga AC, Kavanagh EC, et al. Athletic pubalgia and "sports hernia": optimal MR imaging technique and findings. Radiographics. 2008;28:1415–38.
43. Barile A, Erriquez D, Cacchio A, DePaulis F, Di Cesare E, Masciocchi C. Groin pain in athletes: role of magnetic resonance. Radiol Med. 2000;100:216–22.
44. Leander P, Ekberg O, Sjoberg S, Kesek P. MR imaging following herniography in patients with unclear groin pain. Eur Radiol. 2000;10:1691–6.

Anterior Open Repair of Inguinal Hernia in Adults

Joachim Conze

The last edition of this chapter started out with the question "operation or truss?" The retention and compression of reducible hernias by truss or corsage is at least 4,000 years and to this day remains quite widespread. Notwithstanding their long history, trusses remain an unsafe therapy; they are cumbersome and without any chance of healing. The number of prescriptions for trusses remains amazingly high considering advances in surgery and anesthesia in the last century. There is neither an explanation nor justification for a truss, the threat of a surgical solution blown out of all proportions.

Open repair of a groin hernia does not involve major exploration of a body cavity, manipulation of viscera or hemodynamic hazard. There are no metabolic complications either. Sepsis is rare after groin hernia repair. Wearing a truss does not guarantee that an indirect inguinal or femoral hernia will remain reduced. A truss increases the patient's chance of developing complications; it may obstruct the venous and lymphatic drainage of intra-hernial viscera and precipitate strangulation. In addition, particularly with the large direct hernia, the pressure of the truss leads to atrophy of the muscular and fascial margins of the defect, enlarging the hernial orifice, promoting enlargement of the hernia, and making surgical repair even more difficult.

Sir Geoffrey Keynes, in 1927, commented on the complications of a truss [1]:

> The tissues underlying such a truss will be found to be matted, thinned out and the muscles almost entirely converted to fibrous tissue. It is impossible to look upon the truss as anything but an antiquated piece of apparatus, the very existence of which is a sorry testimonial to progressive surgery, the use of which generally results in gradual injury to the wearer, and the results of which tax the surgeon's best efforts to undo when the time comes that the truss is no longer able to hold up the protrusion.

There is no need for truss treatment, but does every inguinal hernia require surgery? The incidence and prevalence of inguinal hernia are not precisely known [2]. Primatesta and Goldacre reported the cumulative lifetime risk of inguinal hernia repair: at currently prevailing rates they estimated the chance of a person needing to undergo inguinal hernia repair during life at 27% for men and 3% for women [3]. The main reason and motivation for elective inguinal hernia repair has always been the fear and danger of acute incarceration. The Danish and Swedish hernia registers give clear evidence that emergency operation for a strangulated hernia is associated with a mortality rate >5% vs. <0.5% for elective hernia surgery [3–5]. But how often does incarceration occur? There are no accurate data available on the annual rate of hernia incarceration, but it is estimated to be 0.3–3%. The rate of incarceration for indirect inguinal hernias is at least ten times greater compared with direct inguinal hernias. Also the length of history seems to be of importance. In a retrospective study Gallegos et al. studied the cumulative probability of strangulation in relation to the length of history calculated independently for inguinal and femoral hernias at the Middlesex Hospital over a three-year period [6] (439 inguinal, 37 femoral); there were 34 strangulations (22 inguinal, 12 femoral). After three months the cumulative probability of strangulation for inguinal hernias was 2.8%, rising to 4.5% after 2 years. For femoral hernias the cumulative probability for strangulation was 22% at 3 months and 45% at 21 months. They concluded that the rate at which the cumulative probability of strangulation increased was in both cases greatest in the first 3 months. Similar results were reported by Rai et al. that proved a short duration of hernia to be a risk factor predicting complications in an adult with groin hernia [7].

What do we know about the natural course of untreated inguinal hernia? Two level 1B randomized controlled trials have been published, comparing operation versus "watchful waiting." In a trial coordinated by Fitzgibbons, 356 men (over 18 years of age) were assigned to operation and 366 men were assigned to watchful waiting (WW). After 2 years

J. Conze (✉)
Department of General and Visceral and Transplantation Surgery,
University Hospital RWTH Aachen, Aachen, Germany
e-mail: jconze@ukaachen.de

A.N. Kingsnorth and K.A. LeBlanc (eds.), *Management of Abdominal Hernias*,
DOI 10.1007/978-1-84882-877-3_14, © Springer Science+Business Media London 2013

of follow-up there was a 23% crossover from WW to operation, one acute incarceration without strangulation within 2 years and one incarceration with bowel obstruction within 4 years [8].

In a trial coordinated by O'Dwyer, 80 men (over 55 years of age) were randomized to operation and 80 to WW; 23/80 (29%) patients crossed over from observation to operation, and three serious hernia-related adverse events occurred in the WW group after 1 year of follow-up. One crossover patient had a postoperative myocardial infarction and died, one patient had a postoperative stroke, and one patient had an acute hernia. Both patients that had a serious postoperative event had comorbid cardiovascular disease which had deteriorated significantly in the period under observation. Had they been operated on at presentation, such an event may have been avoided [9].

The results of both trials are not conclusive and differ slightly; however, watchful waiting is an acceptable option for men with asymptomatic or minimally symptomatic inguinal hernias. Incarcerations occur rarely. In one trial, it was concluded that (elderly) men with significant comorbidity could benefit from an operation electively in order to reduce the risks of increase in this morbidity and a higher (operative) mortality when operated in an emergency setting.

To estimate the risk of incarceration versus the option for "watchful waiting" Gai reported a study investigating the morphology of the hernial sac by ultrasound. He differentiated three different sono-morphological hernia types: if the hernial orifice and hernial sac appear like a bulge, it's a type A hernia; if the hernial orifice and hernial sac appear like a tube, it is a type B hernia; and if it appears like a sandclock, it is a type C hernia. According to his results the highest risk for incarceration is a type C hernia. Gai used this tool to decide on "watchful waiting" versus elective surgery in asymptomatic hernias [10].

Classification of Inguinal Hernia

[AU1]

Are all hernias the same? Is there a "standard" hernia? Surgeons know that a small lateral hernia is easier to repair with excellent long-lasting results than a large medial hernia. It does make a difference though the majority of publications do not take this into account. Accordingly, a classification of inguinal hernias is required, to facilitate a comparison of the results and to make an evaluation of the different surgical techniques possible. Only by classification and long follow-up investigations will it be possible to find the best therapy for each type of hernia. We are still faced with many uncertainties regarding the optimal treatment of groin hernias and the requirement to develop operative strategies that are generalizable and applicable to every case. In order to achieve this, the requirements in each scenario should be defined.

There have been many attempts to classify hernias, but so far none of the enlisted classifications has reached worldwide acceptance and propagation.

Gilbert Classification

In 1988 Gilbert introduced a classification for inguinal hernia [11]. He proposed a system based on anatomic and functional defects described at operation. He classified inguinal hernias into five classes: types 1, 2, and 3 are indirect and types 4 and 5 direct. Type 1 has a tight internal ring through which passes a peritoneal sac of any size. When this sac is surgically reduced, it will be held within the abdominal cavity by the intact internal ring. Type 2 has a moderately enlarged internal ring which measures no greater than 4 cm. Type 3 has a patulous internal ring, greater than 4 cm, with the sac frequently having a sliding or scrotal component which usually impinges on the direct space. In type 4 hernias occupy the entire posterior wall (floor) of the inguinal canal which is defective. Type 5 consists of a direct diverticular defect in a suprapubic position. His classification was modified by Rutkow and Robbins in 1993 [12]. They added a sixth type to encompass those groin hernias which consist of both indirect and direct components and a seventh for femoral hernias. As in any classification system, there can be numerous variations and combinations which are difficult to account for, and these variables (i.e., primary/recurrent, sliding component, reducible/incarcerated, lipoma) must be noted.

Nyhus Classification

In 1991 Nyhus introduced a further classification [13]. He defined the status of the fascia transversalis in the posterior wall of the inguinal and femoral canal. He recommended minimalist repair of the medial side of the inguinal ring only when this was necessary, and he warned against extensive posterior wall repair at the expense of disrupting a normal inguinal posterior wall. He railed against surgery that resulted in overtreatment of many comparatively simple hernias. Nyhus classified groin hernias into four types, which enabled individualization of surgery to be recommended.

Type I

Type I hernias are indirect inguinal hernias in which the internal abdominal ring is of normal size, configuration, and structure. They usually occur in infants, children, or young adults. The boundaries are well delineated and Hesselbach's triangle is normal. An indirect hernial sac extends variably from just distal to the internal abdominal ring to the middle of the inguinal canal.

Type II

Type II hernias are indirect inguinal hernias in which the internal ring is enlarged and distorted without impinging on the posterior wall (floor in American surgical anatomy) of the inguinal canal. Hesselbach's triangle (the posterior wall of the canal) is normal when palpated through the opened peritoneal sac. The hernial sac is not in the scrotum, but it may occupy the entire inguinal canal.

Type III

Type III hernias are of three subtypes: direct, indirect, and femoral.

1. *Type IIIA* hernias are direct inguinal hernias in which the protrusion does not herniate through the internal abdominal (inguinal) ring. The weakened transversalis fascia (posterior inguinal wall medial to the inferior epigastric vessels) bulges outward in front of the hernial mass. All direct hernias, small or large, are type IIIA.
2. *Type IIIB* hernias are indirect inguinal hernias with a large dilated ring that has expanded medially and encroaches on the posterior inguinal wall (floor) to a greater or lesser degree. The hernial sac frequently is in the scrotum. Occasionally the cecum on the right or the sigmoid colon on the left makes up a portion of the wall of the sac. These sliding hernias always destroy a portion of the posterior wall of the inguinal canal. (The internal abdominal ring may be dilated without displacement of the inferior epigastric vessels. Direct and indirect components of the hernial sac may straddle those vessels to form a pantaloon hernia.)
3. *Type IIIC* hernias are femoral hernias, a specialized form of posterior wall defect.

Type IV

Type IV hernias are recurrent hernias. They can be direct (type IVA), indirect (type IVB), femoral (type IVC), or a combination of these types (type IVD). They cause intricate management problems and carry a higher morbidity than do other hernias.

Zollinger Classification

This system builds upon the traditional indirect, direct, and femoral anatomic locations using a defect sizing and more importantly the competence of the internal ring and integrity of the direct floor as emphasized by Nyhus. Zollinger derived his classification from a survey of 50 North American and 25 European expert hernia surgeons which revealed that four systems were in active use, by these experts: traditional (indirect, direct, and femoral) Nyhus, Gilbert, and in addition the Aachen system (see later) [14]. In the Zollinger system, the following are recognized: (1) Small indirect hernias (Type I) have an intact internal ring, while small direct ones

Table 14.1 EHS groin classification [15]

EHS groin classification			Primary	Recurrent		
	0	1		2	3	x
L						
M						
F						

(Type III) have an intact rim of functioning direct floor. Large indirect hernias (Type II) have loss of internal ring function, while large direct ones (Type IV) have lost the integrity of the entire direct floor. Although the designations small and large correlate with abdominal wall defect sizes, the preservation or loss of function, rather than a precise defect measurement in cm, is the dominant factor in this classification. (2) A combined inguinal hernia (Type V) is defined as one with loss of internal ring competence (Type VA), direct floor integrity (Type VC), or both (Type VB). (3) In addition to femoral hernia (Type VI), an additional category of inguinal–femoral hernia "other" (Type O) is included for those not defined with a category number such as the femoral plus inguinal combinations, the very rare prevascular, and the special circumstances such as massive inguinal hernias.

The EHS Classification

The latest attempt for a practical and user-friendly classification was introduced in 2006 by the European Hernia Society [15]. On the basis of the Aachen classification by Schumpelick, they agreed on the following parameters: anatomical location (indirect = lateral = L/direct = medial = M/femoral = F) and hernial orifice size, graded in three groups (I ≤ 1.5 cm, II = 1.5-3 cm, III ≥ 3 cm) (Table 14.1: EHS classification). According to the Aachen classification, the grading size of 1.5 cm was chosen because that is the average diameter of a surgeon's index fingertip or the length of the branches of laparoscopic scissors, simplifying the practical measurement. Today this classification has become the standard in Europe.

A classification must remain simple and easy to perform. But its use is absolutely mandatory. Only by classification will it be possible to objectively assess the surgical results of all the different procedures.

One Fits All or Tailored Repair?

The existing surgical literature, reinforced by guidelines, dictates that inguinal hernia repair always needs mesh reinforcement. But is this absolute requirement really necessary, irrespective of age, gender, family history, and other possible risk factors?

The results of the Shouldice repair that were performed in 1992 at the Aachen University Hospital were followed up

Table 14.2 Risk factors for inguinal hernia in adult male [16]

Risk factor		Odds ratio	p
Type	Recurrent vs. primary hernia	3.4	0.01
Localization	Medial/combined vs. lateral	1.7	0.27
Hernial orifice size	>3 cm vs. <3 cm	1.5	0.46
Age	>50 years vs. <50 years	9.9	0.01
Gender	Male vs. female	1.8	0.56
Family	Affected vs. not affected	3.9	0.05
Smoking	Smoker vs. nonsmoker	4.0	0.01

over a decade. In 2002 the follow-up with clinical and ultrasound investigations revealed a recurrence rate of 11.2% in 290 procedures. The patients with a recurrence were further investigated for morphological and systematic risk factors. Age above 50 years, smoking and type of hernia had a significant impact on development of recurrence. The results are summarized in Table 14.2.

Also family history proved to be a significant risk factor [16]. This has been confirmed by Lau et al., who investigated the family history of 1,414 male patients with inguinal hernia. Those patients with a positive family history had an eight-times elevated risk for inguinal hernia [17].

As long ago as 1967, McVay and Read presumed some unrecognized connective tissue disorder was involved in the development of inguinal hernia [18]. They continued their research and reported on a large series of veterans with inguinal herniation appearing with a preponderance of bilateral and direct defects. Biochemical investigations revealed a striking loss of collagen and poorly proliferating fibroblasts with decreased collagen synthesis. The collagen fibrils were more cystic with varying diameter and diminished polymerization, differing from the normal structure of collagen. Even more interesting were the findings of similar collagen changes in the skin and pericardium, suggesting a systemic disease of the collagen metabolism [19].

Three decades later it was Klinge et al. who investigated the collagen metabolism of hernia patients in comparison to non-hernia patients, finding a significant increase of collagen Type III in the hernia patients, stating "herniosis" as a systematic disease [20–23]:

> The decision concerning which technique to use should not be driven by the surgeons favorite, standard procedure but should take into account the patient's systemic condition and type of hernia. Therefore a surgeon who operates on inguinal hernias should have several techniques in his surgical arsenal, "tailoring" the surgical procedure to each patient, taking into account the patients personal risk profile and individual hernia anatomy.

Historical Development: Milestones in Open Inguinal Repair

The surgical literature abounds with descriptions of operations for open inguinal hernia (Table 14.3). However, few of

Table 14.3 Techniques for inguinal hernia repair

Single-layered closure
Halsted (1889) [104]
Madden (1971) [105]

Multilayered closure
Bassini–Halsted principle
Bassini (1887) [25]
Ferguson (1899) [106]
Andrews (1895) [107]
Halsted II (1903) [108]
Fallis (1938) [109]
Zimmerman (1938, 1952) [110]
Reinhoff (1940) [111]
Tanner (1942) [112]

Shouldice repair
Glassow (1943) [113]
Griffith (1958) [114]
Lichtenstein (1964, 1966) [115]
Palumbo (1967) [116]

Cooper's ligament repair
Lotheissen–McVay principle
Narath (cited by Lotheissen, 1898) [117]
Lotheissen (1898) [117]
McVay (1942, 1958) [118]

Preperitoneal approach
Cheatle (1920) [119]
Henry (1936) [120]
Musgrove and McReady (1940) [121]
Mikkelson and Berne (1954) [122]
Stoppa (1972) [123]
Condon (1960) [124]
Nyhus (1959) [125]
Read (1976) [126]
Rignault (1986) [127]
Paillier (1992) [128]

Primary repair with prosthetic materials
Koontz (1956) [129]
Usher (1960) [130]
Lichtenstein (1972) [115]
Trabucco (1989) [131]
Valenti (1992) [132]
Corcione (1992) [133]

Plug repair
Lichtenstein (1970) [115]
Bendavid (1989) [134]
Gilbert (1992) [135]
Robbins and Rutkow (1993) [65]
Gilbert (1998) [136]

Laparoscopic repair
Ger (1990) [137]
Corbitt (1991) [138]
Ferzli (1992) [113]

these essays describe new or original principles. The foundations underlying the modern approach to inguinal hernia were laid by Marcy, who observed the anatomy and physiology of the deep inguinal ring and correctly inferred the importance of the obliquity of the canal [24]. Bassini, who had heard Marcy's lecture in 1881, grasped the significance of the anatomic arrangement and, in particular, the role of the fascia transversalis and transversus abdominis tendon [25].

Many surgeons have contributed to the recognition of the essential role of the transversalis fascia in the pathology of groin hernia, resulting from degeneration and change in structure and function [26, 27].

Bassini stressed the importance of dividing the fascia transversalis and reconstructing the posterior wall of the canal by suturing the fascia transversalis and transversus muscle to the upturned, deep edge of the inguinal ligament. In his repair, Bassini included the lower arching fibers of the internal oblique muscle where they form the conjoint tendon with the transversus muscle. He called the upper leaf of his repair the "triple layer," that is, fascia transversalis, transversus abdominis, and internal oblique.

Bassini's original observations about the fascia transversalis and "triple layer" have somehow been lost from the later literature. Many of the failures of "Bassini's operation" occur in cases where the fleshy conjoint tendon only has been sutured to the inguinal ligament.

Division of the cremaster muscle and the posterior wall of the inguinal canal are essential components of the original Bassini hernia operation. Many surgeons, however, still perform the Bassini operation, dividing neither the cremaster muscle nor the posterior wall of the inguinal canal, possibly because Bassini did not actually describe these steps in his original papers. Attilio Catterina, a colleague of Bassini's, later described and depicted the operation in a book illustrated with numerous watercolors. This atlas, although it was published in many languages in the early 1930s in Europe, was never published in North America, nor disseminated widely to European surgeons, possibly accounting for the inaccurate dissemination of Bassini's technique.

Wantz has accurately traced the history of the relationship between Bassini and Catterina, which resulted in the enthusiastic promulgation of Bassini's technique through his atlas, illustrated by the surgeon artist O. Gaigher and numerous lectures across the European continent. Catterina, a protégé and colleague, and latterly Professor of Surgery at Genoa, recognized the importance of Bassini's quantum leap in surgical technique and the fact that Bassini had failed to get the technical points across to his surgical audience. Figure 14.1 indicates specifically that Bassini described dividing the cremaster muscle and the posterior wall of the inguinal canal.

The Bassini operation without these two essential steps gives poor results; hence in America this corrupt Bassini operation was abandoned in favor of the McVay–Cooper's ligament repair, Marcy's simple ring closure, or Nyhus preperitoneal approach. Bassini was also the first surgeon to insist on the use of nonabsorbable suture material to repair his triple layer.

The third person in seminal herniology is Halsted. Halsted's original input was to advise drawing the external oblique

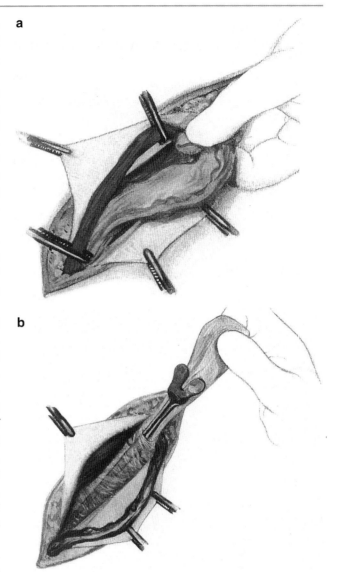

Fig. 14.1 (**a**) Bassini completely isolated and excised the cremaster muscle and its fascia from the cord. He thus ensured complete exposure of the deep ring and all the posterior wall of the inguinal canal, an essential prerequisite to evaluate all the potential hernial sites. (**b**) Bassini stressed the complete exposure and incision of the fascia transversalis of the posterior wall of the inguinal canal. To complete the repair, he sutured the divided fascia transversalis, together with the transversus muscle, and the internal oblique muscle, "the threefold layer," to the upturned inner free margin of the inguinal ligament (from Catterina, The Bassini Procedure, published by H.K. Lewis, 1934)

down behind the cord in order to strengthen the repair. He later abandoned this. His major contribution is really twofold: he insisted on scrupulous atraumatic technique and he emphasized, as Bassini had, the importance of adequate follow-up. In a more general sense, Bassini and Halsted are epoch individuals because they introduced quality control and audit to surgeons. Florence Nightingale's exhortation that "to understand God's will we must study statistics" was translated into surgical science by Bassini and Halsted.

Principles of Open Inguinal Hernia Repair

All surgical procedures in open anterior hernia repair can be divided into two steps: separation and dissection of the hernial sac from adjacent structures, including the cord, followed by repositioning of the contents of the sac into the preperitoneal space or peritoneal cavity. Once this has been achieved, the second step is reconstruction of the inguinal floor by suture or augmentation by prosthetic mesh.

Step I: The Preparation

– Skin incision
– Dissection of the inguinal canal
– Management of the hernial sac

The Skin Incision

The skin incision is performed one finger above and lateral to the pubic tubercle, usually transverse along the skin crease lines with a length of approximately 5 cm. This access provides better cosmetic outcome and facilitates sufficient overview (Fig. 14.2). It is important to keep the knife at right angles to the patient's skin during the incision in order to avoid undercutting the flap in one or the other direction. After skin incision a stepwise sharp dissection of the subcutaneous fatty tissue is performed. Usually the Vasa epigastrica superficialis are encountered and need appropriate ligation. The aponeurotic layer of the m. oblique externus emerges and facilitates medially the exposure of the superficial inguinal ring. This superficial inguinal ring is the first landmark of every open anterior repair (Fig. 14.3). Alternatively, an oblique incision that runs parallel to the inguinal ligament can be chosen. It provides excellent exposure but at the expense of a slightly inferior cosmetic result.

The Dissection of the Canal

The external oblique aponeurosis is opened in the long axis of the inguinal canal. This incision extends down to the external inguinal ring, the margin of which is divided. With the ring opened, the upper medial flap of the external oblique is grasped and lifted up off the underlying cremaster fascia. The incision in the external oblique should commence at the most superior point of the superficial ring along the fiber lines. The optimum site is to divide the external oblique about 2–3 cm cranial to the inguinal ligament; this "high" incision allows maximal tissue for final closure and reconstitution of the inguinal canal (Fig. 14.4). The aponeurosis is gently freed from underlying structures by careful dissection up to its fusion into the lateral anterior rectus sheath. Similarly, the lower lateral leaf of the external oblique is mobilized and freed of the underlying cord coverings down

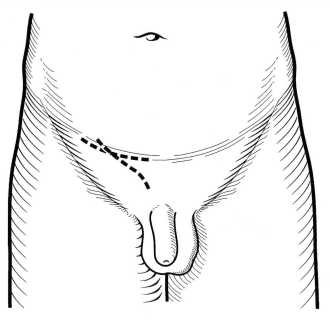

Fig. 14.2 An incision is made 1 cm above and parallel to the inguinal ligament; the incision should expose the superficial inguinal ring. Incision and dissection medial to the pubic tubercle is unnecessary and harmful

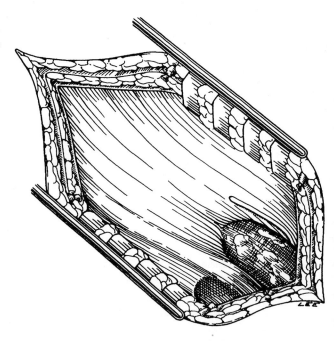

Fig. 14.3 The external oblique aponeurosis exposed

to the upturned deep edge of the inguinal ligament, which is exposed (Fig. 14.5). Thus the whole of the cord is exposed.

Identification of the Fascia Transversalis

After the contents of the cord have been adequately visualized, they are lifted up and the continuation of the fascia transversalis onto the cord at the deep ring is identified. The condensation of the fascia transversalis about the emerging

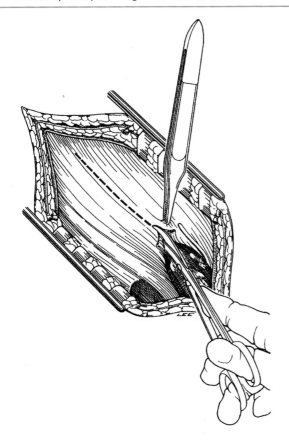

Fig. 14.4 Opening the inguinal canal

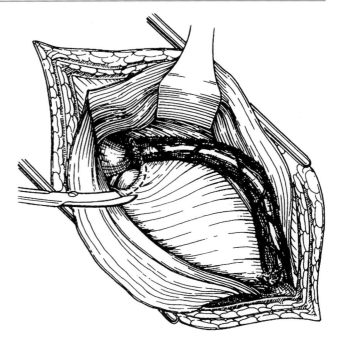

Fig. 14.6 The deep ring is freed from the cord by sharp dissection

cord is the deep ring, and it must be dissected accurately. The correct identification and dissection of the deep ring is crucial to the subsequent repair operation.

The internal spermatic fascia must be dissected off the deep ring all around the cord. Only when the cord is fully dissected like this can the deep ring be assessed.

The medial superior margin of the cord needs careful inspection now to identify any indirect sac. However small—even a tiny crescent of peritoneum entering the cord between the vas and medial margin of the deep ring—such a sac must be dissected cleanly and removed; otherwise, it will enlarge postoperatively and appear later as a fully developed indirect hernia. A peritoneal crescent is the herald of an early recurrence if it is not treated adequately (Fig. 14.6).

It is important to check all the hernial sites at operation. A femoral or a direct inguinal hernia may easily be overlooked if exposure is inadequate. If a hernia is missed, it will either appear postoperatively or later as "a recurrence." Whether the recurrent hernia is through a repaired portion of the inguinal region or not is immaterial to the patient; it is "a recurrence" from the patient's perspective and most importantly necessitates another operation. Careful inspection of all hernial areas must be carried out at each operation.

The Management of the Hernial Sac

The degree of difficulty in locating the hernial sac depends on several factors such as the soft tissues in the canal, the location of the hernia orifice, and the size of the hernial sac.

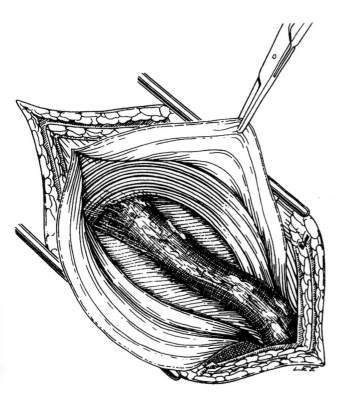

Fig. 14.5 Dissection of the canal

Also the possibility of a combined hernia should always be considered.

Indirect

An indirect hernial sac lies on the anterosuperior aspect of the cord structures and is usually easier to find. In the case of scrotal herniation, with a fixed hernial sac in the scrotum, a transection of the hernial sac at the midpoint of the canal leaving the distal part in situ is recommended to minimize the risk of postoperative ischemic orchitis. The anterior wall of the distal sac can be incised to prevent postoperative hydrocele formation. Further management depends on the presence and nature of the contents of the indirect hernial sac.

No Contents

If the sac is empty and does not extend beyond the pubic tubercle, it is lifted and freed from the adjacent structures by careful dissection. It is traced back to its junction with the parietal peritoneum, transfixed with an absorbable suture, which is tied around it securely, and the redundant sac excised (Fig. 14.7). If an indirect hernial sac extends beyond the pubic tubercle, the sac is transected and the distal sac left in situ (Fig. 14.8).

Small Bowel and/or Omentum, With or Without Adhesions

Unless the hernia is strangulated and the small bowel nonviable, any adhesions are divided and the small bowel is returned to the abdominal cavity. Strangulated omentum or small bowel can be resected at this stage. The diagnostic decision as to what should be done about very adherent and frequently partially ischemic omentum is difficult. If there is any doubt about omentum, it is best excised because to return omentum of doubtful viability to the peritoneal cavity invites the formation of adhesions.

Sliding Hernia

Such a hernia may contain the cecum and appendix (on the right side) in its wall, the sigmoid colon (on the left side), or the bladder (in the medial wall on either side). The following guidelines apply in these circumstances:

1. No attempt should be made to separate cecum or sigmoid colon from the sac wall. This may compromise their blood supply and lead to further unnecessary problems.
2. The appendix must not be removed, as this could introduce sepsis.
3. Appendices epiploicae must never be removed from the sigmoid colon—they may harbor small colonic diverticula, excision of which will precipitate sepsis.
4. On the medial side of a sac there should be no attempt to dissect the bladder clear. If the bladder is inadvertently

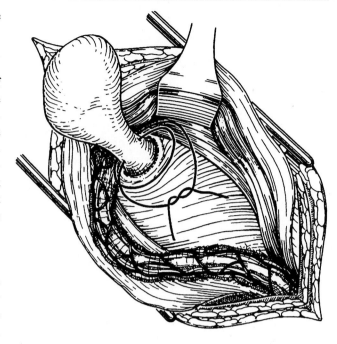

Fig. 14.7 A simple sac is ligated flush to the parietal peritoneum

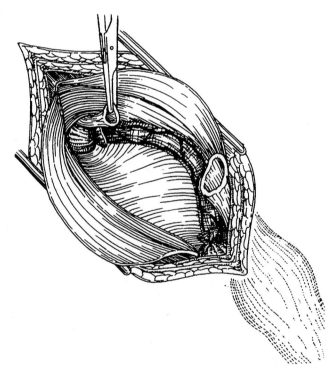

Fig. 14.8 If the indirect sac extends beyond the inguinal canal, it must never be dissected beyond the pubic tubercle; instead, the proximal sac is identified across and ligated flush with the peritoneum at its neck. The distal sac is *left* in situ to preserve the rich anastomosis of vessels that occurs in the cord and prevent ischemia of the testicle

opened, a two-layer closure with absorbable polymer and urethral drainage are required for 7 days at a minimum. Recovery will obviously be delayed.

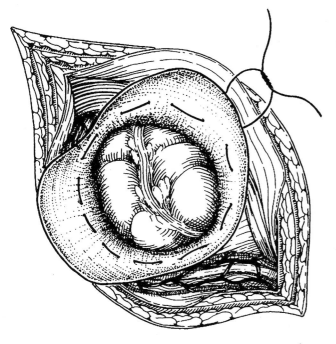

Fig. 14.9 Closing the sac of a sliding hernia

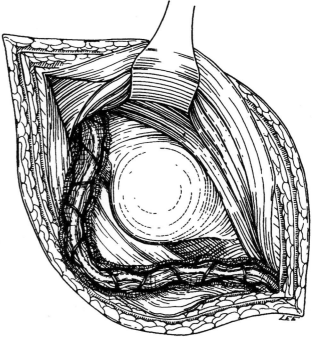

Fig. 14.10 The *dome*-shaped direct bulge; there is no need to open this sac

A sliding hernia is dealt with by excising as much peritoneal hernial sac as possible and then closing it using an "inside out" purse-string suture. When it is closed it is pushed back behind the fascia transversalis (Fig. 14.9).

Direct

The direct sac may be either a broad-based bulge behind and through the fascia transversalis or, less commonly, it may have a narrow neck. In the first type, interference with the peritoneum is not needed—the sac should be pushed behind the fascia transversalis, which will subsequently be repaired (Fig. 14.10). In the case of a narrow-necked hernia, which is usually at the medial end of the canal, the extraperitoneal fat is removed, the sac carefully cleared, the redundant peritoneum excised, and the defect closed with absorbable transfixion suture. Care must be taken to avoid the bladder, which is often in the wall of such a sac (Fig. 14.11).

Combined Direct and Indirect

Lastly, a combined direct and indirect "pantaloon" sac straddling the deep epigastric vessels may be found. In such cases the sac should be delivered to the lateral side of the deep epigastric vessels and dealt with as described for an indirect hernia (Hoguet's maneuver) [28, 29] (Fig. 14.12).

The indirect sac is completely freed from the vas, spermatic vessels, and the adjacent fascia transversalis at the deep ring. It is best then to mobilize the fascia transversalis

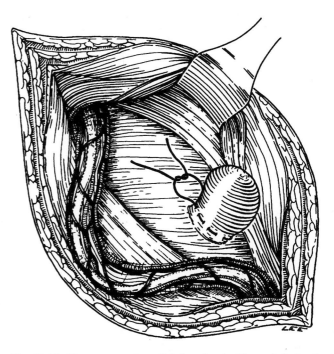

Fig. 14.11 The narrow neck medial direct hernia. The sac is isolated, closed, and excised

medially so that the whole of the sac can be drawn laterally. Whether or not the direct sac should be opened at this stage is a question of judgment. The hazard of wounding the bladder must be acknowledged. Any opening into a direct

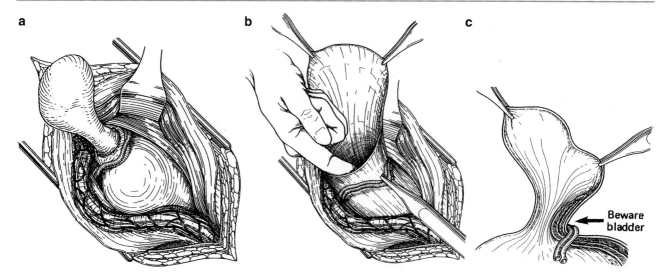

Fig. 14.12 Hoguet maneuver. The combined direct/indirect sac (pantaloon hernia) is delivered lateral to the deep epigastric vessels. Any redundant peritoneum is excised and the sac closed

sac must be commenced laterally; care must be taken to identify the bladder margin medially and any peritoneal incision must stop short of this. Alternatively the direct sac can be opened—a finger inserted into the peritoneal cavity through the indirect sac will identify the dimensions of the direct sac and facilitate dissection and mobilization.

Once the indirect and direct sacs are mobilized, the redundant peritoneum is excised and the peritoneal defect closed.

Step II: The Reconstruction

After the preparation an assessment of the hernial orifice is possible. This is also the moment to look for the femoral orifice to rule out a concomitant femoral hernia.

The repair of the defect can be achieved by an impressive variety of different procedures. The main differentiation is a repair by suture or by augmentation with nonabsorbable mesh prosthesis, in an anterior or posterior position:

– Suture repair
  • Marcy/Zimmermann
  • Shouldice
  • McVay
– Anterior flat mesh repair
  • Lichtenstein
– Anterior plug and patch

Open Suture Technique

In Table 14.3 the most common suture techniques are enlisted. A description of each technique would certainly go beyond the scope of this chapter. Therefore only techniques in common usage will be described.

Marcy/Zimmermann Suture Repair

The first description of a narrowing of the deeper inguinal hernia ring by suture was by Marcy in 1887 [24] and later by Zimmermann [30]. Indications for his simple repair are small, indirect inguinal hernias (EHS classification L1) with a stable fascia transversalis. In these cases a further incision of the posterior wall is neglected and a reduction of the hernial orifice by suture is performed.

A prerequisite for this repair is a sufficient preparation of the internal inguinal ring, with identification of the fascia transversalis, complete dissection of the spermatic cord from the internal inguinal ring, and removal of preperitoneal fatty tissue. The suture repair starts medial to lateral. The narrowing of the internal hernia ring should accomplish a remaining orifice of 5–8 mm, admitting just the tip of a finger, to guarantee a sufficient blood supply for the testis. To standardize the size of the ring, the use of an 11.5 Hegar dilator has proved to be helpful. The closing sutures are placed medial to the spermatic cord. To achieve a secure placement of the sutures, the fascia transversalis, the aponeurosis of the m. transversus, and the caudal fibers of the iliopubic tract are included into the suture.

After sufficient narrowing of the internal hernia ring, the posterior wall of the inguinal canal is augmented by a single continuous suture fixation of the internal oblique and transverse muscles to the inguinal ligament.

Results and Evaluation

Due to the lack of classification and differentiation of the different non-mesh techniques for inguinal hernia repair in adults, an evaluation of this technique is limited. Valenti et al. performed a modified Marcy repair, sparing the cremaster muscle, in over 200 patients with indirect hernias. After a median follow-up of 4.7 years, they did not have a recurrence [31].

Hübner et al. have compared the results of a Marcy repair versus tension-free Lichtenstein repair in small lateral hernias. After a median follow-up period of 56 months, there was no difference concerning recurrence or chronic pain but a clear trend to less neuropathic symptoms in favor of the suture repair [32].

The Marcy/Zimmermann repair is a fast and minimal procedure with reduction of surgical trauma in comparison to other open techniques. The long-term results correlate with careful patient selection. Only small indirect hernias in young patients without risk factors should be considered for this procedure.

One of the advantages of an open approach is the option to switch the procedure according to the intraoperative findings. In case of a weak fascia transversalis or in larger hernias (EHS classification >L1), other open techniques such a complete reduplication of the posterior wall (Shouldice repair) or mesh augmentation (Lichtenstein) can be performed.

Shouldice Repair

In 1945 it was Earl E. Shouldice who described this novel method of inguinal hernia repair. It is an open, transinguinal suture technique to repair defects in the posterior wall of the inguinal canal. In the same year he founded the Shouldice Hospital, but it took until 1952 and the support of his assistants E. A. Ryan and N. Obney that after several modifications of the initial technique led to the development of today's classical "Shouldice repair" also known as the "Canadian repair" [33].

Dissection of Fascia Transversalis

The most essential part of the Shouldice operation is the repair of the fascia transversalis. This structure should

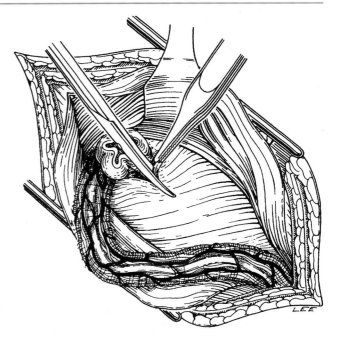

Fig. 14.13 Dissection of the fascia transversalis

already have been identified at its condensation around the cord forming the deep inguinal ring. The condensed medial margin of the deep inguinal ring is freed from the emerging cord by sharp dissection. When this is completed, the medial margin of the ring is grasped in a dissecting forceps or a hemostat and lifted up off the underlying extraperitoneal fat. Dissecting scissors are now passed through the ring between the fascia and the underlying fat. By this maneuver the fascia is separated from the underlying structures, particularly the deep epigastric vessels. If there is no direct herniation and no gross distortion of the deep ring, only the margin of the deep ring, the "sling" of the deep ring, needs dividing; if there is a direct hernia and attenuation of the fascia transversalis, the fascia transversalis is now divided along the length of the canal, beginning at the deep inguinal ring and continuing down to the pubic tubercle. The upper medial flap is lifted up away from the underlying fat. Attention is now turned to the lower flap. If it is penetrated by cremasteric vessels arising from the deep epigastric vessels, these should now be divided and ligated close to their origin. If care is not taken with the cremasteric vessels, they may be torn off the deep epigastric vessels and troublesome hemorrhage will follow. If a direct hernia is present, it will bulge forward at this time and must be pushed back in order to free the lower lateral flap of the fascia transversalis. This flap must be freed down to its continuation as the anterior femoral sheath deep to the inguinal ligament. The lower, condensed fascia transversalis as it merges to the anterior femoral sheath is the iliopubic band. Any grossly attenuated fascia transversalis about a direct sac is excised. With the fascia transversalis

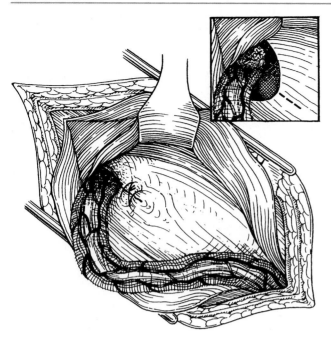

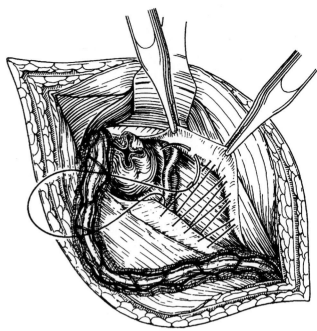

Fig. 14.14 After the neck of the sac has been divided at the deep inguinal ring, the fascia transversalis of the deep opening is identified and assessed. If ring is normal sized the stump of the sac is reduced and no more need be done. If the ring is marginally dilated (*stretched*) it should be carefully dissected and possibly divided slightly (*inset*) and then sutured tightly around the medial side of the cord with polypropylene to reconstitute a competent deep inguinal ring

Fig. 14.15 Suturing the lower lateral flap of fascia transversalis to the undersurface of the upper medial flap along the "*white line*" or "*arch*"

opened and developed, the femoral canal should be checked again (Fig. 14.13).

Repair of Fascia Transversalis

If the previous dissection has been carried out carefully, and if hemostasis is now complete, the repair with the reconstruction of the inguinal floor commences. First, the fascia transversalis is reapproximated and the deep ring is carefully reconstituted using a "double breasting" technique. The posterior wall of the canal must be reconstituted so that all of the peritoneum and the stump of a hernial sac are retained behind it. To do this, the lower lateral flap of the fascia transversalis is sutured to the deep surface of the upper medial flap. The repair is begun toward the medial end of the canal. Where the medial margin of the deep ring only has been divided and the more medial aspect of the posterior wall of the canal shown to be sound, no direct herniation, only the divided fascia transversalis at the medial margin of the deep ring, the "sling," will need careful two-layered reconstruction with a nonabsorbable suture (Fig. 14.14). If there is a direct hernia, the whole of the posterior wall of the canal will have been divided and will need repair, the first suture being placed in fascia transversalis where that structure becomes condensed into the aponeurosis and perios-

teum on the pubic tubercle. The lower lateral flap of the fascia transversalis is then sutured to the undersurface of the upper flap at the point where the upper flap is just deep to the tendon of the transversus abdominus (conjoint tendon). At this point there is a thickening or condensation of the fascia transversalis (the "white line" or "arch"), which holds sutures easily (Fig. 14.15).

Care must be taken with the closure of the fascia transversalis as it approaches the lateral rectus sheath, which must be adequately repaired to the fascia transversalis and the pubic tubercle. The anatomy here is variable, and the falx inguinalis should be included in the repair. The fascia is sutured laterally until the stump of an indirect hernia lies behind it and it has been snugly fitted around the spermatic cord (Fig. 14.16). The direction of suturing is then reversed. The free margin of the upper medial flap is brought down over the lower lateral flap and sutured to the fascia transversalis at its condensation (the iliopubic tract), just above the upturned deep edge of the inguinal ligament in the floor of the canal. Suturing is continued back to the pubic tubercle, where the suture is tied. By this maneuver the fascia transversalis is "double breasted" on itself, the "direct area" of the canal is reinforced, and the internal ring carefully reconstituted and tightened. It is important not to split the fascial fibers. Sutures should be placed about 2–4 mm apart and bites of different depth taken with each so that an irregular "broken saw tooth" effect is produced. The repair of the fascia transversalis is the crucial part of the operation. The fas-

a

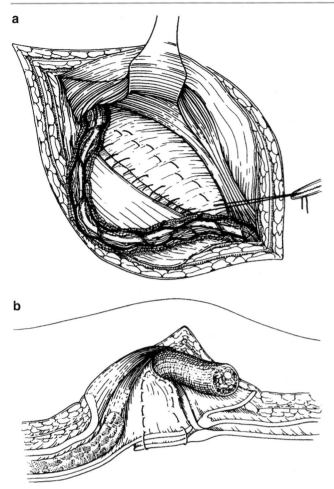

b

Fig. 14.16 Completing the overlap of the fascia transversalis repair. The margin of the upper medial flap is sutured to the anterior surface of the lower lateral flap (**a**). A neat closure up to the cord makes a new deep ring (**b**)

cia must be dissected and handled with care if its structure is to be maintained.

A "trick of the trade" sometimes facilitates this suturing of the fascia transversalis: After the upper medial and lower lateral leaflets of fascia transversalis have been developed to clearly show the "white line" of the transversus tendon through the fascia above and the iliopubic tract below, a loose swab (sponge) is pushed into the dissection to keep the extra-peritoneal fat out of the way when the first sutures are introduced (Fig. 14.17).

When these sutures are loosely in place, the swab is removed and the suture tension adjusted to give tissue closure.

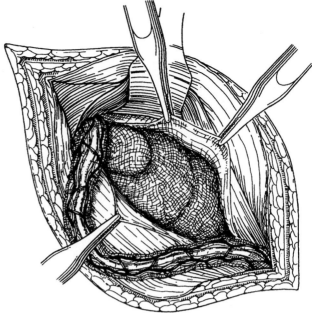

Fig. 14.17 If the subjacent extraperitoneal fat and peritoneum is bulging, a "trick of the trade" is to pack it down with a gauze swab. This must be removed before the sutures are snugged tight

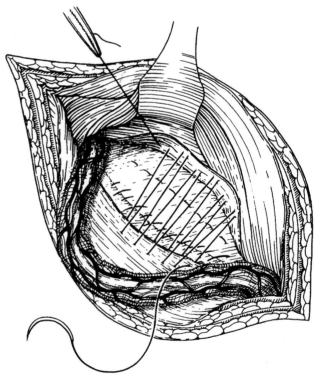

Fig. 14.18 The aponeurotic, *white* part of the internal oblique tendon and the conjoint tendon are used to reinforce the repair

Reinforcement with the Conjoint Tendon

The conjoint tendon is now used to reinforce the repair of the

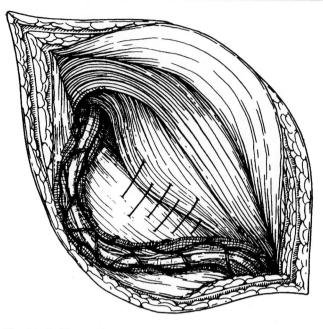

Fig. 14.19 The anterior aponeurotic surface of the internal oblique aponeurosis is loosely sutured to the aponeurosis of the external oblique medially

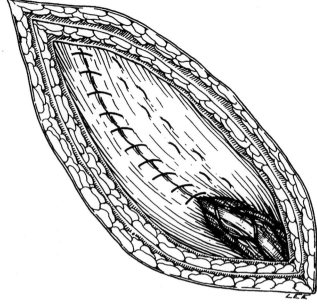

Fig. 14.20 The external oblique aponeurosis is closed, double breasted, anterior to the cord. Thus the inguinal canal is reconstituted with the cord obliquely traversing it

fascia transversalis medially. A suture is started laterally through the upturned deep edge of the inguinal ligament medial to the margin of the reconstituted deep inguinal ring and continued to the deep tendinous surface of the conjoint tendon, which is directly to the medial side of the deep ring. Sometimes, particularly if the cord is bulky, it is easier to proceed in reverse by passing the needle first through the undersurface of the conjoint tendon and then under the cord and through the upturned edge of the inguinal ligament. At the point where this suture is inserted, the deep surface of the conjoint tendon is just beginning to become aponeurotic (the tendon of the transversus muscle), and it should hold sutures easily. The suture is continued in a medial direction, picking up the upturned edge of the inguinal ligament and the under-surface—the aponeurotic part—of the conjoint tendon down to the pubic tubercle (Fig. 14.18). The direction is then reversed, suturing the aponeurotic part of the conjoint tendon, the internal oblique tendon now, loosely to the external oblique aponeurosis about 0.5 cm above the inguinal ligament. The "broken saw tooth" technique previously mentioned is again used, and as it is done the suture is gently pulled snug, not tight, so that the conjoint tendon and rectus sheath are rolled down onto the deep surface of the external oblique aponeurosis. Suturing is continued laterally until the conjoint tendon ceases to be aponeurotic at the medial edge of the emergent spermatic cord. The suture is then tied. The reconstruction of the posterior wall and the floor of the ingui-

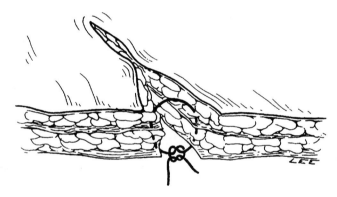

Fig. 14.21 Closure of the subcutaneous tissue

nal canal is now complete. The cord is now placed back in the canal (Fig. 14.19).

External Oblique Aponeurosis

Now that the cord has been replaced, the external oblique aponeurosis can be closed over it. This can be performed as a single continuous suture or a "double breasting" technique. Remembering that aponeurotic wounds are slow to regain strength, nonabsorbable sutures are used for this layer. A new superficial inguinal ring is constructed at the medial end of the canal. Care should be taken during the suturing to spare the ilioinguinal nerve from the suture line. The repair

Fig. 14.22 The skin is closed with a subcuticular continuous absorbable polymer suture

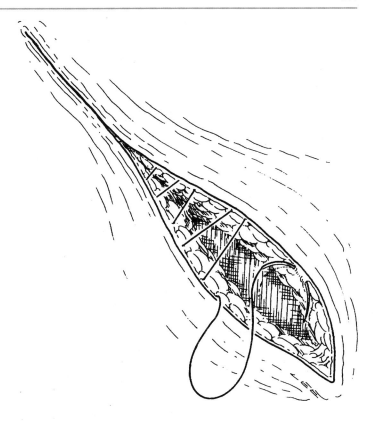

is now complete, and if all the layers have been sutured exactly as described, the loads on the suture lines should be well distributed; there should be no undue tension and no splitting of fiber bundles. Indeed, the structures should have just "rolled together" (Fig. 14.20).

Subcutaneous Tissue and Skin Closure

The subcutaneous tissue is carefully closed with interrupted absorbable sutures. No "dead spaces" should be left and the fat should be closed so that the skin is closely approximated. If there is much tissue trauma or dead space, a closed drain is useful in this layer but seldom necessary (Fig. 14.21). The skin is closed with a subcuticular absorbable suture (Fig. 14.22).

Results and Evaluation

In the 1980s the Shouldice repair has become the standard suture procedure for inguinal hernia repair in Europe. Compared to the customary Bassini repair, it has proved superior. The long-term results with follow-up of 5–10 years showed recurrence rates between 1.3 and 6.7% [16, 34–36]. High recurrence rates of up to 22% occurred in patients with large medial hernias and in recurrent hernias [16, 34] emphasizing the need of meticulous patient selec-

tion, tailoring the surgical therapy to each patient's individual condition.

The Shouldice repair however requires a good detailed anatomical knowledge and surgical experience. It is a more demanding surgical procedure than for example a Lichtenstein repair. The learning curve takes longer, and a higher number of procedures are required to gain competence. Muschaweck reported on 158 reoperations for recurrence after previous Shouldice repair [37]. In less than 20% of the patients could evidence of an actual previously performed Shouldice repair be found, accentuating the urgent need of standardization of our surgical technique. This might also help to understand the wide range of recurrence rates.

In a recent Cochrane review from 2009, the Shouldice technique was compared to other open techniques for inguinal hernia repair. The authors found 16 trials with a total of 2,566 hernias in the Shouldice group and 1,608 other non-mesh techniques. The authors' conclusion found the Shouldice herniorrhaphy the best non-mesh technique in terms of recurrence, though it is more time consuming [38].

McVay: Repair

The initial indication for the McVay/Cooper's ligament repair was for patients with a large direct hernia and an absent cau-

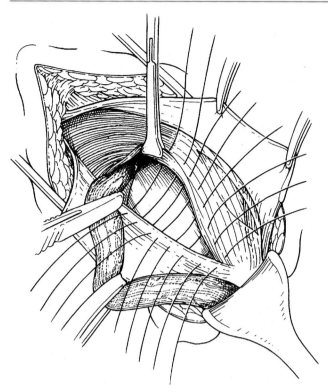

Fig. 14.23 The McVay/Cooper's ligament operation: clearing the anterior femoral sheath

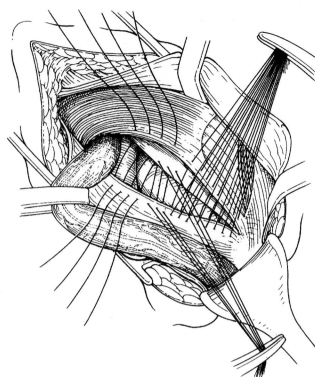

Fig. 14.24 Sutures are placed between the transversalis abdominis arch and Cooper's ligament as far as the femoral vein

dal margin of the fascia transversalis. It is also useful in the management of concomitant femoral and inguinal hernias. Today the McVay repair has lost most of its initial relevance. The advantages of the different mesh techniques have reduced the indication and propagation of this technique.

The McVay repair is therefore described only in summary. The incision, exposure, and dissection of the canal and cord are identical to the above mentioned. The transversalis fascia is incised, preserving the inferior epigastric vessels, and the preperitoneal space opened. The dissection is then taken deeper to expose and free the iliopectineal (Cooper's) ligament. Great care must be taken here to preserve the anastomosis between the obturator and epigastric arteries ("the corona mortis"). The hernial sac can be dissected bluntly away from the superior pubic ligament. The main principle of this procedure is a triple layer repair, attaching the fascia transversalis, the m. transversus abdominis, and the m. oblique internus to Cooper's ligament. To reduce possible tension on the suture line, a relaxing incision is made as medial as possible in the internal oblique aponeurosis—anterior rectus sheath—deep to the external oblique aponeurosis before the two aponeuroses fuse (Fig.14 .23). The repair is now initiated by bringing the transverse abdominis arch down to the inguinal ligament. This is best achieved with a layer of interrupted sutures, beginning at the pubic tubercle and continued laterally to the medial edge of the femoral vein. Each is placed carefully under direct vision and held before serial knotting (Fig. 14.24)

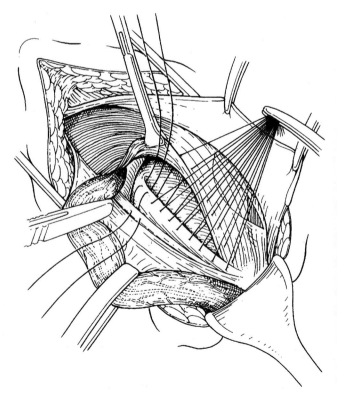

Fig. 14.25 The femoral canal is closed with two or three transition sutures between Cooper's ligament and the anterior femoral fascia

and placed between the transversus arch, the "white line," and the iliopectineal (Cooper's) ligament. The femoral vein is retracted and protected by a retractor. The femoral canal is then narrowed by placement of two or three transition sutures of nonabsorbable sutures between Cooper's ligament and the anterior femoral fascia (sheath). The lateral suture is placed just lateral to the last suture in Cooper's ligament; the medial two or three are medial to this and go between the Cooper's ligament sutures (Fig. 14.25). The repair is now continued laterally between the transversus abdominis arch and the anterior femoral fascia with the line of sutures just displacing the internal ring laterally, but not placing any sutures lateral to the cord. These sutures are of monofilament, nonabsorbable material. The sutures are now tied beginning medially and a new internal ring created such that a hemostat can be inserted between the last tied suture and the cord.

Results and Evaluation

In McVay's experience of the Cooper's ligament repair, a recurrence rate of under 1% in 1,000 cases over 16 years is recorded. In part these excellent results are due to the securing of an adequate viable posterior wall for the inguinal canal (the intact rectus sheath with its blood supply) to the firm anchorage of Cooper's ligament. Rutledge records 906 consecutive primary Cooper's ligament repairs with a recurrence rate of 1.9% overall: 3.5% for direct and 1.1% for indirect inguinal hernia. The patient follow-up was 97%, 80% of patients being examined, and average follow-up was 9 years. The operative technique, however, is extensive, requiring deep retraction. In 13% of patients the repair was combined with a Marlex mesh overlay. With a 5% testicular atrophy rate in skilled hands, this operation might have medicolegal consequences. Rutledge comments that the recurrence rate rises to 5.5% if the cord is brought out straight through the external oblique and transplanted subcutaneously. Testicular atrophy occurred in 7.9% of recurrent hernia repairs [39]

The recurrence rates in the literature seem quite inconsistent, ranging between 0.5 and 20.9%, depending on follow-up time and centers [40–45].

The Open Anterior Mesh Repair

The Lichtenstein Technique

The true tension-free hernioplasty using mesh and no suture closure of the hernial defect was introduced in 1984 by Irving Lichtenstein and colleagues [46].

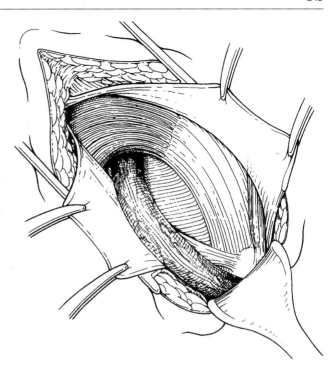

Fig. 14.26 Wide dissection of the posterior wall of the canal

The Lichtenstein Tension-Free Hernioplasty

The incision, exposure, dissection of the canal and cord, and the method of dealing with indirect hernial sacs are identical to that described for the open suture techniques.

The upper leaf of the external oblique aponeurosis needs to be lifted up and dissected from the underlying internal oblique muscle and aponeurosis high enough to accommodate a 6–8-cm-wide patch. Between these two layers the anatomical cleavage is avascular and the dissection can be performed nontraumatic by blunt preparation. In most cases the n. iliohypogastricus and the n. inguinalis can be displayed and if possible preserved. A sufficient overlap is required for Hesselbach's triangle, the pubic tubercle, and laterally beyond the internal ring. Medially this dissection should be taken beyond the pubic tubercle to the midline (Fig. 14.26). The cremaster muscle is preserved to cover the cord as a natural barrier for the mesh contact.

In the case of large direct sacs, in order to flatten the posterior inguinal wall to facilitate placement of the mesh, a running, inverting, absorbable suture is applied to the transversalis fascia.

A nonabsorbable mesh prosthesis precut to 16×8 cm is now tailored to the individual patient's requirements. This will involve trimming 1–2 cm of the patch's width and the upper medial corner so that it will tuck itself between the external oblique and internal oblique muscles without wrinkles.

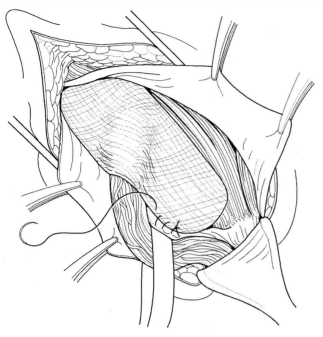

Fig. 14.27 Initial half of continuous suture to allow mesh to overlap pubic tubercle and appose to inguinal ligament

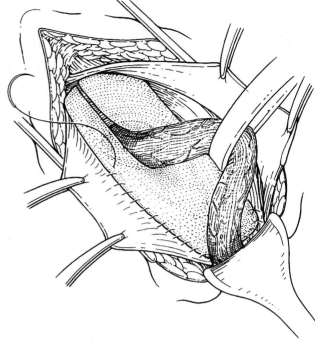

Fig. 14.29 The lower "tail" of the mesh is flipped behind the cord, followed by the continuous suture with needle, and the cord is retracted upward

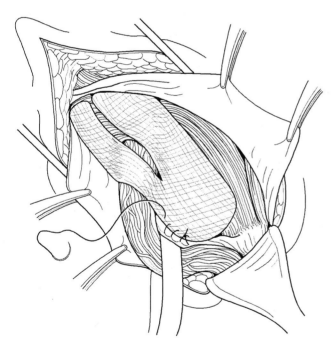

Fig. 14.28 The mesh is slit (one-third below, two-thirds above), up to the medial margin of the internal ring

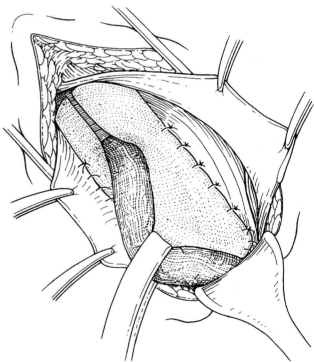

Fig. 14.30 The continuous suture line along the inguinal ligament is now continued to the lateral border of the internal ring

The cord is now retracted downward and the mesh aligned into the inguinal canal such that its inferior border lies parallel with the inguinal ligament, and its medial border overlaps the pubic tubercle by 1–2 cm. Using a nonabsorbable monofilament running suture beginning at the upper, medial, rounded border of the mesh, the suture is placed into the tough aponeurotic tissue of the midline and secured with a knot. This suture then continues around the edge of the mesh

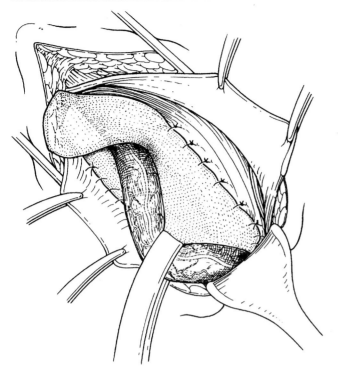

Fig. 14.31 Three or four sutures tack the mesh cranially

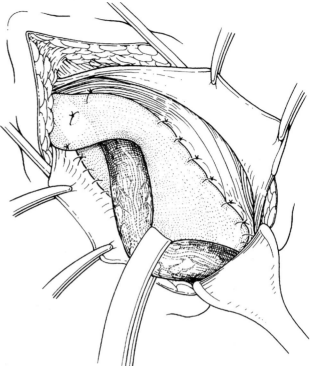

Fig. 14.32 "Tails" are overlapped and crossed and a single suture placed to create a new "internal" ring

taking bites of firm connective tissue under direct vision but avoiding the periosteum of the bone.

As the suture continues it picks up the lower edge of the shelving margin of the inguinal ligament. Having secured the mesh medially and also secured it to 1–2 cm of inguinal ligament, this suturing is temporarily halted (Fig. 14.27). A slit is now made at the lateral end of the mesh, creating two tails, a wider one (two-thirds above) and a narrow one (one-third below) (Fig. 14.28). The lower, narrower tail together with the needle and its running suture is now passed behind the cord, which is then retracted upward (Fig. 14.29). The wider upper tail and the narrow lower tail are overlapped and grasped in a hemostat to retract the mesh and prevent unnecessary wrinkles.

The running suture between the lower edge of the mesh and the shelving margin of the inguinal ligament is now completed to a point just lateral to the internal ring (Fig. 14.30). The upper leaf of the external oblique aponeurosis is now retracted strongly upward, and the upper edge of the mesh is sutured to the underlying internal oblique aponeurosis or muscle with a series of interrupted sutures approximately 2–3 cm apart. Care is taken to avoid underlying blood vessels and sensory nerves, such as the ilioinguinal and iliohypogastric nerves (Fig. 14.31). The mesh should not be completely flattened, but should be seen to have some degree of anterior convexity in order to remain tension-free. The last fixation suture is placed laterally at approximately the same level as the internal ring.

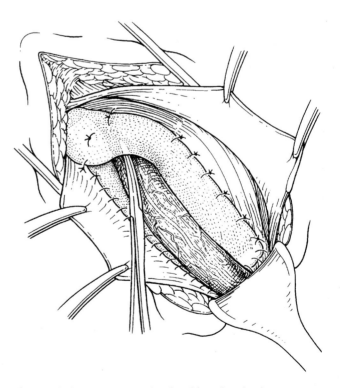

Fig. 14.33 Sutures may now be placed lateral to the ring to prevent shifting and curling. An artery clip is run down between the mesh and new internal ring to ensure an adequate aperture

The lower edges of each of the two tails are now fixed to the inguinal ligament at a point just lateral to the completion knot of the lower running suture. A point is chosen in the lower edge of the upper tail approximately 1 cm beyond the lateral margin of the internal ring to avoid unnecessary buckling of the mesh (Fig. 14.32). Having created a new internal ring with crossover and overlap of the two tails, excess patch on the lateral side is now trimmed in order to leave approximately 3–4 cm of mesh beyond the internal ring. This lateral tail is now tucked underneath the external oblique aponeurosis and may be prevented from movement, curling up, or wrinkling by placing sutures between it and the underlying muscle. The size of the new internal ring is now tested with a hemostat, which should pass easily between the cord and the mesh. If this gap is too wide, it may be closed loosely with a nonabsorbable suture (Fig. 14.33).

Having completed the repair of the posterior inguinal wall with nonabsorbable mesh prosthesis, the cord is placed back into the canal. The wound closure is identical to that described for the suture repairs.

The original Lichtenstein technique as described above has seen many modifications over the years. The main focus is today directed on the mesh and the fixation technique. The advances in mesh technology provide a great variety of different meshes.

Mesh Fixation

Lichtenstein used a nonabsorbable polypropylene suture for mesh fixation. In a recent survey of the Swedish Hernia Registry, different sutures were investigated. The data of over 80,000 Lichtenstein repairs were analyzed in respect of the suture material, nonabsorbable, long-term or short-term absorbable suture. There was no difference in the recurrence rate between the first two groups, but a significant increase in the short-term absorbable suture group [47].

Today there is a great variety of suture- and tack-free mesh fixation options available. In experimental studies the strength of glue or fibrin sealant in comparison to sutures has been demonstrated [48]. Fibrin sealant for mesh fixation was first introduced by Chevrel and Rath in 1997 for the treatment of open onlay meshes in incisional hernia repair and is now also used for inguinal open Lichtenstein repair. Negro and colleagues have performed an observational multicenter study including 520 patients over a 12-month period. They found significantly less intense pain, numbness, and discomfort in the fibrin sealant group [49].

A new mesh modification that addresses the problem of fixation and mesh structure has gained popularity among hernia surgeons. Absorbable microhooks on the fascia-facing side of the mesh induce a "self-gripping" or Velcro-like property, negating any additional type of fixation [50]. Recent publications have shown some advantages in total length of

operation time and less pain, though long-term results need to be awaited.

Results and Evaluation

Lichtenstein reported his personal experience of 6,321 cases in 1987 with a 91% follow-up over a period of 2–14 years and a recurrence rate of 0.7% [51]. At this time apart from the innovation of polypropylene mesh, Lichtenstein had abandoned high ligation and excision of indirect sacs but continued to use single-layer approximation of the transversus abdominis and the inguinal ligament with a relaxing incision. After a period of evolution the perfected tension-free hernioplasty was reported by Lichtenstein, Shulman, Amid, and Montelier in 1989 [52].

Repair of the posterior abdominal layer with a suture line was abandoned, except for a simple imbrication suture for large sacs that aided flattening of the posterior wall before placement of the mesh. The recurrence rate in over 1,000 cases was 0% at 1–5-year follow-up, with no mesh infections, and the authors stated that the technique was simple, rapid, and relatively pain-free, allowing prompt resumption of unrestricted physical activity. This report prompted a campaign of popularization of the tension-free hernioplasty [53].

Like the Shouldice Hospital, the Lichtenstein Institute surgeons have written multiple publications in the surgical literature, repeating their experiences with a gradually enlarging number of patients [54–56]. The authors emphasize that the hernial defect edges are not approximated and the sole strength of the repair is based on placing a synthetic implant over the posterior inguinal wall with a tension-free patch. Many thousands of patients have now undergone repair with this operation at the Lichtenstein Institute, the operation being performed under local anesthesia and patients discharged within a few hours of operation with minimal discomfort, for which mild analgesics are prescribed. Unrestricted activity is encouraged, and patients discharged from the unit are able to resume normal activity in 2–10 days. A postal survey performed by Shulman of 70 surgeons utilizing this technique who did not have a special interest in inguinal hernia surgery indicated similar results in 22,300 repairs [57].

In the UK the Lichtenstein technique was first reported by Kingsnorth and colleagues, and subsequently by a private hernia clinic, The British Hernia Centre [58, 59].

Kark and colleagues, reporting on 1,098 tension-free hernia repairs, found only one recurrence after primary repair and an overall sepsis rate of 0.9% [59]. This report emphasized the cost savings associated with the operation and the rapid return to activity: with 50% of office workers returning to work in 1 week or less, and 60% of manual workers in 2 weeks or less. Nevertheless, the operation can present technical difficulties to the novice, as illustrated by a report from Brussels in which 139 primary inguinal hernias were repaired by tension-free hernioplasty and a 4.6% recurrence rate was reported during a mean follow-up of 12.7 months. The probable technical fault was failure to overlap the pubic tubercle and the entire posterior inguinal wall by a wide margin of mesh [60]. These authors reported a 50% saving of resources by utilization of the tension-free hernioplasty.

The first randomized trial reporting a comparison between the tension-free hernioplasty and the Shouldice operation was reported by Kux and colleagues, verifying the low recurrence rate (one recurrence in the Lichtenstein group over a 30-month period), and a reduced requirement for postoperative pain relief. Patients under the age of 60 years were excluded from this study [61].

The EU Hernia Trialists Collaboration examined all randomized and quasi-randomized trials comparing open mesh with open non-mesh methods for repair of groin hernia [62]. Fifteen eligible trials, which included 4,005 participants, were identified. Return to usual activities was quicker in the mesh group for 7 of the 10 trials (p value not significant). There were fewer reported recurrences in the mesh groups (1.4% compared with 4.4%). Therefore using the powerful statistical methods followed by the Cochrane Collaboration, the currently available literature indicates that mesh repair is associated with 3 times fewer recurrences than non-mesh, in the repair of inguinal hernia. All these studies comparing different surgical procedures are limited in their conclusion due to the missing classification of the hernia included.

Amid published his results of 5,000 Lichtenstein procedures with a recurrence rate of 0.1% after a follow-up of 5–10 years. But the data of multicenter studies show a different recurrence rate of up to 10% [5, 36, 63].

Antibiotic Prophylaxis

The use of prophylactic antibiotic cover in the form of powder instillation or a single perioperative intravenous bolus is a vexed question. The Lichtenstein Institute has used both methods, but has not made a firm recommendation. However, Gilbert and Felton in a cooperative multicenter prospective study of 2,493 inguinal hernia repairs by 65 surgeons found a wound infection rate of less than 1% whether or not biomaterials or antibiotics were used [11]. Moreover, the removal of polypropylene biomaterials from infected wounds was not necessary to eliminate infection and indeed is not recommended because of technical difficulty and inevitable recurrence. The new generation of large-pore low surface meshes also seems to be advantageous in lowering infection. The authors conclude that the expense incurred for routine prophylactic antibiotic cover in inguinal hernia

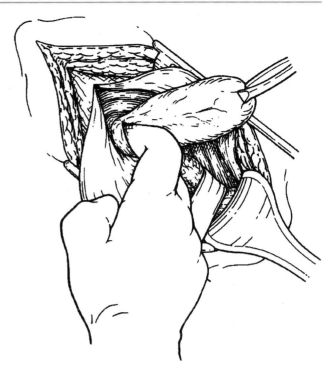

Fig. 14.34 A pocket is created for positioning of the mesh in the preperitoneal space

operation when prosthetic materials are used could not be reconciled by any benefits obtained. The European Guidelines recommend antibiotic prophylaxis in elective open hernia groin surgery only in high risk patients with accordant risk factors for wound infection. Thus a perioperative single shot of antibiotics should be considered in patients with advanced age, immunosuppressive conditions, or in case of a recurrence [64].

Plug-and-Patch Repair

This technique was introduced by Ira Rutkow in 1989, published in 1993 [27]. The procedure consists of two parts: the plug part, placing a cone-shaped alloplastic mesh prosthesis into the defect, filling out the hernial orifice in a cork-like manner; and a second part, placing a flat mesh in the onlay position over the plug. It is therefore a combination of an anterior and posterior repair since the plug extends through the posterior wall into the preperitoneal space.

The essential feature of the mesh plug hernioplasty is minimal dissection. For indirect hernias the sac is approached by separating the cremaster fibers longitudinally along the spermatic cord so as not to destroy the cremaster reflex. The sac is dissected free, down to the preperitoneal fat pad at the level of the internal ring and a pocket created for positioning of the mesh plug (Fig. 14.34). For direct hernias the attenuated transversalis fascia is elevated with an Alice

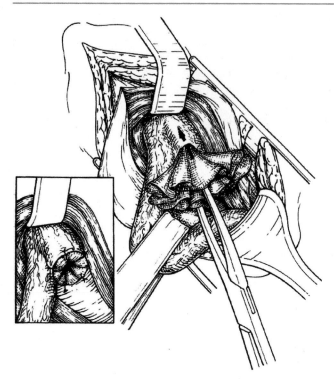

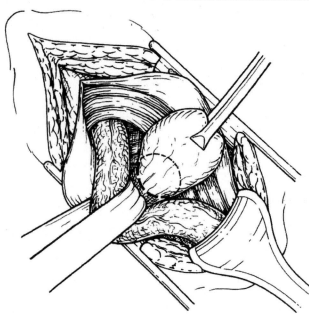

Fig. 14.37 The plug is inserted into the preperitoneal space through the direct hernia defect

Fig. 14.35 The preperitoneal space is entered via an incision in the transversalis fascia at the neck of the sac

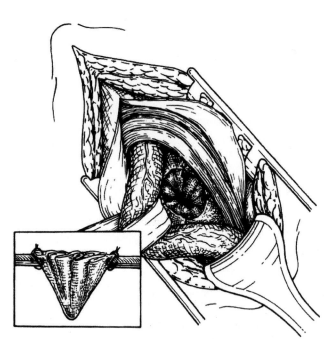

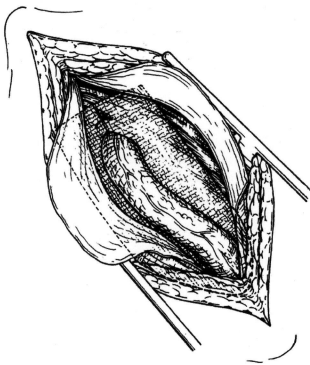

Fig. 14.38 Onlay mesh reinforces the plug repair

Fig. 14.36 The plug is inserted into the preperitoneal space via the internal ring

clamp, and the neck of the sac is completely circumscribed with sharp dissection to allow the preperitoneal fat space to be entered (Fig. 14.35). For both indirect and direct hernias the mesh plug can now be inserted, tapered end first into

either the internal ring (Fig. 14.36) or the defect in the posterior wall (Fig. 14.37). The mesh plug is then secured either to the crura of the ring or to surrounding intact tissue of the posterior wall by several interrupted sutures. This mesh plug repair is then reinforced with an onlay flat patch based on the anterior surface of the posterior wall of the inguinal canal from the pubic tubercle to above the internal ring (Fig. 14.38). A slit in the mesh to accommodate the cord, and the two ends are sutured back together around the cord, and this suture represents the only fixation.

Results and Evaluation

The plug-and-patch repair has become a very popular method of herniorrhaphy. It is a quick procedure that is relatively easily learned.

Rutkow and Robbins report a very low recurrence rate with low postoperative discomfort and rapid return to normal activities [65–67]. They have extended the technique to treat all inguinal hernias, femoral hernias, recurrent groin hernias, and small incisional hernias. In 1,563 cases two recurrences were recorded with an average follow-up of 82% at 2.4 years.

Because of its simplicity and short operation time, this operation is popular in specialized out-patient hernia centers.

The plug-and-patch technique has been criticized because the plug is a three-dimensional semirigid structure, which occludes only part of the posterior wall, combined with an onlay patch. There is some indication that unacceptable rates of postoperative pain occur in up to 5% of patients treated with the plug from studies by several authors [68–71]. Additionally, this plug often tends to shrink, leading to so-called meshomas [72]. Others have described plug migration with organ-related complications, such as sigmoid fistula, obstruction, or strangulation of small intestine [73–80].

On the other hand there is clear evidence from prospective randomized controlled trials comparing the plug-and-patch technique with other open mesh techniques that this technique has equivalent results [75, 76, 81–83]. Dalenbäck et al. found in an RCT no difference between Lichtenstein, Prolene Hernia System (PHS), and mesh and plug repair after a 3-year follow-up [84].

Recurrent Inguinal Hernia

In spite of apparent progress in hernia surgery during the last century, encompassing worldwide changes to the use of meshes in the majority of cases, the overall proportion of surgical repair for recurrent hernia remains high, between 10 and 15% [85]. If the same surgical approach as the previously failed operation is undertaken, reoperation will be carried out through the same scar. This can be sometimes difficult, particularly identifying the hernial sac, with a risk of damaging the vas or testicular vessels. There is little evidence available on this selected patient population, but in one randomized controlled trial, a high re-recurrence rate of

14.1% after 2 years of follow-up was found after open anterior re-operative surgery [63].

Therefore a change of surgical access should be considered. After open anterior inguinal hernia repair, a posterior approach, preferable in a laparoscopic/endoscopic technique, is not more complex than for a primary hernia. Lau had excellent results with TEP repair after recurrent open mesh hernias, although peritoneal tears are more likely [86]. In the NICE recommendations from 2001, it was already advised and is also a component of the European Guidelines [64]: For the repair of recurrent hernias after conventional open hernia repair, endoscopic inguinal hernia techniques are recommended.

Inguinal Hernia in Women

Anatomy and overall incidence is different in women. During the 26-year period 1945–1971, more than 75,000 hernia repairs were performed in the Shouldice clinic, Toronto; of these 1,672 (2.2%) were primary inguinal hernias in women and 414 (0.05%) primary femoral hernias in women. Of the inguinal hernias, 1,548 were indirect and only 124 were direct. Thus primary indirect inguinal hernia is 13 times more common than direct hernias. Direct inguinal hernias in women are very rare, and when they do occur they present usually in the lateral part of the posterior wall close to the deep epigastric vessels rather than in the medial canal as they do in men [87, 88]. In contrast to femoral hernia, pregnancy and vaginal delivery are not risk factors and obesity appears to be protective [89]. Recurrent inguinal hernias in women are more frequently indirect than direct—medial direct recurrences are a complication of previous groin surgery, Pfannenstiel incisions, or the high repair of femoral hernia. Occasionally, this is the result of an overlooked hernia that is missed at the prior operation.

In women, the round ligament should be excised and the inguinal canal closed [87]. The fascia transversalis is sutured down to the iliopubic tract and medially onto the iliopectineal line as in the McVay/Cooper's ligament operation, thus reducing the risk of subsequent femoral herniation (Fig. 14.39).

The long-term follow-up on inguinal hernia repair in women was performed for the European Guidelines in 2009. It was concluded at Level 2c evidence that women have a higher risk for recurrence than men for both inguinal and femoral hernias following an open inguinal hernia operation. Therefore it is mandatory to exclude the existence of a femoral hernia in all cases. For this reason the grade D recommendation proposes a preperitoneal, endoscopic approach in female hernia repair. The role of inguinal meshes and pregnancy has not been sufficiently investigated so far. An inguinal hernia during pregnancy is

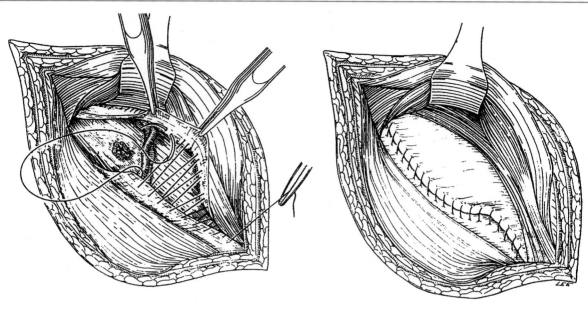

Fig. 14.39 Inguinal hernia in women: the sac and the round ligament are excised and then the canal closed by suturing the fascia transversalis to the iliopectineal ligamen

not an indication for an emergency repair. Buch and colleagues [90] performed a strategy of "watchful waiting" during the pregnancy with a hernia repair performed after delivery. Nevertheless mesh procedures should be avoided in women of child-bearing age.

Bilateral Hernia

Bilateral hernias occur in 10–22% of patients presenting with a unilateral hernia [91]. In the past the indication to perform a bilateral hernia repair simultaneously was cautious. The fear of a translocation of a possible infection or sepsis and the possible limitations in mobilization during the early postoperative period have dissuaded surgeons from operating on bilateral hernias simultaneously.

A small study by Serpell and colleagues investigated 31 patients undergoing bilateral simultaneous inguinal hernia repair, and five patients undergoing bilateral sequential repair, and compared these two groups against 75 patients having unilateral inguinal hernia repair. There were no differences in wound complications, postoperative respiratory complications, or other adverse effects between the three groups [92]. However, operating time and hospital stay were reduced by 2 days in those patients undergoing simultaneous repair. A larger but retrospective study from the Mayo Clinic, of patients undergoing hernia repair, compared 333 patients who underwent sequential unilateral repair against 329 who underwent simultaneous bilateral repair. Although there was greater

morbidity in the bilateral group, these complications for specific events were not significantly different between the two groups, except for urinary retention, which occurred in 6.1% of the unilateral group and 15% for the bilateral group. The Lichtenstein operation and laparoscopic inguinal hernia repair both lend themselves more easily to simultaneous repair of bilateral inguinal hernias [93, 94]. With the Lichtenstein operation the simultaneous repairs can be carried out under local anesthesia, and with the laparoscopic repair there is less pain after operation and a faster return to activity and work. In 2001 the National Institute for Clinical Excellence in the UK published guidance on the use of laparoscopic surgery for inguinal hernia. Laparoscopic surgery was recommended as an option for the repair of bilateral inguinal hernia [95]. Nevertheless simultaneous bilateral open procedure is also a good surgical option with comparable results to the laparoscopic/endoscopical approach [96–103].

Conclusion

We do not have standard patients with standard hernias. Therefore a standard therapy is not really possible. An individualized approach tailoring the surgical procedure to the patient's systemic condition should be considered. There remains a great discrepancy between the results of specialized centers and multicenter studies. Individual protagonists have equally excellent results with their espoused technique: Shouldice had a recurrence rate of 0.6% in over 6,000 suture repairs with a follow-up of 17 years. Lichtenstein's and Amid's recurrence rate for their technique remains below 1%. But in general practice these excellent results have not been achieved so far.

The anterior open approach to inguinal hernias facilitates an intraoperative decision on the choice of mesh or suture repair. In small lateral hernias without multiple risk factors, a suture repair can be considered with excellent results. In larger defects and/or more risk factors, a Lichtenstein repair should be performed. Another advantage is the option to perform the anterior open repair in local anesthesia. But most important of all remains the dedication and surgical education of the surgeon. Not every Shouldice operation is a Shouldice operation and not every Lichtenstein procedure is a Lichtenstein procedure. In a recent questionnaire circulated among hernia surgeons at the Berlin Hernia meeting in 2009, surgeons were asked to reveal the technical steps of their of "Shouldice" repair. Over 16% of the surgeons used absorbable sutures for the repair; more than 47% repaired with just a double row of sutures. Less than one-third did a genuine Shouldice repair according to the original description. Surgical standardization is essential, and quality control with a follow-up of at least 5 years should become mandatory.

References

1. Keynes G. The modern treatment of hernia. BMJ. 1927;1:173–9.
2. Rutkow IM. Epidemiologic, economic, and sociologic aspects of hernia surgery in the United States in the 1990s. Surg Clin North Am. 1998;78(6):941–9,vi.
3. Primatesta P, Goldacre MJ. Inguinal hernia repair: incidence of elective and emergency surgery, readmission and mortality. Int J Epidemiol. 1996;25(4):835–9.
4. Nilsson H, Stylianidis G, Haapamaki M, Nilsson E, Nordin P. Mortality after groin hernia surgery. Ann Surg. 2007;245(4):656–60.
5. Bay-Nielsen M, Kehlet H, Strand L, et al. Quality assessment of 26,304 herniorrhaphies in Denmark: a prospective nationwide study. Lancet. 2001;358(9288):1124–8.
6. Gallegos NC, Dawson J, Jarvis M, Hobsley M. Risk of strangulation in groin hernias. Br J Surg. 1991;78(10):1171–3.
7. Rai S, Chandra SS, Smile SR. A study of the risk of strangulation and obstruction in groin hernias. Aust N Z J Surg. 1998;68(9):650–4.
8. Fitzgibbons Jr RJ, Giobbie-Harder A, Gibbs JO, et al. Watchful waiting vs repair of inguinal hernia in minimally symptomatic men: a randomized clinical trial. JAMA. 2006;295(3):285–92.
9. O'Dwyer PJ, Chung L. Watchful waiting was as safe as surgical repair for minimally symptomatic inguinal hernias. Evid Based Med. 2006;11(3):73.
10. Gai H. [Ultrasound of inguinal hernias: morphological classification for a potentially conservative treatment in asymptomatic patients]. Ultraschall Med. 2010;31(3):258–63.
11. Gilbert AI. An anatomic and functional classification for the diagnosis and treatment of inguinal hernia. Am J Surg. 1989;157(3):331–3.
12. Rutkow IM, Robbins AW. Classification systems and groin hernias. Surg Clin North Am. 1998;78(6):1117–27, viii.
13. Nyhus LM. Iliopubic tract repair of inguinal and femoral hernia. The posterior (preperitoneal) approach. Surg Clin North Am. 1993;73(3):487–99.
14. Zollinger Jr RM. Classification systems for groin hernias. Surg Clin North Am. 2003;83(5):1053–63.
15. Miserez M, Alexandre JH, Campanelli G, et al. The European hernia society groin hernia classification: simple and easy to remember. Hernia. 2007;11(2):113–6.
16. Junge K, Rosch R, Klinge U, et al. Risk factors related to recurrence in inguinal hernia repair: a retrospective analysis. Hernia. 2006;10(4):309–15.
17. Lau H, Fang C, Yuen WK, Patil NG. Risk factors for inguinal hernia in adult males: a case-control study. Surgery. 2007;141(2):262–6.
18. McVay CB, Read RC, Ravitch MM. Inguinal hernia. Curr Probl Surg. 1967;1–50.
19. Read RC. Pervasive co-morbidity and abdominal herniation: an outline. In: Schumpelick V, Kingsnorth AN, editors. Recurrent hernia. Berlin-Heidelberg: Springer; 2007. p. 45–52.
20. Junge K, Klinge U, Rosch R, et al. Decreased collagen type I/III ratio in patients with recurring hernia after implantation of alloplastic prostheses. Langenbecks Arch Surg. 2004;389(1):17–22.
21. Klinge U, Junge K, Mertens PR. Herniosis: a biological approach. Hernia. 2004;8(4):300–1.
22. Klinge U, Binnebosel M, Rosch R, Mertens P. Hernia recurrence as a problem of biology and collagen. J Minim Access Surg. 2006;2(3):151–4.
23. Franz MG. The biology of hernia formation. Surg Clin North Am. 2008;88(1):1–15, vii.
24. Marcy HO. The cure of hernia. J Am Med Assoc. 1887;8:589–92.
25. Bassini E. Nuova technica per la cura dell'ernia inguinali. Societa Italiana di Chirurgica. 1887;4:379–82.
26. Read RC. The development of inguinal herniorrhaphy. Surg Clin North Am. 1984;64:185–96.
27. Rutkow IM, Robbins AW. "Tension-free" inguinal herniorrhaphy: a preliminary report on the "mesh plug" technique. Surgery. 1993;114(1):3–8.
28. Hoguet JP. Direct inguinal hernia. Ann Surg. 1920;72(6):671–4.
29. Qvist G. Saddlebag hernia. Br J Surg. 1977;64(6):442–4.
30. Zimmermann LM, Anson BJ. Anatomy and surgery of hernia. 2nd ed. Baltimore: Williams and Wilkins; 1967. p. 216–27.
31. Valenti G, Baldassarre E, Conforti A. The Marcy repair modified using cremaster muscle sparing. A new and effective method for performing prosthetic hernioplasty. Surg Today. 2005;35(8):645–8.
32. Hubner M, Schafer M, Raiss H, Demartines N, Vuilleumier H. A tailored approach for the treatment of indirect inguinal hernia in adults—an old problem revisited. Langenbecks Arch Surg. 2011;396(2):187–92.
33. Bendavid R. Biography: Edward Earle shouldice (1890-1965). Hernia. 2003;7(4):172–7.
34. Wantz GE. The Canadian repair: personal observations. World J Surg. 1989;13(5):516–21.
35. Arlt G, Schumpelick V. [The Shouldice repair for inguinal hernia—technique and results]. Zentralbl Chir. 2002;127(7):565–9.
36. Arvidsson D, Berndsen FH, Larsson LG, et al. Randomized clinical trial comparing 5-year recurrence rate after laparoscopic versus Shouldice repair of primary inguinal hernia. Br J Surg. 2005;92(9):1085–91.
37. Muschaweck U. How to treat recurrent inguinal hernia. In: Schumpelick V, Fitzgibbons RJ, editors. Recurrent hernia—prevention and treatment. Heidelberg: Springer; 2007. p. 289–97.
38. Amato B, Moja L, Panico S, Persico G, Rispoli C, Rocco N, et al. Shouldice technique versus other open techniques for inguinal hernia repair. Cochrane Database Syst Rev. 2009 Oct 7;(4):CD001543. Review.

39. Rutledge RH. Cooper's ligament repair: a 25-year experience with a single technique for all groin hernias in adults. Surgery. 1988;103(1):1–10.

40. Hay JM, Boudet MJ, Fingerhut A, et al. Shouldice inguinal hernia repair in the male adult: the gold standard? A multicenter controlled trial in 1578 patients. Ann Surg. 1995;222(6):719–27.

41. Lund J, Hvidt V, Kjeldsen-Andersen J. Inguinal and femoral hernioplasty. Five-year follow-up of 284 cases of McVay repair. Acta Chir Scand. 1966;131(1):72–80.

42. Rutledge RH. Cooper's ligament repair for adult groin hernias. Surgery. 1980;87(6):601–10.

43. Panos RG, Beck DE, Maresh JE, Harford FJ. Preliminary results of a prospective randomized study of Cooper's ligament versus Shouldice herniorrhaphy technique. Surg Gynecol Obstet. 1992;175(4):315–9.

44. Burcharth F, Hahn-Pedersen J, Andersen B, Andersen JR. Inguinal hernia repair with silk or polyglycolic acid sutures: a controlled trial with 5-years' follow-up. World J Surg. 1983;7(3):416–8.

45. Ingimarsson O, Spak I. Inguinal and femoral hernias. Long-term results in a community hospital. Acta Chir Scand. 1983;149(3):291–7.

46. Shulman AG, Amid PK, Lichtenstein IL. Patch or plug for groin hernia–which? Am J Surg. 1994;167(3):331–6.

47. Novik B, Nordin P, Skullman S, Dalenback J, Enochsson L. More recurrences after hernia mesh fixation with short-term absorbable sutures: a registry study of 82 015 Lichtenstein repairs. Arch Surg. 2011;146(1):12–7.

48. Schwab R, Schumacher O, Junge K, Binnebosel M, Klinge U, Schumpelick V. Fibrin sealant for mesh fixation in Lichtenstein repair: biomechanical analysis of different techniques. Hernia. 2007;11(2):139–45.

49. Negro P, Basile F, Brescia A, et al. Open tension-free Lichtenstein repair of inguinal hernia: use of fibrin glue versus sutures for mesh fixation. Hernia. 2011;15(1):7–14.

50. Chastan P. Tension free open inguinal hernia repair using an innovative self gripping semi-resorbable mesh. J Minim Access Surg. 2006;2(3):139–43.

51. Lichtenstein IL. Herniorrhaphy. A personal experience with 6,321 cases. Am J Surg. 1987;153(6):553–9.

52. Lichtenstein IL, Shulman AG, Amid PK, Montllor MM. The tension-free hernioplasty. Am J Surg. 1989;157(2):188–93.

53. Peacock EE. Here we are: behind again! Am J Surg. 1989; 157(2):187.

54. Amid PK, Shulman AG, Lichtenstein IL. Critical scrutiny of the open "tension-free" hernioplasty. Am J Surg. 1993;165(3):369–71.

55. Shulman AG, Amid PK, Lichtenstein IL. The safety of mesh repair for primary inguinal hernias: results of 3,019 operations from five diverse surgical sources. Am J Surg. 1992;58(4):255–7.

56. Shulman AG, Amid PK, Lichtenstein IL. Returning to work after herniorrhaphy. BMJ. 1994;309(6949):216–7.

57. Shulman AG, Amid PK, Lichtenstein IL. A survey of non-expert surgeons using the open tension-free mesh patch repair for primary inguinal hernias. Int Surg. 1995;80(1):35–6.

58. Davies N, Thomas M, McIlroy B, Kingsnorth AN. Early results with the Lichtenstein tension-free hernia repair. Br J Surg. 1994;81(10):1478–9.

59. Kark AE, Kurzer M, Waters KJ. Tension-free mesh hernia repair: review of 1098 cases using local anaesthesia in a day unit. Ann R Coll Surg Engl. 1995;77(4):299–304.

60. Rutten P, Ledecq M, Hoebeke Y, Roeland A, Van den Oever R, Croes L. Primary inguinal hernia: Lichtenstein's ambulatory hernioplasty: early clinical results and economic implications. Study of the initial 130 surgical cases. Acta Chir Belg. 1992; 92(4):168–71.

61. Kux M, Fuchsjager N, Feichter A. Lichtenstein patch versus Shouldice technique in primary inguinal hernia with a high risk of recurrence. Chirurg. 1994;65(1):59–62.

62. Mesh compared with non-mesh methods of open groin hernia repair: systematic review of randomized controlled trials. Br J Surg. 2000;87(7):854–9.

63. Neumayer L, Giobbie-Hurder A, Jonasson O, et al. Open mesh versus laparoscopic mesh repair of inguinal hernia. N Engl J Med. 2004;350(18):1819–27.

64. Simons MP, Aufenacker T, Bay-Nielsen M, et al. European Hernia Society guidelines on the treatment of inguinal hernia in adult patients. Hernia. 2009;13(4):343–403.

65. Robbins AW, Rutkow IM. The mesh-plug hernioplasty. Surg Clin North Am. 1993;73(3):501–12.

66. Rutkow IM, Robbins AW. Mesh plug hernia repair: a follow-up report. Surgery. 1995;117(5):597–8.

67. Rutkow IM, Robbins AW. [Hernioplasty with mesh implant]. Chirurg. 1997;68(10):970–6.

68. Marre P, Damas JM, Penchet A, Pelissier EP. [Treatment of inguinal hernia in the adult: results of tension-free procedures]. Ann Chir. 2001;126(7):644–8.

69. Pelissier EP, Marre P. [The use of a plug in inguinal hernia]. J Chir (Paris). 1998;135(5):223–7.

70. Kingsnorth AN, Porter CS, Bennett DH, Walker AJ, Hyland ME, Sodergren S. Lichtenstein patch or Perfix plug-and-patch in inguinal hernia: a prospective double-blind randomized controlled trial of short-term outcome. Surgery. 2000;127(3):276–83.

71. LeBlanc KA. Complications associated with the plug-and-patch method of inguinal herniorrhaphy. Hernia. 2001;5(3):135–8.

72. Amid PK. Classification of biomaterials and their related complications in abdominal wall hernia surgery. Hernia. 1997;1:15–21.

73. Jeans S, Williams GL, Stephenson BM. Migration after open mesh plug inguinal hernioplasty: a review of the literature. Am Surg. 2007;73(3):207–9.

74. Stout CL, Foret A, Christie DB, Mullis E. Small bowel volvulus caused by migrating mesh plug. Am Surg. 2007;73(8):796–7.

75. Chen MJ, Tian YF. Intraperitoneal migration of a mesh plug with a small intestinal perforation: report of a case. Surg Today. 2010; 40(6):566–8.

76. Chuback JA, Singh RS, Sills C, Dick LS. Small bowel obstruction resulting from mesh plug migration after open inguinal hernia repair. Surgery. 2000;127(4):475–6.

77. Liang X, Cai XJ, Yu H, Wang YF. Strangulated bowel obstruction resulting from mesh plug migration after open inguinal hernioplasty: case report. Chin Med J (Engl). 2008;121(2):183–4.

78. Moorman ML, Price PD. Migrating mesh plug: complication of a well-established hernia repair technique. Am Surg. 2004;70(4): 298–9.

79. Murphy JW, Misra DC, Silverglide B. Sigmoid colonic fistula secondary to Perfix-plug, left inguinal hernia repair. Hernia. 2006;10(5):436–8.

80. Rettenmaier MA, Heinemann S, Truong H, Micha JP, Brown III JV, Goldstein BH. Marlex mesh mimicking an adnexal malignancy. Hernia. 2009;13(2):221–3.

81. Armstrong T. Randomized trial comparing the Prolene Hernia System, mesh plug repair and Lichtenstein method for open inguinal hernia repair (Br J Surg 2005; 92: 33-38). Br J Surg. 2005; 92(4):493.

82. Frey DM, Wildisen A, Hamel CT, Zuber M, Oertli D, Metzger J. Randomized clinical trial of Lichtenstein's operation versus mesh plug for inguinal hernia repair. Br J Surg. 2007;94(1):36–41.

83. Nienhuijs SW, van Oort I, Keemers-Gels ME, Strobbe LJ, Rosman C. Randomized trial comparing the Prolene Hernia System, mesh plug repair and Lichtenstein method for open inguinal hernia repair. Br J Surg. 2005;92(1):33–8.

84. Dalenbäck J, Andersson C, Anesten B, Björck S, Eklund S, Magnusson O, et al. Prolene Hernia System, Lichtenstein mesh and plug-and-patch for primary inguinal hernia repair: 3-year outcome of a prospective randomised controlled trial. The BOOP

study: bi-layer and connector, on-lay, and on-lay with plug for inguinal hernia repair. Hernia. 2009;13(2):121–9; discussion 231. Epub 2008 Nov 13.

85. Nixon SJ, Jawaid H. Recurrence after inguinal hernia repair at ten years by open darn, open mesh and TEP–no advantage with mesh. Surgeon. 2009;7(2):71–4.

86. Lau H. Endoscopic totally extraperitoneal inguinal hernioplasty for recurrence after open repair. ANZ J Surg. 2004;74(10):877–80.

87. Glassow F. Inguinal hernia in the female. Surg Gynecol Obstet. 1963;116:701–4.

88. Glassow F. An evaluation of the strength of the posterior wall of the inguinal canal in women. Br J Surg. 1973;60(5):342–4.

89. Liem MS, van der Graaf Y, Zwart RC, Geurts I, van Vroonhoven TJ. Risk factors for inguinal hernia in women: a case-control study. The Coala Trial Group. Am J Epidemiol. 1997;146(9):721–6.

90. Buch KE, Tabrizian P, Divino CM. Management of hernias in pregnancy. J Am Coll Surg. 2008;207(4):539–42.

91. Griffin KJ, Harris S, Tang TY, Skelton N, Reed JB, Harris AM. Incidence of contralateral occult inguinal hernia found at the time of laparoscopic trans-abdominal pre-peritoneal (TAPP) repair. Hernia. 2010;14(4):345–9.

92. Serpell JW, Johnson CD, Jarrett PE. A prospective study of bilateral inguinal hernia repair. Ann R Coll Surg Engl. 1990;72(5):299–303.

93. Amid PK, Shulman AG, Lichtenstein IL. Simultaneous repair of bilateral inguinal hernias under local anesthesia. Ann Surg. 1996;223(3):249–52.

94. Sarli L, Iusco DR, Sansebastiano G, Costi R. Simultaneous repair of bilateral inguinal hernias: a prospective, randomized study of open, tension-free versus laparoscopic approach. Surg Laparosc Endosc Percutan Tech. 2001;11(4):262–7.

95. National Institute for Clinical Excellence: Technology Appraisal Guidance No. 18. Guidance on the use of laparoscopic surgery for inguinal hernia. London, UK.

96. Gilbert AI. Simultaneous repair of bilateral groin hernias using local anaesthesia. Hernia. 2005;9(4):401.

97. Kark AE, Belsham PA, Kurzer MN. Simultaneous repair of bilateral groin hernias using local anaesthesia: a review of 199 cases with a five-year follow-up. Hernia. 2005;9(2):131–3.

98. Kald A, Fridsten S, Nordin P, Nilsson E. Outcome of repair of bilateral groin hernias: a prospective evaluation of 1,487 patients. Eur J Surg. 2002;168(3):150–3.

99. Tocchi A, Liotta G, Mazzoni G, Lepre L, Costa G, Miccini M. [Anterior approach and simultaneous tension-free repair of bilateral inguinal hernia under local anesthesia]. G Chir. 1999;20(10): 429–32.

100. Celdran A, Seiz A. Simultaneous repair of bilateral inguinal hernias under local anesthesia. Ann Surg. 1997;226(1):113–4.

101. Amid PK, Shulman AG, Lichtenstein IL. Simultaneous repair of bilateral inguinal hernias under local anesthesia. Ann Surg. 1996;223(3):249–52.

102. Miller AR, van Heerden JA, Naessens JM, O'Brien PC. Simultaneous bilateral hernia repair. A case against conventional wisdom. Ann Surg. 1991;213(3):272–6.

103. Stott MA, Sutton R, Royle GT. Bilateral inguinal hernias: simultaneous or sequential repair? Postgrad Med J. 1988;64(751):375–8.

104. Halsted WS. The radical cure of hernia. Bull Johns Hopkins Hosp. 1889;1:12–3.

105. Madden JL, Hakim S, Agorogiannis AB. The anatomy and repair of inguinal hernias. Surg Clin North Am. 1971;51:1269–92.

106. Ferguson AH. Oblique inguinal hernia. Typic operation for its radical cure. J Am Med Assoc. 1899;33:6–14.

107. Andrews WE. Imbrication of lap joint method: a plastic operation for hernia. Chic Med Rec. 1895;9:67–77.

108. Halsted WS. The operative treatment of hernia. Am J Med Sci. 1895;110:13–7.

109. Fallis LS. Direct inguinal herniation. Ann Surg. 1938;107:572.

110. Zimmerman LM, Laufman H. Sliding hernia. Surg Gynecol Obstet. 1942;75:76–8.

111. Reinhoff Jr WF. The use of the rectus fascia for closure of the lower or critical angle of the wound in the repair of inguinal hernia. Surgery. 1940;8:326–39.

112. Tanner NC. A slide operation for inguinal and femoral hernia. Br J Surg. 1942;29:285–9.

113. Ferzli GS, Massad A, Albed P. Extraperitoneal endoscopic inguinal hernia repair. J Laparoendosc Surg. 1992;2:281–5.

114. Griffith CA. Inguinal hernia: an anatomical surgical correlation. Surg Clin North Am. 1959;39:531–56.

115. Lichtenstein IL. Hernia repair without disability. St Louis: C.V. Mosby; 1970.

116. Palumbo LT, Sharp WS. Primary inguinal hernioplasty in the adult. Surg Clin North Am. 1971;51:1293–308.

117. Lotheissen G. Zur Radikaloperation der Schenkel-hernien. Centralblatt für Chirurgie. 1898;21:548–9.

118. McVay CB, Anson BJ. Inguinal and femoral hernioplasty. Surg Gynecol Obstet. 1949;88:473–85.

119. Cheatle GL. An operation for radical cure of inguinal and femoral hernia. Br Med J. 1920;2:68–9.

120. Henry AK. Operation for femoral hernia by a midline extraperitoneal approach: with a preliminary note on the use of this route for reducible inguinal hernia. Lancet. 1936;1:531–3.

121. Musgrove JE, McReady FJ. The Henry approach to femoral hernia. Surgery. 1949;26:608–11.

122. Mikkelsen WP, Berne CJ. Femoral hernioplasty: suprapubic extraperitoneal (Cheatle–Henry) approach. Surgery. 1954;35:743–8.

123. Stoppa R, Warlaumont CR, Verhaeghe PJ, Odimba BKFE, Henry X. Comment, pourquoi, quand utiliser les prostheses de tulle de Dacron pour traiter les hernies et les eventrations. Chirurgie. 1982;108:570–5.

124. Condon RE, Nyhus LM. Complications of groin hernia and of hernia repair. Surg Clin North Am. 1971;51:1325–36.

125. Nyhus LM, Condon RE, Harkins HN. Clinical experiences with pre-peritoneal hernial repair for all types of hernia of the groin. Am J Surg. 1960;100:234–44.

126. Read RC. Attenuation of the rectus sheath in inguinal herniation. Am J Surg. 1970;120:610–4.

127. Rignault DP. Properitoneal prosthetic inguinal hernioplasty through a Pfannenstiel approach. Surg Gynecol Obstet. 1986;163:465–8.

128. Paillier JL, Baranger B, Darrieu H, Schill H, Neveux Y. Clinical analysis of expanded PTFE in the treatment of recurrent and complex groin hernias. Postgrad Med J. 1992;4:168–70.

129. Koontz AR. Hernia. New York: Appleton; 1963.

130. Usher FC. Further observations on the use of Marlex mesh. A new technique for the repair of inguinal hernias. Am Surg. 1959;25:792–5.

131. Trabucco EE, Trabucco AF. Flat plugs and mesh hernioplasty in the inguinal box: description of the surgical technique. Hernia. 1998;2:133–8.

132. Valenti G, Capnano G, Testa A, Barletta N. Dynamic self regulating prosthesis (protesi autoregolantesi dinamica—PAD): a new technique in the treatment of inguinal hernias. Hernia. 1999;3:5–9.

133. Corcione F, Cristinzio G, Maresca M, Cascone U, Titolo G, Califano G. Primary inguinal hernia: the held-in mesh repair. Hernia. 1997;1:37–40.

134. Bendavid R. New techniques in hernia repair. World J Surg. 1989;13:522–31.

135. Gilbert AI. Sutureless repair of inguinal hernia. Am J Surg. 1992;163:331–5.

136. Gilbert AI, Graham MF. Symposium on the management of inguinal hernias. 5. Sutureless technique: second version. Can J Surg. 1997;40:209–12.

137. Ger R, Monroe K, Duvivier R, Mishrick A. Management of indirect hernias by laparoscopic closure of the neck of the sac. Am J Surg. 1990;159:371–3.

138. Corbitt JD. Laparoscopic herniorraphy. Surg Laparosc Endosc. 1991;1:23–5.

Martin Kurzer

Introduction

The open preperitoneal mesh repair of groin hernia places nonabsorbable mesh in a bloodless plane that lies outside the peritoneal cavity, between the transversalis fascia and the anterior abdominal wall, in the region of what is known as the myopectineal orifice (MPO) (see below). This is the same space that is developed during laparoscopic repair of a groin hernia. None of the open preperitoneal repairs enter the peritoneal cavity, which means they are in effect open versions of a TEP (totally extraperitoneal) laparoscopic repair, with access to this space gained via an abdominal incision rather than a laparoscope.

Some surgeons would say that in the current era of laparoscopic surgery, an open preperitoneal repair is now only of historical interest. How far this is true, I will let the reader judge. I hope to show that it still does have indications and is a procedure and a skill that should be in the "toolkit" of every surgeon who declares a special interest in hernia surgery.

In this chapter I will review the history and development of this approach, describe the variations, and outline the advantages and indications of each. I will also briefly outline the operative techniques, although more detailed descriptions by their developers are available in the original papers and other textbooks (all well worth reading in the original), and finally will describe the reported results.

The plane in which the mesh lies is outside (extraperitoneal) or in front of (preperitoneal) the peritoneal cavity. George Wantz, and other American surgeons, also used the term "properitoneal."

M. Kurzer (✉)
Department of Surgery, British Hernia Centre,
London, UK
e-mail: m.kurzer@me.com

History

The preperitoneal approach to the groin is historically associated with the names of Annandale, Cheatle, and Henry, who all recognized the excellent access afforded to the posterior aspect of the abdominal wall in the region of the inguinal canal [1, 2]. The interested reader might like to refer to Raymond Read's comprehensive review in a recent textbook [3]. It was seen as an ideal method of dealing with incarcerated or strangulated groin hernias, and although the access and views that it afforded of the posterior aspect of the inguinal canal and femoral region ("The Myopectineal Orifice"—see below) were excellent, it never gained wide acceptance. It is however still regarded by experienced surgeons as the procedure of choice for strangulated femoral hernia.

Nyhus and Read in the USA, and Rives and Stoppa in France, became interested in the preperitoneal approach for recurrent and complex groin hernias in the late 1950s and early 1960s [4–7]. They were all dissatisfied with the results obtained for recurrent hernias when operating through the previous incision and reopening a scarred inguinal canal. In the case of multi-recurrent hernias, often with extensive scarring and tissue loss, and before the introduction of modern meshes, effecting a good long-term repair with a conventional approach was well nigh impossible. Recurrence rates could be well over 50%, and many multi-recurrent hernias were probably deemed "inoperable." In addition, the likelihood of testicular atrophy was high [8].

Using a preperitoneal approach through a transverse lower quadrant abdominal incision allowed Nyhus and his colleagues access to the preperitoneal space, avoiding scar tissue from previous surgery and allowing them to operate in a virtually virgin field. They found that the dissection was straightforward and the defect or defects were easily seen and assessed. However, despite the advantage of easy access and good visualization, Nyhus found that the failure rate (hernia recurrence) was still high—as much as 30%—if the margins of the defect were sutured. He therefore added what he termed a "prosthetic mesh buttress" attached inferiorly to

A.N. Kingsnorth and K.A. LeBlanc (eds.), *Management of Abdominal Hernias*,
DOI 10.1007/978-1-84882-877-3_15, © Springer Science+Business Media London 2013

the superior pubic ramus (Cooper's ligament) in order to "reinforce" his sutured repair. The incidence of re-recurrence dropped dramatically. "There were no re-recurrences after we adopted the routine placement of the prosthetic mesh buttress to bolster the anatomic repair" and this technique rapidly became his routine for virtually all cases. He published a 38-year review of his work in 1993 [9], describing the technique again, and could not understand why general surgeons refused to adopt it. He wrote, "My associates and I were perplexed about the failure of this method to flourish."

At about this time surgeons in France, Rives in Reims [6], and Stoppa in Amiens [7], had also started to use a preperitoneal method for complex, recurrent groin hernias, but from the outset, they used mesh in every case. Rives used a trans-inguinal approach, which meant that with recurrent hernias, he still had to operate through the scar tissue from previous surgery. In addition in the Rives technique, the mesh was cut and shaped in a complex fashion and sutured inferiorly to Cooper's ligament [6]. Other surgeons more recently have also described trans-inguinal techniques for preperitoneal mesh placement with the theoretical advantage of allowing preperitoneal mesh placement under local anesthetic [10, 11].

Stoppa developed his method to deal with complex bilateral hernias, and he accessed the preperitoneal space through a lower midline incision in order to avoid reoperating through scar tissue. Stoppa's genius was in proposing the radical step that no attempt should be made to close the actual defect, thus avoiding any tension. Rignault put it well—"The idea of interposing a large surface of prosthetic mesh between the peritoneum and the deficient inguinal wall instead of 'mending' the defect, represents a radical departure from previous methods of hernia repair…. The mesh must be much larger than the defect, since it is not sutured in place and only intra-abdominal pressure maintains it in place over the hernia defect" [12]. This concept has subsequently been vindicated and is of course now standard practice in laparoscopic repair.

George Wantz in the USA was dissatisfied with what he termed the "properitoneal patch hernioplasty" that had been developed by Raymond Read—a prosthesis that was just sutured to the edges of the defect. He was however impressed with the Stoppa technique and agreed with Stoppa that it was much more logical to use a large piece of mesh covering the whole of the MPO with a wide overlap and no closure of the defect. He modified the bilateral procedure for unilateral recurrent hernias using the Nyhus transverse lower quadrant incision and an innovative way of anchoring the mesh, "hanging" it from above like a sheet on a washing line (see Fig. 15.16). Stoppa had called the procedure "La Grande Prothese Reinforce de Sac Visceral," and this was translated verbatim by Wantz in his seminal article [13] as Giant Prosthetic Reinforcement of the Visceral Sac. Hence, the operation is also known, somewhat cryptically, as GPRVS.

Both the unilateral (Wantz) and bilateral (Stoppa) techniques were particularly well suited to complex and multi-

recurrent defects. Like the Nyhus procedure, they were never widely adopted, possibly because of general surgeons' unfamiliarity with, and reluctance to venture into, the preperitoneal space. Of course, the modern era of laparoscopic surgery started at about this time, and it is interesting to observe that surgeons now seem to have no concerns about entering this space with a laparoscope.

Indeed, the introduction of laparoscopic techniques resulted in a reevaluation of the need for large incisions to position the mesh, and new open methods were developed by two surgeons Kugel and Ugahary to allow access to the preperitoneal space through very small incisions. The intention was to combine the short learning curve and economic advantages of the open approach with the potential for rapid recovery with minimal access surgery [14, 15].

The Myopectineal Orifice

All preperitoneal groin hernia repair are based on the concept of the MPO, first described by Henri Fruchaud, a French anatomist and surgeon [16] who defined groin hernias as "any hernia of the inguino-femoral region that results from failure of the transversalis fascia to retain the peritoneum in the weak area of the groin known as the myopectineal orifice." The borders of the MPO are the internal oblique muscle superiorly, the iliopsoas laterally, the rectus muscle medially, and the superior pubic ramus inferiorly (Figs. 15.1 and 15.2). This bony muscular framework is divided in two by the inguinal ligament, traversed by the spermatic cord above and the femoral vessels below.

To quote George Wantz—"…it [the myopectineal orifice] is bridged in a drumlike fashion by the transversalis fascia only… Protrusion of a peritoneal sac through the myopectineal orifice defines a hernia. Failure of the transversalis fascia to retain the peritoneum then becomes the fundamental cause of all hernias of the groin" [17]. In a preperitoneal prosthetic repair (open or laparoscopic), the prosthesis is sandwiched between the peritoneum and the anterior abdominal wall and substitutes for the defective or weakened transversalis fascia. It is strengthened later by an ingrowth of connective tissue. The peritoneum can therefore no longer push through the MPO; it is effectively held in—like a balloon in a string bag—and formal repair of the MPO, that is, closure of the defect, is not necessary.

Indications for the Open Preperitoneal Technique

1. Recurrent or multiple recurrent groin hernias following a previous open, anterior repair. Operating in the unscarred, virgin preperitoneal plane is simpler and safer, and all potential defects can be inspected.
2. Combination groin hernias where there are multiple defects, for instance, combinations of pre-vascular,

Fig. 15.1 Fruchaud's myopectineal orifice (MPO). *Right side*, anterior view

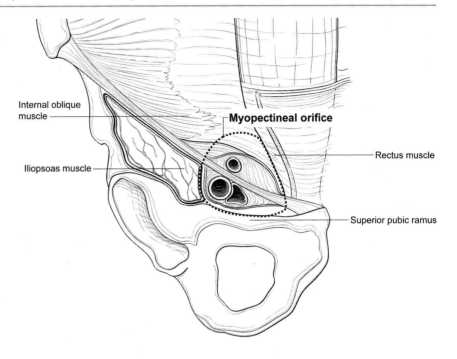

Internal oblique muscle

Myopectineal orifice

Rectus muscle

Iliopsoas muscle

Superior pubic ramus

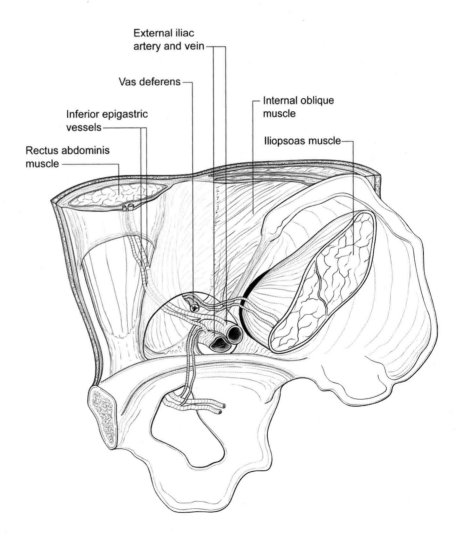

External iliac artery and vein

Vas deferens

Inferior epigastric vessels

Rectus abdominis muscle

Internal oblique muscle

Iliopsoas muscle

Fig. 15.2 Fruchaud's MPO. *Right side*, posterior view

femoral, indirect and direct inguinal, and low Spigelian hernias. All potential defects can be inspected.

3. Giant inguino-scrotal hernias, either unilateral or bilateral, where replacement of abdominal contents through a groin incision alone would be technically difficult. "Pulling" the sac contents back from behind through the defect is simpler and safer than "pushing" from the front.

4. Incisional hernia after, for example, a Pfannenstiel incisions or the rare incisional hernia through the lateral rectus sheath (acquired Spigelian hernia).

5. Hernias associated with connective tissue disorders (Ehlers-Danlos and Marfan's syndrome) where multiple points of weakness may be present.

The Operations

There are essentially five open preperitoneal operations in current use:

1. Bilateral Stoppa procedure
2. Unilateral Wantz procedure
3. Trans-inguinal [6, 18]
4. Kugel procedure [14]
5. Ugahary procedure [15]

They can be grouped as standard incision repairs, Stoppa (bilateral) and Wantz (unilateral); small incision methods, Kugel or Ugahary; and trans-inguinal, Rives and Schumpelik. Apart from the possibility of operating under local anesthesia, the trans-inguinal approach seems to offer no other benefit.

Advantages of a Preperitoneal Approach

The advantages of a preperitoneal approach for recurrent groin hernia are:

(a) Avoiding reoperating through scarred distorted anatomy
(b) Avoiding the risk of damage to the testicular vessels
(c) Permitting inspection of all potential groin hernia sites

The trans-inguinal approach has been advocated by some because of a claimed advantage in terms of post-op pain if mesh is placed in the preperitoneal space. It seems unnecessarily complex for primary hernias and by reopening the inguinal canal, still involves a dissection through scar tissue in recurrent hernias. It therefore loses out on (a) and (b) and confers no real advantage. It has not been widely adopted and will not be described here in detail.

The Kugel and Ugahary operations avoid the scar tissue from previous surgery; but they are carried out through small incisions and do not allow easy visual inspection of the whole area. Only the Stoppa and Wantz procedures combine all three advantages.

Operative Techniques of Open Preperitoneal Repair

Preoperative Preparation

This is standard for all methods. The patient should pass urine immediately preoperatively before coming to the operating room (OR). Some advocate routine urinary catheterization, though this has its own set of complications and I have never found it to be necessary. Venous thromboembolism (VTE) prophylaxis should be used and a single-shot broad-spectrum intravenous antibiotic given intravenously on induction of anesthesia, both according to up-to-date local guidelines. The operating table is tilted 20–30° head down (Trendelenburg position) in order to allow the intra-abdominal contents to fall away from the region of the hernia.

Choice of Anesthesia

In practice general anesthesia is the method of choice for the majority of patients undergoing a Stoppa or Wantz procedure because of the requirement for a relaxed abdominal wall. Regional block (spinal or epidural anesthesia) is an alternative but is likely to result in a high incidence of urinary retention. Local anesthesia (LA) is not really feasible for the Wantz procedure (although Wantz said it was—personal communication) unless the operator is particularly experienced and the patient is slim and cooperative. Both Kugel and Ugahary maintained that their procedures could easily be performed under local anesthesia.

Operative Technique: Stoppa and Wantz

The Bilateral Stoppa Operation
Incision. Stoppa saw little merit in a Pfannenstiel incision [19] and used a lower midline incision routinely. He avoided the problem of subsequent incisional hernia by bringing the mesh up high behind the incision. However, our experience and that of others [11, 20] is that a Pfannenstiel incision gives excellent access, less postoperative discomfort, and a better cosmetic result (Fig. 15.3).

The Pfannenstiel incision is transverse and curvilinear and is made 2 cm above the pubis. After deepening through subcutaneous fat, incise the rectus sheath in a V, with the point of the V 2 cm above the pubis, and raise the sheath off the rectus muscle with a combination of sharp and gentle blunt dissection.

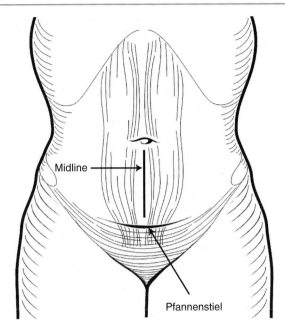

Fig. 15.3 Access to the preperitoneal space through a vertical or Pfannenstiel incision

Identify the midline and gently separate the two rectus muscles. Break through the transversalis fascia and you are in preperitoneal or extravesical fat. Gentle blunt dissection will easily open the spaces behind the pubis (cave of Retzius) and laterally each side of the midline (space of Bogros). Open these spaces widely, down to the superior pubic ramus, below the spermatic cord and pedicle of an indirect hernia sac (if present), and over (above) the iliac vessels. It is usually easier to do this from the opposite side of the patient (Fig. 15.4). Continue the dissection laterally to open up the whole area. At this stage a direct hernia will have reduced easily. There is no need to suture direct defects, but the dead space of a large direct sac can be reduced by withdrawing (inverting) the transversalis fascia and suturing it to the abdominal wall.

Dealing with the Spermatic Cord: "Parietalization"

This involves separating the spermatic cord from that part of the visceral peritoneum that lies against the anterior abdominal wall in the region of the MPO, so that the mesh can be interposed (Fig. 15.5). This separation is of course now a standard maneuver in laparoscopic repair, but a number of earlier descriptions described splitting and then resuturing the mesh to allow passage of the spermatic cord. This is a less elegant technique and one more prone to lead to recurrence. As the dissection proceeds you will see the testicular vessels and the vas diverge, the former passing laterally and the latter passing medially giving a characteristic triangular appearance (Fig. 15.6).

Insertion of the Mesh

Stoppa used a chevron-shaped prosthesis (Fig. 15.7) and a complex arrangement of eight long clamps to insert the mesh (Fig. 15.8), which was held by only one single midline suture (Fig. 15.9). It was important to cleave this space widely because wrinkling or folding of the mesh would occur if an insufficient space had been prepared. Figure 15.10 shows an idealized final mesh position in the bilateral operation. There is however a real risk of mesh displacement in the early postoperative period, and most surgeons who used this technique would anchor the prosthesis at strategic points (Fig. 15.11). An alternative, which I have found easier than the single large prosthesis, is to use two separate meshes, each 15 cm × 15 cm, attached inferiorly at the pectineal ligament, effectively a Wantz operation on each side (see Wantz technique below).

The Unilateral Wantz Operation

This has been clearly described elsewhere in detail by Wantz [13, 17]. Make a transverse incision in the groin (higher than a standard open inguinal approach) well above the deep ring (Fig. 15.12). Incise the rectus sheath transversely, extend onto the external oblique aponeurosis, and retract the rectus muscle medially and elevate it. There is no posterior rectus sheath at this level, and you should see the inferior epigastric vessels. It is important to gently elevate these vessels with the muscle so that you are beneath them at this stage. Preserve them if you can, though they can be divided with impunity if in the way (Fig. 15.13). Break through the transversalis fascia taking care not to open the peritoneum, and widely cleave the preperitoneal space as in the bilateral operation (Fig. 15.14). Parietalize the spermatic cord by separating it from the visceral peritoneum and an indirect sac if present. Wantz used a quadrangular-shaped prosthesis, with an extended inferolateral corner to ensure complete cover of the myopectinal orifice (Fig. 15.15). He had experienced the occasional lateral re-recurrence with his original rectangular shape.

Wantz secured the upper border prosthesis to the anterior abdominal wall with three sutures place at 3 cm intervals above the incision and no attachment inferiorly (Fig. 15.16). The inferior border of the mesh was then passed down below and behind the peritoneum with three long clamps, at points 4, 5, and 6, which grasp the two lower corners and center of the lower border (Figs. 15.17 and 15.18). This is a tricky maneuver, and as with the bilateral procedure, wrinkling or folding of the mesh will occur if an insufficient space has been prepared.

I have found that securing the mesh superiorly is difficult, and my colleagues and I had four early recurrences of direct hernias, where the inferomedial corner of the mesh had moved upward (point D in Fig. 15.19) [19]. We now secure the inferomedial corner to the back

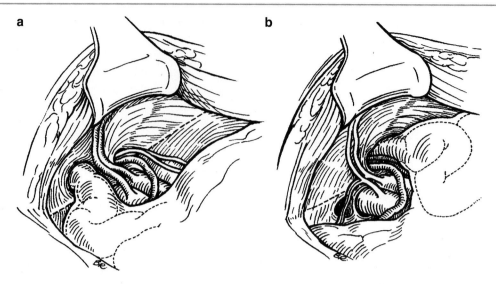

Fig. 15.4 (**a, b**) Preperitoneal view of the right groin (MPO), from the left side of the patient, showing a right indirect inguinal hernia (lateral to the inferior epigastric vessels) prior to its reduction, and note the femoral canal medial to the femoral vein (from Stoppa [36], with permission)

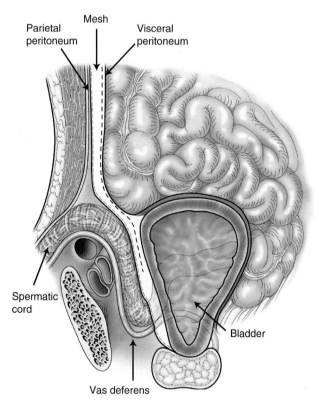

Fig. 15.5 Parasagittal section to demonstrate the mesh in the extraperitoneal or preperitoneal space, lying between the parietal peritoneum and spermatic cord on one side and the visceral peritoneum and bladder on the other

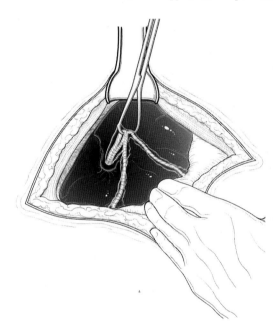

Fig. 15.6 The triangular appearance of the completed dissection on the right side, showing the vas deferens passing medially, testicular vessels passing laterally, and peritoneum. When released, the elements of the cord will fall against the parietal pelvic wall (parietalization)

Choice of Prosthesis

Both Stoppa and Wantz advocated Mersilene (polyester) (*trademark*) mesh claiming that its flexibility allowed it to conform to the complex curvatures of the abdominal wall.

Wantz's criteria for an ideal prosthesis were:
- Flexibility or suppleness to allow it to curve to the shape of the abdominal wall
- "Graininess" to grip the peritoneum and prevent slippage early on

of the pubic bone, almost in the midline (point D in Fig. 15.20 and point 4 in Fig. 15.21), and place one or two sutures to attach the inferior border of the mesh to the superior pubic ramus (point E in Fig. 15.20 and point 5 in Fig. 15.21). The illustrations show the idealized final position of the mesh.

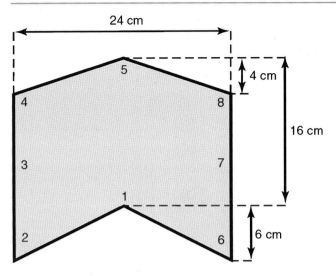

Fig. 15.7 The cardinal points of positioning of the clamps on the single bilateral prosthesis to aid in its insertion

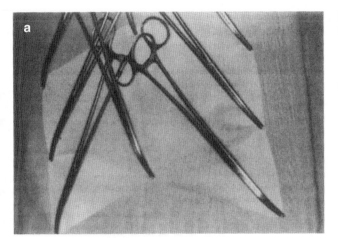

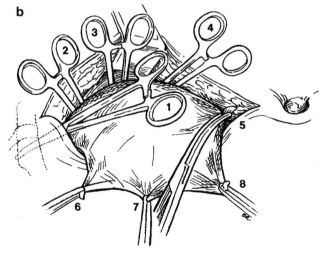

Fig. 15.8 (**a**) The chevron-shaped prosthesis is seized by eight long-curved clamps. (**b**) Operator view of the insertion of the bilateral mesh prosthesis, which is being pushed with clamps nos. 1–5. The numbers show the order in which the clamps have been used. Clamps nos. 6–8 will be used for the placement of the left part of the prosthesis. This is a complex maneuver, requiring the surgeon to have a good 3D appreciation of the space as well as a good assistant (from Stoppa [36], with permission)

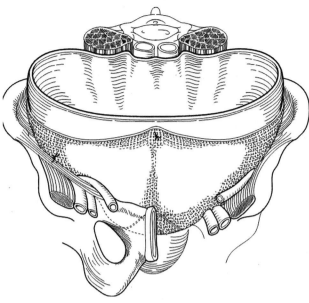

Fig. 15.9 Stoppa's recommended placement of the single suture to fixate the giant prosthesis

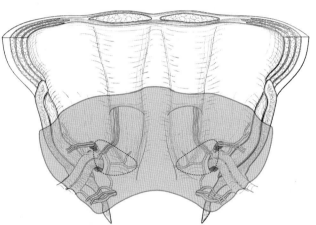

Fig. 15.10 The bilateral prosthesis in position, replacing the endopelvic transversalis fascia and extending far beyond the borders of both MPOs

- Reactive enough to induce a fibroblastic response to ensure rapid fixation

He thought polypropylene too rigid and inflexible, though this has not been our experience, nor that of the exponents of TEP lap repair who are happy with the newer "lightweight" polypropylene meshes.

Operative Technique (Kugel and Ugahary): Open "Minimal Access" Preperitoneal Placement of the Prosthesis

The phrase "open minimal access" might appear at first to be a contradiction in terms, but these two operations were designed specifically to allow access to the preperitoneal

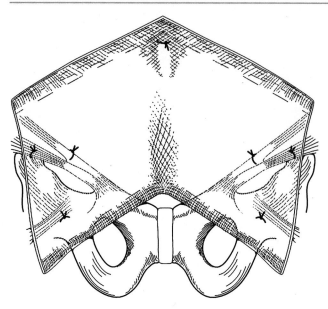

Fig. 15.11 Suture placement for fixation of the bilateral mesh

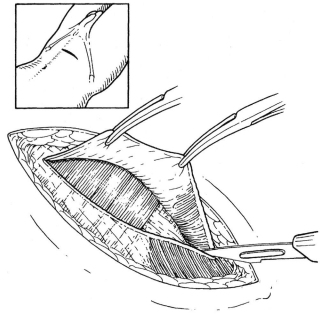

Fig. 15.12 Wantz unilateral procedure makes the transverse incision above the level of the deep inguinal ring, from the midline extending laterally. Incise the rectus sheath and extend laterally into the aponeurosis of the oblique abdominal muscles, and note the yellow fat marking the best entry point into the preperitoneal space

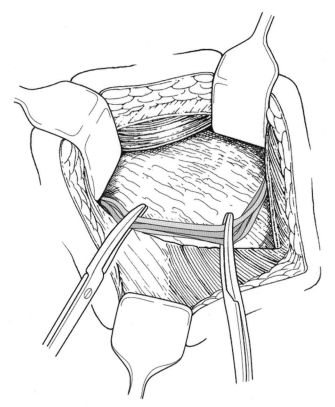

Fig. 15.13 The rectus muscles retracted medially and elevated to expose preperitoneal fat. This is below the arcuate line, so there is no posterior rectus sheath. The transversalis fascia has been incised, and the inferior epigastric vessels are about to be divided. This is not always necessary—they can be elevated and retracted medially with the rectus muscle

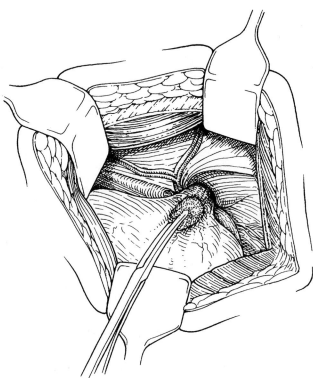

Fig. 15.14 "Teasing" an indirect hernia sac out of the abdominal wall defect

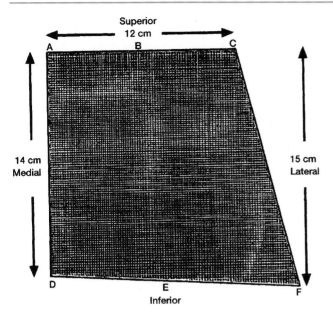

Fig. 15.15 Wantz procedure—trapezoid shape of the mesh to be inserted in preperitoneal space. The letters A–F illustrate the position of the mesh after placement

space through small incisions—perhaps 3–4 cm in length. Their developers maintained that these operations could be performed with local anesthesia, so that in theory, they offered the advantages of a preperitoneal inguinal hernia repair without the need for general anesthesia or expensive laparoscopic equipment. The plane in which the mesh was placed is the same as that used for the Wantz/Stoppa procedures (and for laparoscopic repair), that is, posterior to or below the epigastric vessels and the transversalis fascia. As with all preperitoneal methods, patients are tilted head down to move the intestines away from the lower abdomen and pelvis. With both repairs the location of the incision is critical to the performance of the procedure in an easy fashion. They are also both highly dependent on the surgeon's understanding of the local anatomy of the preperitoneal space in the inguinal area. They are certainly not procedures for the inexperienced trainee.

The Kugel Repair

Kugel designed a mesh patch that incorporated a memory recoil ring that allowed the patch to spring back open after being inserted through a small incision. A number of the larger patches (placed intraperitoneally and used for incisional hernia repair) were found to have faulty memory recoil rings and were recalled around 2005. A modified and improved device is currently in use.

Kugel made a 3-cm transverse, slightly oblique incision at the midpoint between the anterior superior iliac spine and the

pubic tubercle (Fig. 15.22). The external oblique aponeurosis is opened, and the abdominal muscles split in the line of their fibers. The preperitoneal space is entered by incision of the transversalis fascia in a vertical direction. The dissection should allow just enough free space to accommodate the prosthesis. The entrance is small so the space has to be developed with the use of either forceps or other instruments. The cord structures are separated from the peritoneum 3 cm above the internal ring to expose Cooper's ligament and the pubic bone, and great care has to be taken not to injure either the inferior epigastric or testicular vessels.

Having formed the correct size space, the operator's index finger is inserted into the slit that was on one side of the mesh and the prosthesis rolled onto the finger (Fig. 15.23). A malleable retractor is used to maintain the space created by the preperitoneal dissection while the mesh is inserted.

When properly placed, the patch should lie completely flat and open, parallel to the inguinal ligament and covering the entire inguinal floor and the femoral space (Fig. 15.24). A single absorbable suture fixes the lateral edge of the patch.

The Ugahary Operation

Ugahary has described his operation in detail elsewhere, with numerous technical tips [21], and I have summarized the essential steps below. The incision is made approximately 3 cm above and lateral to the internal ring (Fig. 15.25). Because of the location and direction of the incision, it has become known as the gridiron hernioplasty. As with the Kugel repair, the preperitoneal space is entered by a muscle-splitting dissection of the internal oblique and transversus abdominis muscles, followed by incision of the transversalis fascia in a transverse direction.

The space is developed using special long thin retractors, and the cord structures are separated from the peritoneum. A 10×15 cm prosthesis is tightly rolled around a 30-cm forcep with the side that will be facing the inguinal floor on the outside of the roll. The rolled mesh on the forceps is then inserted into the space with the very distal end placed behind the pubis (Fig. 15.26). The retractors are carefully removed, and one is then reinserted into the roll of the mesh. The second retractor is then used to unroll the mesh by a sweeping and rotating motion (Fig. 15.27). The two retractors are used in sequential fashion, one to hold the mesh in place while the other completes the flattening against the anterior abdominal wall in the region of the MPO. Finally, one absorbable suture is used to fix the lateral corner of the mesh to the transversus muscle. In theory the polypropylene mesh should then be lying exactly behind the MPO, similar to its position after a laparoscopic repair or the unilateral open repair of Wantz (Fig. 15.28).

Fig. 15.16 Arrange the mesh so it stretches transversely. Its width is cut equal to the distance between the midline and the anterior superior iliac spine minus 1 cm, and its length is made approximately equal to 12 cm. Wantz had an innovative way of attaching the mesh, drawing it into place underneath the rectus muscle and superior abdominal wall with three slowly absorbable sutures at 1, 2, and 3

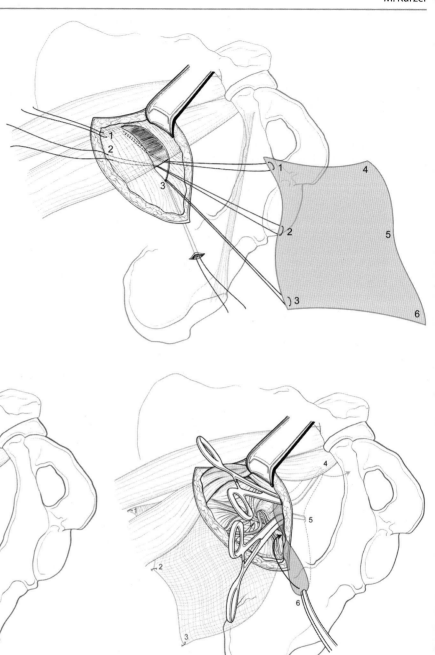

Fig. 15.17 The abdominal wall is retracted and the properitoneal space exposed. The superior portion of the prosthesis (1–3) is depicted indistinctly to illustrate its position after placement beneath the muscles of the abdomen in the preperitoneal space. Clamps nos. 4, 5, and 6 along the distal margins of the prosthesis are poised, ready to implant the mesh inferiorly

Fig. 15.18 Clamp no. 4 is placed medially deep into the space of Retzius in the midline and is steadied by an assistant. A very large curved or right-angled clamp helps keep point 4 at the midline. Next, clamp no. 5 positions the middle of the inferior edge deep into the pelvis, followed by clamp 6 pushing laterally. Again, a complex maneuver

Personal Comment (MK)

Both Kugel and Ugahary maintained that their respective procedures were easy to perform, and indeed in skilled hand they were.

As with most things in life, things are easy when you know how, and when proficiently carried out, these two operations did yield excellent results. But they required a detailed knowledge of the local anatomy and were unforgiving of technical errors. The correct plane had to be entered with the minimum of unnecessary dissection. Trying to control excess bleeding in a deep hole

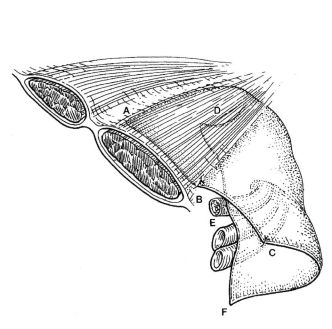

Fig. 15.19 Slightly different view of the position of the Wantz prosthesis. Points D, E, and F are equivalent to 4, 5, and 6 in this figure

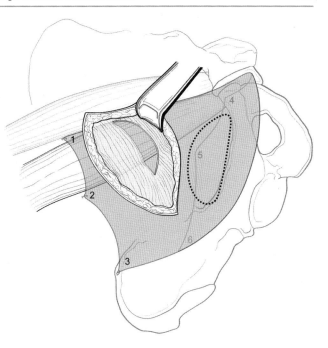

Fig. 15.20 Final position of the prosthesis in unilateral GPRVS. The prosthesis extends far beyond the borders of the dotted outline of the MPO

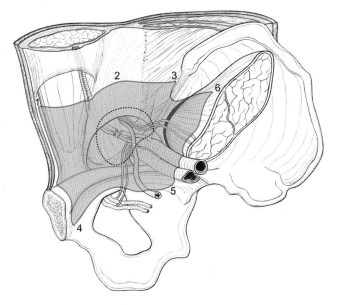

Fig. 15.21 View from within the pelvis of the final position of the prosthesis in unilateral GPRVS. This is essentially the same as the position of the mesh in laparoscopic repair, extending far beyond the borders of the MPO

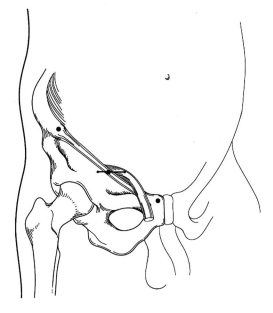

Fig. 15.22 Location of the small incision for the Kugel repair of inguinal hernia. The *left* and *right dots* denote the pubic tubercle and the anterior iliac spine. The incision is positioned between these two structures

through a small incision could be problematic. The presence of even a small hematoma was likely to prevent the mesh from sitting properly and would compromise the repair. The learning curve is possibly less than for laparoscopic repair, but most surgeons will still not wish to, or have the opportunity to, invest the time in attaining technical proficiency. The procedures have efficacy, but probably not much effectiveness, as can be seen from some of the results below, and in this era of laparoscopic surgery, one might question whether they have any use in the hands of anyone apart from their original developers.

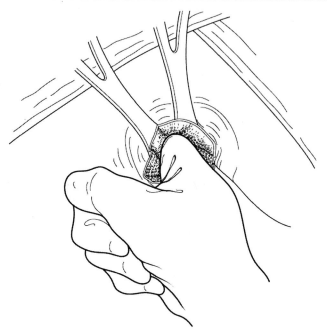

Fig. 15.23 Insertion of the patch is simplified by using a malleable retractor as a shoehorn

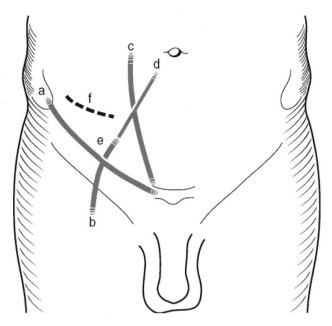

Fig. 15.25 The skin incision (*f*) for Ugahary's operation. Surface anatomy: (*a*) inguinal ligament, (*b*) femoral artery, (*c*) lateral border of the rectus muscle, (*d*) line perpendicular to the inguinal ligament from the femoral artery, and (*e*) the deep or internal ring

Results

Nyhus, reporting his preperitoneal approach and prosthetic buttress repair for recurrent hernia, assessed 203 operations in 195 patients [9]. Regional anesthesia was used in most patients, no perioperative antibiotics were given, and

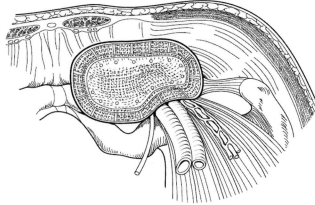

Fig. 15.24 Preperitoneal view showing final position of the Kugel patch (reprinted from Am J Surg. 1999;178:298–302 with permission)

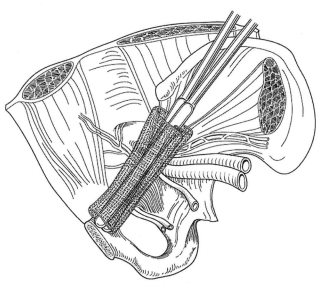

Fig. 15.26 Ugahary operation—insertion and positioning of the rolled up prosthesis

long-term follow-up was available for 115 hernias (56%) in 102 patients (52%) over a period of 6 months to 10 years. Eight patients had repeat recurrences at a mean of 30 months after repair, but only two of these (1.7% of those who followed up) have recurred after sutured repair supplemented with mesh buttress. The other six recurrences occurred in an earlier experience when no mesh buttress was being used. This was just before the start of the laparoscopic era, and the authors felt strongly that the preperitoneal approach for recurrent groin hernia with reinforcing mesh buttress should be the procedure of choice for all recurrent groin hernias.

Stoppa et al. published an early report of the GPRVS procedure in English in 1975 [22], and more detailed reports from the Amiens group appeared in 1984 and 1986 [23, 24]. The initial report was of 255 operated patients, with 218 (84.2%) having a completely uncomplicated postoperative course. The hematoma rate was 7.9%, and the local sepsis

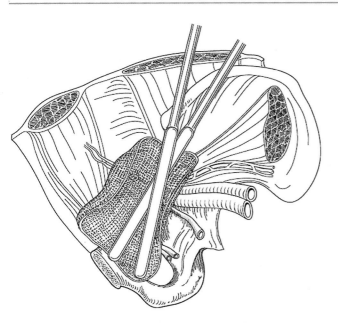

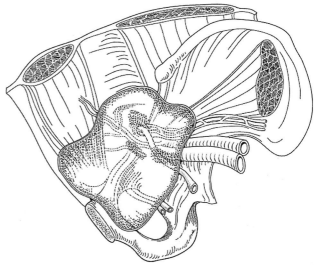

Fig. 15.28 Final position of the mesh

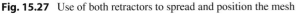

Fig. 15.27 Use of both retractors to spread and position the mesh

rate was 5.8%. These were excellent results, especially for that era, particularly when one realizes that many of these early patients were elderly or poor risk and had undergone multiple previous operations. Later results in a larger series, with a follow-up of 91.3% at 2–10 years, revealed a recurrence rate of 2.5%. These figures were probably an order of magnitude better than the general results obtained by general surgeons at that time. Stoppa's reported recurrence rate using this technique eventually fell to an amazing 1.4% [25]. In general it seemed that the recurrences tended to occur during the first postoperative year, indicating that the pattern of recurrence does not follow the same course as anterior repairs, and is likely to be related to technical problems [26]. Very few of the infections were deep and related to the prosthesis, and almost all resolved with antibiotics without the need for mesh removal. Rignault, utilizing a large piece of mesh without closure of hernial defects, reported similar results; during a 14-year period, 767 patients, of which 239 were recurrent, underwent preperitoneal prosthetic inguinal hernia repair with a 2% sepsis rate and a 1.2% recurrence rate [12]. Once again, most recurrences were seen within the first postoperative year and were related either to sepsis or to technical mistakes made by inexperienced surgeons. Wantz's results were equally impressive. An early series of 358 patients with recurrent hernias revealed a recurrence rate of 4.4% [13]. Wantz felt that most of the recurrences were related to technical problems and inadequately sized mesh, and modified these accordingly [17].

Other groups have reported similar results. Mozingo and colleagues treated 100 recurrent hernias in 84 men, with three re-recurrences occurring within 6 months of surgery at a follow-up of 6 months to 5 years. They reported few complications and no testicular complications [26]. Two randomized trials have compared laparoscopic with open preperitoneal mesh for bilateral [26] and a mixed group [27] of groin hernias and found no significant difference in short-term recurrence rates. Beets et al. [28] compared laparoscopic repair with open preperitoneal mesh for recurrent hernia in 75 patients with 150 hernias (24 primary and 126 recurrent) using Marlex mesh. Recurrence rates were 2% for open and 12% for laparoscopic, and the authors commented that, of the two, they found the open repair an easier procedure with a shorter learning curve. Kurzer [20] reported the results of its use in recurrent hernia only—101 consecutive patients with 114 recurrent inguinal hernias—and reassessed the patients 4 years postoperatively. There were five recurrences in total, all occurring within 6 months of surgery. Four of the recurrences were in the first 20 cases, prompting a modification of the technique. Hoffman [29] used the technique in 175 patients with 152 primary and 52 recurrent inguinal hernias. There was one recurrence, and wound complications occurred in 12 patients (5.9%). It is important however to carry out the operation correctly. One retrospective study of 112 patients found a recurrence rate of 32% [30]. In the main, virtually all studies of the open preperitoneal mesh repair have confirmed the short learning curve and excellent results of the open preperitoneal mesh repair.

Ugahary's gridiron operation has not been widely adopted, though the Kugel hernioplasty was supported by a number of recent publications from other surgical groups (see below). Ugahary himself reported on 427 hernia repairs in 364 patients operated over a 3-year period [21]. There were seven recurrences, though we are not told the length of follow-up, and four of the recurrences were technical problems occurring in the first week after surgery.

Kugel's own results were excellent. As originally reported, he had a recurrence rate of 0.62%, (five recurrences in 808 patients) though a later study gave an overall recurrence rate of 0.4% [14]. In all cases recurrence was due to the lower edge of the mesh lifting away from the posterior abdominal wall allowing the hernia to recur underneath the patch, all within the first 6 months. Because of this, the prosthesis was placed in a more posterolateral position. Other surgeons did adopt this procedure and maintained that it was a safe and effective operation, with short operative times, low complication rates, "minimal" post-op pain, and a rapid return to normal activities [31, 32]. Fenoglio reported a large retrospective series—a recurrence rate of 0.47% in 1,072 hernias with a follow-up of 2–47 months—and van Nieuwenhove's was a multicenter prospective study in 450 patients with a 1.9% recurrence at a mean follow-up of 18 months. The claimed advantages are a preperitoneal inguinal hernia repair without the need for general anesthesia or expensive laparoscopic equipment [33] and possibly less discomfort than the Lichtenstein repair [34].

The Ugahary procedure is however a technically demanding procedure, and one study of 355 patients with six surgeons revealed an overall re-recurrence rate of 18%, almost 30% for recurrent hernias, and an estimated learning curve of at least 36 cases [35]. The authors concluded, understandably, that the recurrence rate was "unacceptably high" and that the procedure "may not be suitable for repair of recurrent inguinal hernias or primary large direct inguinal hernias."

Conclusion

The open preperitoneal approach provides excellent access to, and views of, the MPO. It thus permits inspection of all potential groin hernia sites. It avoids reoperating through the distorted anatomy and scar tissue that are present after a failed anterior operation, and the risk of damage to the testicular vessels is minimized. Does it have a place in the laparoscopic era?

- The learning curve is probably shorter than for laparoscopic repair, and major vessel or visceral injury is less likely.
- It requires no expensive specialized equipment and therefore has significant economic advantages.
- It can be used in patients unfit for general anesthesia—Kugel or Ugahary.
- It remains arguably the best operation for strangulated femoral hernia.
- It is probably the best procedure for dealing with incarcerated recurrent hernias and large sliding inguinal hernias.

- It is probably the best procedure for repairing large recurrent inguinal hernias with tissue loss, for example, absent inguinal ligament.
- It serves as an excellent "stepping stone" to laparoscopic TEP repair, providing a means of familiarizing trainees with the complex anatomy of the preperitoneal space.

While the majority of preperitoneal mesh hernia repairs will admittedly be carried out laparoscopically, the open preperitoneal repair of groin hernia remains an important and useful technique and should have a place in the armamentarium of every surgeon who professes an interest in hernia surgery.

References

1. Cheatle GL. An operation for radical cure of inguinal and femoral hernia. Br Med J. 1920;2:68–9.
2. Henry AK. Operation for femoral hernia by a midline extraperitoneal approach: with a preliminary note on the use of this route for reducible inguinal hernia. Lancet. 1936;1:531–3.
3. Read RC. Use of the preperitoneal space in inguinofemoral herniorrhaphy. In: Bendavid R, et al., editors. Historical considerations. Abdominal wall hernias. Principles and management. New York: Springer-Verlag; 2001. p. 11–15.
4. Nyhus LM, Condon RE, Harkins HN. Clinical experience with preperitoneal hernia repair for all type of hernia of the groin. Am J Surg. 1960;100:234.
5. Read RC. Preperitoneal exposure of inguinal herniation. Am J Surg. 1968;116:653.
6. Rives J. Surgical treatment of the inguinal hernia with Dacron patch: principles, indications, technique and results. Int Surg. 1967;47:360–2.
7. Stoppa RE, Petit J, Henry X. Unsutured Dacron prosthesis in groin hernias. Int Surg. 1975;60:411–2.
8. Wantz GE. Testicular atrophy as a sequela of inguinal hernioplasty. Int Surg. 1986;71:159–63.
9. Nyhus LM. Iliopubic tract repair of inguinal and femoral hernia: the posterior preperitoneal approach. Surg Clin North Am. 1993; 73:487.
10. Arlt G, Schumpelick V. [Transinguinal preperitoneal mesh-plasty (TIPP) in management of recurrent inguinal hernia]. Chirurg. 1997;68:1235–8.
11. Pelissier E, et al. Inguinal hernia: a patch covering only the myopectineal orifice is effective. Hernia. 2001;5:84–7.
12. Rignault DP. Properitoneal prosthetic inguinal hernioplasty through a Pfanenstiel approach. Surg Gynecol Obstet. 1986;163:465–8.
13. Wantz GE. Giant prosthetic reinforcement of the visceral sac. Surg Gynecol Obstet. 1989;169:408–17.
14. Kugel RD. Minimally invasive, nonlaparoscopic, preperitoneal, and sutureless inguinal herniorrhaphy. Am J Surg. 1999;178:298–302.
15. Ugahary F, Simmermacher RKJ. Groin hernia repair via a gridiron incision: an alternative technique for preperitoneal mesh insertion. Hernia. 1998;2:123–5.
16. Fruchaud H. Anatomie chirurgicale des hernies de l'aine. Paris: G. Doin; 1956.
17. Wantz GE. Prosthetic repair groin hernioplasties. In: Wantz GE, editor. Atlas of hernia surgery. New York: Raven Press; 1991. p. 94–151.
18. Schumpelick VCJKU. [Preperitoneal mesh-plasty in incisional hernia repair. A comparative retrospective study of 272 operated incisional hernias] [German]. Chirurg. 1996;67:1028–35.

19. Stoppa R, et al. The use of dacron in the repair of hernias of the groin. Surg Clin North Am. 1984;64:269–85.
20. Kurzer M, Belsham PA, Kark AE. Prospective study of open preperitoneal mesh repair for recurrent inguinal hernia. Br J Surg. 2002;89:90–3.
21. Ugahary F. The gridiron hernioplasty. In: Bendavid R, Abrahamson J, Arregui M, et al., editors. Abdominal wall hernias. Principles and management. New York: Springer-Verlag; 2001. p. 407–11.
22. Stoppa R, et al. Prosthetic repair in the treatment of groin hernias. Int Surg. 1986;71:154–8.
23. Stoppa R. The preperitoneal approach and prosthetic repair of groin hernias. In: Nyhus LM, Condon RE, editors. Hernia. Philadelphia: Lippincott; 1995. p. 188–210.
24. Lowham A, et al. Mechanisms of hernia recurrence after preperitoneal mesh repair. Ann Surg. 1997;225:422–31.
25. Mozingo D, et al. Properitoneal synthetic mesh repair of recurrent inguinal hernias. Surg Gynecol Obstet. 1992;174:33–5.
26. Velasco J. Preperitoneal bilateral inguinal herniorrhaphy; 1996.
27. Champault GG, Rizk N, Catheline J-M. Totally preperitoneal laparoscopic approach versus Stoppa operation: randomized trial of 100 cases. Surg Laparosc Endosc. 1997;7:445–50.
28. Beets GL, et al. Open or laparoscopic preperitoneal mesh repair for recurrent inguinal hernia? Surg Endosc. 1999;13:323–7.
29. Hoffman H, Traverso A. Preperitoneal prosthetic herniorrhaphy; one Surgeon's Successful Technique. Arch Surg. 1993;128: 964–70.
30. Schaap HM, van de Pavoordt HDWM, Bast TJ. The preperitoneal approach in the repair of recurrent inguinal hernias. Gynecol Obstet. 1992;174:460–4.
31. Fenoglio ME, et al. Inguinal hernia repair: results using an open preperitoneal approach. Hernia. 2005;9:160–1.
32. van Nieuwenhove Y, et al. Open, preperitoneal hernia repair with the Kugel patch: a prospective, multicentre study of 450 repairs. Hernia. 2007;11:9–13.
33. Baroody M, Bansal V, Maish G. The open preperitoneal approach to recurrent inguinal hernias in high-risk patients. Hernia. 2004;8:373–5.
34. Nienhuijs S, et al. Pain after open preperitoneal repair versus lichtenstein repair: a randomized trial. World J Surg. 2007;9:1751–7.
35. Schroder D, et al. Inguinal hernia recurrence following preperitoneal Kugel patch repair. Am Surg. 2004;70:132–6.
36. Stoppa R. Reinforcement of the visceral sac by a preperitoneal bilateral mesh prosthesis in groin hernia repair. In: Bendavid R, Abrahamson J, Arregui ME, Flament JB, Phillips EH, editors. Abdominal wall hernias: principles and management. New York: Springer; 2001. p. 428–36.

Laparoscopic Inguinal Hernia Repair

Karl A. LeBlanc, Brent W. Allain Jr., and William C. Streetman

Introduction

The first report of a hernia repair using laparoscopy was made by Ralph Ger in 1982 [1]. In a patient with right indirect inguinal hernia the neck of the sac was closed with a series of staples using an operating laparoscope and a cannula placed in the right iliac fossa. Although this procedure was carried out in November 1979, Ger states that the first patient to be treated by laparoscopic closure of the neck of the sac was under the care of Dr Fletcher of the University of West Indies, Jamaica.

The use of prosthetic material for laparoscopic repair of an inguinal hernia was introduced by Corbitt and Schultz in 1991 [2, 3]. These repairs involved the use of a polypropylene plug, patch, or both to close the inguinal canal in a tension-free manner. Because of unacceptably high early recurrence rates these approaches were abandoned in favor of laparoscopic placement of a preperitoneal prosthetic biomaterial. This repair follows the same principles as the open Stoppa repair [4]. After reducing the hernia sac a large piece of mesh is placed in the preperitoneal space covering all potential hernia sites in the inguinal region. The mesh becomes sandwiched between the preperitoneal tissues and the abdominal wall and, provided it is large enough, is held there by intra-abdominal pressure until such time as it becomes incorporated by fibrous tissue.

The intraperitoneal placement of mesh was introduced by Fitzgibbons and colleagues as a method of laparoscopic hernia repair [5]. This operation is performed using minimal dissection by leaving the hernia sac in situ and covering the defect with mesh, which is stapled to the surrounding peritoneum. The major concerns with this repair are the risk of injury to underlying structures from staples and of obstruction or fistula formation as a result of adhesions between bowel and exposed mesh. These concerns had resulted in this repair being performed in only a few centers. Other materials, such as expanded polytetrafluorethylene, are thought less likely to cause adhesions and were also being investigated with this repair [6, 7]. Currently, however, this technique is seldom utilized in inguinal hernia repair.

The laparoscopic approach for the repair of inguinal hernias is achieving success and there are many areas of the world where this is the preferred method of repair. However, it does not seem that this methodology will become the standard of care for all inguinal hernias. In skilled hands the laparoscopic approach is also effective for incarcerated inguinal hernias [8] and recurrent inguinal hernias after a prior laparoscopic repair [9]. There seems to be a trend to limit the use of this technique in those inguinal hernias that are bilateral and/or recurrent. This trend, however, does not take into account patient preference, surgical training, and the need to maintain a good level of skill or performance for those already undertaking the operation. Conversely, the laparoscopic hernioplasty for incisional and ventral hernias is increasing in popularity. It might possibly become the standard of care for this problem given the results that have been seen thus far.

Extraperitoneal Operation

Anesthesia

Although totally extraperitoneal hernia repair can be performed using either local or epidural anesthesia, it is our preference to use general anesthesia with complete muscle relaxation and mechanical ventilation. This ensures that the

K.A. LeBlanc(✉) • B.W. Allain Jr. • W.C. Streetman
Surgeons Group of Baton Rouge/
Our Lady of the Lake Physician Group,
Baton Rouge, LA, USA
e-mail: Karl.LeBlanc@ololrmc.com

A.N. Kingsnorth and K.A. LeBlanc (eds.), *Management of Abdominal Hernias*,
DOI 10.1007/978-1-84882-877-3_16, © Springer Science+Business Media London 2013

respiratory and cardiovascular changes that occur with extraperitoneal CO_2 insufflation are minimized. These changes are similar to or less than those observed with intraperitoneal CO_2 insufflation, and may be related to the size of the space created during the preperitoneal dissections [10]. All patients undergoing totally extraperitoneal hernia repair receive DVT prophylaxis. Use of antibiotic prophylaxis is controversial in this situation with little evidence for or against their use, however, the authors prefer a preoperative dose of a first-generation cephalosporin in most cases.

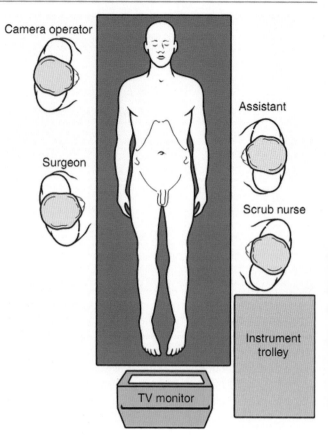

Fig. 16.1 Position of operator, assistants, and television monitor at the operating table for repair of a left inguinal hernia

Position of the Patient on the Table

Before attempting totally extraperitoneal hernia repair, it is important to ensure that the patient's bladder is empty. This can be achieved by asking the patient to micturate before entering the operating theatre. Alternatively, a urinary catheter could be inserted but this is generally unnecessary. The patient should be placed on the operating table in the supine position with a 15° Trendelenburg tilt. Ideally both hands should be placed by the patient's side to allow the operator and the assistant to stand opposite each other at the patient's epigastric level. Care must be taken to correctly pad all pressure points. The operator stands on the side opposite of the hernia being repaired. When bilateral repairs are to be done, the operation can be started by standing on the side of the patient opposite the larger hernia defect. The video monitor should be placed at the foot of the table (Fig. 16.1). If two monitors are being used, one should be placed at either side of the lower end of the operating table.

Trocars and Trocar Position

One 10 mm cannula and two 5 mm cannulas are generally used for this operation. The 10 mm cannula should have a blunt-nosed trocar as it is inserted using an open technique. The 5 mm cannulas should have built-in fixation threads to prevent them from moving in and out of the extraperitoneal space as instruments are passed through. In addition, because of the confined operating space, the 5 mm cannulas should be short (60 mm). All the cannulas can be placed in the lower midline. In this instance, the 10 mm cannula is placed in a sub-umbilical position, one of the two 5 mm cannulas is placed one-third of the way between the symphysis pubis and the umbilicus and the other half way between the symphysis pubis and the umbilicus (Fig. 16.2).

Alternatively, many physicians prefer the two smaller trocars to be placed laterally near the anterior axillary line above the iliac crest on either side of the patient. These latter trocars will usually be positioned after the dissection is nearly completed through the larger midline trocar. This will frequently be accomplished with the use of the laparoscope itself.

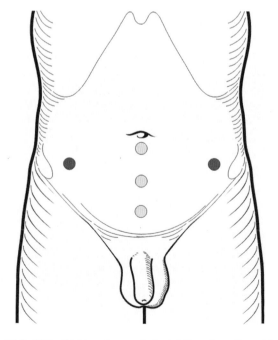

Fig. 16.2 Sites of trocar placements for totally extraperitoneal hernia repair. The mark on either side of the abdomen indicates the alternate location for the 5 mm trocars

Fig. 16.3 (**a**) The deflated PBD2 balloon for dissection of the preperitoneal space. (**b**) The inflated PBD2 balloon for dissection of the preperitoneal space. (**c**) Spacemaker Plus Dissector System

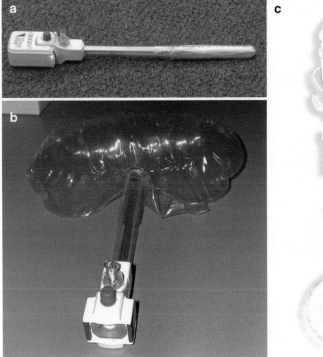

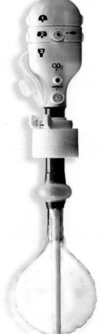

Laparoscope

Some surgeons substitute the 0° laparoscope for a 30 or 45° laparoscope after developing the extraperitoneal space. We find that this is not necessary and that the operation can be completed satisfactorily with a 0° laparoscope. Currently either the 5 or 10 mm laparoscope can be used for the entire procedure. In particularly difficult cases, the 5 mm laparoscope is preferred as this can be placed in the lateral ports to visualize the anatomy from the contralateral aspect.

Developing the Extraperitoneal Space

A transverse incision of 1–1.5 cm, starting in the lower half of the umbilicus and extending laterally is made. The tissues are then separated with scissors or hemostats and retracted with two retractors to expose the anterior rectus sheath on the side of the hernia to be repaired. The sheath is opened with a #11 bladed scalpel through a small transverse incision. The midline and rectus muscle are identified and the space between the rectus muscle and the posterior rectus sheath space is developed using hemostats and blunt dissection. A large right angled retractor (to retract the rectus muscle anteriorly to allow the insertion of a blunt-nosed 10 mm trocar and cannula) is then inserted into this space and moved medially, laterally, and posteriorly to develop the preperitoneal space. Insufflation with CO_2 can commence with insufflation pressure being kept between 10 and 12 mmHg.

A 0° laparoscope is then inserted through the 10 mm cannula and can be gently used as a blunt dissector to further enlarge the space. It is important to feel the pubic symphysis, and stay in the midline and immediately posterior to the rectus muscle with the laparoscope during this dissection. Once the pubic arch is visible, two 5 mm cannulas are inserted under direct vision in the positions previously described.

The preperitoneal space may also be developed using balloon dissection. A deflated balloon on the end of a cannula, of which many different types are available (Fig. 16.3), is placed in the preperitoneal space using the access described. The balloon is then filled with air and the space developed under direct vision using a 0° laparoscope. This method is helpful in the learning period when surgeons are still unfamiliar with the preperitoneal anatomy. While balloon dissection is slightly more rapid, it has the disadvantage of adding additional expense to the operation. In addition, it is associated with bladder and bowel injury in patients who have had previous lower abdominal surgery [11]. In those patients that have had prior lower abdominal surgery or prostatectomy, it is preferred to either perform the entire operation without the use of a balloon dissector or performing a transabdominal preperitoneal operation. Some surgeons will occasionally merge the two techniques. In these cases, the surgeon will enter the abdomen above the umbilicus with a 5 mm port and inspect the lower abdominal contents. If there are no adhesions, which occur frequently, the dissection can be converted to the totally extraperitoneal operation either with or without the use of the balloon dissection.

Dissection

Two atraumatic dissectors, which will grasp but not tear the peritoneum are important for this part of the procedure. A sharp pair of scissors will sometimes be used but is seldom necessary. It is important to identify the anatomical landmarks in an ordered fashion. The pectineal (Cooper's) ligament on the same side as the hernia should be exposed first. At this stage, in thin patients, you may see the external iliac vein laterally and accessory obturator vessels, if present, will be found crossing the pectineal ligament. Separation of the perivascular and extraperitoneal fat is performed in the avascular plane between both using gentle blunt dissection, and is aided by the CO_2 insufflation. Characteristic filamentous tissue, which breaks down easily, will be observed between the two planes.

The retropubic space can now be developed in the midline and on the side of the hernia to above the level of the obturator nerve and vessels (it is not unusual to dissect this far into the pelvis). The inferior epigastric vessels should next be identified and the space between them and the extraperitoneal fat developed. During this part of the dissection, it is important to keep the epigastric vessels up against the rectus muscle using one dissector while the other is used to separate the tissues. If this is not done, the epigastric vessels will come down into the operating field and small branches between them and the rectus muscles will be torn, giving rise to troublesome bleeding. Between the inferior epigastric vessels and extraperitoneal fat, a fascial layer is encountered. This represents the deep layer of the fascia transversalis (Fig. 16.4; see color insert) and should be divided using a combination of blunt and sharp dissection to open up the space lateral to it. This may not always be necessary if the dissection allows the complete separation of these structures.

Much of this will be accomplished with the dissection balloon if this is the chosen technique. The choice of the use of the balloon or blunt dissection has been shown to be equally effective in creating the space necessary to perform this operation [12]. The attention to the epigastric vessels is limited when this is used because the unfurling of the balloon will sometimes pull these vessels down rather than leaving them in situ. This may limit the insufflation of the balloon whereupon the surgeon must complete the dissection manually. Also, for those surgeons that prefer the lateral location of the 5 mm trocars, some of the dissection will usually be necessary with the laparoscope and/or one of the dissection graspers that would be inserted through one of the lateral or midline trocars.

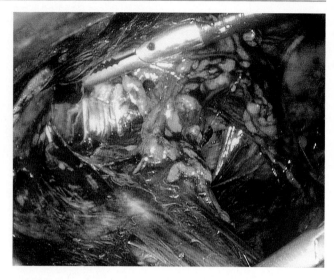

Fig. 16.4 Laparoscopic appearance of the deep layer of fascia transversalis

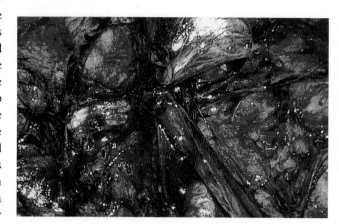

Fig. 16.5 Laparoscopic appearance of an right indirect hernia

Indirect Inguinal Hernias in Males

At this stage it should be possible to identify the sac of an indirect inguinal hernia (Fig. 16.5; see color insert). The sac will be found immediately lateral to the inferior epigastric vessels as it enters the internal ring. The sac should be grasped at the internal ring and reduced by retracting and dissecting the adhesions between it and the inguinal canal. Tension needs to be kept on the sac during this part of the dissection by using both dissectors in a stepwise fashion; otherwise, as the sac is released to regrip it, it will return to the inguinal canal because of its elasticity and inguinal attachments. It is important to dissect all the tissues around the sac down to the peritoneum. These tissues represent attenuated transversalis fascia (see Chap. 2) which invests the cord and indirect sac as it enters the internal ring. Once this has been achieved the sac can be lifted up and the vas deferens will be visible at its posterior border and may be dissected off it along with the testicular vessels. The vas runs medially and crosses over the iliac vessels as it descends into the pelvis, while the testicular vessels take a course slightly lateral to the iliac vessels. In small to moderately sized indirect inguinal hernias, the apex of the sac can be identified and the sac completely reduced into the extraperitoneal space. If the sac is large and entering the scrotum, it may be wise to divide and ligate it at a convenient point as one would do with open hernia repair. This, of course, will be done with intracorporeal suturing. The testicular vessels and vas deferens should be completely skeletonized of any lipomatous material that may be in the inguinal canal. Not infrequently, a small hole may be made in the sac during its reduction. This should not impair the ability to complete the dissection and such defects can usually be ignored. However, it should be noted that great care must be exercised to avoid a large tear of the peritoneal sac during these maneuvers. This will result in the insufflation of the intra-abdominal space, which will limit the available preperitoneal space and subsequent "working room" for the operation to continue. Additionally, this could expose the patch material to the intestinal contents of the abdomen with resulting adhesions. If a large tear occurs and cannot be closed with sutures, there are two options. One may convert to the transabdominal preperitoneal technique and use a tissue separating prosthesis as used in the incisional hernia repair or abandon the laparoscopic approach altogether.

Posteriorly the peritoneal dissection should be taken back until the vas can be seen descending into the pelvis. Laterally it should go to at least to the level of the anterior superior iliac spine while medially dissection should cross the midline and go well below the pectineal ligament (Fig. 16.6). This is to ensure complete exposure of the myopectineal orifice and that there is adequate space for insertion of the mesh.

Lateral to the testicular vessels the femoral branch of the genitofemoral nerve and the lateral cutaneous nerve of the thigh can be identified in patients with little adipose tissue (Fig. 16.7). Care should be taken not to damage these or a small branch of the deep circumflex iliac artery, which lies lateral to the cutaneous nerve of thigh. These structures all lie beneath the iliopubic tract. Therefore, any fixation of the meshes must be placed above this line to assure that these nerves are not in harm's way. Also in thin patients the external iliac vessels will be easily identified, the artery appearing between the testicular vessels and the vas and the vein lying medial to the artery. In all patients the characteristic pulsation from the external iliac vessels will be observed in this position. Small peritoneal branches arising from the iliac artery may also be noted during the dissection and as these

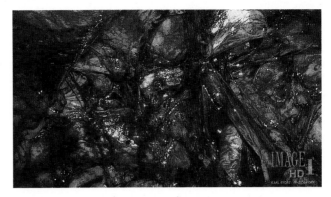

Fig. 16.6 Extent of dissection required with details of anatomy observed at laparoscopy. A left direct inguinal hernia is seen as the right inguinal hernia from Fig. 16.5

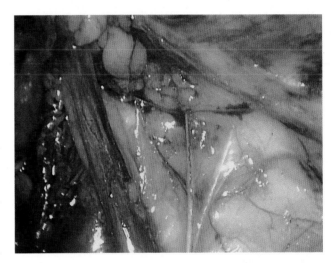

Fig. 16.7 Laparoscopic appearance of femoral branches of genitofemoral nerve and lateral cutaneous nerve of thigh

are usually at the posterior limit of the dissection they can be preserved. As all dissection is carried out in an avascular plane there should be only a limited need to use electrocautery during the operation. Most dissection is performed by gentle separation of tissues using atraumatic dissecting forceps. If an injury to larger vessels such as the epigastric artery or vein, then the use of hemostatic clips or suture ligation will be necessary. If this fails, then one could place transfascial absorbable sutures to maintain hemostasis of these vessels.

Indirect Inguinal Hernias in Females

The approach to these hernias is similar to that of the indirect inguinal hernias in the male patient. Once the sac is reduced the round ligament can be left in situ or divided and ligated at the internal ring depending on the surgeon's preference.

Direct Inguinal Hernias

A direct inguinal hernia will be encountered during the dissection to expose the pectineal ligament. The defect lies laterally to the border of the rectus muscle and is medial to the inferior epigastric vessels except when a combined direct and indirect hernia is present. Sometimes a direct defect can appear to encroach on the femoral canal and in this circumstance may be confused with a femoral hernia. Patients with a direct hernia will also occasionally be found to have a femoral hernia. The direct hernia sac and preperitoneal fat are usually easy to reduce by grasping the sac with atraumatic forceps and simple pulling gently. While the hernia is being reduced the characteristic appearance of a pseudosac, which is attenuated transversalis fascia, will be displayed. This should be allowed to retract into the defect. As with indirect hernias, the sac is reduced into the extraperitoneal space and no attempt is made to open or ligate it. The vas deferens and testicular vessels need to be exposed to exclude a synchronous indirect hernia. The extent of the dissection should be identical to that of the indirect hernia repair. It is important to be careful during this part of the operation as the peritoneum is easily torn at the internal ring in patients with a direct hernia. It is generally best if the peritoneum is pushed with the laparoscopic forceps rather than pulled at this location so that this tear will not occur.

Femoral Hernias

As the pectineal ligament is exposed as far lateral as the external iliac vein in all patients, a femoral hernia should not be missed during totally extraperitoneal hernia repair. This can be reduced in the same manner as for direct hernias. One should be attentive to the possibility of the inclusion of an organ such as the bladder or ovary into the hernia contents. When found these structures should be carefully reduced to avoid injury. Once this has been done dissection should proceed as for other groin hernias.

Recurrent Hernias

A reasonable amount of experience with totally extraperitoneal hernia repair is required before dealing with recurrent hernias following an open repair and even more if subsequent to a laparoscopic approach. This is because the anatomical landmarks are often distorted due to the previous repairs. The inferior epigastric vessels may have been divided and thus be in part absent or visible as a much smaller vessel. Dense adhesions form between the neck of the recurrent sac and the previous repair and because of this it is wise to use careful sharp dissection to free it from these adhesions. Elsewhere the peritoneum is often very thin and easily torn, as stitches may have gone through it from the previous repair. Because of the frequent use of a prosthetic biomaterial in the prior repair, the occurrence of a tear in the peritoneum should be expected during the dissection. This is especially frequent in the patient that has had a prior plug-and-patch repair.

Because of these reasons, it is probably best to use a transabdominal approach (TAPP) if a mesh product resides in the preperitoneal space. This will allow the surgeon the ability to dissect the peritoneum under direct vision and allows the assurance that there are no adhesions from an intra-abdominal organ. This is particularly recommended when the patient has had a previous repair that utilized a polypropylene biomaterial (which is invariably the case).

Bilateral Hernias

Bilateral hernias can be repaired using the same access as for unilateral hernias and additional trocars are not required. Once dissection has been completed on one side the operator simply switches to the other side and reduces the contralateral hernia. Although one large piece of mesh can be used for bilateral hernia repair, it is our preference to use two pieces of 10 cm by 15 cm. In this circumstance it is helpful to fixate one to the pectineal ligament before the contralateral mesh is placed into position. Larger hernias will require even larger meshes of 15 × 15 cm.

For all indirect hernias and most direct hernias, a heavy weight mesh does not need to be tacked, stapled, or sutured in place. If, however, a large direct defect encroaches upon the femoral canal or there is a femoral hernia, the mesh should be stapled or sutured to the pectineal ligament to prevent the inferior border of the mesh from slipping upwards and into the defect. The mesh does not need to be divided to fit around the cord or, indeed, sutured or tacked around the cord.

An exception to the above statement has come about in the last several years. The lighter weight macroporous meshes are very supple and soft, an advantage in their use. However, this characteristic makes fixation necessary so that the product does not protrude into the hernia defect. The type of device will vary according to surgeon preference.

On desufflating the extraperitoneal space it is important to ensure that the inferior fold of the mesh does not roll up with the peritoneum. If an adequate dissection has been carried out, this will be unlikely to occur. After desufflation all cannulas are removed and the rectus sheath at the sub-umbilical incision is closed with 2/0 or 0 Vicryl, while skin is closed with interrupted absorbable subcuticular stitches and/or adhesive tapes.

Fixation of the Mesh

To secure the mesh a fastener device is generally used, however, there is some evidence that fixation may not be necessary [13]. Two or three tacks are usually placed only in the pectineal ligament in the situations previously mentioned. Some surgeons secure the mesh to the rectus muscle medially and the transversus abdominis laterally. Fixation at this position provides no additional support for properly positioned mesh and can be avoided in all but the large inguinal or femoral hernia repairs. Alternatively the mesh can be sutured to the pectineal ligament with a hernia stapler or 2/0 polypropylene or CV-2 ePTFE suture.

When placing these fixation devices, it is often easier to insert them into the pectineal ligament if the instrument is inserted via an ipsilateral trocar. The angle of the ligament is such that a firm grasp of the ligament is best afforded if this approach is used. This will prevent the slippage off of the ligament that is common as the instrument is fired. The contralateral trocar is used for placement of the additional fixators along the muscle above the iliopubic tract.

Newer absorbable fasteners now are available and are becoming increasingly popular. In general, they last approximately 1 year and they are completely absorbed. There are obvious benefits to this concept but there are no long-term studies to prove their efficacy. However, given the ingrowth of the respective mesh products, there is little reason to be concerned see Chap. XX-prosthetics.

Recent randomized prospective studies have shown that it may be efficacious to use a biocompatible fibrin sealant to secure the mesh rather than metal tacking devices [14–17]. This has the obvious advantage that the risk of injury to vascular or neural structures during the repair is virtually eliminated. The subsequent reduction in postoperative neuralgia is thought to lead to quicker return to normal daily and work-related activity. Additional controlled studies in such products are warranted and forthcoming, and will continue to influence the field of herniology in the future.

Conversion to Open Repair

It is necessary in approximately 1% (or as few as 0.23%) of cases to convert to open preperitoneal repair [18]. This usually occurs as a result of a large tear in the peritoneum or, when a very large (estimated defect of 5 cm or greater) direct hernia is encountered. In the latter circumstance a 15×15 cm piece of mesh is required and may be more easily placed at open surgery by some surgeons. If the hernia is unilateral, a small transverse incision is placed over the ipsilateral rectus muscle at the level of the lower 5 mm cannula and the preperitoneal space entered lateral to the rectus muscle. If there are bilateral hernias, a Pfannenstiel incision is made at the same level to gain access to the preperitoneal space.

In the majority of instances when the prospect of conversion becomes a reality, one may convert instead to the transabdominal preperitoneal repair. With this approach the entire abdominal cavity will allow a much larger working space and usually obviates the need for conversion to the open approach. The larger piece of mesh can be inserted and placed. The remainder of the procedure will proceed as the traditional TAPP repair.

Contraindications to Totally Extraperitoneal Hernia Repair

Although there are no absolute contraindications to totally extraperitoneal hernia repair in the elective setting, large inguinoscrotal or irreducible hernias are relative contraindications. Previous lower midline or ipsilateral paramedian incisions also come into this category. Extraperitoneal endoscopic repair is difficult and time-consuming in these circumstances such that it is difficult to justify attempting it in the first place. In these instances, one may elect to attempt a TAPP repair and convert to the open operation if it is obvious that this, too, is not feasible. If there is a concern in regards to the possibility of adhesions that may make the extraperitoneal approach risky, a small laparoscope is inserted into the abdominal cavity and the areas of suspicion are visually inspected. This is done through an infra-umbilical skin incision with the abdominal entry moved to above the potential site for fascial incision for placement of the 10 mm trocar. If there are no adhesions in the area or none that involve the bowel, the 5 mm port can be removed after the abdomen is evacuated of the carbon dioxide. The larger 10 mm port is then inserted via the infra-umbilical incision whereupon the extraperitoneal procedure will be performed with assurance that there is no more than the expected risk of injury to the bowel during the creation of this space.

Transabdominal Hernia Repair

This differs from the totally extraperitoneal approach in that the preperitoneal space is entered through a transverse peritoneal incision made above the hernia defect. The abdomen is entered using either closed or open laparoscopy and two additional cannulas are placed lateral to either rectus muscle at the level of the umbilicus. These can be two 5 mm cannulas or a 5 mm and 12 mm cannula if staples are to be used. Typically, however, the use of all 5 mm ports is possible. The peritoneal incision should extend from the medial umbilical ligament medially to the level of the anterior superior iliac spine laterally. If the patient has a direct hernia, it is wise to divide the medial umbilical ligament, which carries the obliterated umbilical artery (see Chapter 2) to ensure adequate exposure of the pectineal ligament and retro-pubic space beyond the midline.

Once the preperitoneal space has been entered, dissection is as for totally extraperitoneal hernia repair. One of the important aspects of transabdominal hernia repair is adequate closure of the peritoneum after the repair. Suturing or stapling the peritoneum can accomplish this closure effectively. Care must be used if the peritoneum is closed with the helical tacks or the newer absorbable fasteners. These devices are of such a size that it can be difficult to effect an adequate closure of the peritoneum especially if there is a paucity of preperitoneal fat. A defect left between tacks, staples or sutures forms a potential source for internal herniation of the small bowel. Any port site larger than 5 mm should be closed to prevent the development of port site hernias.

As with the totally extraperitoneal approach there are no absolute contraindications to this repair; indeed as noted earlier, it can sometimes be easier to perform for patients with large inguinoscrotal hernias or with extensive lower abdominal adhesions.

Results

There have been many studies that have examined the efficacy of laparoscopic inguinal hernia repair compared to the various open methods that are available today. A few of these are listed in Table 16.1. In several of these papers, the methodology of data collection and the patient selection make firm and accurate comparisons difficult between the series. In fact, in many cases the data cannot be compared directly. Nevertheless, as shown in these series, it appears that the rate of complications in the laparoscopic patients does not exceed that of the open patients. Additionally, the rate of recurrence is not statistically different between the various methods. What is not shown in this table is the indisputable fact that the laparoscopic repair requires a general anesthetic in most cases and the hospital costs are more expensive. Most of these series are consistent in finding that laparoscopic patients return to normal activities and work sooner. This saving in costs to the community makes the overall costs of the laparoscopic operation less than the open operation. However, there are a few centers that forgo the balloon dissection trocars and disposable instruments. This, along with the considerable experience of these surgeons has dropped the hospital costs to levels comparable to that of the open method.

While the majority of information in the literature reveals that the laparoscopic repair is associated with less pain, Picchio found that the tension-free open hernia repair is superior to the TAPP in terms of postoperative pain with no important differences in recovery [19]. This finding is in the minority, however, as most studies consistently show that the pain is less with the minimally invasive approach particularly if an objective analysis such as measured treadmill walking is used as a measure of return-to-physical-work comparing open hernia repair to laparoscopic repair. Rosen found that the laparoscopic repair offered an early advantage to the open repair by this measure [20]. This study reaffirms the clinical setting regarding the laparoscopic repair. Other reports have found similar findings regarding the lessening of postoperative pain with this repair [21–28].

The trend in most centers around the world is for the laparoscopic repair to be limited to bilateral and recurrent inguinal hernias. The results for this indication are excellent. A few studies reported no recurrences with the laparoscopic approach as compared to the open approach [28, 29]. Another study found that the incidence of recurrence after bilateral repair was 0.6% [30] Felix recommends this repair for recurrent hernias following laparoscopic repair [9]. However, Eklund reports no long-term differences in repair of recurrent hernias with the laparoscopic or open approach [27]. Nevertheless, the results for primary repair are impressive. Kapris reported a 0.62% recurrence rate over a 7-year period. Past the learning curve the recurrence rate was 0.16% after 45 months. The total complication rate exclusive of recurrence was 3.68% (2% were due to urinary retention) [18].

When there is no proven superiority of one surgical method over another, the cost-effectiveness of the operations is an important consideration. Due to longer operative times and more expensive equipment, there is little question that the laparoscopic method is more expensive than an open approach for the index operation. Many patients who undergo an open repair are able to do so under local or regional blocks whereas most laparoscopic procedures are done under general anesthesia which increases the cost also. Most studies do not include post operative visits, sick leave, and community costs into the total expense of an operation. Eklund reported upon the total hospital cost of the index operation, costs associated with recurrences and complications, and community costs associated with sick leave. He found that the index operation was significantly more expensive for the TEP repair vs. open (Lichtenstein) and that the TEP repair was associated with more complications and recurrence. This led to increased cost as well. However, the TEP patients returned to work 3 days earlier than the open repair patients, which reduced the cost difference [31]. Hynes et al. reported the cost-effectiveness of all laparoscopic vs. open inguinal hernia repairs. They reported the day of surgery costs for laparoscopic vs. open was significantly more (US$1,589 vs. US$773). They then followed these patients out to 2 years and the total health care use was not significantly different (US$9,564 vs. US$8,926) per patient. In subgroup analyses, the laparoscopic approach was found to be cost-effective for unilateral primary and recurrent hernias. On cost-effectiveness

Table 16.1 Randomized trials of inguinal herniorraphy

Author and year	Method	Median follow-up (years)	Number of hernias	Rate of complications (%)	Rate of recurrence (%)
Payne (1994) [40]	TAPP	N/A	48	12.0	N/A
	Lichtenstein		52	18.0	N/A
Stoker (1994) [41]	TAPP	0.6	75		0
	Lichtenstein		75		0
Maddern (1994) [42]	TAPP	N/A	44	40.0	N/A
	Double Darn		42	47.0	N/A
Barkun (1995) [43]	TAPP	1.2	43	22.0	2.0
	Darn/Lichtenstein		49	12.0	0
Leibl (1995) [8]	TAPP	1.3	54	N/A	0
	Shouldice		48	N/A	0
Lawrence (1995) [44]	TAPP	N/A	58	12.0	N/A
	Darn		66	2.0	N/A
Vogt (1995) [45]	IPOM	0.7	30		0
	Multiple types		31		0
Schrenk (1996) [46]	TAPP	N/A	28		5.0
	TEP		24		16.7
	Shouldice		34		2.9
Liem (1997) [47]	TEP	2.0	493		3.0
	Open		509		6.0
Johansson (1997) [48]	TEP	1.7	179		1.0
	Open mesh		168		3.0
	Anterior repair		177		0
Champault (1997) [49]	TEP	3.0	51	4.0	6.0
	Stoppa		49	29.5	2.0
Beets (1998) [33]	TAPP	1.8	42	67.0	12.5
	GPRVS		37	62.0	1.9
Wellwood (1998) [50]	TAPP	N/A	200		N/A
	Tension-free		200		N/A
Cohen (1998) [51]	TAPP	N/A	78		1.9
	TEP		67		0
Khoury (1998) [52]	TEP	3.0	150		2.5
	Plug and Patch		142		3.0
Johansson (1999) [53]	TAPP	1.0	604		No statistical significance
	Open preperitoneal mesh				
	Tissue repair				
MRC Laparoscopic Hernia Trial Group (1999) [21]	Laparoscopic	1.0	468	29.9	1.9
	Open		433	43.5	0
Lorenz (2000) [22]	TAPP	2.0	86	11.0	2.3
	Shouldice		90	9.0	1.1
Sarli (2001) [29]	TAPP		20	34.7	0
	Tension-free		23	35.0	4.3
Wright (2002) [54]	TEP	5.0	149	N/A	2.0
	Tension-free		107		0
	Stoppa		32		9.4
	Sutured		12		0
Bringman (2003) [23]	TEP	2.0	92	9.8	2.2
	Plug and Patch		104	15.4	1.9
	Lichtenstein		103	20.4	0
Liem (2003) [24]	TEP	3.7	487	4.9	4.3
	Open		507	13.6	8.5
Andersson (2003) [25]	TEP	1.0	80	N/A	2.5

(continued)

Table 16.1 (continued)

Author and year	Method	Median follow-up (years)	Number of hernias	Rate of complications (%)	Rate of recurrence (%)
	Lichtenstein		86		0
Lal (2003) [26]	TEP	1.1	25	N/A	0
	Lichtenstein		25		0
Neumayer (2004) [55]	TAPP/TEP	2.0	989	39.0	10.1
	Lichtenstein		994	33.4	4.9
Eklund (2007) [27]	TAPP	5.1	73	13.6	19.0
	Lichtenstein		74	19.0	18.0
Hallen (2008) [56]	TEP	7.3	73	26.0	4.1
	Lichtenstein		81	33.3	4.9
Pokorny (2008) [57]	Laparoscopic	3.0	129	10.9	5.0
	Open		236	14.6	2.8
Eklund (2009) [58]	TEP	5.1	665	N/A	2.4
	Lichtenstein		705		1.2
Kouhia (2009) [28]	TEP	5.3	49	8.2	0
	Lichtenstein		47	27.7	6.4

GPRVS giant prosthetic reinforcement of the visceral sac (Open)
IPOM intraperitoneal onlay mesh repair (Laparoscopic)
TAPP transabdominal preperitoneal repair (Laparoscopic)
TEP totally extraperitoneal repair (Laparoscopic)

alone, the authors found that the open repair was superior for bilateral inguinal hernias. This could be attributed to greater health care cost for reasons other than their hernia repair over that 2 year follow-up [32]. Beets et al. found that the costs associated with the giant prosthetic reinforcement of the visceral sac (GPRVS) repair were similar to that of the laparoscopic TAPP repair (US$1150 vs. US$1179). In Beets' report, the TAPP patients returned to work 10 days sooner than those with the GPRVS [33]. As shown in Table 16.1, however, there were approximately six times as many recurrences with the laparoscopic procedure but these operations were performed with relatively inexperienced surgeons. Many patients who undergo hernia repairs are still an integral part of the workforce, and it is important to consider the cost of an operation to the community as well.

A summary of all of these comments can be found in the follow-up report by Fingerhut at a European consensus conference [34]. This conference convened in 1994 and again in 2000. At that time, there were more than 60 clinical trials and more than 12,500 patients entered into them. The members of this conference concluded that laparoscopic inguinal repair was associated with less postoperative pain, more rapid return to normal activities but took longer to perform, was more costly and might increase the risk of rare complications. A meta-analysis of all randomized trials by the EU Hernia Trialists Collaboration Group found, in addition to the above, that laparoscopic patients had less chronic pain and numbness, while hernia recurrence was similar to that observed with open mesh repair. While some of these findings could be disputed in experienced centers, they are consistent with the current literature.

The choice between the TAPP and the TEP is merely a matter of personal preference, however. There is no clinical difference between the conversions to open, the complications seen, or the recurrence rates between these two operations in experienced hands [35]. The only difference noted in this study was that the TAPP took 32 min longer to complete than did the TEP. This was due to the need to close the peritoneal flap. This would indicate, then, that the TEP may be the more expeditious and less costly procedure based upon the operating room expenses. The MRC Trial Group did not find any clinical difference between the use of the TAPP versus the TEP operation [21]. McCormack et al. looked at all published reports on TAPP versus TEP. They found only one randomized controlled trial and nine additional non-randomized, observational studies comparing the TAPP operation to the TEP operation. The one randomized trial, found no difference in terms of length of stay, recurrence, hematomas, length of the , and return to normal activities between the two operations. The non-randomized studies reported an increased number of port-site hernias and visceral injuries in the TAPP operation [36].

Disadvantages of Laparoscopic Hernia Repair

One of the drawbacks of laparoscopic surgery has been the steep learning curve associated with its use. This was particularly evident in the early stages of development of the operative procedure. In large part, the surgeons that were attempting to perform this operative procedure had limited experience with the laparoscopic methodology, the laparoscopic anatomy or an adequate understanding of the need to cover the entire myopectineal orifice. As with other forms of hernia repair, recurrence rates and complications were notably higher in this learning period. Such recurrences are often not true recurrences but failure to repair the hernia in the first instance; for example, an indirect sac may be missed or inadequately reduced, mesh size may be too small or incorrectly placed. If any of these circumstances arise, a persistent hernia will usually be apparent within days or weeks of the attempted repair. In a study by Liem et al., evaluating the learning curve for four laparoscopic surgeons inexperienced in totally extraperitoneal repair, the actuarial recurrence rate was 10% at 6 months postoperatively [37]. Over 50% of recurrences were due to overlooking or insufficiently reducing an indirect hernia sac.

We estimate that it may take as many as 100 laparoscopic hernia repairs before an inexperienced laparoscopic surgeon can bring the operating time for laparoscopic hernia repair into a range similar to that for open hernia repair. On the other hand, the surgeon that is experienced with other advanced laparoscopic operations will take approximately 30–50 cases to build an adequate experience and a decreased operative time [38]. Since operating time is expensive this has significant cost implications. Added to this, laparoscopic hernia repair is already more costly than open repair, principally because of the use of disposable instruments. These costs, however, can be brought into a range similar to that of open repair by using reusable rather than disposable instruments and by suturing rather than stapling or tacking when indicated. A hidden cost, often not considered, is use of the laparoscopic equipment itself, which is currently less durable and more expensive than conventional instruments. These costs can be minimized by frequent use and extra care by nursing and medical staff during their use.

The relative difficulty in performing laparoscopic hernia repair using local anesthesia is often cited as a drawback of this operation. This only applies, however, when safe general anesthesia is not available at an institution. Despite its many proponents, there is no evidence that use of local anesthetic is safer than general anesthesia for hernia repair. Edelman, however, has reported satisfactory results using local anesthesia with a laryngeal mask for the TEP as compared to the open repair of inguinal hernias. Perhaps, such a method may become more popular in the future [39].

Conclusions

Laparoscopic hernia repair is technically more demanding than open anterior approaches. This, combined with a poor knowledge of the preperitoneal anatomy by many, will limit its use to surgeons with a special interest in laparoscopic or hernia surgery. Nevertheless, it has advantages in terms of reduced postoperative pain, lower wound morbidity, a more rapid return to normal activity, and less chronic pain and numbness than open repair. The benefits that are realized to the individual patients can be expanded into the societal advantages because these patients are returned to the work force more rapidly. Many surgeons are finding this technique more beneficial for the patients with bilateral and/or recurrent hernias. These advantages need to be balanced against increased costs and a high recurrence rate in the learning curve period. Results from large randomized clinical trials evaluating laparoscopic hernia repair have shown it to be an effective method for the repair of the inguinal hernias.

References

1. Ger R. The management of certain abdominal herniae by intra-abdominal closure of the neck of the sac. Ann R Coll Surg Engl. 1982;64:342–4.
2. Corbitt JD. Laparoscopic herniorrhaphy. Surg Laparosc Endosc. 1991;1:23–5.
3. Schultz L, Graber J, Pietraffita J, et al. Laser laparoscopic herniorrhaphy: a clinical trial. Preliminary results. J Laparoendosc Surg. 1991;1:41–5.
4. Stoppa RE, Rives JL, Warlaumont CR, Palot JP, Verhaeghe PJ, Delattre JF. The use of Dacron in the repair of hernias of the groin. Surg Clin North Am. 1984;64:269–85.
5. Fitzgibbons RJ, Camps J, Cornet DA, et al. Laparoscopic inguinal herniorrhaphy. Results of a multicenter trial. Ann Surg. 1995;221:3–13.
6. LeBlanc KA. Two phase in vivo comparison study of adhesion formation of the Goretex Soft Tissue Patch, Marlex Mesh and Surgipro using a rabbit model. In: Arregui ME, Nagan RF, editors. Inguinal hernia: advances or controversies. Oxford, England: Radcliffe Medical Press Ltd; 1994. p. 515–7.
7. LeBlanc KA, Booth WV, Whitaker JM, Baker D. In vivo study of meshes implanted over the inguinal ring and external iliac vessels in uncastrated pigs. Surg Endosc. 1998;12:247–51.
8. Leibl B, Schwarz J, Däubler P, Ulrich M, Bittner R. Standardisierte laparoskopische hernioplastik versus shouldice-reparation. Chirurg. 1995;66:895–8.
9. Felix EL. A unified approach to recurrent laparoscopic hernia repairs. Surg Endosc. 2001;15:969–71.
10. Welsh DRJ. Sliding inguinal hernias. J Abdom Surg. 1964;6:204–209.
11. Hass BE, Schrager RE. Small bowel obstruction due to Richter's hernia after laparoscopic procedures. J Laparoendosc Surg. 1993;3:421–3.
12. Bringman S, Ek Å, Haglind E, Heikkinen T-J, Kald A, Kylberg F, Ramel S, Wallon C, Anderberg B. Is a dissection balloon beneficial in bilateral, totally extraperitoneal, endoscopic hernioplasty? A randomized, prospective, multicenter study. Surg Laparosc Endosc Percutan Tech. 2001;11(5):322–6.
13. Khajanchee YS, Urbach DR, Swanstrom LL, Hansen PD. Outcomes of laparoscopic herniorrhaphy without fixation of mesh to the abdominal wall. Surg Endosc. 2001;15:1102–7.
14. Kathouda N, Mavor E, Friedlander MH, Mason RJ, Kiyabu M, Grant SW, Achanta K, Kirkman EL, Narayanan K, Essani R. Use of fibrin sealant for prosthetic mesh fixation laparoscopic extraperitoneal inguinal hernia repair. Ann Surg. 2001;233(1):18–25.
15. Lau H. Fibrin sealant versus mechanical stapling for mesh fixation during endoscopic extraperitoneal inguinal hernioplasty: a randomized prospective trial. Ann Surg. 2005;242(5):670–5.

16. Lovisetto F, Zonta S, Rota E, Mazzilli M, Bardone M, Bottero L, Faillace G, Longoni M. Use of human fibrin glue (Tissucol) versus staples for mesh fixation in laparoscopic transabdominal preperitoneal hernioplasty: a prospective, randomized study. Ann Surg. 2007;245(2):222–31.

17. Olmi S, Scaini A, Erba L, Guaglio M, Croce E. Quantification of pain in laparoscopic transabdominal preperitoneal (TAPP) inguinal hernioplasty identifies marked differences between prosthesis fixation systems. Surgery. 2007;142(1):40–6.

18. Kapris SA, Brough WA, Royston CMS, O'Boyle C, Sedman PC. Laparoscopic transabdominal preperitoneal (TAPP) hernia repair. Surg Endosc. 2001;15:972–5.

19. Picchio M, Lombardi A, Zolovkins A, Mihelsons M, La Torre G. Tension-free laparoscopic and open hernia repair: randomized controlled trial of early results. World J Surg. 1999;23:1004–9.

20. Rosen M, Garcia-Ruiz A, Malm J, Mayes JT, Steiger E, Ponsky J. Laparoscopic hernia repair enhances early return of physical work capacity. Surg Laparosc Endosc Percutan Tech. 2001;11(1):28–33.

21. MRC Laparoscopic Groin Hernia Trial Group. Laparoscopic versus open repair of groin hernia: a randomized comparison. Lancet. 1999;354:185–90.

22. Lorenz D, Stark E, Oestreich K, Richter A. Laparoscopic hernioplasty versus conventional hernioplasty (Shouldice): results of a prospective randomized trial. World J Surg. 2000;24:739–45.

23. Bringman S, Ramel S, Heikkinen TJ, Englund T, Westman B, Anderberg B. Tension-free inguinal hernia repair: TEP versus mesh-plug versus lichtenstein. a prospective randomized controlled trial. Ann Surg. 2003;237(1):142–7.

24. Liem MSL, Van Duyn EB, Van der Graff Y, Van Vroonhoven TJMV. Recurrences after conventional anterior and laparoscopic inguinal hernia repair: a randomized comparison. Ann Surg. 2003;237(1):136–41.

25. Andersson B, Hallen M, Leveau P, Bergenfelz A, Westerdahl J. Laparoscopic extraperitoneal inguinal hernia repair versus open mesh repair: a prospective randomized controlled trial. Surgery. 2003;133(5):464–72.

26. Lal P, Kajla RK, Chander J, Saha R, Ramteke VK. Randomized controlled study of laparoscopic total extraperitoneal vs. open Lichtenstein inguinal hernia repair. Surg Endosc. 2003;17(6):850–6.

27. Eklund A, Rudberg C, Leijonmarck CE, Rasmussen I, Spangen L, Wickbom G, Wingren U, Montgomery A. Recurrent inguinal hernia: randomized multicenter trial comparing laparoscopic and Lichtenstein repair. Surg Endosc. 2007;21(4):634–40.

28. Kouhia STH, Huttunen R, Silvasti SO, Heiskanen JT, Ahtola H, Uotila-Nieminen M, Kiviniemi VV, Hakala T. Lichtenstein hernioplasty versus totally extraperitoneal laparoscopic hernioplasty in treatment of recurrent inguinal hernia—a prospective randomized trial. Ann Surg. 2009;249(3):384–7.

29. Sarli L, Iusco DR, Sansebastiano G, Costi R. Simultaneous repair of bilateral inguinal hernias. Surg Laparosc Endosc Percutan Tech. 2001;11(4):262–7.

30. Schmedt C-G, Däubler P, Leibl BJ, Kraft K, Bittner R. Simultaneous bilateral laparoscopic inguinal hernia repair. Surg Endosc. 2002;16:240–4.

31. Eklund A, Carlsson P, et al. Long-term cost minimization analysis comparing laparoscopic with open (Lichtenstein) inguinal hernia. Br J Surg. 2010;97(5):765–71.

32. Hynes D, Stroupe K, et al. Cost effectiveness of laparoscopic versus open mesh hernia operation: results of a department of veterans affairs randomized clinical trial. J Am Coll Surg. 2006;203(4):447–57.

33. Beets GL, Dirksen CD, Go P, Geisler FEA, Baeten CGMI, Kotstra G. Open or laparoscopic preperitoneal mesh repair for recurrent inguinal hernia? Surg Endosc. 1999;13:323–7.

34. Fingerhut A, Millat B, Bataille N, Yachouchi E, Dziri C, Boudet M-J, Paul A. Laparoscopic hernia repair in 2000. Update of the European Association for Endoscopic Surgery (E.A.E.S.) consensus conference in Madrid, June 1994. Surg Endosc. 2001; 15:1061–5.

35. Van Hee R, Goverde P, Hendrick L, Van der Schelling G, Totte E. Laparoscopic transperitoneal versus extraperitoneal inguinal hernia repair: a prospective clinical trial. Acta Chir Belg. 1998;98:132–5.

36. McCormack K, Wake B, et al. Transabdominal pre-peritoneal (TAPP) versus totally extraperitoneal (TEP) laparoscopic techniques for inguinal hernia repair: a systematic review. Cochrane Database Syst Rev. 2005;25(1):CD004703.

37. Liem MS, Van Steensel CJ, Boelhouwer RU, et al. The learning curve for totally extraperitoneal laparoscopic inguinal hernia repair. Am J Surg. 1996;171:281–5.

38. DeTurris SV, Cacchione RN, Mungara A, Pecoraro A, Ferzli GS. Laparoscopic herniorrhaphy: beyond the learning curve. JACS. 2002;194(1S):65–73.

39. Edelman DS, Misiakos EP, Moses K. Extraperitoneal laparoscopic hernia repair with local anesthesia. Surg Endosc. 2001;15:976–80.

40. Payne JH, Grininger LM, Izawa MT, Podoll EF, Lindahl PJ, Balfour J. Laparoscopic or open inguinal herniorrhaphy? A randomized prospective trial. Arch Surg. 1994;129:973–81.

41. Stoker DL, Spiegelhalter DJ, Singh R, Wellwood JM. Laparoscopic versus open inguinal hernia repair: randomized prospective trial. Lancet. 1994;343:1243–5.

42. Maddern GJ, Rudkin G, Bessell JR, Devitt P, Ponte L. A comparison of laparoscopic and open hernia repair as a day surgical procedure. Surg Endosc. 1994;8:1404–8.

43. Barkun JS, Wexler MJ, Hinchley EJ, Thibeault D, Meakins JL. Laparoscopic versus open inguinal herniorrhaphy: preliminary results of a randomized controlled trial. Surgery. 1995;118: 703–10.

44. Lawrence K, McWhinne D, Goodwin A, Doll H, Gordon A, Gray A, Britton J, Collin J. Randomized controlled trial of laparoscopic versus open repair of inguinal hernia: early results. Br Med J. 1995;311:981–5.

45. Vogt DM, Curet MJ, Pitcher DE, Martin DT, Zucker KA. Preliminary results of a prospective randomized trial of laparoscopic onlay versus conventional inguinal herniorrhaphy. Am J Surg. 1995;169: 84–90.

46. Schrenk P, Bettelheim P, Woisetschläger R, Reiger R, Wayand WU. Metabolic responses after laparoscopic or open hernia repair. Surg Endosc. 1996;10:628–32.

47. Liem MSL, Van der Graaf Y, Van Steensel CJ, et al. Comparison of conventional anterior surgery and laparoscopic surgery for inguinal hernia repair. N Engl J Med. 1997;336:1541–7.

48. Johansson B, Hallerback B, Glise H, Anesten B, Smedberg S, Roman J. Laparoscopic mesh repair vs. open w/wh mesh graft for inguinal hernia (SCUR hernia repair study)—preliminary results. Surg Endosc. 1997;11:170.

49. Champault GG, Rizk N, Catheline J-M, et al. Inguinal hernia repair. Totally preperitoneal laparoscopic approach versus stoppa operation: randomized trial of 100 cases. Surg Laparosc Endosc. 1997;7(6):445–50.

50. Wellwood J, Sculpher MJ, Stoker D, Nicholls GJ, Geddes C, Whitehead A, Singh R, Spieghalter D. Randomized controlled trial of laparoscopic versus open mesh repair for hernia: outcome and cost. BMJ. 1998;317:103–10.

51. Cohen RV, Alvarez G, Roll S, Garcia ME, Kawahara N, Schiavon CA, Schaffa TD, Pereira PR, Margarido NF, Rodrigues AJ. Transabdominal or extraperitoneal laparoscopic hernia repair? Surg Laparosc Endosc. 1998;8:264–8.

52. Khoury N. A randomized prospective controlled trial of laparoscopic extraperitoneal hernia repair and mesh-plug hernioplasty: a study of 315 cases. J Laparoendosc Adv Surg Tech A. 1998; 8:367–72.

53. Johansson B, Hallerback B, Glise H, Anesten B, Smedberg S, Roman J. Laparoscopic mesh versus open preperitoneal versus open conventional technique for inguinal hernia repair: a randomized multicenter trial (SCUR hernia repair study). Ann Surg. 1999;230:225–31.

54. Wright D, Paterson C, Scott N, Hair A, Grant A, O'Dwyer PJ. Five-year follow up of patients undergoing laparoscopic or open groin hernia repair—a randomized controlled trial. Ann Surg. 2002;235:333–7.

55. Neumayer L, Giobbie-Hurder A, Jonasson O, Fitzgibbons R, Dunlop D, Gibbs J, Reda D, Henderson W. Open mesh versus laparoscopic mesh repair of inguinal hernia. N Engl J Med. 2004;350(18):1819–27.

56. Hallen M, Bergenfelz A, Westerdahl J. Laparoscopic extraperitoneal inguinal hernia repair versus open mesh repair: long-term follow up of a randomized controlled trial. Surgery. 2008;143(3):313–7.

57. Pokorny H, Klingler A, Schmid T, Fortelny R, Hollinsky C, Kawji R, Steiner E, Pernthaler H, Fugger R, Scheyer M. Recurrence and complications after laparoscopic versus open inguinal hernia repair: results of a prospective randomized multicenter trial. Hernia. 2008;12(4):385–9.

58. Eklund A, Montgomery A, Rasmussen IC, Sandbue RP, Bergkvist LA, Rudberg CR. Low Recurrence Rate After Laparoscopic (TEP) and Open (Lichtenstein) Inguinal Hernia Repair: A Randomized, Multicenter Trial With 5-Year Follow-Up. Ann Surg. 2009;249(1):33–8.

Femoral Hernia

Patrick J. O'Dwyer

A femoral hernia is a protrusion of a peritoneal sac, covered with extraperitoneal fat, into the femoral sheath. The most common femoral hernia enters the femoral canal, which is that "space" in the sheath medial to the femoral vessels as they proceed from the abdomen into the thigh. A femoral hernial sac may contain all or part of an abdominal viscus, including the ureter [1].

Femoral hernias occur much less frequently than inguinal hernias and account for about 2–4% of groin hernia repairs [2, 3]. Femoral hernias are more frequent in females than males with a ratio of 4:1 [4]. Male patients with femoral hernias have frequently undergone an inguinal hernia repair [5]. Femoral hernias are more frequent on the right than left side in a ratio of 2:1 and are bilateral in 1 in 15 persons. The incidence of femoral hernias in children is very low, but it appears that this is twice as common in females than males [6]. In females the incidence increases with age as 42% of femoral hernias are in women aged over 65 years [7]. In the elderly, emergency herniorrhaphy is necessary in 44% of patients with femoral hernias [8]. In general, an emergency operation for femoral hernias is fraught with greater rates of complications and mortality [3]. In tropical Africa, femoral hernias are very rare; it is postulated that the frequency of inguinal lymphadenitis involving Cloquet's node in the femoral canal protects tropical Africans from femoral hernia [9].

One study that evaluated the value of diagnostic laparoscopy during the repair of hernias found that the diagnosis of a femoral hernia that was present at the time of operation was unsuspected preoperatively in 11% of the 253 patients that were studied [10]. This raises several questions regarding the actual incidence of these hernias in the hernia patient population. However, even the authors felt that this high rate of a femoral component may have reflected a bias in patient selection because of the predominance of bilateral hernias in this series. Seventy-two percent of the patients with unsuspected femoral hernias had bilateral hernia, which may signify a diffuse fascial weakness as the etiology of these newly discovered hernias. The use of diagnostic laparoscopy in the pediatric patient population appears to offer benefits as well [11]. Similarly, the use of diagnostic laparoscopy for undiagnosed chronic pain can reveal unsuspected femoral hernias [12].

The etiology of femoral hernia is poorly defined. In contrast to inguinal hernia, there is no easy embryological explanation. The fact that femoral hernias are most frequently found in middle-aged and elderly females and the disparity in incidence between parous and nulliparous women suggests that intra-abdominal pressure and the stretching of aponeurotic tissue consequent on pregnancy are important factors. Chronic cough, intestinal obstruction, constipation, and excessive physical labor may also contribute to raised intra-abdominal pressure. Weight loss in the elderly female is also associated with femoral hernia. Nurses are said to be more prone to femoral hernia. Ten percent of femoral hernias follow a previous operation for an inguinal hernia; indeed, femoral hernias in men almost always occur after an operation for an inguinal hernia [5, 13].

A very rare congenital femoral hernia in males is associated with descent of the testicle through the femoral canal into the thigh. Four well-documented cases are recorded in the literature. Absence of the ipsilateral testicle from the scrotum and an incompletely reducible femoral hernia should arouse suspicion [14].

Anatomy

Femoral hernia has a sinister reputation because of the unyielding anatomy of the femoral canal. The whole canal (i.e., the space between the pubis and the iliopsoas muscle) is bounded anteriorly by the inguinal ligament, posteriorly by

P.J. O'Dwyer (✉)
Department of Surgery, Western Infirmary,
Glasgow, Scotland, UK
e-mail: pjod2j@clinmed.gla.ac.uk

A.N. Kingsnorth and K.A. LeBlanc (eds.), *Management of Abdominal Hernias*,
DOI 10.1007/978-1-84882-877-3_17, © Springer Science+Business Media London 2013

Fig. 17.1 Boundaries of the femoral canal

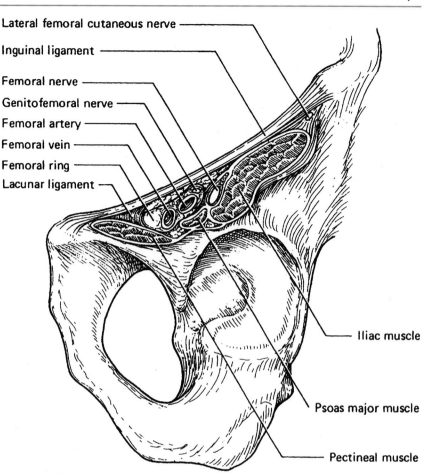

Lateral femoral cutaneous nerve

Inguinal ligament

Femoral nerve

Genitofemoral nerve

Femoral artery

Femoral vein

Femoral ring

Lacunar ligament

Iliac muscle

Psoas major muscle

Pectineal muscle

the pectineal (Cooper's) ligament at its attachment to the iliopectineal line of the pubic bone, medially by the sharp lateral margin of the lacunar ligament, and laterally by the iliopsoas muscle with its overlying fascia (Fig. 17.1).

The canal is divided into two compartments, the lateral being occupied by the femoral artery and femoral vein and the smaller medial by areolar tissue, some lymphatics, and a lymph node. The femoral vessels are encased in the femoral sheath of fascia transversalis. Anteriorly, the sheath is continuous with the fascia transversalis deep to the inguinal ligament; posteriorly, the femoral sheath fuses with the pectineal ligament. The sheath extends into the thigh. From the abdomen the sheath resembles a funnel extending down to the fossa ovalis where the saphenous vein penetrates the cribriform fascia (anteroinferior femoral sheath). It is through this small medial compartment or funnel that the usual femoral hernia penetrates into the thigh [15–17].

Once in the thigh the sac pushes anteriorly onto the relatively weak cribriform fascia—the anterior femoral sheath that surrounds the fossa ovalis opening for the saphenous vein. It carries the stretched cribriform fascia before it and bulges into the thigh. The fundus is then forced upward to lie over the inguinal ligament. Two factors combine to make it turn superiorly: these are the fusion of the femoral sheath

with the deep fascia of the thigh and the repeated flexion of the hip joint (Fig. 17.2) [16]. Because of the upward turn toward the inguinal ligament, the femoral hernia can be misdiagnosed as an inguinal hernia.

In its advancement into the thigh, the hernial sac carries with it some extraperitoneal fat about its fundus, and it may draw the extraperitoneal anterolateral wall of the bladder down with it on its medial aspect. Once the sac is entrenched in the thigh, the medial wall of the hernia, consisting of peritoneal sac, extraperitoneal fat, and fascia transversalis, is pressed up against the sharp margin of the lacunar ligament medially, the unyielding pectineal fascia and pubic bone posteriorly, the inguinal ligament anteriorly, and the femoral vein laterally. As the hernia emerges from the saphenous opening, the sharp upper margin of the cribriform fascia also contributes to the structuring of the sac [17, 18].

The compression of the sac leads to fibrosis in it at its neck so that it constricts any contents, omentum, or intestine. This stricturing of the sac neck is an important factor in the mechanism of strangulation. Very often, the strictured sac neck is the confining structure in a strangulated hernia rather than the lacunar or pectineal ligaments.

Compression of the femoral vein and the saphenous vein by a femoral hernia may occur; indeed, visible distension of

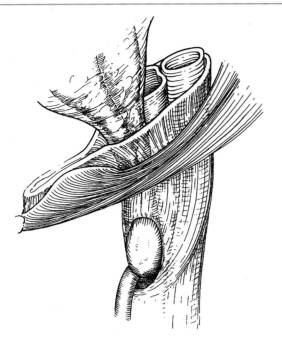

Fig. 17.2 Anatomy of a femoral hernia. The hernial sac progresses down the femoral sheath "funnel" to present in the thigh. In the thigh the fundus of the hernia carries the attenuated cribriform fascia before it

these veins is a diagnostic sign in the differential diagnosis of a femoral hernia from other groin swellings. Saphenous vein distension is particularly pronounced in cases when the femoral hernia has progressed through the cribriform fascia into the thigh and in doing so has compromised the saphenous vein at its termination into the femoral vein [19].

Presentation

Population-based studies demonstrate that 35–40% of femoral hernias present as an emergency [2, 3]. Emergency presentation is more common in women than in men and is associated with a tenfold increase in mortality rate. Bowel resection for strangulation is required in around 1 in 5 patients presenting as an emergency. The next most common method of presentation is a painful lump in the groin that is irreducible. This is sometimes mistaken for painful lymphadenopathy, and it is only on exploration that a femoral hernia is diagnosed. In some patients the lump may not cause pain, and the differential diagnosis with and enlarged lymph node can often be resolved by ultrasound or CT scanning. CT is also helpful in the small group of patients who present with groin pain and no clinical evidence of a femoral hernia or those who present with intermittent or complete small bowel obstruction with similar findings.

Femoral hernias are reducible or often misdiagnosed as an inguinal hernia particularly in men. In a study by Mikkelsen et al. [20] they demonstrated a 15-fold greater incidence of femoral hernia after inguinal herniorrhaphy compared with the spontaneous incidence. These hernias occurred earlier than an inguinal recurrence suggesting that they were overlooked at the primary operation. One reason for misdiagnosis is that finding the femoral canal particularly in obese patients can be difficult. Palpating the adductor longus tendon at the medial end of the groin crease and following the crease laterally until a fingerbreadth from the femoral artery is helpful in these patients. Occluding the canal and asking the patient to cough should differentiate a reducible femoral from an inguinal hernia and allow the rapid surgical management required for these patients. This can be very difficult in the pediatric population especially [21].

Differential Diagnosis

This subject is discussed in Chap. 12.

Management of Femoral Hernias

Operation should always be advised for two reasons:
1. The incidence of strangulation in these hernias is high. Many femoral hernias occur in elderly women, and a strangulated femoral hernia in the elderly woman carries a considerable mortality.
2. It is impossible to make and fit an adequate truss to control such a hernia.

Many femoral hernias present with incarceration or strangulation. The ratio of elective to emergent operations for these hernias varies anywhere from 1.3:1 or 1.5:1 to 5:1 [22–24]. In some other reports, the emergent cases outnumbered the elective ones by 10:1 [25]. The ratio of elective to emergent femoral hernias compared to that of inguinal hernias is approximately 6.4:1 [11]. In other words, the need for an emergent operation for a femoral hernia is over six times greater than that of an inguinal hernia. The female patients incur 76.7% of the incidence of strangulated femoral hernias than the male patients [23]. In this latter series, the frequency of strangulation of femoral hernias was 43% (vs. only 5% of inguinal hernias), but others have reported an incidence of 50% [26]. This demonstrates the need to repair all of these hernias when the diagnosis is made. Additionally, there is an increased frequency of comorbidities in the elderly patients thereby making the nonelective operations more risky [27].

When a patient presents with intestinal obstruction and a femoral hernia, reduction by taxis, should not be employed. A partial enterocele (Richter's hernia) is common in femoral hernias. These patients may have confusing symptoms and signs; a high index of diagnostic suspicion should always be maintained. Urgent operation after adequate resuscitation and cardiorespiratory management in elderly shocked patients needs emphasizing.

Tingwald and Cooperman have emphasized the problems presented by the elderly with groin hernias [25]. Due to the increased risk of postoperative complications, some surgeons are becoming increasingly reluctant to perform elective procedures on these patients [28]. However, with femoral hernias, delay only increases the likelihood of incarceration, and then emergency surgery in a more ill patient will be required. Elective repair of a femoral hernia is an urgency; these patients are at considerable hazard of strangulation if they have to wait for surgery. The National Confidential Enquiry in England has repeatedly warned of the high mortality of emergency surgery for strangulated femoral hernias in the female [29, 30]. All these facts are confirmed by the most recent series from North Tees; the coexisting medical morbidities in the emergency cases included respiratory disease, chronic obstructive airway disease (19%), coronary artery disease (40%), neurological disease (10%), and diabetes mellitus in 8%. The morbidity following emergency operation was also higher than elective operation, with pulmonary embolism occurring only in the emergency cases [27].

Operative Approaches to Femoral Hernia

A femoral hernia is a variety of groin hernia—a defect in the fascia transversalis which is exploited by a peritoneal sac traversing the muscular weakness of the myopectineal orifice of Fruchaud—exactly similar to a patent processus vaginalis in an indirect inguinal hernia exploiting the deep ring in the fascia transversalis posterior wall of the inguinal canal or a direct hernial peritoneal sac expanding into an acquired defect of the fascia transversalis. This being so, repair of a femoral hernia inexorably follows the same canons of repair as an inguinal hernia repair. Isolate and excise the peritoneal sac, repair the fascia transversalis defect, and then reinforce this repair by adjusting the local aponeurotic attachments.

In sequence, a femoral hernia occurs when the femoral sheath, a funnel of fascia transversalis enclosing the femoral vessels beneath the inguinal ligament, becomes dilated. A peritoneal sac enters the femoral funnel and then, as a plunger, causes it to dilate. As the fascia transversalis pushes onto the ligament, it becomes scarred and often strictured around its neck and in doing so pushes the attachment of the transversus abdominis aponeurosis medially along the pectineal line until the medial margin of the femoral sheath abuts on the inguinal ligament anteriorly, the lacunar ligament medially, and the pectineal ligament posteriorly. After excision of the peritoneal sac, the femoral sheath must be repaired medially, and the hernioplasty must prevent further herniation; to do this, the attachment of the fascia transversalis to the pectineal ligament must be broadened. This recon-struction of the medial femoral sheath can be reinforced by suturing the tendon of transversus abdominis to the pectineal line (McVay/Cooper's ligament repair) or from below by turning up a flap of pectineus fascia to close the medial femoral canal or finally by plugging it with a mesh prosthesis [31, 32].

As an alternative, the entire operation can be conducted in the extraperitoneal (preperitoneal) layer and a mesh repair of the canal constructed in this layer [33, 34].

Eponyms really confuse the surgeon here and are best discarded temporarily. Three approaches that apply a tissue repair to femoral hernioplasty are described; because none of these is universally applicable, the surgeon must be acquainted with all three:

1. The abdominal [35], suprapubic [36], retropubic [37], preperitoneal [38], or extraperitoneal [33, 39, 40] operation. This approach, developed by Henry, is often known as the McEvedy approach, although Henry used a midline incision and McEvedy a pararectus incision [41]. A Pfannenstiel incision enables bilateral hernias to be operated simultaneously by this approach (Eponyms: Cheatle [39], Henry [40], McEvedy [41]).
2. The inguinal or "high" operation (Eponyms: Annandale [42], Lotheissen [43], Moschowitz [44]).
3. The crural or "low" operation (Eponyms: Bassini [45], Lockwood [46]).

The open extraperitoneal approach gives excellent access to the femoral canal and to the general peritoneal cavity should that be necessary to deal with a strangulated viscus. However, this approach to the pelvis is unfamiliar to most surgeons and, therefore, not to be recommended to the inexperienced surgeon operating on his first strangulated femoral hernia at the dead of night [47].

The open inguinal approach is familiar but has the twin drawbacks of disrupting the inguinal canal mechanism and not providing adequate access to a strangulated viscus. If this approach is used, an excellent repair of the fascia transversalis (Shouldice technique) must be employed to avoid the complicating inguinal hernia. This is particularly so in women, in whom direct inguinal hernia is almost unknown … except as a complication of this operation.

The open crural approach to the femoral sac is good and bloodless, and repair of the hernia is easy by this method. Its most significant disadvantage is that access to a strangulated viscus is often very inadequate. The crural approach is recommended for elective operation and to the occasional or novice surgeon. This is the quickest and least traumatic operation to perform [27, 48, 49]. If a visceral strangulation is present, it is best to perform either a lower midline or Pfannenstiel incision and deal with the crisis through an incision which is familiar to most abdominal operators. With an emergency situation, or for the inexperienced surgeon, this is no place for an anatomical extravaganza.

The "Low" or Crural Operation

Preoperative Management

In the uncomplicated case no special preoperative management is required. The bladder is frequently a sliding component of the medial wall of a femoral hernia, and preoperative catheterization is a sensible precaution, which will lessen the likelihood of bladder injury.

If the hernia is strangulated or obstructed, preoperative nasogastric aspiration and adequate fluid replacement is mandatory. The patient must be fully resuscitated, and comorbidities, especially in the elderly, adequately managed.

Anesthesia

General anesthesia is preferred, but local anesthesia can be employed. Local infiltration with extra injection around the sac neck will suffice.

The Operation

Position of Patient

The patient is placed supine on the operating table, which is tilted head down 15°.

Draping

If the hernia is not strangulated, draping to allow access to the groin only is required. If strangulation or obstruction is present or suspected, towels should be placed to enable easy access to the lower abdomen if a laparotomy becomes necessary. A sterile adhesive drape can be used.

The Incision

A skin incision is made over the hernia. The incision is about 6 cm long and parallel to the inguinal ligament.

After the skin is divided, it is easy to separate the subcutaneous fat down to the coverings of the hernial sac. Hemostasis should be secured before the sac is mobilized.

Mobilization of Sac

The sac, having emerged from the femoral canal, carries before it fascia transversalis and extraperitoneal fat in front of which are the attenuated cribriform fascia and the femoral

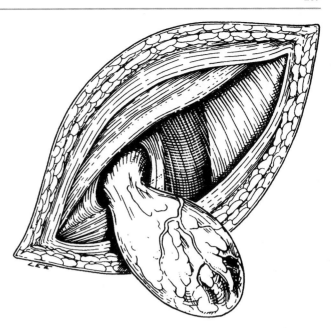

Fig. 17.3 The sac mobilized

fascial layer of the thigh. Because of these fascial layers, the sac usually makes a forward upward turn in its path at the fossa ovalis; thus, its fundus will be found lying over the inguinal ligament. It is important to appreciate this before mobilization is attempted. Once the sac is identified, the fascial layers are cleaned from it by blunt dissection, which is best achieved by breaking up the adherent scar tissue and fat with a hemostat and then wiping the fascia off with a gauze swab. These extraperitoneal coverings of the sac are frequently quite thick and fibrosed and are most often the real constricting layer when strangulation has occurred (Fig. 17.3).

Identification of Femoral Opening

The neck of the sac is now cleared of fat and fascia so that the boundaries of the femoral canal can be identified. It is best to identify the medial and anterior margins of the canal first. The medial margin is the lacunar ligament and is easily seen as it sweeps around from the inguinal ligament to the subjacent pubic bone. Anteriorly, the rolled-over edge of the inguinal ligament can readily be separated from the sac underneath it. The sac should next be lifted up. The fascia on the pectineus muscle is easily recognizable, and if this is traced back to the ramus of the pubis, the posterior margin of the canal—the pectineal ligament—can be recognized.

Attention is now turned to the lateral boundary of the canal—the femoral vein. This is the most vulnerable structure in this area and is difficult to identify because it is covered with a quite opaque fascial sheath. One maneuver is to identify the femoral artery by touch;

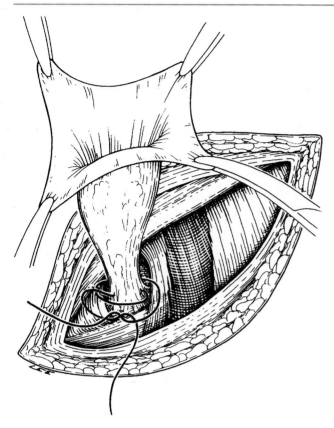

Fig. 17.4 Closure of the sac

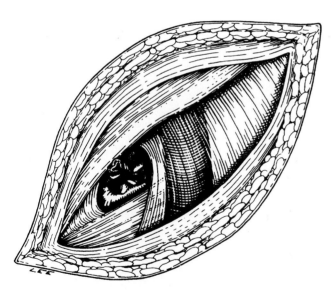

Fig. 17.5 The canal after closure of the sac

the artery lies immediately lateral to the vein, so the vein must be in any space between the sac and the palpable artery. A careful dissection is made on the lateral side of the sac, preferably using Metzenbaum scissors and keeping close to the sac. The dissection of the sac is only complete when the entire circumference of its neck has been clearly defined (Fig. 17.4).

Inspection of Contents of Sac

The lateral side of the fundus of the sac should now be opened. The medial side should be avoided, as it may be partly formed by the bladder. There is always much adherent extraperitoneal fat on the fundus which generally contains many distended veins. If these bleed, they can confuse the anatomy, so the fat should be gently broken through with a hemostat point and the bleeding carefully controlled.

Inside the extraperitoneal fat, the true peritoneal hernial sac will be found. It is grasped in a hemostat and then opened.

Any contents of the sac can now be gently freed, adhesions divided, and the contents reduced back into the general peritoneal cavity. If strangulation is present, an alternative approach to the remainder of the operation may be necessary. Often, a small nubbin of strangulated dead omentum may be discovered; this should be isolated, its blood supply ligated, and then excised.

Closure and Excision of Sac

When it is certain that the neck of the sac is isolated and that the sac is empty, it can be closed and excised. Traction is applied to the open sac, and, using metric 3.5 braided absorbable polymer on a 40-mm round needle (0 or 00 suture on a soft tissue needle), a transfixion suture should be securely tied around the neck. The redundant sac is cut off, leaving a generous cuff beyond the transfixion suture. The stump of the sac will now recede through the femoral canal and out of sight (Fig. 17.5).

Repair of Canal

The canal is repaired using a single figure-of-eight suture of metric 3 (0 or 00) polypropylene (or other nonabsorbable suture) on a J-shaped (or round) needle.

The femoral vein is retracted laterally, and the pectineal ligament clearly identified on the superior ramus of the pubic bone. The first suture is placed through this ligament from its deep aspect at the point where the medial margin of the femoral vein would lie if it were not retracted. It is necessary to experiment with the retractor and identify this point correctly. If the suture is placed too far laterally, the vein will be compromised, and if placed too far medially, the repair will be unsound (Fig. 17.6).

The next bite must pick up the inguinal ligament and iliopubic tract of fascia transversalis at a corresponding distance from its pubic attachment, so that the suture forms the base of an isosceles triangle. Next, the pectineal ligament is picked up, again from deep to superficial, halfway between the first

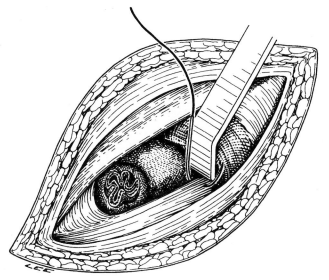

Fig. 17.6 Retraction of the femoral vein laterally enables visualization of the pectineal (Cooper's) ligament. The first suture is not introduced

pectineal suture and the lacunar ligament, and finally the inguinal ligament is picked up, again halfway between the first suture and the attachment of the ligament to the pubis.

Now, the free end of the suture is passed deep to the two loops, and the two ends are tied securely. When the suture is pulled tight, the medial 0.75 cm or so of the inguinal ligament will be approximated to the pectineal line and the femoral canal closed. Furthermore, if the knot is placed at the medial side, it will be away from the femoral vein which will not be damaged by it (Fig. 17.7).

Comment on Crural Operation

Although the primary defect is in the fascia transversalis at the wide part of the femoral canal (the open funnel), this operation does not primarily address itself to this defect. This is the major negative feature of the operation. The fascia transversalis is, inevitably, tangled up when the sac is originally closed, the stump of sac and extraperitoneal fat blocks the medial part of the funnel, and the attachment of the inguinal ligament to the pectineal ligament reduces the potential size of the femoral canal.

The skin and subcutaneous tissues are closed as before. Disadvantages of the "low" approach, which are important in obstructed patients, are as follows:

1. Difficulty in delivering obstructed bowel for review. This is most relevant in Richter's hernia (partial enterocele) where the involved loop is especially liable to slip back into the abdomen and be irretrievable.
2. It is impossible to put an anastomosis, which is bulky, back into the abdomen through the femoral canal. A separate laparotomy is needed if bowel resection is necessary.

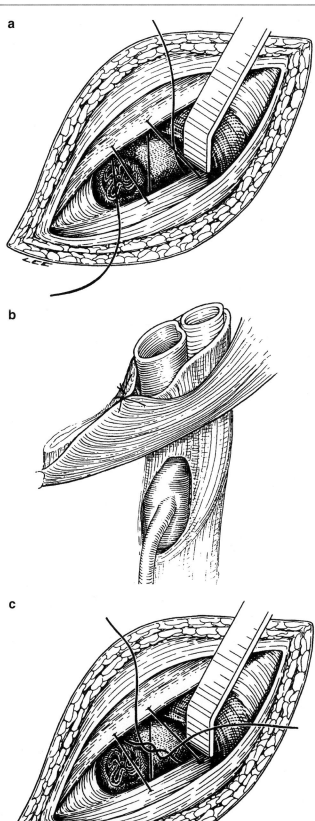

Fig. 17.7 (**a**, **b**) The next suture picks up the inguinal ligament and subjacent iliopubic tract of fascia transversalis. Care must be taken to avoid the cord structures in the wall. The suture is placed to form the base of an isosceles triangle with the apex at the pubic tubercle. (**c**) The knot is tied deeply at the medial side away from the femoral vein

This may lead to contamination of the main peritoneal cavity unless great care is taken.

3. The crural operation provides inadequate exposure if there is difficulty reducing and mobilizing the contents of a hernial sac.

4. It can be difficult to excise a thickened fibrous sac down to flush with the parietal peritoneum.

5. In long-standing hernia, access for an adequate repair is limited.

Inguinal Operation

This operation achieves the same objective of closing the medial portion of the femoral canal which has been described using the crural approach. However, in the inguinal approach, the femoral canal is exposed by opening the posterior wall—the fascia transversalis—of the inguinal canal and achieving initial closure, using the fascia transversalis, of the femoral cone. Approximating the inguinal to the pectineal ligaments, if the inguinal ligament is grossly stretched, can reinforce this repair.

The incision and dissection for this operation are exactly the same as those employed in the Shouldice operation for inguinal hernia. After the fascia transversalis in the posterior wall of the inguinal canal has been opened, the extraperitoneal fat on the neck of the femoral hernia can be identified and removed by blunt dissection (Fig. 17.8).

The sac can now either be delivered above the inguinal ligament or opened below the ligament, and its contents reduced. The neck of the sac is then transfixed and ligated (Fig. 17.9).

The medial extremity of the inguinal ligament is now sutured to the pectineal ligament by figure-of-eight nonabsorbable sutures. In this instance, care must be taken to insure that the deep closure does not impinge upon the femoral vein. In this operation these are inserted from above, that is, through the incision in the posterior wall of the inguinal canal.

The inguinal canal is then repaired using the Shouldice (or Bassini) technique, care being taken to reinforce the femoral repair with the overlapped fascia transversalis at the medial part of the canal. It is advisable, particularly in women with a broad pelvis, to reinforce the medial repair by suturing the insertion of the transversus muscle tendon (conjoint tendon) to the pectineal ligament (Cooper's ligament repair). In the era of mesh repair, the inguinal canal may also be reinforced with an open weave polypropylene mesh after closure of the transversalis fascia in a manner similar to that described by Lichtenstein for inguinal hernia repair.

Comment on Inguinal Operation

The inguinal approach for the repair of femoral hernia is not recommended as the operation of choice because it is technically more difficult and more time consuming than the crural

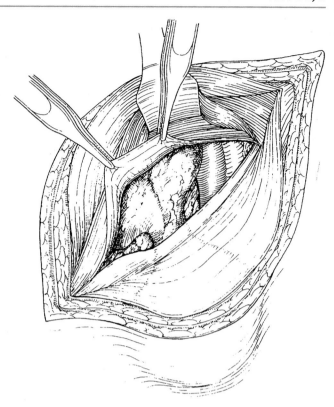

Fig. 17.8 Extraperitoneal fat on the neck of the femoral hernia can be identified and removed by blunt dissection

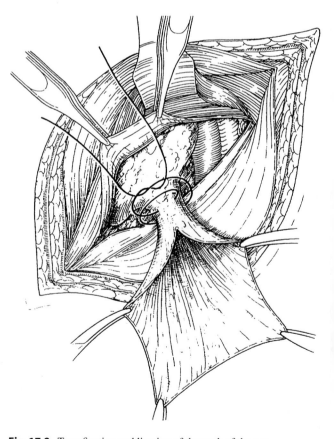

Fig. 17.9 Transfixation and ligation of the neck of the sac

operation and because it disrupts an otherwise normal inguinal canal.

However, some experts, notably Tanner in Britain [50] and Glasgow in Canada [51], recommend this operation strongly. If this approach is used, the repair of the transversalis/transversus layer to the pectineal ligament must be adequate and must extend the tendinous attachment of the transversus muscle laterally along the pectineal ligament as far as the femoral vein. Often, to do this without tension, a generous "medial slide" of the lateral rectus sheath/conjoint tendon must be made. Others have good results either with the tissue repair or with the use of mesh in this approach [52, 53].

Extraperitoneal (Preperitoneal) Operation

This operation illustrates the genius of an expert surgical anatomist exploiting fascial plane dissection at its most elegant. Henry's extraperitoneal approach to the anterior pelvis gives an excellent exposure of both femoral canals simultaneously, but it is not an operation for the novice. In the hands of an expert, it is a fine operation enabling bilateral femoral hernia to be dealt with simultaneously through one incision [40, 54].

The patient is placed on the operating table, and the bladder emptied by catheterization. A vertical midline suprapubic incision is made, the aponeurotic layer is opened vertically in the midline, and the peritoneum is exposed.

Alternatively, a Pfannenstiel incision, with a suprapubic side-to-side opening of the anterior rectus sheath and separation of the rectus muscles, gives good access and a much more acceptable skin scar.

The recti are retracted to either side, and the space between the peritoneum and the abdominal wall muscles is opened by gentle blunt dissection in order to approach the femoral canal on either side. If only a unilateral hernia is present, a pararectal vertical (McEvedy) [41] or skin crease (Ogilvie) [55] incision can be used.

Femoral sacs are dealt with by reduction of their contents, transfixion of their necks, and resection of redundant sac (Fig. 17.10). If strangulation is present, the subjacent peritoneum can easily be opened, the contents of the sac inspected, and so forth (Fig. 17.11).

The femoral canal is repaired using a nonabsorbable suture, as described in the inguinal operation. The anterior abdominal wall is closed layer by layer.

Comment on Extraperitoneal Operation

The extraperitoneal operation has advantages but also disadvantages:

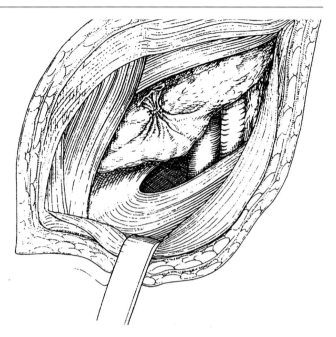

Fig. 17.10 An adequate approach to a unilateral hernia can be made through an oblique or vertical pararectus incision

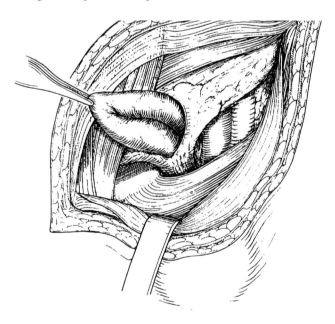

Fig. 17.11 Opening a femoral hernial sac

1. An extensive mobilization of the lower abdominal wall is required.
2. It cannot easily be performed using local anesthesia.
3. With mobilization there is a risk of bleeding and hematoma formation between the peritoneum and the endopelvic fascia.
4. Unless an adequate repair of the abdominal wall is made, an abdominal incisional hernia can ensue.

The Three Open Approaches

The femoral hernia surgeon should ideally be familiar with all three approaches:

1. The low approach is recommended for the easily reducible uncomplicated femoral hernia especially in the thin patient and in the frail ASA class 3 or 4 patient, when it can be undertaken electively using local anesthesia.
2. The inguinal approach is best used when there is a concomitant primary inguinal hernia on the same side which can be repaired simultaneously.
3. The extraperitoneal approach is used when obstruction or strangulation are present, in patients who have undergone previous groin surgery, when inguinal and femoral hernias occur together, and in bilateral cases where both sides can be repaired simultaneously [37, 53].

Open Prosthetic Repair

The above tissue repairs are becoming much less common in the developed nations of the world. The use of prosthetic biomaterials is becoming the preferred method. This is especially true for recurrent repairs in which the recurrence rate is 22% as reported by the Shouldice Clinic in Toronto, Canada. Approximately 20% of primary and 50% of recurrent femoral hernias are repaired with mesh at that institution [56]. Other retrospective studies have identified a reduction in the rate of recurrence from 2–10% to 0–1.1% with the use of prosthetic materials [57, 58]. The use of a bilayer mesh device has been used with success in the repair of femoral hernias [59]. With this method, most surgeons will excise the majority of the overlay portion of the product and utilize the underlay in the preperitoneal space and secure the connecting portion to the tissues (see the prosthetic chapter for a description of this product).

Plug and Patch

The concept of the plug-and-patch repair is based upon the prior "umbrella plug" and "dart" repairs of the inguinal hernia. The development of the preformed plug for the inguinal hernia repair has resulted in its use for the femoral hernia. The open approach to the femoral hernia is similar to that of the inguinal approach above, or one can use the femoral approach directly. The inguinal incision does have the advantage of an easier inspection of the entire inguinofemoral area should the preoperative diagnosis be anatomically incorrect. The sac will be identified and the neck dissected accordingly. In this repair, unlike the tissue repairs described above, the sac is not ligated. The dissection is carried into the preperito-

neal space so that the neck of the sac is also dissected. This is necessary so that the sac can be fully imbricated into the preperitoneal space. If this is not carried out satisfactorily, there will be a higher risk of recurrence. After this dissection is completed, the defect is then filled with the plug. It is important that the inner petals of the plug are removed so that the plug will fill this area with ease, as it is usually too firm to be placed into this site as manufactured. This can result in a permanently palpable mass effect at the site of the former femoral hernia site. Additionally, there is a risk of causing a relative area of venous obstruction as the plug may occupy too much space and impinge upon the femoral vein.

It is important to fixate the plug after it is positioned in the defect. Several absorbable sutures are required such as polyglactin 910. This will prevent the migration that has been reported with the use of the plug. The scarification that will eventuate will secure the plug and repair the hernia defect. The closure of the subcutaneous tissue and skin will usually be performed with an absorbable suture.

There have been few reports in the published literature regarding the use of the plug and patch in the repair of femoral hernias. Because of the very nature of the infrequency of the femoral hernia, the numbers of patients have always been small. One of these early reports included only 24 cases and represented less than 1% of the patients in that series. There were no apparent complications or recurrences in these few patients [60]. Other reports have shown similar results [24, 61, 62]. Recent literature appears to show that the preperitoneal repair is preferred over the plug-and-patch method, as there are fewer instances of seroma formation, sensation of foreign body, and a lower recurrence rate [63].

Laparoscopic Femoral Hernia Repair

The repair of the femoral hernia with the laparoscopic placement of a preperitoneal mesh is identical to the transabdominal preperitoneal or the totally extraperitoneal inguinal operations [64]. These are described in Chap. 14. There is no difference in technique because the exposure of the myopectineal orifice by these two procedures will provide an excellent visualization of the femoral hernia. The identified sac and the frequently encountered prevascular fat will easily be reduced by the laparoscopic approach. It is important to carefully inspect the femoral hernia so that any incarcerated fat will be identified and removed. These defects can be quite small, and this could sometimes be overlooked. Any associated inguinal hernias could also be identified at that time. This has been successfully performed in the pediatric population [65].

The repair would proceed as would the chosen inguinal repair, but one should ensure that the prosthetic mesh is of sufficient size to provide an adequate coverage of the entire inguinal and femoral areas. It is critical that this mesh provides enough overlap to prevent the presentation of an inguinal hernia in the future postoperative period.

Unfortunately, because the repair of femoral hernias with the laparoscopic method is identical to that of the inguinal hernia repair, most series do not differentiate between the two hernioplasties. The actual incidence of isolated femoral hernia repair with the laparoscope may be 1.5%, but the identification of an additional 13.7% of unsuspected femoral hernias in this series suggests that there may be a significant number of "missed" hernias during the anterior approach to inguinal herniorrhaphy [66].

The postoperative care of the patient will be similar to that of the inguinal hernia repair patients. As can occur with the latter group, the site of the prior herniation can frequently fill with seromatous fluid and continue to present as a mass at the site of the former hernia. This is so common that this should be explained to the patient preoperatively to avert the concern that will be forthcoming if this had not been addressed in the office.

Strangulation

Strangulation is very uncommon in patients aged under 40 years old. Strangulation is more frequent in females than males and reaches its highest incidence and greatest morbidity in women in their seventh and eighth decades.

If strangulation is suspected, it is prudent to avoid the laparoscopic totally extraperitoneal repair. As already stated an open preperitoneal approach usually through a pararectal vertical incision is the approach of choice as it allows access to the peritoneal cavity for small bowel resection should it be required [67]. An alternative approach to avoid a lower abdominal incision is to perform a laparoscopy. If the bowel is incarcerated rather than strangulated or the content is omentum only, this can be reduced by adding two 5-mm operating trocars: one in the midline and one in the ipsilateral iliac fossa. An experienced laparoscopic surgeon should be able to perform a TAPP repair or close the defect by suturing the iliopubic tract and inguinal ligament to the pectineal ligament with a nonabsorbable suture. If the surgeon cannot do this, the hernia can now be repaired using a low approach. If there is doubt about the viability of the bowel at laparoscopy, the patient should be converted to an open approach to avoid the risk of peritoneal contamination.

The sac should be opened on the lateral aspect of its fundus and the contents inspected. Once the sac is identified, it will contain blood-stained fluid if strangulation has occurred. A variety of intra-abdominal viscera may be found in the femoral hernial sac. Waddington, in 1971, reviewed 128 patients with strangulated femoral hernia; the most fre-

quently strangulated viscera were, in rank order, small bowel, then small bowel and omentum, then omentum alone, and then appendix, colon, bladder, and lastly fallopian tube [68]. No viscus should be returned to the peritoneal cavity unless it is definitely viable. Viability of any viscus can only be assessed after its blood supply has been normalized by removing the constriction at the neck of the sac.

Any blood-stained fluid in the sac is sampled for microbiological culture, and the remainder sucked out. The contents of the sac are gently manipulated so that the neck of the sac is revealed clearly. It is very important to be careful with a strangulated loop of gut, as operative perforation can seriously hazard the patient's recovery. Quite frequently, careful dissection of the neck of the sac and removal of edematous extraperitoneal fat about it are all that is required to release the strangulation. The constricting agent is usually the thickened transversalis fascia and peritoneal neck of the sac and the edematous extraperitoneal fat about it, rather than the ligamentous structures which form the anterior, posterior, and medial margins of the sac. The femoral vein is very rarely involved in the strangulation process, which confirms that the neck of the sac itself is most usually the constricting agent.

After the strangulation has been released, any contained viscera are wrapped in warm saline packs and left alone for a full 5 min before being inspected. Omentum of doubtful viability is best excised. Small intestine must only be returned to the peritoneal cavity if it has all been inspected and shown to be vital. Often, there is a linear necrosis of the bowel where it has been compressed by the neck of the sac; this should be oversewn.

If the surgeon is unfamiliar with the preperitoneal approach, a lower midline incision can be made, and bowel resected through a synchronous groin wound (to avoid contamination of the peritoneal cavity). Anastomosis is then carried out through the main peritoneal cavity. It is worth stressing the importance of not contaminating the main peritoneal cavity and not returning nonviable bowel into it. The use of a lower midline incision for all cases of difficulty is strongly recommended.

Waddington recommends the low, crural approach, and this was used in 119 of his 128 cases. In only one out of 14 patients needing a bowel resection and anastomosis was a paramedian incision needed for supplementing peritoneal cavity access [68].

Wheeler reports typical results for the UK from the University Hospital, Cardiff. In an 11-year study period, 78 patients underwent a total of 80 operations for femoral hernia. In 44 instances the operations were for acute strangulation; the remaining 36 operations were elective [69].

In the Cardiff series, three approaches were used—the low approach gave the least recurrences, whereas the inguinal (high) and the extraperitoneal (preperitoneal),

Table 17.1 Femoral hernia operations undertaken at Cardiff, 1963–1973[a] (after which Wheeler [69])

Procedure	No. of operations	No. of recurrences	Percentage recurrence
Abdominal pararectal incision (McEvedy)	32 (20)	4	12.5
Midline (Cheatle)	3 (2)	1	33.3
Inguinal (Lotheissen)	7 (3)	3	43.0
Crural (Bassini)	23 (7)	1	4.4

[a]Figures in parenthesis indicate emergency procedures for strangulation

using a midline incision, approaches were the least satisfactory (Table 17.1). The choice of the high approach in strangulation is interesting; this choice confirms "traditional" British teaching that the high approach offers advantages if resection is necessary. On the other hand, the poor results with the inguinal approach demand unfavorable comparison with other series in which this approach has given excellent results.

The more recent series from Stockton-on-Tees represents English district surgical practice in 11 years, 1976–1987; during this period 145 patients (38 male, 107 female) with 146 hernias (99 right, 47 left) underwent femoral hernia repair. In the elective group all but one patient had been aware of the lump for over a month before surgery, in contrast to the emergency group in which 27 (43%) had been aware of the lump for over 1 month. The most significant difference between the emergency and elective groups was age: 43 (68%) of patients in the emergency group were aged over 65 years compared with only 25 (30%) of those having an elective operation ($p < 0.0001$). Both groups had similar incidences of coexisting medical pathology. The preferred operation technique was the low crural (Bassini–Lockwood) operation. There were no deaths in the elective group, but five in the emergency group—an overall death rate of 3.4% (8% in the emergency group). The morbidity was also significantly higher in the emergency group. The most common cause of death was pulmonary embolism. At a median follow-up of 5 years, five patients had a recurrence (3.4%). Three of the recurrences were direct inguinal hernias after the use of the inguinal operation [70].

This study highlighted the problems of patients who delay in seeking medical advice and the difficulties general practitioners have in making a correct diagnosis of femoral hernia; only 35% of femoral hernias were correctly diagnosed by general practitioners in this series [27].

Ponka and Brush report that the crural low repair gives the fewest recurrences in their experience [71]. Likewise, Duvie from West Africa reports that the low approach gives a low recurrence rate (0%) and a shorter operation time and postoperative stay—although it must be commented that this report was of a very small study with no recurrences in either the "high" or the "low" group [48].

Unusual Variants of Femoral Hernia

So far we have considered the commonest variety of femoral hernia; there are, however, six rare variants, all of which pass from the abdomen into the thigh through the space bounded anteriorly by the inguinal ligament, posteriorly by the pectineal ligament and the origin of the pectineus muscle, medially by the lacunar ligament, and laterally by the fusion of the femoral sheath (fascia transversalis) with the iliac investing fascia. These variants are:

1. The hernia associated with maldescent of the testis through the femoral canal (cruroscrotal hernia). This is discussed on page 199.
2. The prevascular hernia (Narath's hernia), in which the sac emerges from the abdomen within the femoral sheath but lies anteriorly to the femoral vein and artery. This hernia can be either medial or lateral to the deep epigastric vessels. Narath described this condition associated with congenital dislocation of the hip. He reported six hernias in four patients, each hernia appearing on the same side as the dislocated hip (there were two bilateral cases). Importantly, the hernias did not appear until after the dislocations were reduced by manipulation. The same condition has been described as a complication of an innominate osteotomy for congenital dislocation of the hip [72]. Similar hernias develop in adults after previous groin surgery or after vascular operations on the external iliac vessels. Repair by an extraperitoneal approach is recommended [73, 74].
3. When the neck of the sac lies lateral to the femoral vessels—the external femoral hernia of Hesselbach and Cloquet [75, 76].
4. The transpectineal ligament femoral hernia when the sac traverses the pectineal part of the inguinal ligament and lacunar ligament (Laugier's hernia) [77].
5. When the sac descends deep to the femoral vessels and pectineal fascia (Callisen's or Cloquet's hernia) [78].
6. When the sac, instead of progressing anteriorly and superiorly through the cribriform fascia, proceeds into the thigh deep to the investing fascia—this hernia is always multilocular and may be mistaken for an obturator hernia. A variant described by Astley Cooper in 1804 and sometimes referred to as Cooper's hernia [79].

All these variants are best managed using either the extraperitoneal mesh prosthetic operation described in Chap. 13 or the laparoscopic methods described in Chap. 14.

With all methods of femoral hernia repair, it is important for the surgeon to be aware of the risk of vascular injury during these operations. The risk of injury to the femoral vein or artery is several fold higher than that for inguinal repair [80]. This may be related to the high rate of emergency presentation with this hernia and the fact that relatively inexperienced surgeons often undertake repair without senior supervision.

Conclusions

Femoral hernia is a common clinical problem, which warrants urgent elective repair to avoid the complication of strangulation.

The mechanism of femoral herniation, a distension and failure of the fascia transversalis in the femoral sheath, is described.

Methods of repair are outlined—the low, crural operation is least traumatic and gives lower recurrence rate. The laparoscopic method has proven to be a viable alternative to the surgeon that is proficient with that technique.

The crural operation is not suitable in multiple hernias or when resection of gut is required. In these circumstances, the surgeon must have the ability to perform the appropriate operation for the patient. The options include a formal laparotomy or either the extraperitoneal or inguinal operations as described above. Laparoscopy is well suited for the patient with multiple hernias, bilateral hernias, or a recurrent femoral herniation.

Strangulated femoral hernia carries a high morbidity and mortality in the elderly. Early diagnosis and repair by an experienced surgeon are required to reduce such unfavorable outcomes.

References

1. Colville JAC, Power RE, Hickey DP, Lane BE, O'Malley KJ. Intermittent anuria secondary to a stone in a ureterofemoral hernia. J Urol. 2000;164:440–1.
2. Bay-Nielsen M, Kehlet H, Strand L, et al. Quality assessment of 26304 Herniorrhaphies in Denmark: a prospective nationwide study. Lancet. 2001;358:1124–8.
3. Dahlstand U, Wollert S, Nordin P, Sandblom G, Gunnarsson U. Emergency femoral hernia repair. A study based on a National Register. Ann Surg. 2009;249:672–6.
4. Devlin HB. Hernia. In: Russell RCG, editor. Recent advances in surgery II. Edinburgh: Churchill Livingstone; 1982.
5. Glassow F. Femoral hernia following inguinal herniorrhaphy. Can J Surg. 1970;13:27–30.
6. Ollero Fresno JC, Alvarez M, Sanchez M. Femoral hernia in childhood: review of 38 cases. Pediatr Surg Int. 1997;12:520–1.
7. Rutkow IM, Robbins AW. Demographic, classificatory, and socioeconomic aspects of hernia repair in the United States. Surg Clin North Am. 1993;73:413–26.
8. Gunnarsson U, Degerman M, Davidsson A, Heuman R. Is elective hernia repair worthwhile in old patients? Eur J Surg. 1999;165:326–32.
9. Cole GJ. Strangulated hernia in Ibadan. Trans R Soc Trop Med Hyg. 1964;58:441–7.
10. Crawford DL, Hiatt JR, Phillips EH. Laparoscopy identifies unexpected groin hernias. Am Surg. 1998;64(10):976–8.
11. Lee SL, Du Bois JJ. Laparoscopic diagnosis and repair of pediatric femoral hernia. Surg Endosc. 2000;14:1110–3.
12. Hernandez-Richter T, Schardey HM, Rau HG, Schildberg FW, Meyer G. The femoral hernia: an ideal approach for the transabdominal preperitoneal technique (TAPP). Surg Endosc. 2000;14:736–40.
13. Ponka JL, Brush BE. Problems of femoral hernia. Arch Surg. 1971;102:417–23.
14. Stirk DI. Strangulated inguino-femoral hernia with descent of the testis through the femoral canal. Br J Surg. 1955;43:331–2.
15. Fruchaud H. Anatomie Chirurgicale des Hernies de l'Aine. Paris: G. Doin; 1956.
16. Lytle WJ. Femoral hernia. Ann R Coll Surg Engl. 1957;21:244–62.
17. Zimmerman LM, Anson BJ. Anatomy and surgery of hernia. 2nd ed. Baltimore: Williams and Wilkins; 1967. p. 216–27.
18. Aird I. Companion in surgical studies. 2nd ed. Edinburgh: Churchill Livingstone; 1957.
19. Gaur DD. Venous distension in strangulated femoral hernia. Lancet. 1967;1(7494):816.
20. Mikkelsen T, Bay-Nielsen M, Kehlet H. Risk of femoral hernia after inguinal herniorrhaphy. Br J Surg. 2002;89:486–8.
21. Wright MF, Scollay JM, Mccabe AJ, Munro FD. Paediatric femoral hernia—the diagnostic challenge. Int J Surg. 2011;9(6):472–4.
22. Devlin HB. Management of abdominal hernias. London: Butterworth; 1988.
23. Henry X, Bouras-Kara Terki N. Should prostheses be used in emergency hernia surgery? In: Bendavid R, Abrahamson J, Arregui M, Flament JB, Phillips E, editors. Abdominal wall hernias: principles and management. New York: Springer-Verlag; 2001. p. 557–9.
24. Gianetta E, DeCian F, Cuneo S, et al. Hernia repair in elderly patients. Br J Surg. 1997;84:983–5.
25. Tingwald GR, Cooperman M. Inguinal and femoral hernia repair in geriatric patients. Surg Gynecol Obstet. 1982;154:704–6.
26. Palot JP, Flament JB, Avisse C, et al. Utilisation des prothèses dans les conditions de la chirurgie d'urgence. Chirurgie. 1996;121:48–50.
27. Nicholson S, Keane TE, Devlin HB. Femoral hernia: an avoidable sense of surgical mortality. Br J Surg. 1990;77:307–8.
28. Daum R, Meinel A. Die operative Behandlung der kindlichen Leistenhernie: Analyse von 3 Fällen. Chirurgica. 1972;43:49–54.
29. Buck N, Devlin HB, Lunn JN. The report of a confidential enquiry into perioperative deaths. London: Nuffield Provincial Hospital Trust and the King Edward's Hospital Fund for London; 1987.
30. National confidential enquiry into perioperative deaths. London; 1995.
31. Barron J. Pectineus fascia for femoral hernia repair. Quoted by Ponka JL, Brush BE, Problems of femoral hernia. Arch Surg. 1971;102:417–23.
32. McVay CB. The anatomic basis for inguinal and femoral hernioplasty. Surg Gynecol Obstet. 1974;139:931–45.
33. Stoppa R, Warlaumont CR, Verhaeghe PJ, Odimba BKFE, Henry X. Comment, pourquoi, quand utiliser les prostheses de tulle de Dacron pour traiter les hernies et les eventrations. Chirurgie. 1982;108:570–5.
34. Wantz GE. Atlas of hernia surgery. New York: Raven Press; 1991.

35. Tait L. A discussion on treatment of hernia by median abdominal section. Br Med J. 1891;2:685–91.

36. Koontz AR. Hernia. New York: Appleton; 1963.

37. Walters GAB. A retropubic operation for femoral herniae. Br J Surg. 1965;52:678–82.

38. Nyhus LM, Condon RE, Harkins HN. Clinical experiences with pre-peritoneal hernial repair for all types of hernia of the groin. Am J Surg. 1960;100:234–44.

39. Cheatle GL. An operation for inguinal hernia. Br Med J. 1921;2:1025–6.

40. Henry AK. Operation for femoral hernia by a midline extraperitoneal approach: with a preliminary note on the use of this route for reducible inguinal hernia. Lancet. 1936;1:531–3.

41. McEvedy PG. Femoral hernia. Ann R Coll Surg Engl. 1950;7:484–96.

42. Annandale T. Reducible oblique and direct inguinal and femoral hernia. Edinb Med J. 1876;21:1087–91.

43. Lotheissen G. Zur Radikaloperation der Schenkel-hernien. Centralblatt Chir. 1898;21:548–9.

44. Moschowitz AV. The rational treatment of sliding hernia. Am J Surg. 1966;112:52.

45. Bassini E. Neue operations–Methode zur Radicalbehandlung der Schenkelhernie. Arch Klin Chir. 1894;47:1–25.

46. Lockwood CB. The radical cure of femoral and inguinal hernia. Lancet. 1893;2:1297–302.

47. Nyhus LM, Harkins HN. Hernia. London: Lippincott; 1965. Also ibid., 2nd edn. Condon RE, editor. Philadelphia: Lippincott; 1978.

48. Duvie SO. Femoral hernia in Ilesa, Nigeria. West Afr J Med. 1988;8:246–50.

49. Thomas D. Strangulated femoral hernia. Med J Aust. 1967;1:258–60.

50. Tanner NC. A slide operation for inguinal and femoral hernia. Br J Surg. 1942;29:285–9.

51. Glassow F. Femoral hernia: review of 1143 consecutive repairs. Ann Surg. 1966;163:227–32.

52. Chan G, Chan CK. Longterm results of a prospective study of 225 femoral hernia repairs: indications for tissue and mesh repair. J Am Coll Surg. 2008;207(3):360–7.

53. Alimoglu O, Kaya B, Okan I, Dasiran F, Guzey D, Bas G, et al. Femoral hernia: a review of 83 cases. Hernia. 2006;10(1):70–3.

54. Andrews WE, Topuzlu C, Mackay AG. Special indications for pre-peritoneal hernioplasty. Arch Surg. 1968;96:25–6.

55. Ogilvie H. Hernia. London: Edward Arnold; 1959.

56. Chan CK. Femoral hernia repairs: the Shouldice experience in the 1990's. In: Presented at the meeting "Hernia in the 21st century", sponsored by the American and European Hernia Societies, Toronto, June 2000.

57. Bendavid R. Femoral hernias: primary versus recurrence. Int Surg. 1989;74:99–100.

58. Bendavid R. Femoral hernias: why do they recur? Probl Gen Surg. 1995;12(2):147–9.

59. Uen YH, Wen KH. An improved method for deploying the polypropylene underlay patch of the prolene hernia system. Am Surg. 2007;73(5):468–71.

60. Rutkow IM, Robbins AW. Groin hernia. In: Cameron JL, editor. Current surgical therapy. St. Louis: Mosby; 1995. p. 41–486.

61. Rutkow IM, Robbins AW. Mesh plug repair and groin hernia surgery. Surg Clin North Am. 1998;78(6):1007–23.

62. Millikan K, Cummings B, Doolas A. A prospective study of the mesh-plug hernioplasty. Am Surg. 2001;67:285–9.

63. Chen J, Lv Y, Shen Y, Liu S, Wang MA. Prospective comparison of preperitoneal tension-free open herniorrhaphy with mesh plug herniorrhaphy for the treatment of femoral hernias. Surgery. 2010;148(5):976–81.

64. Garg P, Ismail M. Laparoscopic total extraperitoneal repair in femoral hernia without fixation of the mesh. JSLS. 2009;13(4):597–600.

65. Adibe OO, Hansen EN, Seifarth FG, Burnweit CA, Muensterer OJ. Laparoscopic-assisted repair of femoral hernias in children. J Laparoendosc Adv Surg Tech A. 2009;19(5):691–4.

66. Kavic MS. Laparoscopic hernia repair. Amsterdam: Harwood Academic Publishers; 1997. p. 33–40.

67. Sorelli PG, El-Masry NS, Garrett WV. Open femoral hernia repair: one skin incision for all. World J Emerg Surg. 2009;4:44.

68. Waddington RT. Femoral hernia: a recent appraisal. Br J Surg. 1971;58:920–2.

69. Wheeler MH. Femoral hernia: analysis of the results of surgical treatment. Proc R Soc Med. 1975;68:177–8.

70. Nielsen DF, Bulow S. The incidence of male hermaphroditism in girls with inguinal hernia. Surg Gynecol Obstet. 1976;142:875–6.

71. Ponka JL, Brush BE. Experiences with the repair of groin hernia in 200 patients aged 70 or older. J Am Geriatr Soc. 1974;22:18–24.

72. Salter RB. Innominate osteotomy in the treatment of dislocation and subluxation of the hip. J Bone Joint Surg. 1961;43-B:518–39.

73. Cox KR. Bilateral pre-vascular femoral hernia. Aust N Z J Surg. 1962;31:318–21.

74. Narath A. Ueber eine Eigenartige Form von Hernia Cruralis (prevascularis) im Anschlusse an die unblutige Behandlung angeborener Hüftgelenksverrenkung. Arch Klin Chir. 1899;59:396–424.

75. Cloquet J. Recherches anatomiques sur les hernies de l'abdomen. These, Paris; 1817. p. 133, 129.

76. Hesselbach FK. Neueste Anatomisch-Pathologische Untersuchungen über den Ursprung und das Fortschreiten der Leisten- und Schenkelbrüche. Warzburg: Baumgartner; 1814.

77. Laugier S. Note sur une nouvelle espece de hernie de l'abdomen a travers le ligament de Gimbernat. Arch Gen Med Paris. 1833;2:27–37.

78. Callisen H. Herniorum rariroram bigna acta societas medicae hafniae. Haanniae. 1777;2:321.

79. Cooper A. The anatomy and surgical treatment of inguinal and congenital hernia I. London: T. Cox; 1804.

80. Hair A, Duffy K, McLean L, et al. Groin hernia repair in Scotland. Br J Surg. 2000;87:1722–6.

Umbilical, Epigastric, and Spigelian Hernias

18

Benjamin S. Powell and Guy R. Voeller

Introduction

Primary anterior abdominal wall defects such as Spigelian, epigastric, and umbilical hernias are less common than their inguinal counterparts. However, a thorough knowledge of the causes and treatment of these hernias is paramount for any practicing general surgeon. These primary abdominal wall hernias oftentimes need to have a high index of suspicion especially epigastric and Spigelian hernias. Umbilical hernias typically account for approximately 10% of all hernias and are more likely to be frequently seen by the general surgeon. This chapter will discuss the presentation of these hernias as well as causes and the different treatments that are currently available.

Embryology

A thorough understanding of the development of the abdominal wall is necessary to appreciate the nature of the hernia defects this chapter discusses. Abdominal wall development and bowel development happen conjointly from the third week of gestation until the 12th week. At the third week, the embryo has cephalic, caudal, and lateral folds (Fig. 18.1). The cephalic fold is anterior and contains the foregut, stomach, and mediastinal contents. Somatic layer defects in the cephalic fold can give rise to diaphragmatic, thoracic wall, cardiac or pericardial defects. The caudal fold contains the colon, rectum, bladder, and the hypogastric abdominal wall. Defects in the caudal fold can cause bladder exstrophy. The lateral folds become the lateral abdominal wall and future umbilical ring. Defects in the lateral fold typically give rise to umbilical hernia or an omphalocele. Umbilical herniation

of the abdominal contents occurs around week 6–7 due to the fact that the embryonic abdominal wall is too small to hold the abdominal contents at this point. At weeks 10–12 the abdominal viscera undergo a counterclockwise rotation and return to the abdominal cavity. Typical abdominal wall defects encountered at birth include omphalocele as well as gastroschisis. Omphalocele by definition is herniation of abdominal contents into the umbilical cord, typically greater than 4 cm in size. Gastroschisis is a full-thickness abdominal wall defect almost always to the right of the umbilicus without a covering membrane. A bridge of skin separates the defect from the umbilicus. These congenital defects are discussed further in other chapters.

Anatomy of the Abdominal Wall

Abdominal wall anatomy is fairly complex and a good understanding of the layers and insertions of the musculature as well as aponeurosis is the key to performing hernia surgery.

The abdominal wall is a hexagonal configuration and is bordered caudally by the pelvic wall and pubic symphysis, cranially by the costal margin and xiphoid, and laterally by the midaxillary line. The rectus abdominis runs vertically from the costal margin to the pubis surrounding the linea alba in the midline (Fig. 18.2). Each rectus muscle has its origin on the fifth, sixth, and seventh rib and the xiphoid. The rectus abdominis inserts onto the pubic bone via a 3-cm band inserting at the pubis. The three-layer lateral portion of the abdominal wall is made up of the external oblique, internal oblique, and the transversus abdominis. Each layer of these muscles runs in different directions with the fibers of the external oblique running downward and forward; the internal oblique runs forward and upward and the transversus abdominis runs horizontally (Fig. 18.3). Primary hernias are very uncommon through these muscle groups; typically they occur through the linea alba or the semilunar line for obvious reasons. Each of these muscles is surrounded by a wide

B.S. Powell, MD (✉) • G.R. Voeller
Department of Surgery, University of Tennessee Health Science Center–Memphis, Memphis, TN, USA
e-mail: grvoeller@gmail.com

A.N. Kingsnorth and K.A. LeBlanc (eds.), *Management of Abdominal Hernias*,
DOI 10.1007/978-1-84882-877-3_18, © Springer Science+Business Media London 2013

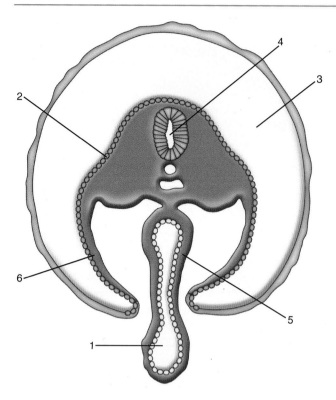

Fig. 18.1 Formation of ventral abdominal wall. *1*. Yolk sac *2*. Surface endoderm *3*. Amniotic cavity *4*. Neural tube *5*. Splanchnic mesoderm *6*. Somatic mesoderm

aponeurosis. However the transversus abdominis is surrounded by both an anterior and posterior aponeurosis.

The linea alba is formed from the aponeurosis of the rectus sheath. It also represents the insertion point in the midline of the lateral flat muscles. It is a median raphe running vertically through the abdominal wall. It is by far the most common site of hernias on the anterior abdominal wall. Most open operations use a midline incision for access to the abdominal cavity leading to most incisional hernias being in the midline. Most primary anterior abdominal wall hernias occur through the linea alba as well. Above the umbilicus the linea alba is typically wider than below it, hence the higher incidence of primary midline hernias such as epigastric hernias in this position. Its average width in cadaver studies is approximately 1.7 cm above and about 0.7 cm below.

The semilunar (Spigelian) line is a semiconcave line that runs lateral to the rectus muscle on either side of the abdomen. It is classically described as a boundary between transversus abdominis muscle body and its aponeurosis. The Spigelian line is not a true line due to the fact the myoaponeurotic borders of the external oblique and the internal oblique do not intersect like the linea alba. The intersection of the Spigelian line and the arcuate line (line of Douglas) is a point of weakness in the abdominal wall. This area is often referred to as the Spigelian hernia belt (Fig. 18.4). The inferior epigastric vessels run in the lateral rectus sheath at this point in

the abdominal wall and many anatomists propose that this contributes to the relative weakness. A triangle is formed by the inferior epigastric vessels medially, the Spigelian line laterally, and the arcuate line superiorly.

Spigelian Hernia

Definition and Epidemiology

Spigelian hernias occur through slit-like defects along the Spigelian (semilunar line) lateral to the rectus sheath. These hernias for the most part typically present below the umbilicus where there is absence of the posterior sheath; however, there are reports of the hernia above the umbilicus as well. The semilunar line as described previously runs from the ninth costal cartilage to the pubic bone inferiorly along the lateral border of the rectus muscle. It has a semiconcave shape; hence, it was given the semilunar nomenclature. Anatomists say that the semilunar line is formed from the branching of the internal oblique aponeurosis with reinforcement anteriorly by the external oblique aponeurosis. The upper two thirds of the abdominal wall is reinforced with the transversus abdominis posteriorly; hence, hernias above the umbilicus are subsequently extremely rare. Spigelian hernias are typically found below the line of Douglas in the lower abdomen [1, 2].

The incidence of Spigelian hernias in children is very low. Occasionally they are caused by trauma and abdominal wall surgery and are typically repaired primarily in this age group. Spigelian hernias are most frequently found in adults from ages 40 to 70. It has been theorized that these hernias may be related to the stretching of the abdominal wall caused by previous surgery, collagen disorders, obesity, COPD, or pregnancy. The most likely cause is due to weaknesses (due to whatever reason) in the internal oblique muscle that allow interdigitations of fat that act as a lead point for the hernia. The male to female ratio is 1:1.8 and some authors estimate that it comprises about 0.12% of all abdominal wall hernias. The hernia is typically a well-defined hernia sac in the transversus aponeurosis. These hernias rarely penetrate the thick external oblique fascia. Usually it is an intraparietal hernia into the rectus muscle, which can make diagnosis very difficult; hence, a good clinical suspicion is necessary to diagnose these patients. Ultrasound and CT scan are useful aids in diagnosis, but as shown by the Mayo study below, there are false negatives with these tests.

History

The Spigelian or semilunar line was first described by Adriaan van den Spieghel in the seventeenth century as the medial concave line that is the boundary between the

Section above arcuate line

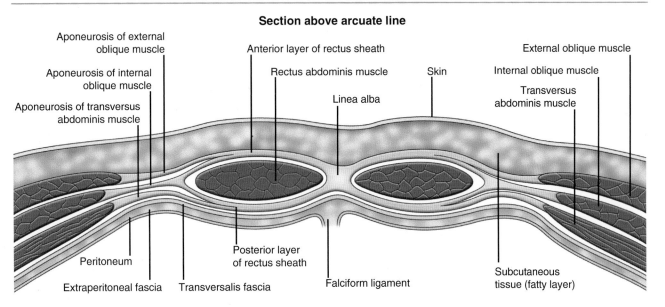

Fig. 18.2 The rectus abdominis surrounding the linea alba in the midline where epigastric and umbilical hernias arise

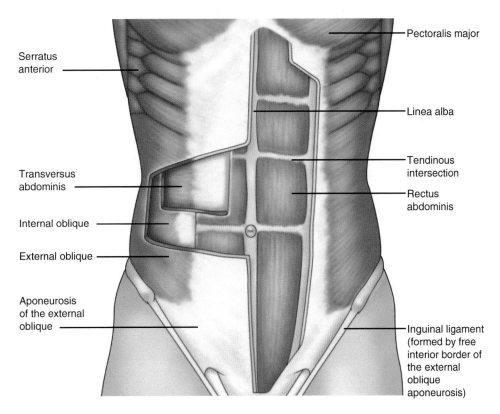

Fig. 18.3 Orientation of the internal oblique, external oblique fibers, and the transversus abdominis of the abdominal wall

muscle and the anterior aponeurosis of the transversus abdominis. Klinkosch however first described the Spigelian hernia in 1764. In the early nineteenth century Sir Astley Cooper had described 23 hernias that occurred along the Spigelian line. Some historical terminology to describe these defects is "spontaneous ventral hernia" or "hernia of the semilunar line" [3, 4].

Current Literature

Literature on Spigelian hernias tends to be limited to small case series and the types of repairs that have been performed to fix these somewhat rare hernias. Most papers on Spigelian hernia started appearing in the 1930s. Louis River wrote a paper in 1942 that discussed

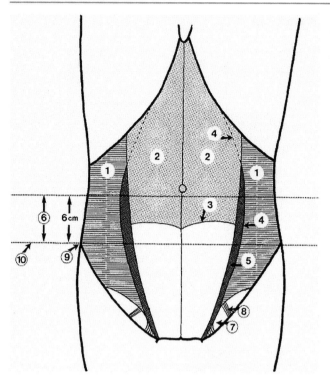

Fig. 18.4 Spigelian hernia belt. External and internal oblique are cut away in this figure. *1*: Transversus abdominis. *2*: Dorsal lamella of the rectus sheath. *3*: Semicircular line of Douglas. *4*: The semilunar line. *5*: Spigelian aponeurosis. *6*: Spigelian hernia belt. *7*: Hesselbach's triangle. *8*: Inferior epigastric vessels. *9*: anterior superior iliac spine. *10*: Interspinal plane

the associated anatomic defects and symptoms that are associated with this hernia. He also presented five cases and described in detail each patients' clinical course and operation. Watson, Read, and Weiss all published papers discussing patient presentations as well as repair of these hernias. All of the repairs were performed prior to the commonplace use of mesh, and each of the hernias was repaired primarily. Current controversies in management of these hernias tend to center around exactly what type of repair to perform. Some authors favor the laparoscopic approach while others favor an open approach. Some papers suggest not using mesh to fix these hernias. Hsieh recently published a paper out of Taiwan in which 11 cases of Spigelian hernias were reviewed [5]. Four of the patients underwent open preperitoneal repair with mesh while the other seven had open primary repair. Mean follow-up was 8.5 years for the non-mesh group, and the follow-up for the mesh group was 6.7 years. They found no recurrences in either group. The paper unfortunately illustrates the low number of these hernias repaired by any one group, so it is difficult to say one repair is superior to another. One of the larger series was published from Turkey in 2006. It was a prospective multicenter study with 34 patients [6]. The most common method of

repair was open intraperitoneal mesh placement. The most common presenting symptom was painful abdominal mass and preoperative diagnosis could be made in 31 of the patients. The largest series of Spigelian hernias was reported by Larson from the Mayo clinic in 2002. There were 81 hernia repairs over a 20-year time period. Mass, pain, or bowel obstruction were the most common symptoms. Preoperative imaging was done in 21 patients and was positive in 15. Suture repair was used in 75 patients, mesh repair in 5, and laparoscopic in one. Mean follow-up for 76 patients was 8 years and 3 hernias recurred, all in the suture repair group [7].

Spigelian hernia does lend itself to a laparoscopic extraperitoneal hernia repair as published by Koksal et al. [8]. They describe an approach in which the trocar setup is virtually identical to a traditional TEP inguinal hernia repair. The preperitoneal space is dissected and used to allow space for mesh placement. The mesh is placed a little more cephalad than when done for an inguinal hernia. We have repaired 17 Spigelian hernias found during TEP inguinal hernia repair in this fashion with no known recurrences to date.

Moreno-Egea et al. showed that laparoscopic repair might be more beneficial to patients in regard to morbidity and length of stay in the hospital [9]. Twenty two patients in their study underwent elective repair of Spigelian hernia; 11 had open preperitoneal repair while the other 11 had laparoscopic repair. In the laparoscopic group eight were performed via the TEP method while the other three underwent intra-abdominal mesh placement. Average length of stay in the open group was 5 days while the laparoscopic approach was one day, with a *p* value <0.001. There were no postoperative complications in the laparoscopic approach, but the conventional method had four patients with hematomas. This chapter makes a strong case for laparoscopic repair due to the fact many of these can be done as an outpatient procedure with less morbidity. An approach we have also used is a combined laparoscopic and open approach. We place a 5 mm scope to evaluate the hernia and then make a small incision over the hernia and repair it with a Ventralex-type patch. This allows excision of the hernia sac and closure of the fascia over the patch. This approach is excellent for the large hernia sac that may lead to seromas and bulging if not excised.

Epigastric Hernia

Definition and Epidemiology

Epigastric hernias are primary hernias found in the anterior abdominal wall between the xiphoid and umbilicus. They are usually in or near the linea alba, linea semilunaris, or one of the linea transversus of the rectus sheath [10]. Most of these hernias are single in nature and quite small in size. However, they can be multiple in number and on occasion quite large. Initially epigastric hernias start out with preperitoneal fat protruding through the linea alba; however, they can grow to include a hernia sac which becomes subcutaneous in the midline or interstitial in the rectus sheath. The incidence of epigastric hernias is largely unknown and they are typically infrequent in children. Usually they are found in adults with a male to female ratio of around 3:1. In the few studies that are available they account for approximately 1–5% of abdominal wall hernias. One autopsy series of 10,000 hernias found that only 116 were epigastric hernias with 105 being in males. Another autopsy series found epigastric hernias in 5–10% of the bodies examined. They often are found in young men such as athletes or soldiers who do a large amount of strenuous exercise.

Several theories regarding the cause of epigastric hernias have been put forward since the early 1900s. Originally it was theorized by Witzel that a small defect in the deep fascia of the abdominal wall leads to preperitoneal tissue protruding through the defect. This tissue can lead to peritoneum being forced through defect and having a hernia sac. Most authors now believe that preperitoneal fat penetrates the fascial openings where the vessels and nerves of the abdominal wall penetrate. Continued intra-abdominal pressure leads to sac formation and a hernia. This also explains why these hernias are multiple in up to 20% of patients.

Heredity and smoking might share some importance as well in the formation of these hernias, but increased intra-abdominal pressure is a definite factor. This coupled with diminished resistance of the abdominal wall fibers can play an important role in their production. Hence, these hernias can be seen in young active males as well as obese relaxed females. Askar dissected a large number of cadavers and emphasized the importance that fibers crossing the midline play in reinforcing the linea alba. He showed that epigastric hernias were more likely in those where fiber decussation was minimal [11].

Epigastric hernias can have symptoms out of proportion to their relative size. Historically patients can have vomiting after meals, indigestion, colic, and occasionally constipation. Other symptoms involving depression, neurasthenia, and other nervous symptoms have been related to epigastric hernias. Curiously, these symptoms resolve after repair. Preperitoneal fat can become incarcerated causing strangulation of this fat. With strangulation of this fat it becomes tender and edematous. Patients will often have severe abdominal pain at this point due to compression of the contents and/or the neurovascular bundle. Patients do need a full examination to rule out other causes of abdominal pain as well. Epigastric hernias can mimic other intra-abdominal pathology such as symptomatic cholelithiasis and peptic ulcer disease. Often patients, especially thin women, desire repair for cosmetic reasons.

History

Epigastric hernias were first described in 1285 by Arnaud de Villeneuve in France, but not until 1742 did Rene' de Garengeot clearly define the hernia. He first theorized that the hernias were due to pathology from the abdominal organs. Leveille first used the term epigastric hernia in 1812 and the first successful repair of an epigastric hernia was described in 1802. The procedure was abandoned for a time due to the iatrogenic injury of intra-abdominal viscera. Not until 1885 did Terrier operate for the cure of the epigastric hernia. His first publication and elimination of the pain associated with epigastric hernias called attention to the treatment of these hernias.

Literature

There are relatively few recent studies looking at just pure epigastric hernias. Stabilini recently published a study comparing suture repair against open preperitoneal mesh placement with polypropylene mesh [12]. The mean hernia defect size was 2.5 cm (range of 0.5–10 cm). Recurrence rate was 14.7% in the suture repair group vs. 3.1% in the mesh group. There were a few more local wound complications with the mesh group; however, this does not seem to offset the recurrence risk in the suture group. Unfortunately most other data on epigastric hernias in the last 20 years is isolated to interesting case reports [13, 14]. There are studies that lump epigastric hernias into papers addressing all anterior wall hernias and laparoscopy [15]. These will be discussed later.

Umbilical Hernia

Definition and Epidemiology

Umbilical hernias are frequent pathology seen by most general surgeons. Not nearly as common in frequency as inguinal hernias they nonetheless can cause significant morbidity. They are obviously related to our embryological development and are not that uncommon in the pediatric population.

As discussed earlier, the embryology of the abdominal wall is fairly complicated. Umbilical hernias form through defects in closure of the abdominal orifice where the umbilical cord emerges after the celomic sac is obliterated. Three weeks into development, the skin and fascial coverings of the abdominal wall form to cover the intra-abdominal contents. The intestines and other abdominal viscera are extruded into the celomic sac, and then they subsequently return to the abdominal cavity. Failure of this process leads to numerous abdominal wall defects. The lower portion of the umbilicus has the vitelline duct, paired umbilical arteries, and the umbilical vein. These structures leave the inferior portion of the umbilicus fairly well protected from changes in intra-abdominal pressure and hernia. The superior portion of the umbilicus has a thinner aponeurosis, which makes it more vulnerable to hernia and changes in intra-abdominal pressure. The advent of laparoscopic surgery coupled with a typical periumbilical incision can lead to incisional hernias at the umbilicus. These port-site hernias tend to be amenable to surgical repair similar to an umbilical hernia.

The female to male ratio in adults for umbilical hernias is typically 3:1, mostly due to the increased pressure caused from pregnancy. Other factors that can contribute to umbilical hernia are malignancies, ascites, and of course obesity. There does not appear to be a strong relationship between childhood and adult umbilical hernias. Typically only about 10% of adults with umbilical hernias had them as children.

History

Stoser performed the first umbilical hernia repair in the United States in 1894. Cheselden reported an early repair in 1740, and initially the surgical repair included ligation and fixation of the hernia sac. This often led to necrosis and further advancements were made in the late 1800s. Mayo described his technique of overlap in 1898, called the "vest-over-pants" technique [16]; this operation was widely done and was seen as a technical breakthrough since it significantly reduced the morbidity over earlier approaches. Most surgeons tend to favor a tension-free repair with mesh at this point in time.

Umbilical Hernia and Cirrhosis

Umbilical hernia in a patient with cirrhosis and ascites bears special mentioning. These patients are difficult treatment dilemmas due to the inherent operative risk in these patients, coupled with ascites and possible chance of hernia recurrence [17, 18]. Figure 18.5 shows a picture of what an epigastric hernia occasionally looks like in a cirrhotic. Traditional dogma has been that umbilical hernias in Child's C cirrhotics or patients with ascites should be watched due to the risk of general anesthetic in these patients. There are several case reports of complications after elective hernia repair in these patients, including emergency liver transplantation [19]. There are also multiple reports of bowel evisceration in patients that do not undergo repair [20–24]. There are several studies looking at the optimal time to repair these hernias, if at all. Telem recently published a retrospective review of 21 umbilical herniorrhaphies done from 2002 through 2008 [25]. Fifteen of the patients pre-

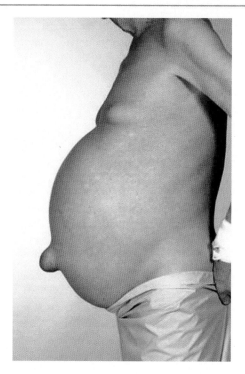

Fig. 18.5 Umbilical hernia in a cirrhotic patient with ascites

sented with incarceration, while six had umbilical rupture. They found that their mortality rate was 5% with a morbidity rate of 71%. In conjunction with the hernia repair they did TIPS preoperatively in six patients and postoperatively in two patients. Due to the low number of patients, it was difficult to draw any definitive conclusions about how to lower complication rates in this population since all of the patients in this study had emergent repairs. Gray et al. performed a study in 2008 from the VA National Surgical Quality Improvement Program looking on the outcomes of cirrhotic patients vs. non-cirrhotic patients with either elective or emergent umbilical herniorrhaphies [26]. A number of cases (1,421) were reviewed with 127 of the patients having cirrhosis (8.9%). Cirrhotics were much more likely to undergo emergent repair (26.0% vs. 4.8%) along with higher rates of bowel resection, return to the OR, and increased postoperative stay. From this data they found that cirrhosis was not a significant predictor of postoperative complications overall. Cirrhosis was strongly predictive of postoperative complications in emergent repairs. They theorized that earlier elective repair may improve overall outcomes for patients with cirrhosis. Marsman et al. also reported their data on patients with umbilical hernia and cirrhosis [27]. Their group searched their hospital database over a 14-year period and 34 patients with an umbilical hernia and cirrhosis were identified. Half of the patients had elective repair, while 13 others had conservative therapy. Four other patients underwent hernia repair during liver transplantation. Of the patients with elective hernia repairs,

4 of the 17 had recurrences. In the conservative therapy group, 10 of the 13 went on to have incarceration; two patients in this group died from complications of the hernia. Other groups have even advocated laparoscopic repair of these hernias electively and shown decent results in a small cohort of patients [28]. From these studies it can be shown that emergent repair of umbilical hernias is laden with complications. Obviously careful patient selection in these patients is the key since this is a difficult patient population with which to deal.

Current Literature

Current discussion in regard to umbilical hernias deals mainly with mesh placement vs. suture repair along with when laparoscopic repair is appropriate. Most of the data currently available shows that the recurrence rates with mesh use are less than suture repair of the hernia. This has to be balanced with the potential complications of mesh placement.

Asolati looked at predictors of recurrence for patients with umbilical hernias. It was a retrospective study looking at all umbilical hernia repairs in a VA over a 6-year span [29]. Two hundred and twenty nine patients were followed with 97 undergoing suture repair and the others receiving mesh repair. Seven patients in the suture repair group had recurrences vs. four in the mesh repair group (7.7% vs. 3%). In their patient population African-American gender, diabetes, and hyperlipidemia were found to be the factors that were significant for recurrence. Smoking, obesity, type of hernia, nor size were found to be significant in their study. Eryilmaz looked at their experience of repairing umbilical hernias with either mesh or suture repair [30]. Over a five-year span they did suture repair on any hernia less than 3 cm and polypropylene mesh repair on any hernia larger than 3 cm. Primary repair was performed in 63 patients, with mesh repair in 48 patients. The recurrence rate in the suture repair group was 14% vs. 2% in the mesh group. They concluded that mesh should be used in all umbilical hernias.

Arroyo in 2001 and Sanjay in 2005 [31, 32] both showed lower recurrence rates with the use of mesh for repair of umbilical hernia. Sanjay had a follow-up of 4.5 years.

Schumacher [33] in 2003 found that in patients with a BMI >30 the recurrence rate of umbilical hernia was 32% vs. only 8% in those with a BMI <30. He also found that the larger the hernia, the higher chance of recurrence if the repair was done without mesh.

In 2008 we published a paper looking at the use of Ventralex mesh in umbilical and epigastric hernia repairs [34]. It was a retrospective review of our experience of eight-eight patients. The average BMI was 32 in our patients. Twenty-two percent of the patients were females and the

mean age was 52. Our average OR time was 52 min and the f/u at that time ranged from 8 days to 3 years. No hernia recurrences were found in follow-up. Two patients had mesh infection requiring removal. From our experience with this composite patch we concluded it has a valuable role in epigastric and umbilical hernia repairs. In addition, we compared this experience to our experience with a similar number of umbilical hernia repairs using the laparoscope. The laparoscopic group had no recurrences and no mesh infections but was $1200 more expensive than the open approach using the Ventralex patch.

Presentation and Diagnosis of Anterior Abdominal Wall Hernias

Patients can present with a variety of different symptoms when they have primary anterior abdominal wall hernias depending on hernia location and hernia contents. Umbilical hernias tend to be the most common anterior abdominal wall hernias and often are easier to diagnose than their Spigelian and epigastric hernia counterparts. Typically they present with a reducible bulge at the umbilicus that can at times be tender. If patients have an acute incarceration/strangulation of omentum, they can present with pain and erythema, but more frequently it is a chronic incarceration without signs of strangulation. Incarcerated small intestine can present as a bowel obstruction or perforation. If the hernia is very large, it can contain multiple viscera with a variety of related symptoms.

Epigastric hernias can at times be difficult. Often a thorough history is the best clue with patients complaining of a bulge and/or pain in the epigastrium. Physical exam is helpful if the defect is large enough to palpate and confirms the diagnosis. If there is still concern about the true etiology of the pain, an abdominal ultrasound or CT scan can be helpful in the diagnosis [1, 35, 36]. Most epigastric hernias are small in nature and often only have preperitoneal fat in the hernia. However, the size of the hernia can vary widely and contain a variety of tissues including preperitoneal fat, omentum, stomach [37], liver [38], colon, or small intestine. There have even been reported epigastric hernias causing pancreatitis [39]. Due to this fact, a variety of symptoms can be present.

Spigelian hernias are often difficult to diagnose due to their relative rarity and low clinical suspicion, especially in obese patients. Presentation is often similar to the above-mentioned hernias except they are found along the Spigelian line and not in the midline. Patients' presentations will be different depending on hernia sac contents as well. Once again ultrasound and CT scan have aided in the diagnosis, but there are false negatives with these methods, and diagnostic laparoscopy is an excellent diagnostic tool in the patient with pain in this area and a negative work-up.

Preoperative Planning

Most anterior abdominal wall hernias can be repaired with similar techniques that are applicable to each type. As with most hernias, a tension-free repair is ideal so mesh is usually used unless there is a clear contraindication to doing so. The next question is should the repair be done open or with the laparoscope. We tend to recommend open repair in most primary anterior abdominal wall defects due to our success using the Ventralex-type patch with most of these hernias. The patients have similar or less pain than their laparoscopic counterparts; it is less expensive and it is an easy repair to perform. These patches allow a sublay repair through a small incision with minimal morbidity. For larger hernias we typically favor the laparoscopic approach due to wider overlap of the hernia and decreased wound infection and mesh infection rates.

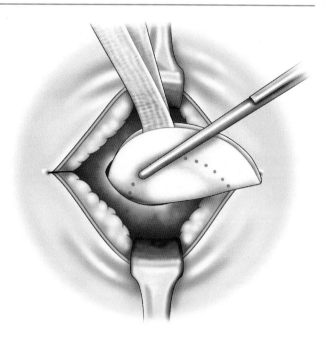

Fig. 18.6 Placement of the Ventralex patch into the hernia defect

Treatment of Anterior Abdominal Wall Hernia

Open hernia repair has long been the mainstay of treatment for anterior abdominal wall hernias. Before Mayo began his "vest-over-pants" repair there was a high morbidity and mortality with this defect. The trend in recent repairs of umbilical hernias has been continued evolution to tension-free techniques due to high recurrence rates with primary closure. Most authors advocate fixing the hernia with mesh if the defect is larger than 2 cm with mesh. Other authors fix all defects with mesh.

Patients undergoing a typical open anterior abdominal wall hernia repair at our institution receive a cephalosporin or vancomycin if they are penicillin allergic. We use an Ioban to minimize the contact of the mesh with the skin if mesh is to be used. The appropriate incision is made and the hernia sac is dissected from the subcutaneous tissues and transected at fascial level. The skin and fat are then dissected off of the fascia for 2–3 cm to get back into good, healthy fascia (Fig. 18.6). The appropriate size circular patch is selected to provide a good amount of sublay beyond the hernia defect. It is placed into the peritoneal cavity, and the surgeon makes sure it is completely opened and abuts the peritoneal surface of the abdominal wall 360° without any viscera interposed between the patch and the abdominal wall. We use 2–0 double-armed Prolene sutures to place U-stitches at the 12, 3, 6, and 9 o'clock positions. These sutures include the polypropylene part of the Ventralex patch only and then a good purchase back into good fascia (Fig. 18.7). We use stitches at the 12 and 6 o'clock positions only for the small patch. The fascia is then closed over the mesh to add another barrier of protection from possible wound infections (Fig. 18.8). The skin is closed based on

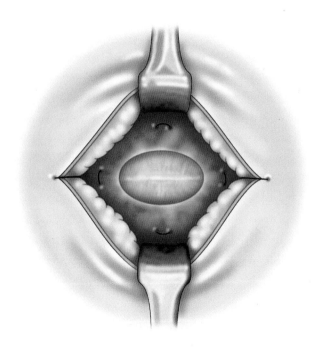

Fig. 18.7 After the Ventralex patch has been placed with four Prolene U-stitches securing it in place

the type of hernia repaired. We use a compression dressing to help with hemostasis and to decrease seroma formation and have the patient wear an abdominal binder postoperatively. We do not routinely leave drains unless there is a large dead space. If there is evidence of ischemic bowel at any point of the procedure, synthetic mesh should not be used. The surgeon should decide whether to use a biologic mesh or perform a primary repair.

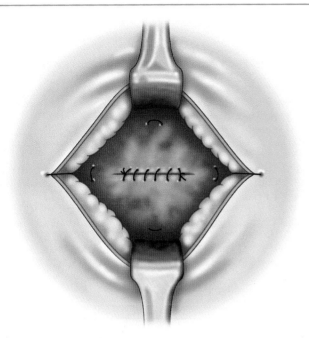

Fig. 18.8 Fascial closure over the mesh to reinforce repair and separate mesh from subcutaneous fluid collection

Laparoscopic Anterior Abdominal Wall Hernia Repair

Laparoscopic anterior abdominal hernia repair is essentially identical to ventral hernia repair as mentioned in previous chapters. The patient will receive antibiotics prior to the skin incision. A Veress needle in the left upper quadrant at the costal margin is an ideal way to insufflate the abdomen safely. Alternatively one can use a Hasson trocar, but this makes a large hole that can lead to hernia formation. Most of the primary abdominal wall hernias can be repaired using all 5-mm trocars and we place two of these laterally on each side of the abdomen (Fig. 18.9). The contents of the hernia sac are reduced. Specifically with these hernias, it is the key to take down the peritoneum and reduce the preperitoneal fat that can still be felt if left in situ. For epigastric hernias it is important to remove the falciform ligament from the peritoneal surface of the abdominal wall. Once the fascial defect is clearly delineated, it is measured and a 5-cm overlap is typically used to estimate the size of mesh needed. Four transfascial sutures are used to fix the mesh superiorly, inferiorly, and laterally on each side. A laparoscopic tacker is then used to tack the mesh circumferentially to help with fixation and prevent internal hernias. If the hernia is very large, additional transfascial sutures should be used. We also use a compression bandage for the laparoscopic repair and an abdominal binder. Patients should be advised to be aware of postoperative seroma that is commonly seen after the laparoscopic approach.

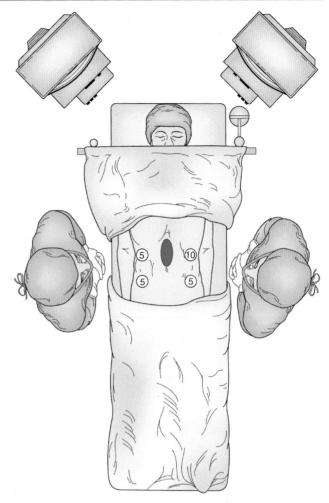

Fig. 18.9 Trocar placement and tower setup for most laparoscopic anterior abdominal wall hernia repairs. Four trocars are placed, two in either flank laterally with video towers at both sides at the head of the bed

Complications

Complications involving all of these hernias are relatively similar. Small hematomas and ecchymoses are not uncommon and will resolve if observed. Seromas can be seen in larger repairs. Typically they will slowly resolve over weeks to months. The desire to aspirate the seroma should be placed on hold if possible to decrease the chance of infecting it. If patients do get wound infections, they should be treated accordingly. The decision to remove infected mesh will depend on the judgment of the practitioner. Depending upon the type of mesh used and whether the infection communicates with the mesh will determine whether the mesh should be removed. Usually a simple cellulitis will resolve with antibiotics.

Postoperative Activities

We do not restrict the patient's activity postoperatively. They will limit any strenuous activity for awhile due to discomfort from the repair. This policy can be adjusted to each individual patient depending on body habitus, age, type of repair, and job requirements.

References

1. Sutphen JH, Hitchcock DA, King DC. Ultrasonic demonstration of Spigelian hernia. AJR Am J Roentgenol. 1980;134(1):174–5.
2. Read RC. Observations on the etiology of Spigelian hernia. Ann Surg. 1960;152:1004–9.
3. River LP. Spigelian hernia: spontaneous lateral ventral hernia through the semilunar line. Ann Surg. 1942;116(3):405–11.
4. Weiss Y, Lernau OZ, Nissan S. Spigelian hernia. Ann Surg. 1974;180(6):836–9.
5. Hsieh HF, Chuang CH, Lin Ch YJC, Hsieh CB. Spigelian hernia: mesh or not? Rev Esp Enferm Dig. 2007;99(9):502–4.
6. Malazgirt Z, Topgul K, Sokmen S, Ersin S, Turkcapar AG, Gok H, et al. Spigelian hernias: a prospective analysis of baseline parameters and surgical outcome of 34 consecutive patients. Hernia. 2006;10(4):326–30.
7. Larson DW, Farley DR. Spigelian hernias: repair and outcome in 81 patients. World J Surg. 2002;26:1277–81.
8. Koksal N, Altinli E, Celik A, Oner I. Extraperitoneal laparoscopic approach to Spigelian hernia combined with groin hernias. Surg Laparosc Endosc Percutan Tech. 2004;14(4):204–6.
9. Moreno-Egea A, Carrasco L, Girela E, Martín JG, Aguayo JL, Canteras M. Open vs laparoscopic repair of spigelian hernia: a prospective randomized trial. Arch Surg. 2002;137(11):1266–8.
10. Hotchkiss LW. VI. Epigastric hernia. Ann Surg. 1911;54(1):78–82.
11. Bendavid R, Abrahamson J, Arregui ME, Flament JB, Phillips EH. Abdominal wall hernias: principles and management. New York: Springer; 2001.
12. Stabilini C, Stella M, Frascio M, De Salvo L, Fornaro R, Larghero G, et al. Mesh versus direct suture for the repair of umbilical and epigastric hernias. Ten-year experience. Ann Ital Chir. 2009;80(3):183–7.
13. McCaugham JJ. Epigastric hernias: results obtained by surgery. AMA Arch Surg. 1956;73:972.
14. Muschaweck U. Umbilical and epigastric hernia repair. Surg Clin North Am. 2003;83(5):1207–21.
15. Wright BE, Beckerman J, Cohen M, Cumming JK, Rodriguez JL. Is laparoscopic umbilical hernia repair with mesh a reasonable alternative to conventional repair? Am J Surg. 2002;184(6):505–8. discussion 508–9.
16. Mayo WJ. VI. An operation for the radical cure of umbilical hernia. Ann Surg. 1901;34(2):276–80.
17. Runyon BA, Juler GL. Natural history of repaired umbilical hernias in patients with and without ascites. Am J Gastroenterol. 1985;80(1):38–9.
18. Telem DA, Schiano T, Divino CM. Complicated hernia presentation in patients with advanced cirrhosis and refractory ascites: management and outcome. Surgery. 2010;148(3):538–43.
19. Reissfelder C, Radeleff B, Mehrabi A, Rahbari NN, Weitz J, Büchler MW, et al. Emergency liver transplantation after umbilical hernia repair: a case report. Transplant Proc. 2009;41(10):4428–30.
20. Choo EK, McElroy S. Spontaneous bowel evisceration in a patient with alcoholic cirrhosis and an umbilical hernia. J Emerg Med. 2008;34(1):41–3.
21. Ginsburg BY, Sharma AN. Spontaneous rupture of an umbilical hernia with evisceration. J Emerg Med. 2006;30(2):155–7.
22. Carbonell AM, Wolfe LG, DeMaria EJ. Poor outcomes in cirrhosis-associated hernia repair: a nationwide cohort study of 32,033 patients. Hernia. 2005;9(4):353–7.
23. Lemmer JH, Strodel WE, Knol JA, Eckhauser FE. Management of spontaneous umbilical hernia disruption in the cirrhotic patient. Ann Surg. 1983;198(1):30–4.
24. Klosterhalfen B, Klinge U, Schumpelick V. Functional and morphological evaluation of different polypropylene-mesh modifications for abdominal wall repair. Biomaterials. 1998;19(24):2235–46.
25. Cobb WS, Burns JM, Peindl RD, Carbonell AM, Matthews BD, Kercher KW, et al. Textile analysis of heavy weight, mid-weight, and light weight polypropylene mesh in a porcine ventral hernia model. J Surg Res. 2006;136(1):1–7.
26. Gray SH, Vick CC, Graham LA, Finan KR, Neumayer LA, Hawn MT. Umbilical herniorrhaphy in cirrhosis: improved outcomes with elective repair. J Gastrointest Surg. 2008;12(4):675–81.
27. Marsman HA, Heisterkamp J, Halm JA, Tilanus HW, Metselaar HJ, Kazemier G. Management in patients with liver cirrhosis and an umbilical hernia. Surgery. 2007;142(3):372–5.
28. Belli G, D'Agostino A, Fantini C, Cioffi L, Belli A, Russolillo N, et al. Laparoscopic incisional and umbilical hernia repair in cirrhotic patients. Surg Laparosc Endosc Percutan Tech. 2006;16(5):330–3.
29. Farrow B, Awad S, Berger DH, Albo D, Lee L, Subramanian A, et al. More than 150 consecutive open umbilical hernia repairs in a major Veterans Administration Medical Center. Am J Surg. 2008;196(5):647–51.
30. Eryilmaz R, Sahin M, Tekelioglu MH. Which repair in umbilical hernia of adults: primary or mesh? Int Surg. 2006;91(5):258–61.
31. Arroyo A, García P, Pérez F, Andreu J, Candela F, Calpena R. Randomized clinical trial comparing suture and mesh repair of umbilical hernia in adults. Br J Surg. 2001;88(10):1321–3.
32. Sanjay P, Reid TD, Davies EL, Arumugm PJ, Woodward A. Retrospective comparison of mesh and sutured repair for adult umbilical hernias. Hernia. 2005;9:248–51.
33. Schumacher OP, Peiper C, Lorken M, Schumpelick V. Long-term results after Spitzy's umbilical hernia repair. Chirurg. 2003;74:50–4.
34. Martin DF, Williams RF, Mulrooney T, Voeller GR. Ventralex mesh in umbilical/epigastric hernia repairs: clinical outcomes and complications. Hernia. 2008;12(4):379–83.
35. Yeh H, Lehr-Janus C, Cohen C, et al. Ultrasonography and CT of abdominal and inguinal hernias. J Clin Ultrasound. 1984;12:479–86.
36. Hodgson TJ, Collins MC. Anterior abdominal wall hernias: diagnosis by ultrasound and tangential radiographs. Clin Radiol. 1991;44:185–8.
37. Arowolo OA, Ogundiran TO, Adebamowo CA. Spontaneous epigastric hernia causing gastric outlet obstruction: a case report. Afr J Med Med Sci. 2006;35(3):385–6.
38. Gupta AS, Bothra VC, Gupta RK. Strangulation of the liver in epigastric hernia. Am J Surg. 1968;115(6):843–4.
39. Lankisch PG, Petersen F, Brinkmann G. An enormous ventral (epigastric) hernia as a cause of acute pancreatitis: Pfeffer's closed duodenal loop model in the animal, first seen in a human. Gastroenterology. 2003;124(3):865–6.

Maciej Śmietański

Anatomy

The lumbar area is bounded above by the 12th rib, below by the iliac crest, behind by the erector spinae (sacrospinalis), and in front by the posterior border of the external oblique (a line passing from the tip of the 12th rib to the iliac crest). Within this area two triangles are described: the superior lumbar triangle (of Grynfelt) and the inferior lumbar triangle (of Petit). The superior lumbar triangle is an inverted triangle, its base is the 12th rib, its posterior border is the erector spinae and its anterior border the posterior margin of the external oblique, and its apex is at the iliac crest inferiorly. The base of the inferior lumbar triangle is the iliac crest, its anterior border is the posterior margin of the external oblique muscle, its posterior border is the anterior edge of the latissimus dorsi muscle, and its apex is superior. Both the superior and the inferior lumbar triangles vary in size depending on the attachments of muscles to the iliac crest (Fig. 19.1). The floor of both triangles is the thoracolumbar fascia incorporating the internal oblique and the transverses abdominis to a variable degree.

The T12 and L1 nerves both cross the superior lumbar triangle. The abdominal wall musculature (rectus abdominis, external and internal oblique, and transverses abdominis) and overlying skin are supplied by the 7th through 11th intercostal nerves and subcostal nerve (12th intercostal equivalent). It is described that the 11th intercostal nerve divides into two branches (at the tip of the 11th rib). The posterior branch supplies motor innervation of the transverses abdominis and internal oblique muscles and the anterior branch supplies motor innervation of the external oblique and sensory innervation of the overlying skin [1]. This is important to mention that if the nerve will be injured proximal to its division (e.g., intraoperatively), motor innervation for entire segment of the muscles would be compromised.

The cutaneous sensory nerves of the abdomen overlap with adjacent sensory nerves to provide the innervation in the dermatomal distribution. In contrast minimal overlap exists between adjacent motor nerves. Segments of each abdominal muscles are innervated by a single intercostals nerve. So the loss of a single spinal level of motor nerves results in paralysis of a full-thickness segment of the abdominal musculature, what can lead to postoperative flank bulging, often diagnosed as a type of lumbar herniation [2].

Another important finding for the surgical anatomy is that the segmental nerves and vessels are situated between the internal oblique and transverse muscles, so to avoid possible nerve irritation or injury (possibly leading to pain and functional impairment of the lateral abdominal wall) this layer should not be used for surgical procedures.

Clinical Features

Congenital lumbar hernia does occur and can be bilateral [3]. Such congenital hernias present as a bulge in the loin maybe associated with intestinal symptoms. Lumbar hernias may be acquired, following sepsis in the retroperitoneal tissues [4] as a result of osteomyelitis or tuberculosis of the vertebral bodies or iliac crest which disrupts the lumbodorsal fascia [5], or following surgical operations on the kidneys [6], aortic aneurysm, but also following iliac bone harvest and latissimus dorsi myocutaneous flap [7, 8]. Traumatic lumbar hernias occur following direct blunt trauma [9] and seat-belt injuries in vehicle accidents [10, 11]. During the vehicle crash poorly applied seat belt tends to migrate above the iliac crest exposing the full abdominal musculature to the forces of deceleration. This results in anterior rotation of the pelvis with a shearing action that predisposes the patient to tearing of the musculofascial structures [12] In this cases even large disruption of the posterolateral abdominal wall from the level of T12 vertebra to the iliac crest can occur, causing large lumbar hernia involving sigmoid and descendent colon and/ or the kidney [13].

M. Śmietański (✉)
Department of General and Vascular Surgery,
Ceynowa Hospital in Wejherowo, Wejherowo, Poland
e-mail: smietanski@herniaweb.org

A.N. Kingsnorth and K.A. LeBlanc (eds.), *Management of Abdominal Hernias*,
DOI 10.1007/978-1-84882-877-3_19, © Springer Science+Business Media London 2013

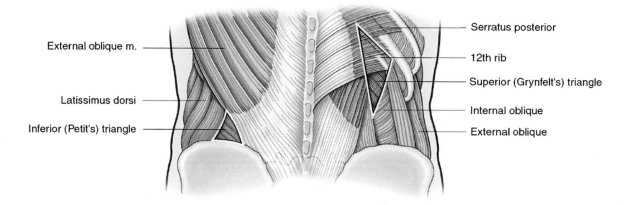

Fig. 19.1 Dissection of the lumbar region to illustrate the anatomy of the *inferior lumbar triangle* (*left*) and the *superior lumbar triangle* (*right*)

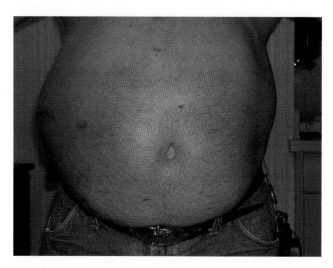

Fig. 19.2 Preoperative appearance of a "denervation hernia" after a right nephrectomy

Lumbar hernia is also described following the anterior approach to the lumbar spine for vertebral interbody fusion for lumbar disc disease. These are usually not true hernias as there is no true fascial defect. In some cases a fascial defect may be demonstrable but, in the majority, this is not the case. These abdominal wall deformities result from the injury to the nerves that innervate the upper portions of the external oblique, internal oblique, transverses abdominus. and rectus muscles. The path of the T11 and T12 nerves can be traversed during the dissection of open space for the above operation as well as during the exposure for a nephrectomy or aortic aneurysm operation. The development of a permanent flank bulge as a consequence of flank incision for radical nephrectomy is underestimated and can occur in almost half of the patients [14] The deformity can be progressive as the protrusion of the upper portions of the paralyzed muscles will cause an outward protrusion of the normal portions of these muscles (Fig. 19.2). Bulge can increase in the time causing pain and discomfort especially during the Valsalva maneuver and walking [2].

Lumbar hernias may contain a variety of intra-abdominal organs; hernias of the colon are most frequent but small intestine, stomach, and spleen are also likely candidates for herniation. A particular curiosity is the sliding hernia of the colon, which causes intermittent obstructive symptoms.

Differential diagnosis must include tumors of the muscles, lipoma, hematoma associated with blunt trauma, and abscess andrenal tumors. Small fatty protrusions of retroperitoneal fat through the lumbodorsal fascia have been implicated as a cause of low back pain [15, 16].

Backache radiating to the groin, presumably due to irritation of lateral cutaneous branches of the 10th, 11th, and 12th intercostal nerves, has been recorded. Tiny fatty hernias along the tracks of cutaneous nerves through the lumbar fascia give rise to severe low back pain with radiation to the buttocks and thigh. These hernias are palpable and tender. They are similar to the fatty hernias that occur through the linea alba and anterior aponeurosis. Local anesthetic infiltration abolishes the pain and confirms the diagnosis. Local excision and closure of the defect cures the condition. The diagnosis is made/confirmed by CT scan, which will delineate the defect [10, 17].

The patients that have the "denervation" injury that leads to the protrusion of the flank will frequently complain of back pain that is related to the defect. It is difficult to explain the source of this complaint as many of these patients will have had a long preexisting complaint of back pain requiring the disk surgery. The most common presentation is the acknowledgement of the significant cosmetic deformity that is caused by the musculature paralysis. This will cause asymmetry to the contour of the abdomen.

The Operation

Operative treatment of lumbar hernia varies in above mentioned different clinical situations. Primary lumbar hernias rarely extend over 7–10 cm and many alternative operations have been described giving a positive result in short- and medium-term follow-up. Different methods and approaches should be used in the "denervation" hernias. Acute traumatic hernias with comorbid injures create many clinical situations, so the time and extension of the procedure should be the point of consideration.

Elective treatment of primary lumbar hernia could be performed via open and laparoscopic approach. Small hernias (diameter less than 5 cm) have been successfully treated without synthetic implant using simple closure of the defect with nonabsorbable sutures. In this cases open access parallel to the 12th rib was performed, sac identified and reduced. If only the preperitoneal fatty mass was found in the hernia orifice excision after ligature was performed to reduce the content. No recurrences were found in this series of patients in the mean 8-month follow-up [18]. However this treatment option could be taken into consideration and most of the authors believe that the synthetic material implanted in the sublay position will improve the results. Small hernia was cured successfully with open implantation of a plug (Bard Mesh Dart) in one described case [19]. In other series (10 patients) an open approach was used (incision over the hernia typically in the parailiac location) to place the implant in the preperitoneal space. Mesh should extend the defect with an overlap of minimum 5 cm to secure the repair. In the area of iliac crest when the overlap was not sufficient (hernia orifice extended to the bone) fixation to the bone with double suture-armed bone anchor (Mitek GII titanium anchor) was performed [20]. In the recent years laparoscopic approach seems to dominate over open techniques due to better visualization of the defect, its simplicity and proven good results [8, 21, 22]. Also for incisional lumbar hernias transperitoneal approach allows dissection of the omental adhesions from the previous surgery, careful extraction of the hernia content, and exposure of the hernia orifice [8, 23]. Even if the open repair must be performed due to the hernia size, laparoscopic exploration of the abdominal cavity is advised to assess the clinical situation [13]. In this method the approach and technique is similar to that of the incisional hernia repair (described in chapter on ventral hernias) . A significant difference is that the patient must be turned in the lateral decubitus position (Fig. 19.3). The use of transfascial sutures and fixation devices is identical to the incisional hernia operation. Mesh could be placed intraperitoneally (composite anti-adhesive material) or retroperitoneally after hernia sac extraction [24]. In this cases polypropylene or partially absorbable lightweight mesh is used. The peritoneum is closed over the mesh to avoid contact with the bowel unless a tissue-separating product is used [8, 23].

One paper considering the totally extraperitoneal approach shows the possibility of that repair. That author believes that retroperitoneoscopy allows more safe dissection of the space and tension-free placement of the mesh. However only one

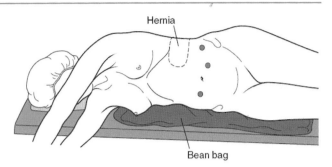

Fig. 19.3 Position of patient to repair a lumbar hernia of the left side. This position is also used for the repair of the "denervation hernia." The three *dark circles* connote the approximate location of the trocar sites

case was described, but this method is similar to the TEP in inguinal hernia repair and could be a valuable alternative in the future [25].

In the acute traumatic situation, where full laparotomy to exclude intraperitoneal bleeding is mandatory, the abdomen should be explored through a midline abdominal incision.

Extensively damaged, ischemic colon in the hernia will need resection with the formation of a stoma if indicated. The defect in the lumbodorsal fascia should be sutured with nonabsorbable sutures. The defect in the fascia is best reinforced with a prosthetic biomaterial in addition to primary closure. However, the acute repair of the traumatic lumbar hernia is associated with a high recurrence rate. In recently described series, 50 % of patients developed a recurrence. Due to this data delayed repair was proposed. The authors believe that even if the patient requires abdominal exploration for other injuries, the repair of traumatic lumbar hernia is not mandatory at that time and should be individualized. At that time, it may be best to defer to an expeditious, elective repair once the other acute issues have resolved. Repair in high-risk patients with associated injuries and contaminated wounds may lead to wound infection and, eventually, failure of the repair thereby making any subsequent repair more difficult [13].

In the situation of the denervation injury, the repair is more problematic. Because no fascial defect is present many surgeons are reluctant to repair what is reasonably believed to be a cosmetic problem [26]. As mentioned, according to the recent follow-up studies the flank bulge leads very often to persistent pain and limits the daily activity [14]. Because of this many such patients have a strong desire to undergo a reparative operation. The difficulty lies not only in the decision to operate but also in the type of repair that can be done in these patients. The data on any of these choices is sparse. There are three basic options in which to approach this problem. The first is seemingly a very simple procedure. The involved flank muscles can be exposed and sutured in the form of a plication. Several layers of these sutures can be applied which will result in a very appreciable improvement in the appearance of the contour of the abdomen at the time of surgery and shortly thereafter. Unfortunately, the denervated muscle cannot be cured nor does the plication provide a final solution. The muscle adjacent to the plication is still paralyzed and will bulge as before within several months to a few years. Because of this failure, the use of a prosthetic material is recommended. The surgeon must provide for a very wide overlap of the prosthetic to effect a long-term result. The prosthetic can be placed in the extraperitoneal position or over the external oblique muscle. The muscles are divided and the extraperitoneal space is dissected. A large piece of material is placed in that location. It is important to ensure that the mesh extends from above the ribs to the level of the iliac crest. Only in this manner will all of the denervated muscle be covered. The difficulties lie in the dissection of the preperitoneal space, as this area will be densely scarred. There are two proposed approaches to the preperitoneal space. A lateral approach through the previous incision and a medial approach through incision of the rectus sheath and placement of the mesh also on the unaffected site to overlap the defect. In a small series (7 lateral vs. 8 median) the lateral approach to the denervation area did not provide satisfactory long-term results. Conversely the median approach resulted in the maintenance of the proper shape of the flank in long-term observation [27].

The results achieved can be even more satisfying when plication of the muscles is performed concomitantly. Because the fibers of the abdominal muscles are orientated in opposing directions, the forces that the muscles exert are in opposition. The anatomical repair restores these opposing forces through plication of the lateral muscles transversally. In these cases implanted mesh additionally reinforces the strength of the repair [2].

Another, less favored, method, is the prefascial (onlay) method. In this case, the denervated muscles are plicated. A large piece of a prosthetic material is then placed from above the ribs to below the iliac crest. This can be sutured with permanent sutures in an interrupted or continuous fashion. The theoretical disadvantage of this approach is that the denervated muscle is supported from above rather than behind the fascia. On contrary this repair seems to be easier to perform, does not increase the possibility of intra-abdominal injury. Evidence favoring onlay or extraperitoneal approach are still lacking.

Another option is a hybrid operation. In this instance, an open approach begins the operation. The muscles are incised to allow placement of an intraperitoneal mesh product, which is then fixed to the abdominal wall and diaphragm. Laparoscopic trocars are placed prior to completion of the mesh coverage. The muscles are then plicated over the mesh to restore the normal contour of the flank. Finally, laparoscopy is performed to completely fixate the mesh with fasteners and transfascial sutures. There are no reported long-term results but studies are ongoing (KAL).

Conclusions

- The incidence of lumbar hernias is low.
- The use of prosthetic reinforcement is recommended.
- Laparoscopic approach is beneficial for small and middle size hernias and even in the cases of open repair of the large hernias allows better assessment of the clinical intra-abdominal situation.
- The problem of the denervation flank bulge needs an extended approach and complex repair. A large prosthesis should be used in this cases. The new concept of a hybrid approach may provide the best long-term outcomes.

References

1. Gardner GP, Josephs LG, Rosca M, et al. The retroperitoneal incision. An evaluation of postoperative flank bulge. Arch Surg. 1994;129:753–6.
2. Hoffman RS, Smink DS, Noone R, et al. Surgical repair of the abdominal bulge: correction of a complication of the flank incision for retroperitoneal surgery. J Am CollSurg. 2004;199:5.
3. Adamson RJW. A case of bilateral hernia through Petit's triangle with two associated abnormalities. Br J Surg. 1958;46:88–9.
4. Myers RN, Shearburn EW. The problem of recurrent inguinal hernia. Surg Clin North Am. 1973;53:555–8.
5. Watson LF. Hernia: anatomy, etiology, symptoms, diagnosis, differential diagnosis, prognosis, and the operative and injection treatment. 2nd ed. London: Harry Kimpton; 1938.
6. Geis WP, Saletta JD. Lumbar hernia. In: Nyhus LM, Condon RE, editors. Hernia. 3rd ed. Philadelphia: Lippincott; 1989.
7. Stumpf M, Conze J, Prescher A, et al. The lateral incisonal hernia: anatomical considerations for a standardized retromuscularsublay repair. Hernia. 2009;13:293–7.
8. Yavuz N, Ersoy YE, Demirkesen O, et al. Laparoscopic incisional lumbar hernia repair. Hernia. 2009;13:281–6.
9. Kretschmer HL. Lumbar hernia of the kidney. J Urol. 1851; 65:944–8.
10. Esposito TJ, Fedorak I. Traumatic lumbar hernia. Case report and review of the literature. J Trauma. 1994;37:123–6.
11. McCarthy MC, Lemmon GW. Traumatic lumbar hernia: a seat belt injury. J Trauma Injury Infect Crit Care. 1996;40:121–2.
12. Burt BM, Afifi HY, Wanz GE, et al. Traumatic lumbar hernia: reports of cases and comprehensive review of the literature. J Trauma. 2004;57:1361–70.
13. Bathla L, Davies E, Fitzgibbons RJ, et al. Timing of traumatic lumbar hernia repair: is delayed repair safe? Report of two cases review of the literature. Hernia. 2011;15:205–9.
14. Chatterjee S, Nam R, Fleshner N, et al. Permanent flank bulge is a consequence of flank incision for radical nephrectomy in one half of patients. Urol Oncol Seminars Orig Invest. 2004;22:36–9.
15. Copeman WSC, Ackerman WL. Fibrositis of the back. Q J Med. 1944;13:37–40.
16. Faille RJ. Low back pain and lumbar fat herniation. Am Surg. 1978;44:359–61.
17. McCarthy MP. Obturator hernia of the urinary bladder. Urology. 1976;7:312–4.
18. Zhou X, Nve JO, Chen G. Lumbar hernia: Clinical analysis of 11 cases. Hernia. 2004;8:260–3.
19. Solaini L, di Francesco F, Gourgiotis S, et al. A very simple technique to repair Grynfeltt-Lesshaft hernia. Hernia. 2010;14:439–41.

20. Carbonell AM, Kercher KW, Sigmon L, et al. A novel technique of lumbar hernia repair using bone anchor fixation. Hernia. 2005;9:22–6.

21. Aird I. Companion in surgical studies. 2nd ed. Edinburgh: Churchill Livingstone; 1957.

22. Akita K, Niga S, Yamato Y, Munata T, Sato T. Anatomic basis of chronic groin pain with special reference to sports hernia. Surg Radiol Anat. 1999;21:1–5.

23. Iannitti DA, Biffl WL. Laparoscopic repair of traumatic lumbar hernia. Hernia. 2007;11:537–40.

24. Palanivelu C, Rangarajan M, John SJ, et al. Laparoscopic transperitoneal repair of lumbar incisional hernias: a combined suture 'double-mesh' technique. Hernia. 2008;12:27–31.

25. Habib E. Retroperitoneoscopic tension-free repair of lumbar hernia. Hernia. 2003;7:150–2.

26. Salameh JR, Salloum EJ. Lumbar incisional hernias: diagnostic and management dilemma. JSLS. 2004;8:391–4.

27. Zieren J, Menenakos C, Taymoorian K, et al. Flank hernia and bulging after open nephrectomy: mesh repair by flank or median approach? Report of a novel technique. Int Urol Nephrol. 2007;39:989–93.

Michael S. Kavic, Stephen M. Kavic, and Suzanne Marie Kavic

There are several large openings in the bony pelvic girdle, including its floor that can allow for intestine or viscera to pass through and develop a hernia. However, the near vertical walls of the pelvis mitigate against the development of hernia—mitigate—but not completely deny hernia formation. Although rare, hernias of the deep pelvic structures can occur and cause debilitating symptoms. Unfortunately, physicians often ignore these symptoms because hernias in the pelvic areas are difficult to see and to palpate. For the most part, pelvic wall hernia is not even considered in females with vague abdominal or pelvic symptoms. Nonetheless, general surgeons need a thorough knowledge of pelvic anatomy, particularly, potential hernia sites in women, to avoid inadequate diagnostic workup and examination. Patients, usually older female patients, suffer the consequences of our inattention.

A good example of disease neglected by the general surgeons is chronic pelvic pain in females. Chronic pelvic pain is a common gynecologic problem in women accounting for 10–30% of all gynecological visits. It is considered the principle indication for 20% of hysterectomies performed for benign disease and approximately 40% of gynecological laparoscopies [1]. About 78,000 hysterectomies are performed each year in the United States for chronic pelvic pain [2]. It has been estimated that 70% of female patients who have chronic pelvic pain have disease in the reproductive genital tract; however, 10% of patients with chronic pelvic pain had gastrointestinal tract disorders, 8% had musculoskeletal neurologic disease, 7% had myofascial abnormalities and 5% had urologic causes

of chronic pelvic pain [3]. Chronic pelvic pain can have many etiologies, and the general surgeon must not shirk from actively participating in the evaluation of these patients.

Chronic pelvic pain has three main dimensions: (1) duration—pelvic pain lasting 6 months or more; (2) anatomic—pain in the pelvis defined by physical findings at laparoscopy; and (3) affective/behavioral—pelvic pain accompanied by significant alterations in physical activity such as work, recreation and sex, as well as changes in mood related to the chronic pain [3]. Most standard laboratory and imaging studies such as complete blood count, abdominal and pelvic ultrasound and computed tomographic studies are often within normal limits.

Frequently referred to as "female trouble," chronic pelvic pain has resisted intensive efforts to determine its cause. Chronic pelvic pain can have many etiologies, and a multidisciplinary approach is frequently necessary for proper patient evaluation [4]. Nevertheless, chronic pelvic pain is a real entity and it is now appreciated that obscure, rare conditions such as sciatic, obturator, supravesical, and perineal hernia may cause chronic pain in women. A case in point is the seldom diagnosed sciatic hernia.

Sciatic Hernia

Sciatic hernia, one of the rarest of abdominal and pelvic wall hernias, was first described by Verdier in 1753 [5, 6]. It is the protrusion of peritoneal sac and content through the greater or lesser sciatic foramen. The hernia may occur superior to the piriformis muscle (suprapiriformis), inferior to the piriformis (infrapiriformis), or through the lesser sciatic notch (subspinous) (Fig. 20.1). Known variously as sacrosciatic hernia, ischiatic hernia, ischiocele, hernia incisurae ischiadicae or gluteal hernia, the hernia sac may contain ovary, tube, or intestine. Entrapment of these organs may cause chronic pelvic pain or bowel obstruction.

There were only 39 cases of sciatic hernia reported in the world literature up to 1958 [5, 6]. However, in 1998, Miklos and colleagues reported 20 cases of sciatic hernia diagnosed

M.S. Kavic (✉)
Department of Surgery, St. Elizabeth Health Center,
Youngstown, OH, USA
e-mail: Mkavic@aol.com; mkavic@sls.org

S.M. Kavic
Department of Surgery, University of Maryland School of Medicine,
Baltimore, MD, USA

S.M. Kavic
Division Reproductive Endocrinology and Infertility Associate
Professor of OB/GYN and Medicine Loyola University Medical
Center 630-953-6669, Maywood, IL 60153

A.N. Kingsnorth and K.A. LeBlanc (eds.), *Management of Abdominal Hernias*,
DOI 10.1007/978-1-84882-877-3_20, © Springer Science+Business Media London 2013

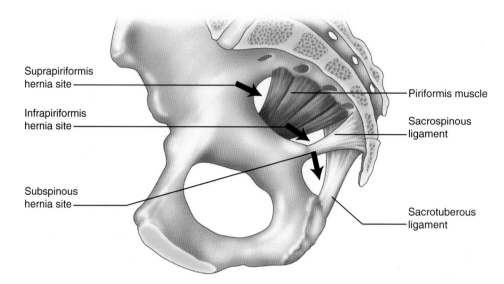

Fig. 20.1 Sciatic hernia. The hernia may occur superior to the piriformis muscle (suprapiriformis), inferior to the piriformis (infrapiriformis), or through the lesser sciatic notch (subspinous)

in a series of 1,100 female patients who had diagnostic laparoscopy for chronic pelvic pain. All of these cases had the ipsilateral ovary alone or fallopian tube contained within the hernia sac. If this incidence of sciatic hernia in patients who required diagnostic laparoscopy for chronic pelvic pain (1.8%) is carried over into the general population, sciatic hernia cannot be as rare as previously thought [7].

Anatomy

The sacrospinous ligament converts the greater sciatic notch into the greater sciatic foramen which is filled with the piriformis muscle. In addition to the piriformis muscle, the greater sciatic foramen transmits the gluteal vessels and nerves, internal pudendal vessels and nerve, and nerves to the obturator internus and quadratus femoris muscles. Above the piriformis muscle, the suprapiriformus area allows for passage of the superior gluteal artery, vein and nerve. Below the piriformis muscle, lies the infrapiriformis space which transmits the inferior gluteal vessels, posterior femoral cutaneous nerve, nerve to the obturator internus, internal pudendal vessels and nerves and sciatic nerve.

The lesser sciatic notch is transformed into a foramen by the sacrospinous ligament superiorly and the sacrotuberous ligament inferiorly. The lesser sciatic foramen transmits the tendon of the obturator internus, its nerve and the internal pudendal vessels [5]. In females, the abdominal opening of a sciatic hernia is posterior to the broad ligament. In males, the opening lies in the lateral pelvis between the urinary bladder and rectum. Hernias below the sacrotuberous ligament are considered to be perineal hernias [8].

Clinical Presentation

Sciatic hernias are rarely noted on physical examination as the large gluteal muscles cover and overlap the sciatic foramen. To further complicate matters, openings in the sciatic foramen are small and many of these cases present with incarceration and obstruction. Frequently, the diagnosis is only revealed at laparotomy. Even so, the pain of chronic sciatica may call attention to the gluteal area where physical examination may suggest a bulge that is more pronounced on standing. Compression of the sciatic nerve can cause muscle weakness of the lower leg with pain radiating down the posterior thigh made worse with dorsiflexion. Herniography can be helpful in delineating a sciatic hernia, however, a computerized tomography (CT) scan is the initial diagnostic imaging of choice.

Treatment

Sciatic hernias have been repaired by a transabdominal or transgluteal approach [9, 10]. A transabdominal approach is usually recommended as these hernias are difficult to diagnose, and most surgeons are more comfortable performing an exploration for possible bowel obstruction in an open manner. Laparoscopic access, however, can offer satisfactory visualization of a sciatic hernia [7] (Fig. 20.2).

After the abdomen has been opened or pneumoperitoneum established for laparoscopic access, a thorough intra abdominal examination is performed. The liver, gallbladder, stomach, intestine , appendix, uterus, tubes, ovaries and peritoneal surfaces are examined [11]. The entire pelvis is inspected for hernias, adhesions and endometriosis.

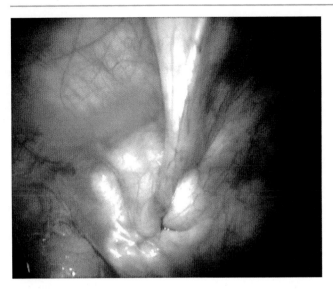

Fig. 20.2 Laparoscopic view of a sciatic hernia

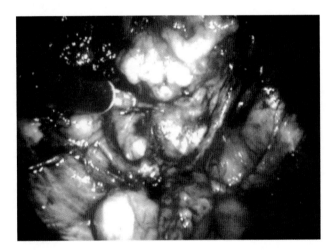

Fig. 20.3 Sciatic hernia sac reduction

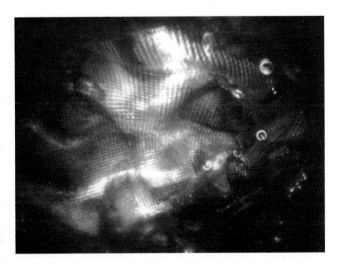

Fig. 20.4 Mesh repair of a sciatic hernia

If a sciatic hernia is found, its content are reduced. Dusky bowel should be observed for 5–10 min to see that adequate circulation is reestablished. Non-viable bowel should be resected with primary anastomosis. If the bowel is viable, a preperitoneal incision is made superior to the hernia defect and the hernia sac reduced (Fig. 20.3). The sciatic foramen is visualized and completely covered with non absorbable synthetic mesh. There should be a 2.5–3.0 cm overlap of the hernia defect with mesh circumferentially. The mesh is secured with endohernia tacks or fasteners to the obturator internus fascia laterally and coccygeus medially (Fig. 20.4). The area is reperitonealized by closing the peritoneal incision with intracorporeal suture, tacks or fasteners. The laparoscopic trocar sites or abdominal incision are then closed in the standard manner.

Obturator Hernia

An obturator hernia is an abnormal protrusion of preperitoneal fat or intestine through the obturator canal. These hernias are rarely visualized and are usually not found preoperatively unless a palpable bulge is noted on rectal or bimanual pelvic examination [12, 13]. An obturator hernia may contain a "pilot tag" of preperitoneal tissue, large or small bowel, appendix, uterus, tube or ovary [14]. Herniation through the obturator canal is rare, occurring in 0.073% of all hernias in one series [15]. Two broad groups of patients have been described who most frequently suffer obturator hernia [14–16].

1. Elderly patients, usually women, with a history of chronic disease, weight loss, increased intra abdominal pressure, and attenuation of the obturator membrane.
2. Women of childbearing age.

Anatomy

The obturator foramen is the largest bony foramen in the human body (Fig. 20.5). It is roughly circular in shape and shielded by the obturator membrane. The internal opening of the obturator canal is about 1 cm diameter and sited in the superior midsection of the obturator membrane. The obturator canal itself is a fibro osseous tunnel about 2–3 cm in length whose roof is formed by the obturator sulcus of the pubic bone and its floor by the internal and external obturator muscles and their fascia. The obturator nerve, artery and vein pass through the obturator canal with the nerve typically superior to the artery and vein (Fig. 20.6). After passing through the obturator canal, the obturator nerve divides into an anterior and posterior branch. The anterior branch courses over the superior border of the obturator externus muscle to supply the adductor longus, gracilis and adductor brevis muscles. The posterior branch pierces the obturator externus muscle to supply the adductor magnus and adductor brevis.

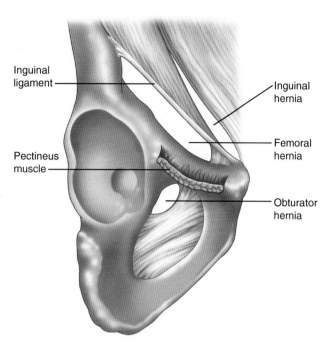

Fig. 20.5 Obturator anatomy

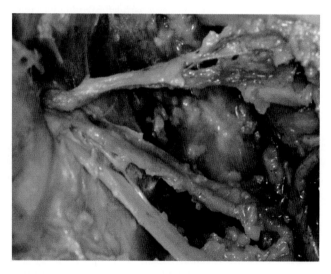

Fig. 20.6 Obturator nerve, artery, and vein

Obturator hernia sacs that follow the anterior division of the obturator nerve pass between the pectineus and above the obturator externus muscle. Hernia sacs that follow the posterior division of the obturator nerve pass through the obturator externus muscle.

Clinical Presentation

Historically, obturator hernia has been associated with four signs or symptoms [14].

1. Intestinal obstruction (elderly females, frequently intermittent)

2. Howship-Romberg sign
3. History of previous attacks
4. Palpable mass (rare)

Although the first two are the most common signs, the nature of intestinal obstruction is usually unclear and the Howship-Romberg sign only recalled after exploration has revealed the presence of obturator hernia.

A palpable mass is occasionally noted on rectal or pelvic examination. However, since obturator hernia is rarely considered in a differential diagnosis of vague abdominal pain, the presence of a mass in the obturator region is rarely sought.

John Howship first noted the pain characteristic of obturator hernia in 1840. He described this pain as extending down the inner surface of the involved thigh, exacerbated by thigh extension, adduction or medial rotation [17] (Fig. 20.7). Howship's sign was independently described by Moritz Romberg in 1848 [18]. Although the Howship-Romberg sign is pathognomonic of obturator hernia, by no means is it invariably present. About 50% of patients will complain of this pain down the inner aspect of their thigh caused by compression of the cutaneous branch of the obturator nerve in the narrow confines of the obturator canal [14, 19].

Some have suggested that an obturator hernia develops over several stages. It first begins as a prehernia with a plug of preperitoneal connective tissue or "pilot tag" entering the obturator canal [14] (Fig. 20.8). This concept was supported by a post mortem study of female cadavers. In this report, a "pilot tag" was found in 64% of female cadavers that were examined [20]. The second stage of obturator hernia formation continues with dimpling of the peritoneum over the obturator canal and progresses to invagination of a peritoneal sac (Fig. 20.9). Finally in the evolution of an obturator hernia, bowel, uterus, tube or ovary may enter the peritoneal sac and pass along the obturator canal.

Chronic pelvic pain can result from incarceration of tube or ovary in the obturator hernia. Symptomatic intestinal obstruction can result from incarceration of small or large bowel in the obturator canal. Delay of diagnosis, however, is common as an obturator hernia is usually not visible or even palpable because of its deep location between the pectineus and adductor longus muscles.

More recently, computerized tomography has developed into a reliable diagnostic tool for evaluation of patients with possible obturator hernia. In two small series, CT scans detected the presence of an obturator hernia in 87 and 100% of the cases studied [12, 13].

Treatment

Despite advances in imaging technology, the mainstay of diagnoses and treatment remains abdominal exploration. Exploration may be via open laparotomy or with laparoscopic visualization. Regardless of the method used to obtain

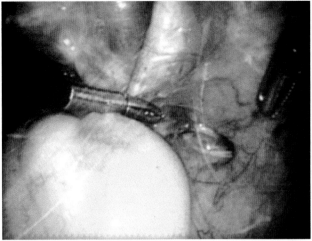

Fig. 20.9   Reduction of an obturator canal hernia

access, the entire pelvis must be examined and evaluated. If bilateral obturator defects are found, both hernias should be repaired.

After an obturator hernia has been identified, contents of the sac are reduced and a preperitoneal dissection is done to expose the internal obturator opening and obturator canal. At this point, the internal opening of the obturator canal can be closed with permanent monofilament suture securing periosteum of the symphysis pubis to fascia of the internal obturator muscle. It is necessary to take care not to injure the obturator nerve or obturator vessels. An alternative method to repair obturator hernia is to use permanent synthetic mesh to secure the breach in the obturator membrane. Polypropylene, polyester, or expanded polytetrafluoroethylene mesh can be used. Mesh must cover the entire defect with a 2.5–3.0 cm overlap circumferentially and secured with adequate fixation. In addition to the obturator opening, it is usual to cover the entire myopectineal orifice—femoral and inguinal orifices—with mesh (Fig. 20.10).

After the mesh has been secured, the operative area is reperitonealized . Typically, the peritoneal incision is closed with an intracorporeal running suture of 2-0 absorbable suture; polydioxanone or polyglactin 910 are suitable choices (Fig. 20.11).

Perineal Hernia

Perineal hernias are very rare hernias that insinuate themselves through muscle and fascia of the pelvic floor (pelvic diaphragm) into the perineum (Fig. 20.12). Perineal hernias have also been called ischiorectal hernias, subpubic hernias, pudendal hernias, posterior labial hernias, hernias of the pouch of Douglas and vaginal hernias. Perineal hernias are

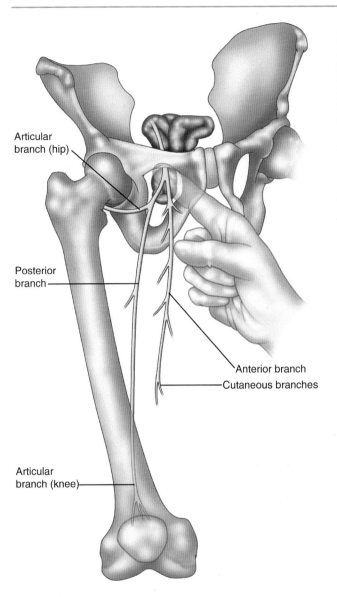

Articular branch (hip)

Posterior branch

Anterior branch
Cutaneous branches

Articular branch (knee)

Fig. 20.7   Howship-Romberg sign in obturator hernia

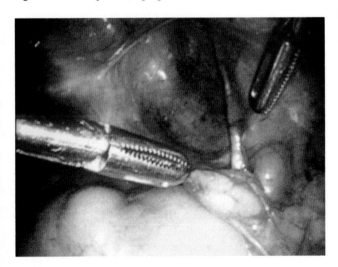

Fig. 20.8   Obturator canal pilot tag

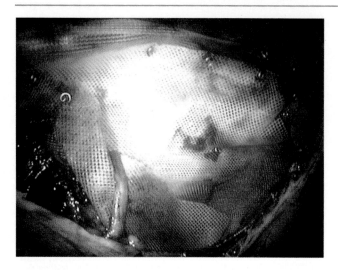

Fig. 20.10 Obturator hernia mesh repair with tacks

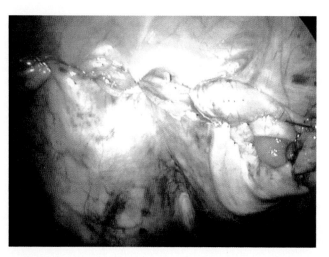

Fig. 20.11 Closure of the peritoneum in obturator hernia repair

commonly found in women and are true hernias with a distinct peritoneal sac.

Factors thought to contribute to perineal hernia include the broad female pelvis, childbirth, injuries incident to childbirth, obesity, exenteration procedures for pelvic cancer, abdominal perineal resection, and, in men, perineal prostatectomy. Perineal hernias may present anterior or posterior to the superficial perineal muscle, though the levator ani, or between the levator ani and coccygeus muscle.

Anatomy

A pudendal hernia is an anterior perineal hernia that occurs only in females. This hernia is also known as a labial hernia and may protrude into the labium majus as an overt mass. A pudendal hernia exits the pelvis through a triangle bounded by the bulbocavernosus, ischiocavernosus and transversus

perineal muscles [20]. A posterior perineal hernia may emerge between fibers of the levator ani or between the levator ani and coccygeus muscles, [21, 22]

Presentation

Perineal hernias are bounded by compliant muscle and soft tissue and, as such, rarely cause intestinal obstruction. They can, however, cause chronic pelvic pain. Typically, perineal hernia present as a palpable, soft bulge in the perineum that is easily reducible or reduces itself when the patient is recumbent. If an overt perineal bulge is not evident, herniography with intrabdominal instillation of radio opaque dye may be used to further refine a diagnosis of perineal hernia (Figs. 20.13, 20.14, 20.15 and 20.16).

Treatment

The only definitive treatment for perineal hernia is surgical repair. Access to a perineal hernia can be obtained via a perineal incision, or transabdominally using open laparotomy or laparoscopic techniques. Traditionally, these hernias have been repaired by closure of the perineal defect with non absorbable suture and the patient's own tissues. This procedure, while grounded in the principles of classic open surgery, has the disadvantage of using attenuated muscle and fascia to secure the repair.

Another approach that is gaining favor for the evaluation of abdominal and pelvic wall hernias has been that of laparoscopy [11]. A transabdominal laparoscopic examination offers the benefit of minimal access with maximum visualization of potential hernia sites in the abdominal and pelvic cavities. Once a perineal hernia has been visualized, its contents are reduced and a preperitoneal dissection carried out to define the borders of the hernia defect. Permanent synthetic mesh is used to cover and overlap the hernia defect with a 3 cm margin. Laparoscopic suture, staples or tacks are used to fix the mesh and the operative area is reperitonealized closing the peritoneal incision with intracorporeal absorbable suture.

Supravesical Hernia

Supravesical hernias are herniation of abdominal content through a supravesical fossa of the anterior abdominal wall. They are classified as either external or internal supravesical hernias [22]. External supravesical hernias pass inferiorly through the supravesical fossa to present medially as direct inguinal hernias or intraparietal hernias of the anterior inferior abdominal wall. Internal supravesical hernias pass downward to enter the retropubic space of Retzius (Fig. 20.17).

Fig. 20.12 Perineal hernia

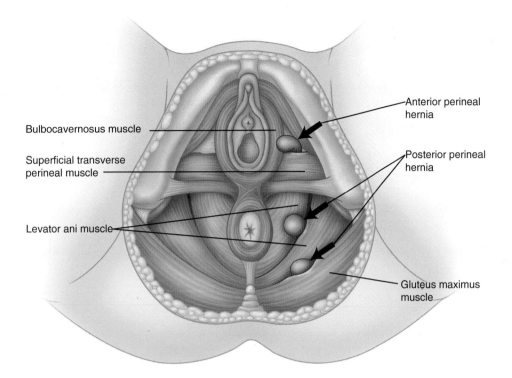

Bulbocavernosus muscle

Superficial transverse
perineal muscle

Levator ani muscle

Anterior perineal
hernia

Posterior perineal
hernia

Gluteus maximus
muscle

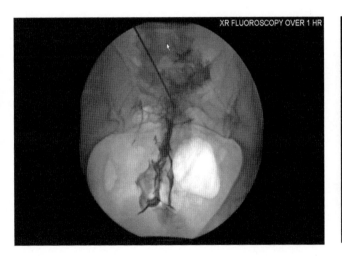

Fig. 20.13 Perineal herniography (Note: the *arrow* is an X-ray mark and is irrelevant to the present discussion)

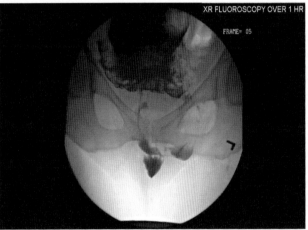

Fig. 20.14 Perineal herniography

The diagnosis of supravesical hernias that exit through the posterior inguinal wall or femoral canal may be obvious. However, an internal supravesical hernia that passes into the retropubic space of Retzius is usually more difficult to diagnose. Although a small bowel series, ultrasound or computed tomography may aid in the workup, diagnosis is usually made at abdominal exploration.

Management of supravesical hernia is that of operative repair. Hernias that present as external supravesical hernias (i.e. as direct hernias) may be managed with traditional Bassini or Shouldice herniorrhaphy techniques or Lichtenstein anterior hernioplasty with mesh. Hernia in the retropubic space of Retzius—internal supravesical hernia—may be better served with a transabdominal laparoscopic approach that permits a complete visualization of abdomen and pelvis. As with other hernias of the abdomen and pelvic wall, a preperitoneal dissection is performed after reduction of hernia content. Hernioplasty with appropriate synthetic mesh and adequate overlap of hernia margins is followed by reperitonealization of the operative site.

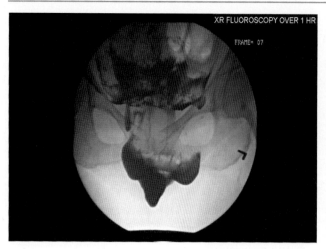

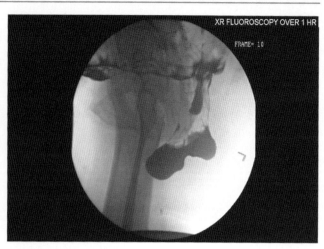

Fig. 20.15 Perineal herniography. If an overt perineal bulge is not evident, herniography with intraabdominal instillation of radiopaque dye may be used to further refine a diagnosis of perineal hernia

Fig. 20.16 Perineal herniography: X-ray fluoroscopy over 1 h

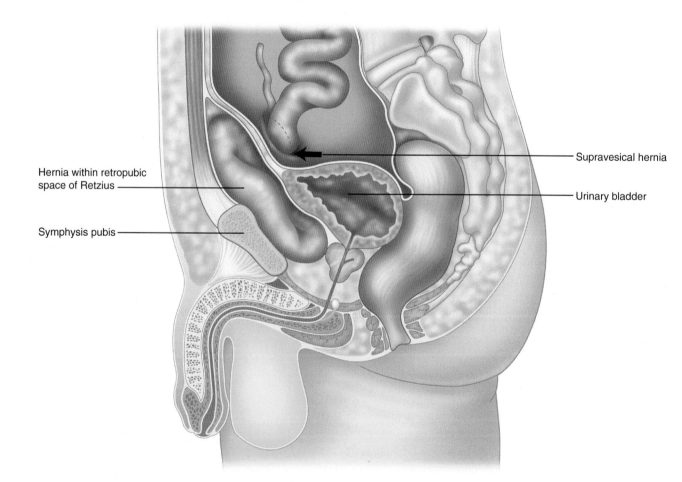

Fig. 20.17 Supravesical retropubic hernia

Conclusion

In years past, diagnosis of hernia was only seriously entertained when a mass was seen or a bulge was palpable at a hernia's point of presentation. This mindset did not include the possibility of non-visualized, non-palpable symptomatic hernias that were evident only at their site of origin [23–26]. All the same, non palpable, clinically significant occult hernias do exist and in one series constituted 8% of those hernia cases repaired [23].

Occult symptomatic abdominal and pelvic wall hernias can be visualized at their site of origin with advanced imaging and during laparoscopic exploration. The use of laparoscopic visualization allows for the diagnosis and repair of common and rare abdominal and pelvic wall hernias at their site of origin rather that at their point of presentation. A principle of hernia repair that was first clearly articulated by Henri Fruchaud in his 1956 insightful discussion of groin anatomy and description of an abdominal myopectineal orifice [26].

References

1. Howard FM. The role of laparoscopy in chronic pelvic pain: promise and pitfalls. Obstet Gynecol Surg. 1993;48(6):357–87.
2. Kloch SC. Psychosomatic issues in obstetrics and gynecology. In: Ryan KJ, Berkowitz R, Barberi RL, editors. Kistner's gynecology. Principles and practice. 6th ed. St. Louis: Mosby Yearbook Inc; 1995. p. 391–411.
3. Carter JE. Surgical treatment for chronic pelvic pain. JSLS. 1998;2(2):129–39.
4. Rapkin AJ, Mayer EA. Gastroenterologic causes of chronic pelvic pain. Obstet Gynecol Clin North Am. 1993;20(4):663–83.
5. Black S. Sciatic hernia. In: Nyhus LM, Condon RE, editors. Hernia. 2nd ed. Philadelphia: JB Lippincott; 1978. p. 443–52.
6. Watson LF. Hernia: anatomy, etiology, symptoms, diagnosis, differential diagnosis, prognosis and treatment. 3rd ed. St Louis: CV Mosby; 1948.
7. Miklos JR, O'Reilly MJ, Saye WB. Sciatic hernia: a cause of chronic pelvic pain in women. Obstet Gynecol. 1998;91(6):998–1001.
8. Cali RL, Pitsch RM, Blatchford GJ, et al. Rare pelvic floor hernias: report of a case and review of the literature. Dis Colon Rectum. 1991;25:604–12.
9. Gaffney LB, Schand J. Sciatic hernia: a case of congenital occurrence. Am J Surg. 1958;95:974.
10. Losanoff J, Kjossen K. Sciatic hernia. Acta Chir Belg. 1995;95(6):269–70.
11. Kavic MS. Laparoscopic hernia repair. Amsterdam: Harwood Academic Publishers; 1997. p. 33–40.
12. Haraguchi M, Matsuo S, Kanetaka K, Tokai H, Azyma T, Yamaguchi S, Kanematsu T. Obturator Hernia in an Aging Society. Ann Acad Med Singapore. 2007;36(6):413–5.
13. Nakayama T, Kobayashi S, Shiraishi K, Nishiumi T, Mori S, Isobe K, Furuta Y. Diagnosis and treatment of obturator hernia. Keio J Med. 2002;51(3):129–32.
14. Gray SW, Skandalakis JE. Strangulated obturator hernia. In: Nyhus LM, Condon RE, editors. Hernia. 2nd ed. Philadelphia: JB Lippincott; 1978. p. 427–42.
15. Bjork KJ, Mucha P, Cahill DR. Obturator hernia. Surg Gynecol Obstet. 1988;167(3):217–22.
16. Ritz TA, Deshmukh N. Obturator hernia. South Med J. 1990;83:709–12.
17. Howship J. Practical remarks on the discrimination and appearances of surgical disease. London: John Churchill; 1840.
18. Romberg MH. Die Operation des singeklemmten Bruches des eirunden Loches. Operatio hernia foraminis ovales incarceratae. In: Dieffenbach JF, editor. Die operative chirurgie, vol. 2. Leipzig: F.A. Brockhaus; 1848.
19. Chung CC, Mok CO, Kwong KH, Ng EK, Lau WY, Li AK. Obturator hernia revisited: a review of 12 cases in 7 years. J R Coll Surg Edinb. 1997;42:82–4.
20. Singer R, Leary PM, Hofmeyer NG. Obturator hernia. S Afr Med J. 1955;29:74.
21. Koontz AR. Perineal hernia. In: Nyhus LM, Condon RE, editors. Hernia. 2nd ed. Philadelphia: J.B. Lippincott; 1978. p. 453–62.
22. Gray SW, Skandalakis JE, McClusky DA. Atlas of surgical anatomy. Baltimore: Williams & Wilkens; 1985. p. 326–7.
23. Herrington JK. Occult inguinal hernia in the female. Ann Surg. 1995;181:481–3.
24. Fodor PB, Webb WA. Indirect inguinal hernia in the female with no palpable sac. South Med J. 1974;64:15–6.
25. Bascom JU. Pelvic pain. Perspect Colon Rectal Surg. 1999;11(2):21–40.
26. Fruchaud H. The Surgical Anatomy of Hernias of the Groin. (Translated and edited by Robert Bendavid, 2006). France: Gaston Doin & Cie; 1956. Printed in Canada by University of Toronto Press, First printing 2006.

Andrew N. Kingsnorth

Historical Note

Incisional hernia is iatrogenic and its incidence has increased with each increment of abdominal surgical intervention. An incisional hernia is the most perfect example of a "surgeon-dependent variable." The introduction of continuous ambulatory peritoneal dialysis was followed by its own unique harvest of incisional hernias [1, 2]. Laparoscopic surgery also added a new entity: "port site" hernia (Chap. 18) [3]. Although it was hoped that the latter would become infrequent with the advent of smaller ports, the overall incidence of abdominal wall herniation in the CLASICC trial of laparoscopic vs. open surgery for colorectal cancer revealed that there was no reduction in the incidence of abdominal wall hernias (9.2% in the laparoscopic group vs. 8.6% in the open group) comparing open resection vs. laparoscopic surgery [4].

The development of abdominal surgery in the nineteenth century—the excision of an ovarian cyst by McDowell in 1809 [5], partial gastrectomy by Billroth in 1881 [6], and cholecystectomy by Langenbuch in 1882 [7]—has been followed by operations to manage the incisional hernias which followed as complications. Gerdy repaired an incisional hernia in 1836 and Maydl another in 1886 [8]. Judd in 1912 [9] and Gibson in 1920 [10] both described repair techniques based on extensive anatomic dissection of the scar and adjacent tissues. Prosthetic materials were introduced early on: autografts of fascia lata by Kirschner in 1910 [11] and fascial strips by Gallie and Le Mesurier in 1923 [12]. Tendons, cutis, and whole skin grafts, both homografts and heterografts, have been advocated and found to have problems. Nonbiological prosthetics that have been used in the past include stainless steel and tantalum gauze. More recently polypropylene (Marlex, Prolene), polyester (Mersilene), and

ePTFE (DualMesh Plus) have been introduced and are the materials of choice for many surgeons (these are reviewed in Chap. 7).

The ideal prosthetic material has yet to be discovered. The visionary Theodor Billroth stated more than a century ago, "If we could artificially produce tissues of the density and toughness of fascia or tendon, the secret of radical cure of hernia would be discovered" [13]. The currently available products, however, are generally excellent alternatives to the native tissues when the repair of these hernias is undertaken.

Symptoms and Signs

An incisional hernia is defined by Pollock and his colleagues as "a bulge visible and palpable when the patient is standing and often requiring support or repair" [14].

Sixty percent of patients with incisional hernias do not experience any symptoms; however, symptoms that predicate medical advice include difficulty in bending, cosmetic deformity, discomfort from the size of the hernia, persistent abdominal pain, and episodic subacute intestinal obstruction. Incarceration persisting to acute intestinal obstruction and strangulation necessitate emergency surgery.

Spontaneous rupture of incisional hernia is an unusual but life-threatening complication (Fig. 21.1). This complication is more likely in infra-umbilical hernia. It may be exacerbated by friction of clothes or corsetry [15]. Hernias after gynecological and obstetric interventions are most at risk [16].

The demonstration of small incisional hernias may be very difficult. Patients with tiny protrusions of extraperitoneal fat and a small peritoneal sac may complain of a tender lump, which is not always there, but which causes quite severe localized pain when it is present. Physical examination of the patient supine and relaxed usually reveals the cause. Ultrasound examination is a useful diagnostic test and will often reveal an impalpable defect, particularly in the obese patient. However, the sonographic

A.N. Kingsnorth (✉)
Department of Surgery, Peninsula College of Medicine & Dentistry, Plymouth, Devon, UK
e-mail: andrew.kingsnorth@nhs.net

A.N. Kingsnorth and K.A. LeBlanc (eds.), *Management of Abdominal Hernias*,
DOI 10.1007/978-1-84882-877-3_21, © Springer Science+Business Media London 2013

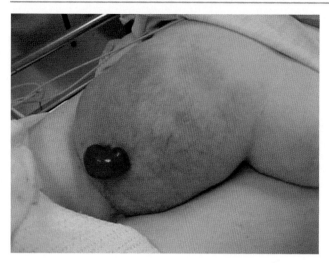

Fig. 21.1 Spontaneous rupture of an incisional hernia

examination of the abdominal wall is dependent upon a skilled interpreter. It is sometimes difficult to differentiate between a hernia and subcutaneous fat or small bowel in the hernia vs. in close proximity to a weakened anterior fascia. In most situations and particularly for massive complex incisional hernias, CT scan may be much more efficient and accurate in defining the defect and planning the preoperative preparation of the patient and the operation chosen. CT scan is particularly helpful in obesity and in patients with extensive laparotomy scars as it defines the contents of the sac especially if the abdominal wall hernias are clinically occult. In addition it distinguished them from other diseases such as hematoma, abscess, and neoplasia [17].

Incidence

The overall incidence of incisional hernias is difficult to estimate. Homans, in 1887, reported that 10% of abdominal operations were followed by incisional hernias [18]. The reported incidence of this complication has not fallen in recent years, even though major sepsis has diminished, monofilament, nonabsorbable sutures have been introduced, and the technique of wound closure has been emphasized. Incisional hernias are slightly more frequent in males than females (55:45).

Until recently there were very few studies with adequate follow-up of laparotomy wounds to determine the real incidence of incisional hernia. Stanton, in 1916, reported 500 consecutive laparotomies followed up for 5–7 years. Over this period a total of 24 postoperative hernias were found (4.8%). In 260 clean cases only three incisional hernias developed, whereas in 186 contaminated cases 18 hernias developed [19].

Although the incidence of burst abdomen has been reduced by the use of high-tensile sutures, incisional hernia remains an important problem. The strength of the abdominal wall resides in the aponeurotic layers, the linea alba, and the rectus sheath. These layers are slow to heal and only regain adequate strength after 120 days from wounding [20]. On a theoretical basis, most incisional hernias would be expected to be apparent before this healing is complete. The reports of onset of incisional hernia which occur in the standard textbooks are usually based on the information gleaned from patients having repair operations for symptomatic incisional hernias; hence, they probably overemphasize these large and early onset hernias. For instance, Akman estimated that 97% of incisional hernias were apparent at 5 years [21].

Long-term prospective studies of laparotomy wounds were unknown until Hughes and Ellis separately raised the question of late wound failure in the early 1980s. Ellis and colleagues from the Westminster Hospital followed up 363 patients who had undergone laparotomy but who had sound wounds without herniation when examined at 1 year. When reviewed between $2^1/_2$ and $5^1/_2$ years later, 21 patients (5.8%) had developed incisional hernias [22–26].

Mudge and Hughes from Cardiff have published an important continuation of their study of incisional hernia [26]. During the years 1972–1973, 831 patients aged over 40 years undergoing major abdominal surgery were entered into a long-term study. Of 564 patients surviving and being willing to enter the study at the end of 1 year, 337 patients were followed up for a further 9 years. Of the remainder, 128 patients had died and 99 patients had an incomplete follow-up for various reasons. All the patients were questioned regarding symptoms and incapacity.

Of the 564 patients 62 (11%) had developed incisional hernias by the definition of Pollock. Of these 62 patients developing incisional hernias, details of the original operative closure technique were known for 52 and for 408 patients who did not develop hernias. The incidence of hernia in patients having nylon closure to both peritoneum and linea alba was 11 of 143 (7.7%); for catgut to peritoneum and nylon to linea alba, 24 out of 196 developed incisional hernia (12%); for catgut to both layers, 14 out of 100 developed incisional hernias (14%); of four patients having nylon through-and-through tension sutures, two developed incisional hernias. When the 337 completing the 10-year follow-up are scrutinized, 37 (11%) developed an incisional hernia, and 13 of these (35%) first appeared at 5 years or later. One in three of these hernias caused symptoms.

More than half the incisional hernias first appeared more than 1 year after the initial operation. These 10-year results confirm that there is a continued attrition of the healed laparotomy wound, with incisional hernias developing up to and after 10 years. When the distress and disability of the hernias is considered, those that develop in the first 3 years after laparotomy cause the most symptoms; they are also the larger hernias and are more likely to require repairs [24].

These findings from two independent groups in London and Cardiff confirm each other, the failure rate of abdominal wounds being about 6% at 5 years rising to 11% at 10 years.

Akman's earlier statement that 97% of incisional hernias are apparent at 1 year after the original surgery is not confirmed by these long-term studies. Moreover, without full-scale prospective follow-up the incidence of incisional hernia will be underestimated. Fortunately not all incisional hernias warrant an operation.

Currently it is believed that up to 13% of laparotomy incisions will eventually develop hernias. In a systematic review of et al. (see Chap. 6) [27], it was concluded that abdominal fascial closure of midline laparotomy wounds with a continuous, nonabsorbable suture results in a significantly lower rate of incisional hernia than using either nonabsorbable or interrupted techniques.

Etiologic Factors

The important causative factors include sepsis (60% of patients developing an incisional hernia within the first year after surgery have had significant wound infection), the placement of drainage tubes through the original incision, a previous operation through the same incision within 6 months, initial closure with catgut alone ("inept methods of suture") [28, 29], steroid and other immunosuppressant therapy, and inflammatory bowel disease. Obesity is an important risk factor both for the occurrence of the original incisional hernia and for the likelihood of recurrence of the hernia after repair [22, 30]. Early wound dehiscence is frequently followed by incisional herniation. Needle puncture incisional hernias are described as "satellites" of a main wound failure or "button-hole" hernias. These hernias may be related to the sawing effect of nonabsorbable sutures on the aponeurosis [31]. Less significant factors include age and gender, anemia, malnutrition, hypoproteinemia, diabetes, type of incision, postoperative intestinal obstruction [32], and postoperative chest infection. Two recent retrospective reviews which included multifactorial regression analysis of putative risk factors, such as sex, age, smoking, chronic lung disease, obesity, sight, surgeon's experience, closure method, and suture material, have found that size of the hernia and obesity were the prime factors involved in recurrence after incisional hernia repair [32, 33]. Many of these hernias recurred early with remedial time between the primary operation and the first symptoms of hernia being within a year. Other centers with a large experience have added further risk factors which include age over 60 years, a previous attempt at repair of the hernia, and postoperative complications [34]. With time the lateral abdominal wall shortening occurs and

atrophy of the oblique musculature. This combined with pathological fibrosis due to myopathic disuse atrophy of the rectus abdominis muscles results in an increased transfer of load forces to the midline at the time of repair increasing the likelihood of recurrence [35]. Fifty-five percent of incisional hernias occur in men. Incisional hernias are infrequent under the age of 40 years and their incidence increases with age. There is an association between the development of incisional hernias and the occurrence of the post-thrombotic syndrome [36].

Of particular importance as an etiologic factor is the wound drain. Ponka records that of 126 patients with herniation through a subcostal incision for biliary surgery all had drains delivered through the wound at the time of the initial operation [30].

Midline incisions are at greater risk than paramedian incisions [37]. However, no matter which anatomic type of incision is made, the choice of suture material is crucial. Kirk compared paramedian incisions closed with two layers of catgut with midline incisions closed with nylon; the crucial difference was not the anatomy of the incision but the choice of suture—the nylon-closed incisions were significantly better than those closed with catgut [38].

Lower midline incisions seem to be at greater risk than upper midline incisions (but this may be a faulty finding; inadequate suture techniques as well as physiological factors need assessment). Many of the lower midline incisions are done for gynecological interventions, and the subsequent hernias are often not included in purely "surgical" follow-up data; hence, there may be under-recording of the true overall incidence of this problem. The location of incisional hernias has changed during recent years with the new generation of laparoscopic operations that have evolved [39].

Mass suture with wire is a secure method, and no late incisional hernias developed in the cases closed with interrupted wire [40]. The newer absorbable polymer sutures polyglactin (Vicryl) and polyglycolic acid PGA (Dexon) have been subjected to trial and are reported as less good than nonabsorbables for fascial closure. The longer life polymer polydioxanone (PDS) is under evaluation. A controlled trial of PDS vs. polyamide (nylon) in the closure of 233 major laparotomy wounds failed to show any statistically significant difference. The patients were randomized to either suture, a mass-closure technique was used, and patients were followed up to 6 months. There were two wound failures in the PDS group and more sepsis in the PDS group. There were no wound sinuses in either group [41].

Late hernias occur just as frequently in patients whose wounds are sutured with an absorbable polymer or nonabsorbable monofilament. At present there is no explanation of why mature collagen should yield to form hernia so long after healing has occurred. There is no etiological factor to account for these late hernias [24, 26] although the concept of collagen failure, metastatic emphysema, may offer an explanation (see page 69).

Epigastric incisional hernias are recently reported as a complication of median sternotomy wounds for cardiac surgery. The risk factors identified include male sex, obesity, wound infection, aortic valve replacement, and left ventricular failure [42].

In children, either a layered or a mass closure with polyglycolic acid sutures gives acceptable results and a low failure rate. Nonabsorbable sutures are unnecessary in children [43]. For some unknown reason the risk of failure in children is greatest in those undergoing pyloromyotomy (Ramstedt's) operation for hypertrophic pyloric stenosis [44]. Early incisional hernias in children are likely to resolve spontaneously. The late development of incisional hernias occurs rarely in children [45].

Principles of Open Repair

The following principles should be followed:

1. Whenever possible the normal anatomy should be reconstituted, prior to placement of prosthetic mesh. In midline hernias this means the linea alba must be reconstructed; in more lateral hernias there should be layer-by-layer closure as far as possible. The use of sutures alone for the repair of incisional hernias is associated with a rate of recurrence that is at least as high as 43% [46].
2. Only tendinous/aponeurotic/fascial structures should be brought together. In situ darning over the defect without adequate mobilization and apposition of the aponeurotic defect gives a 100% recurrence rate [24].
3. The suture material must retain its strength for long enough to maintain tissue apposition and allow sound union of tissues to occur. A nonabsorbable or slowly absorbable material must, therefore, be used.
4. The length of suture material is related to the geometry of the wound and to its healing. Using bites at not more than 0.5-cm intervals, the ratio of suture length to wound length must be 4:1 and not more than 5:1 [47, 48].
5. Repair of an incisional hernia inevitably involves returning viscera to the confines of the abdominal cavity with a resultant rise in intra-abdominal pressure. It is important to minimize this. Preoperative weight reduction is the first precaution. This, unfortunately, is generally not possible. If the linea alba cannot be reconstituted without undue tension, steps must be taken to perform a relaxing incision such as an external oblique release (Ramirez procedure, see below). This is almost always required with very large hernias.
6. Every care must be taken to prevent abdominal distension due to adynamic ileus, which will lead to additional stress on repair suture lines. For this reason, handling of the viscera should be minimized.
7. Postoperative coughing can put an additional unwarranted strain on the suture lines. Hence, pulmonary collapse, pulmonary infection, and pulmonary edema must be avoided. Restriction of preoperative smoking, chest exercises, weight reduction, and avoidance of excessive blood or fluid replacement (and their hemodynamic effects on the heart) are important components in the successful repair of an incisional hernia.
8. The repair must be performed aseptically; inoculated bacteria, traumatized tissue, and hematoma should not be features of these wounds.

Drawing these eight points together, appropriate preparation for operation includes measures to reduce the risk of subsequent infection: all skin lesions and erosions should be resolved before surgery and pulmonary function should be optimized. A carefully planned procedure using a repair with prosthetic reinforcement is recommended in appropriate patients [49].

Two more points should be considered:

1. The use of antibiotics. A randomized trial comparing the use of antibiotic prophylaxis against no antibiotic in incisional hernia repair using a prosthesis has never been carried out. Nevertheless most surgeons consider it best practice to administer a systemic dose of antibiotics preoperatively. When combined with a second dose of antibiotics, a significant reduction in wound infection occurs even in the context of a clean operation without contamination [50]. When there are other risk factors such as diabetes, obesity, and previous wound infection, the need for antibiotic prophylaxis becomes imperative. The use of prosthetic materials and in particular biological tissue grafts will be addressed elsewhere in this book (Chap. 7).
2. The use of prosthetic synthetic or biological meshes. There are limited clinical data and short-term follow-up for only a few of the many biological tissue grafts, and additional clinical studies are required [51]. Prosthetic, synthetic meshes are designed to withstand the theoretical maximum intra-abdominal pressure of 20 kPa at an average human body diameter of 32 cm. From this it is calculated that the maximum required tensile strength of any material to maintain abdominal wall closure is 16 N/cm. All synthetic prosthetic materials used for incisional hernia repair are designed to this standard, and the choice is left to the individual surgeon. In a contaminated or potentially contaminated field a biological mesh is favored, and there are many new products to choose from [52].

A meta-analysis of randomized control trials with a Jadad quality score of greater than 3 revealed that the lowest occurrence of incisional hernia occurred when nonabsorbable sutures were used for abdominal wall closure and the suture technique favored a continuous suture rather than interrupted stitches [27]. More recently a further meta-analysis indicated that there was no difference in rate of incisional hernia with midline laparotomy closure between a nonabsorbable suture and a slowly absorbable suture material. This analysis also revealed similar outcomes with continuous and interrupted suture techniques [53]. The continuous suture method may be more effective since it requires half as much time and less suture material [54]. The meta-analysis by these authors also confirmed previous findings that braided suture materials increased the incidence of infection, suture sinus formation, and postoperative abdominal wall pain. More recently two groups have challenged the dogma of big-bite closure. Using small stitches with small suture differences (a 0.5-cm bite with a 0.5-cm stitch interval), the suture length/wound length ratio can be maintained at 4:1, but at the same time in an experimental animal model increasing the tensile strength across the wound from 534 to 787 N. The small sutures are placed 4–6 mm from the wound edge and cut through the aponeurosis and not through the rectus abdominis muscle [55]. In the clinical scenario this short stitch length resulted in a greatly reduced incidence in incisional hernia from 18 to 5.6% and reduction of wound infection by half from 10.2 to 5.2% [56].

In epigastric incisional hernia repair it should be remembered that the linea alba is broad in the epigastrium—at least as broad as the xiphoid cartilage is wide—therefore, efforts to draw the rectus muscles close together are unanatomic and doomed to disruption. Most of the side-to-side tension in the linea alba in the epigastrium is generated in the anterior rectus sheath which consists of two laminae, the anterior lamina being the external oblique arising from the lower ribs. The short span of this muscle makes this layer relatively inelastic and unstretchable to the midline for repair [57]. For this reason, on occasion the epigastric midline cannot be closed even with an external oblique release, and an inlay prosthetic graft is required.

Incisional Hernia Following Appendectomy

Incisional hernias related to open appendectomy are reported in all series. Etiological factors include severe postoperative wound sepsis and the placement of a drain through a gridiron appendectomy wound. These hernias occurring through the red muscle in the flank are difficult to repair adequately. If there is a well-developed fibrous margin to the defect, this can be used as the basis of a Mayo-type overlap repair, prior to supplementary prosthetic mesh. Direct suture of these hernias, suturing red muscle, often fails, and if an adequate overlap cannot be constructed, extraperitoneal mesh (page 337) or mesh reinforcement of the external oblique aponeurosis is advised.

Table 21.1 A grading system for abdominal wall injury that can be helpful in predicting the potential for future abdominal wall herniation at the site of injury [60]

Clinical presentation	Type
Subcutaneous tissue contusion	I
Abdominal wall muscle hematoma	II
Single abdominal wall muscle disruption	III
Complete abdominal wall muscle disruption	IV
Complete abdominal wall muscle disruption with herniation of abdominal contents	V
Complete abdominal wall muscle disruption with evisceration	VI

Traumatic Abdominal Wall Hernia

Abdominal wall injury may result in hernia that is not be immediately recognized at the time of injury [58]. Clinically apparent anterior traumatic abdominal wall hernias have a high rate of associated intra-abdominal injuries requiring laparotomy. Occult traumatic abdominal wall hernias are diagnosed only with CT scan and usually do not require urgent laparotomy or hernia repair. The mechanism of injury should be considered when deciding if urgent laparotomy is required. Diaphragmatic lumbar and extrathoracic hernias are also well-described complications of blunt trauma [59]. Early recognition of these hernias can be a diagnostic challenge and delayed presentation is common. The surgical treatment for these hernias is evolving and a variety of options are available to the surgeon. On the basis of a review of all available abdominal and pelvic CT scans of 1,549 patients presenting to a trauma unit over an 18-month period, 9% of patients were shown to have an abdominal wall injury and a grading system was devised (Table 21.1).

The incidence of these was found to be as follows: I (53%), II (28%), III (9%), IV (8%), V (2%), and VI (0.2%). There was no association between abdominal wall injury and seat belt use or injury severity score. This large study concluded that abdominal wall injury occurs in 9% of blunt trauma patients having CT scan, the incidence of herniation at presentation was only 0.2%, and the incidence of future herniation was 1.5% [60].

Pneumoperitoneum as an Aid in Surgical Treatment of Giant Hernias

Management of giant incisional hernia is often compromised by obesity, intrahernial adhesions, and contraction in the volume of the abdominal cavity—the hernial contents have lost their "right of domain." Long operations to free the adhesions and brutal reduction of the contents can lead to ileus, pulmonary restriction, and cardiac compromise. After these operations, if the patient does not succumb to the cardio-respiratory complications, the persistent ileus will lead to disruption of the repair.

The use of pneumoperitoneum before attempting definitive repair of giant hernias was originally suggested by Moreno in 1940 [61]. The advantages of the technique are:

- Stretching of the abdominal wall, creating a larger cavity into which the hernial contents can be replaced
- Reduction of edema in the mesentery, omentum, and viscera in the hernial sac, creating less mass to be reduced
- Stretching of the hernial sac leading to elongation of adhesions, making dissection and reduction easier [62]
- Increased tone of the diaphragm, allowing preoperative respiratory and circulatory adaptation to the elevation of the diaphragm [63]

The technique of pneumoperitoneum is simple: under local anesthetic an epidural catheter, an intracath or a ureteric pigtail catheter, is introduced into the peritoneal cavity. The site of puncture should be kept well away from the hernia or its margins to avoid damaging viscera fixed by adhesions. The optimum site is probably through the linea alba. Successful abdominal puncture is marked by a lessening of the pressure required to advance the needle. The catheter can then be easily threaded into the peritoneal cavity and its position checked radiologically after injection of a small quantity of contrast medium [64]. The catheter is fixed into position and about 500 mL of gas or air is injected via a micropore filter [65]. Graduated amounts of gas or air are injected on successive days, 500 mL at a time once, twice or thrice a day, until a daily volume of about 2.5 L is obtained. Caldironi and colleagues used nitrous oxide in 41 patients with giant incisional hernias. A laparoscopic insufflator was used to top up the pneumoperitoneum every other day for a mean of 5.5 days, a total volume of 23.2 L of nitrous oxide being injected. The volume introduced at each session was 1,000/1,500 mL greater than the previous session and the procedure was well tolerated in all but one patient. The good results of the subsequent repairs (only two recurrences in 40 repairs at a mean 25 months follow-up) attest to the success of this technique [66]. The abdomen will inevitably be blown up like a balloon and much patient reassurance may be needed. If the patient develops discomfort, shoulder tip pain, tachycardia, or dyspnea, the rate of insufflation can be reduced; indeed, if severe symptoms occur, gas or air can be withdrawn. No attempt is made to prevent the hernial sac distending; distension of the hernial sac is helpful, stretching adhesions and allowing contents to reduce spontaneously prior to operation. Unfettered distension of the peritoneal sac may reveal subsidiary hernial protrusions, enabling a more adequate surgical repair to be planned and undertaken. There is a need for this technique in the surgical armamentarium, but while this has been found to be of significant benefit in South America and some parts of Europe, the experience with this technique in the United States is limited.

Due to the failure of most clinicians to adopt pneumoperitoneum, few advances have been made in its application [67]. However, recently a simpler technique using a double lumen intra-abdominal catheter inserted through a Veress needle in the left hypochondrium has utilized the daily insufflations of ambient air [68]. Over a period or an average of 9.3 days between 1,000 and 4,000 cc were insufflated depending on patient comfort to reach a maximum intra-abdominal pressure of 15 mm of mercury (measured by sphygmomanometer). Subsequent successful hernia repair was carried out in all patients.

In practice, the patient is ready for operation at about a 2 weeks after induction of the pneumoperitoneum, the end point being judged by the tension of the abdominal wall, which should feel as tight as a drum, especially in the flanks [69]. The patient should be operated on at this stage—if possible most of the dissection should be performed with the hernial sac unpunctured and distended. Puncture of the sac at operation will allow easy reduction of contents and the slack parietes will facilitate repair. Air is only slowly absorbed from the peritoneal cavity, and often after the first 2 or 3 days absorption is so reduced as to become inconsequential.

Contraindications to pneumoperitoneum include abdominal wall sepsis, prior cardiorespiratory decompensation, and strangulation of hernial contents. Complications, which are very rare, include visceral puncture, hematoma, and the risk of an embolism into a solid organ if the liver or spleen is needled prior to insufflation. Mediastinal and retroperitoneal surgical emphysema are rare complications.

Indications for Operation

Incisional hernias produce symptoms of disfigurement, discomfort, and pain, and often recurrent colic if subacute obstructive episodes occur. Such symptoms are reason enough for operative intervention. Irreducibility and a narrow neck are further indications for surgery. Obstruction and strangulation are absolute indications.

Contraindications to Elective Operation

Extreme obesity can be a contraindication to surgery. Obese patients frequently have cardiorespiratory decompensation and diabetes, making weight reduction essential prior to surgery [70]. Subcutaneous and intra-abdominal obesity make the open repair more difficult and postoperative complications more likely. In the particularly high-risk patients, the use of invasive monitoring such as a Swan-Ganz catheter and the monitoring that the intensive care units provide will allow such patients to undergo these operations without undue risk.

Continuing deep sepsis in the wound is also a contraindication to repair surgery. Such cases frequently have a history of more than one repair attempt, and the wound may be indurated with many sinuses in it. If the sepsis is long standing, calcification may be present. Usually wounds with continuing infection contain buried and heavily infected nonabsorbable material; it is best to open these wounds, remove all the foreign material, and drain all the pockets of pus. The wound is then left to granulate over. Only when the wound has been without deep sepsis for 6–9 months should repair surgery be undertaken.

Skin infections and intertrigo beneath a vast incisional hernia are common and require vigorous preoperative treatment. Operation should be delayed until the skin is sound.

Biological meshes can be used in infected situations if surgery cannot be delayed until the infected areas have been fully treated. The long-term results of such usage of biologic products are still under investigation.

Choice of Operative Technique

It is usually preferable to make an accurate assessment of the anatomy of the hernia prior to surgery. How big is the defect? Does the size of the defect increase or decrease on movement? Are the contents easily reducible? If the hernia contents are incarcerated, this may not be possible. If the hernia is reducible, the sac and fibrous margins of the sac are examined with the patient supine and at ease and then standing erect.

Finally the patient is laid flat again, and as much of the sac as possible is reduced and held reduced by the examining surgeon. The patient is then asked to sit up while the surgeon continues to hold the hernia reduced. In some hernias, particularly upper midline ones, the margins of the defect close together on movement and the contraction of the abdominal wall will then hold the sac reduced (Fig. 21.1). These maneuvers may provide the surgeon with the information necessary to decide upon the operation that should be used and if there is a possibility that the laparoscopic method (smaller defects of up to 10–15 cm) should be performed rather than the open repair.

Prosthetic Mesh Operation

Due to the poor results of tissue repairs, it is mandatory that a prosthesis is used in all incisional hernia repairs. Even if the fascial defect is less than 4 cm, a prosthesis is recommended. The prosthetic materials that are available are described in Chap. 7.

The tissue repair or Mayo procedure for repair of abdominal incisional hernia gives unacceptable results with recurrence rates of up to 84% with 5.7 years of follow-up [71]. When suture repair for incisional hernia is compared with mesh repair, the incidence in incisional hernia at 36 months is reduced from 43% (suture) to 24% (mesh) in patients with a vertical midline incision of less than 6 cm in length [46]. However, in this study patients only received 2-cm overlap of mesh which currently would be considered inadequate, and the 10-year cumulative rate for recurrence was 32% for the mesh repair, a figure that would now be highly unacceptable [72]. Further insight into the benefit of mesh came from a comparative retrospective study of 421 incisional hernias on 348 patients undergoing 241 Mayo repairs and 180 mesh repairs over a 25-year period [73]. The total recurrence rate following Mayo repair was 37% in contrast to 15% after mesh implantation. In the mesh repair group the only significant prognostic factor concerning quality of life and recurrence was the size of the mesh implanted. There were more wound-related complications in the mesh repair group and recurrences occurred at the upper and lower edges of the mesh where there had been insufficient overlap.

The choice of mesh material today is generally between a prosthesis of polypropylene and polyester. There are many designs and configuration of weave, thickness of weave, and strand and size of pore [74]. The effect that these differences between the various weaves and knits, organic polymers, spinning an extrusion of yarns, and conversion to mesh and the properties of the final product is complex. Some materials shrink, but additionally some mesh studies reveal that no shrinkage takes place. Polyester was developed in 1939 and introduced in the USA in 1946 then marketed by Ethicon in 1950 under the trade name of Mersilene and is still used and is widely popular in France. Polypropylene products resulted from further advances in polymerization techniques and introduced into hernia surgery in the 1950s. Explantation of meshes shows that they remain intact but that minor flaking and fissuring occurs. In experimental studies the reduction in area due to shrinkage is shown to be at a maximum of between 3 and 6 months of approximately 30–45%. In reality this would result in the reduction in area of a 10 cm × 10 cm mesh (100 cm^2) to an area of 8 cm × 8 cm (64 cm^2) or a 36% reduction in area and a reduction in width from 10 to 8 cm leaving sufficient overlap to prevent recurrence, if the mandatory 5 cm (each side of the repaired defect) is adhered to. It is therefore not necessary to have an overlap of more than 5 cm as long as peripheral fixation is secure [75, 76]. This rate of shrinkage has been confirmed in humans with ventral hernias by Vega-Ruiz [77]. In 23 patients radiological follow-up was undertaken in patients who underwent surgery for midline ventral hernias with diameter of at least 5 cm. The polypropylene mesh was marked with titanium clips at the ends of the longest transverse and longitudinal axes. X-rays performed at 1, 3, 6, and 12 months measured the distance between the clips and the area of the mesh was calculated. In patients receiving both onlay and sublay mesh repairs, the maximum reduction in calculated area occurred between 6 and 12 months and was between 29 and 34%.

Several attempts have been made to classify synthetic meshes that are used in abdominal wall hernia surgery [78]. However, these are not of particular practical use to the surgeon. Four types of mesh have been identified depending on pore size (greater or less than 75 µm), the larger pore meshes tending to admit macrophages and fibroblasts to a greater degree allowing new blood vessel formation and collagen synthesis, and pore size of less than 10 µm delivers a microporous mesh with greater anti-adhesive properties and suitable for intraperitoneal implantation. Although it was originally intended that lightweight meshes may improve abdominal wall compliance after incisional hernia repair, a randomized controlled trial comparing lightweight composite meshes with polyester or polypropylene [79] showed no difference in abdominal wall compliance between the two groups of patients. The lightweight mesh also had a more than two times increased incidence of recurrence of the incisional hernia occurring at the edges of the mesh [80].

Classification

Incisional hernias are a diverse and heterogeneous problem because of the multiplicity of incisions used to gain access to the abdominal cavity. Therefore it is not easy to produce a classification system that covers all eventualities. Nevertheless classifications are useful for comparison of results of new methods of repair to enable comparisons to be made. Important factors, which should be taken into account for a classification system, include localization of the previous incision (vertical, transverse, oblique, or combined), the size of the defect (horizontal and transverse stratified into less than 5 cm, 5–10 cm, greater than 10 cm), number of times the hernia has recurred, reducibility, and symptoms [81]. Since 98% of vertical midline incisional hernias can be closed primarily (with or without separation of components) the most important dimension of the abdominal wall defect is vertical length, when the fascia has been completely closed, prior to mesh placement.

Anesthesia

Unless there is a strong contraindication to general anesthesia, even small incisional hernias without a tissue defect should be repaired using a general anesthetic because of the unexpected finding of an occult hernia that may escalate the complexity of the operation. Muscle relaxants will assist in reducing the contents of the sac, and drawing together the

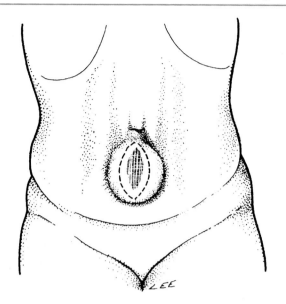

Fig. 21.2 Elliptical incisions are made on either side of the hernial cicatrix

margins of the defect during the repair and full cooperation of an anesthetist is required at this critical stage of the operation. In some circumstances, the use of spinal or epidural anesthesia may be considered, but this would depend upon the location of the hernia site and the surgeon's familiarity with the choice of that anesthesia method.

The Open Operation

Position of Patient

If the hernia is located in the midline or lateral aspects of the anterior abdominal wall, the patient is placed in the supine position on the operating table.

The Incision

A wide elliptical incision is made to enclose the cutaneous scar. The incision must generally be extended at either end to give adequate access to all the margins of the defect. The direction of this initial incision will depend on the shape of the original scar through which the hernia has come. Care should be taken not to excise too much skin: at this stage the minimum excision of cutaneous scar tissue is done (Fig. 21.2).

Removal of Overlying Redundant Tissue

The redundant skin and scar are separated from the underlying hernial sac, which is often just subcutaneous especially

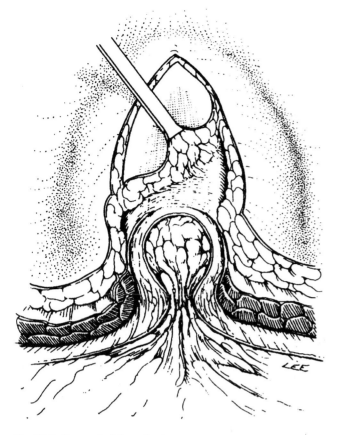

Fig. 21.3 Removal of the redundant scar

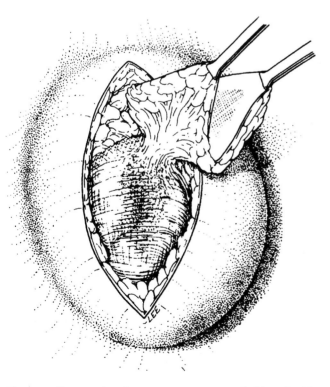

Fig. 21.4 Care must be taken not to remove too much skin and not to damage the hernial sac. The cutaneous cicatrix is often closely adherent to the sac

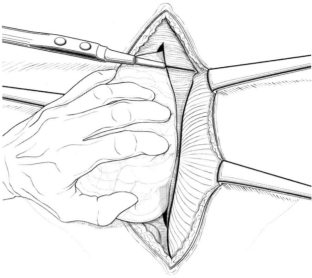

Fig. 21.5 Skin flaps are raised in order to fully dissect out the sac and allow placement of the mesh, with or without "components separation." A 4–5-cm exposure of the anterior rectus sheath is required on each side for an onlay (prefascial) repair; less exposure is required for a sublay (retrorectus) repair

near the fundus of the hernia. Redundant skin and scar tissue are removed (Fig. 21.3). This is a significant advantage of the open approach compared with the laparoscopic method because a better cosmetic result is achieved.

If the hernia is very large, the skin and underlying peritoneal sac may be virtually fused into one layer near the fundus of the hernial protrusion. When removing the redundant skin, care is necessary to avoid damage to the hernia contents which may be adherent over wide areas inside the sac (Fig. 21.4).

Exposure

The hernia is dissected from the surrounding subcutaneous fat by raising skin flaps (Fig. 21.5). The surgeon may choose to use the scalpel blade, scissors, electrocautery pencil and/or the ultrasonic dissection device for this dissection. The coverings of the hernia are stretched scar tissue merging into the stretched abdominal wall aponeurosis at the circumference of the protrusion and a variable amount of extraperitoneal fatty tissue.

The hernia sac is now dissected out completely following the contours carefully until the neck of the sac is reached circumferentially, which in a large hernia will require the elevation of large skin flaps (Fig. 21.6). These large areas of pannus should be removed later by horizontal panniculectomy (see later) to lessen the incidence of seroma formation collecting in loose folds of skin.

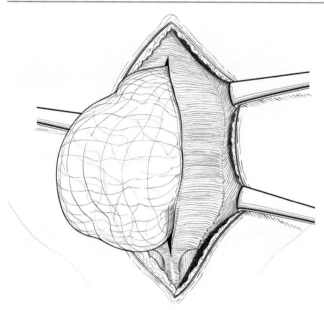

Fig. 21.6 Circumferential exposure of the neck of the sac is achieved

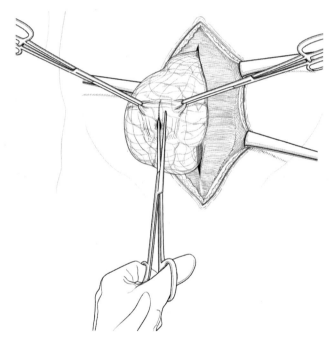

Fig. 21.7 The sac is opened at a point where it is judged that bowel is not adherent beneath it, usually at the fundus

Managing the Peritoneal Sac

The hernia sac is now opened carefully avoiding damage to the visceral contents of the sac, either at the fundus or by an elliptical incision around the hernia neck, where it merges with the stretched aponeurosis (Fig. 21.7).

It is recommended that the hernia sac is completely resected in all cases because intra-sac adhesions and sac compartmentalization can be a potent cause of intestinal obstruction if the sac is merely inverted and pushed into the

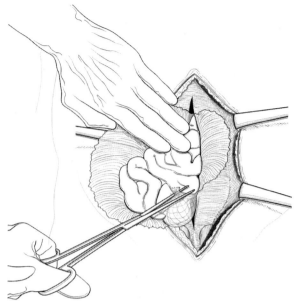

Fig. 21.8 Adhesions between the bowel and sac are divided, and bowel is returned to the peritoneal cavity

abdominal cavity. The advent of laparoscopic techniques for incisional hernia repair has revealed that at least one-third of hernia sacs contain visceral contents which are adherent to the sac itself. After opening the sac, adhesions of the contents are divided (Fig. 21.8), the viscera returned to the peritoneal cavity, and then the sac is completely excised to the edge of the rectus fascia on each side (Fig. 21.9). Since the peritoneal layer will not be sutured separately (it is too weak to retain sutures), complete excision of the sac allows the medial fascial edges of the rectus sheath to be seen clearly for accurate suture placement when closing the abdomen.

Contents of the Sac

The sac may contain almost any intraperitoneal viscus, but usually omentum, small bowel, and transverse colon are found.

Unless the hernia is strangulated and the small bowel nonviable, any adhesions are divided and the small bowel is returned to the abdominal cavity. Strangulated small bowel or omentum can be resected at this stage. The diagnostic decision is now made as to what should be done about very adherent and frequently partially ischemic omentum. If there is any doubt about omentum, it is best excised; to return omentum of doubtful viability to the peritoneal cavity invites the formation of adhesions.

Particular care must be taken in manipulating and dissecting any colon in the sac. Any densely adherent hernial sac should be trimmed and left adherent to the bowel and returned to the peritoneal sac rather than risk perforating the bowel in

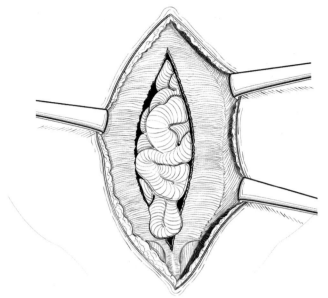

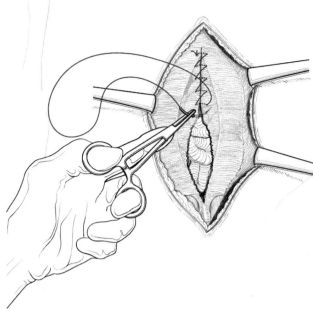

Fig. 21.9 Completion of excision of the sac, laying bare the medial margins (linea alba) of the rectus sheath in preparation for midline fascial closure

Fig. 21.10 Construction of a neo-linea alba by approximation of the medial edges of the rectus sheaths. This should be achieved with negligible tension utilizing a nonabsorbable or slowly absorbable continuous suture of 1 gauge suture material to achieve 4:1 suture length/wound length (<10 mm bites at <10 mm intervals). Suture bites do not include muscle

a tedious dissection. The greatest care must be taken to avoid puncturing the colon. If the colon is punctured, a minor injury could generally be closed with sutures. A substantial injury must be treated by creation of a colostomy, the re-anastomosis of the colon and repair of the hernia can be performed at a later operation after full patient evaluation and colon antibacterial preparation.

Closure of Aponeurotic Layer

For the onlay (prefascial, Chevrel) method fascial closure is achieved by placing a running suture of a strong nonabsorbable or slowly absorbable suture into the anterior rectus sheath (without taking a bite of the rectus muscle) taking bites of 5–10 mm, with a stitch interval of 5 mm, to achieve a suture length/wound length of 4:1 (Fig. 21.10). The author uses a nonabsorbable suture that is started at each end of the defect, and the two ends are tied together at the midpoint of the closure. The repair of large defects of the abdominal wall in this manner will result in a significant amount of tension on the fascia in the midline and also the risk of abdominal compartment syndrome. If this situation is likely to occur, a Ramirez "components separation" technique is recommended (see below), and surgeons operating on such large hernias should have this technique in their armamentarium.

For the sublay (retrorectus, Rives) method fascial closure of the posterior rectus sheath is achieved after bilateral, medial opening of the rectus fascia which exposes the medial edges of the rectus muscles and the bloodless plane behind the muscles (see later). After mesh placement, the anterior

rectus sheath is closed in a similar fashion to that described for the onlay method.

Panniculectomy if required is carried out after complete fascial closure at this stage. Depending upon local custom, the subcutaneous fat is either left unclosed or is closed in layers with absorbable sutures. The skin margins are now approximated. Skin closure must be effected without any tension. This may be accomplished with sutures and/or skin staples.

Postoperative Care

Immediate active mobilization is the key to rapid convalescence. In the absence of extensive handling of the intestines there is no postoperative adynamic ileus and no need for encumbrances such as nasogastric suction or intravenous drips. The patient is made to take deep breaths; breathing exercises and, where necessary, chest percussion are given. As soon as possible the patient gets up and walks. Fluids are given for the first day, and then a light diet is started. These patients may experience a significant amount of pain, which will require parenteral analgesia. If this can be controlled with oral analgesics and the patient does not experience a significant ileus, a minimal hospital stay can be expected. Generally, the length of stay will be 3–5 days depending upon the size of the hernia, the amount of dissection required, and the number of comorbid conditions of the patient.

The Choices of Technique in Open Prosthetic Repair

The choice is between the onlay (prefascial, Chevrel) technique and the sublay (retrorectus, Rives) technique. The use of unprotected intraperitoneal mesh in open surgery is not considered appropriate because it leads to adhesion formation between the mesh and bowel and the risk of fistulation. A survey in Sweden revealed that when using mesh for incisional hernia repair 54% of surgeons employed the onlay, prefascial technique and 44% the sublay, retrorectus technique. Recurrence rates did not differ significantly [82]. The onlay technique is technically simpler to perform, it is applicable to all quadrants of the abdominal wall, and there is no risk of contact between the bowel and mesh, which can occur with the sublay technique, particularly when the mesh is placed in the lower midline where a tear in the peritoneum below the arcuate line risks contact between mesh and bowel. Moreover, the posterior rectus sheath is frequently a thin and fragile layer, which tears easily when under minimal tension.

For very complex abdominal wall reconstruction techniques of tissue expansion, vacuum-assisted closure devices, abdominal component separation, local and distant muscle flaps, and free tissue transfer can be adopted [83]. However, for the general surgeon performing incisional hernia repair such advanced surgical techniques should only be attempted in collaboration with a plastic surgeon unless he or she is familiar with these techniques. In general small hernias below 10 cm in size are amenable to laparoscopic repair (see Chap. 16) although they are satisfactorily repaired by the open technique with the additional benefit of achieving cosmesis of the anterior abdominal wall skin. Hernias between 10 and 15 cm in size are best repaired by open techniques although advanced laparoscopic surgeons can achieve good results. Hernias over 15 cm in size usually require a Ramirez "component separation" of parts repair because of significant loss of domain [84].

A Cochrane database of systematic reviews in 2008 concerning open surgical procedures for incisional hernia included eligible studies if they were randomized controlled trials comparing different techniques for open incisional repair. Eight trials were identified of which one was excluded and 1,141 patients had been enrolled into the studies. Three trials concerned suture vs. mesh repair (onlay or sublay), which revealed that the recurrence and wound complications were more frequent after sutured repair. Two trials compared the onlay (prefascial) vs. the sublay (retrorectus) technique and found no difference in outcome except for a shorter operative time for the onlay method indicating its ease of use. Finally comparison between lightweight and standard mesh showed a trend for more recurrence in the lightweight group.

An onlay vs. intraperitoneal mesh trial showed no differences in outcomes except for increased pain in the intraperitoneal group [85]. The review concluded that open mesh was superior to suture techniques for recurrence and reduction in wound infection, but there was insufficient evidence as to which type of mesh or which mesh position (onlay or sublay) should be used. In addition the study also found insufficient evidence to advocate the use of components separation technique and clearly this requires further study. A quasi-randomized study allocating patients alternately to either a sublay or an onlay arm for meshplasty in ventral hernias, excluding patients with defects greater than 10 cm found a more favorable outcome for the onlay technique with complications recurring in 22.5% (sublay) vs. 15% (onlay) with similar wound complications [86]. Hospital stay was similar and there were no recurrences.

The Onlay (Prefascial, Chevrel) Technique for Open Prosthetic Repair

Chevrel popularized the onlay, prefascial technique more than 30 years ago [87]. Reporting 257 prosthetic repairs, Chevrel reported a morbidity of 10.5% including 6.3% seroma, two wound infection, and 4.9% recurrence and favoring the use of polypropylene mesh. In addition Chevrel advocated the use of fibrin glue and relaxing incisions in approximately half of his patients. Relaxing incisions were placed in the anterior rectus sheath, which was a favored technique prior to the introduction of the component separation, which places the relaxing incisions in the external oblique aponeurosis. Similar results have been reported in smaller series which advocate a significant overlap of mesh after the midline fascial closure and extensive suturing of the mesh to the anterior abdominal wall in order to prevent shifting, curling, or movement of the mesh allowing recurrence [88–90]. Recurrence rates in the series ranged from 3 to 16%, which is a satisfactory outcome for large incisional hernias.

Panniculectomy is an important adjunct to surgery of the anterior abdominal wall to allow removement of large flaps of skin, which are redundant, once the large underlying hernia sac has been removed and reduced [91]. Failure to remove a large pannus or skin flap can result in a troublesome chronic seroma requiring multiple aspirations or surgery if it forms a pseudocyst on the abdominal wall.

The onlay technique is the ideal operation to combine with components separation in patients with very large incisional hernias with loss of domain [92]. In a series of 116 large hernias treated in a 2-year period, 21 patients required component separation in order to achieve fascial closure avoiding abdominal compartment syndrome. Only 9.5% of patients experienced seroma and 1.7% deep wound infections with no requirement for mesh removal, and four patients

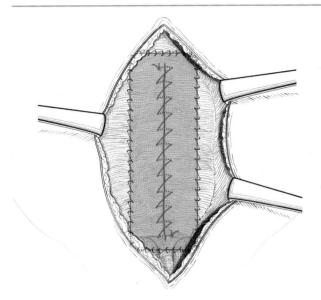

Fig. 21.11 The onlay (prefascial) technique. After construction of the neo-linea alba, a strip of prosthetic mesh 8–10 cm in width and 3–4 cm longer than the abdominal wall closure is placed and secured with a continuous peripheral suture of nonabsorbable suture material and a continuous suture to attach the mesh to the midline closure

experienced recurrent hernias. In a telephone follow-up at 2 years 82% of patients were pain-free, 9% had occasional pain, and 8% had pain limiting some daily activity indicating not only a good anatomical outcome but an excellent physiological outcome with return of function of the abdominal wall musculature.

The mesh should be approximately 10 cm in width in order to get a 5 cm either side of the midline fascial closure. If the midline fascial closure cannot be achieved without tension, then a components separation may be required. The mesh is secured with a continuous suture with nonabsorbable or slowly resorbable material around the periphery of the mesh with an additional reinforcing suture down the midline to fix it to the fascial closure (Fig. 21.11).

Incision and Dissection

An elliptical incision removing the previous scar is used. In order to perform the panniculectomy triangular wedges of skin and subcutaneous fat are removed at the lower end of the midline scar, which will eventually produce an inverted T-shaped incision which requires closure with care and accuracy. Beginning at the fundus of the sac, the entire sac is carefully dissected down to its neck in order to expose it completely without opening. At this stage the skin flap should only be minimally dissected in order to mobilize the sac and clearing an area of not more than 5 cm beyond the edge of the rectus muscle. The sac is now opened, and any adhesions between the bowel, peritoneum,

and the sac are divided and abdominal contents returned to the peritoneal cavity. In all cases the sac should now be completely excised.

In all cases the surgeon should be able to completely close the midline without tension. Where the width of the gap between the rectus muscles is relatively small, the anterior rectus sheath on each side may be closed with a strong running suture of nonabsorbable or slowly resorbable suture material. Prior to doing this the anterior rectus sheath is dissected from the subcutaneous fat for 5–7 cm to accommodate the onlay mesh. The mesh is now cut to size being a width of 10 cm and allowing for 3–4-cm overlap superiorly and inferiorly. If the polypropylene or polyester mesh is allowed to be in direct contact with intestine, there is a risk of adhesion formation and fistulation. There is also a risk of mesh erosion into the bowel with these types of meshes. In open prosthetic mesh repair there is no place for the use of newer meshes with incorporated anti-adhesive agents placed over the bowel as an inlay method without midline fascial closure. These dual meshes are specifically for use by laparoscopic surgeons when placed over a defect from inside the abdomen and in which contact with viscera is inevitable. There are no long-term studies to verify absence of complications seen many years after the insertion of such meshes. However, the use of such products has been longer than 15 years.

The Sublay (Retrorectus, Rives) Repair

The sublay repair places the mesh in the retromuscular space. Rives originally described this technique more than 30 years ago [93]. Placement of the prosthesis in the retromuscular plane requires opening of the rectus sheath near the linea alba to gain access to this space on both sides. After closure of the posterior rectus sheath the mesh is placed on top of this behind the rectus muscles, and conclusion of the abdominal wall closure is achieved by suture of the anterior rectus sheaths in the midline. Leaving a gap in the anterior or posterior rectus sheath achieves poor results and a high recurrence rate, and the relaxing incision in the external oblique of "components separation" should be applied in order to gain complete midline closure. The mesh overlap achieved is similar to the onlay technique with 5–6 cm in all directions and gives good results [94, 95]. This repair also gives good results in patients with large hernias with significant loss of domain [96].

Each rectus sheath is incised along its medial border and opened in the midline to expose the anterior and posterior aspects of the rectus muscle (Fig. 21.12). With blunt dissection the entire width of the muscle is exposed on its undersurface superficial to the posterior rectus sheath (Fig. 21.13). The posterior rectus sheath is now closed with a continuous

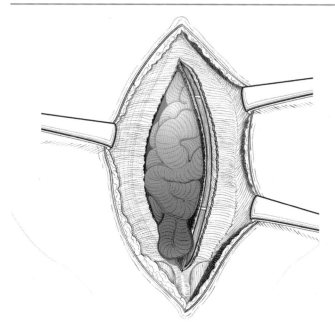

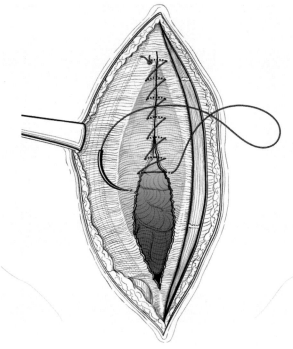

Fig. 21.12 The medial border of the rectus sheath is incised along the length of the fascial defect on both sides

Fig. 21.14 The posterior rectus sheath is closed with a nonabsorbable suture. This should be achieved with negligible tension

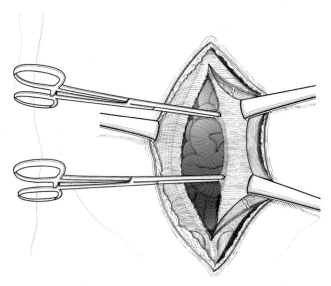

Fig. 21.13 The bloodless plane behind the rectus muscle and anterior to the posterior rectus sheath is dissected to the lateral limit of the rectus muscle

running suture of nonabsorbable or slowly resorbable material and the mesh placed in the posterior retrorectus position to occupy the width of the rectus muscles on both sides (Fig. 21.14). A prosthetic mesh approximately 10 cm in width and long enough to achieve a 3–4-cm overlap superiorly and inferiorly is now placed in the retrorectus space (Fig. 21.15). To prevent migration or movement of the mesh, a few absorbable sutures are placed between the mesh and the posterior rectus sheath or peritoneum. It may be advisable to place a suction drain in the retrorectus position prior

to closure of the anterior rectus sheath, which is achieved by a continuous suture of nonabsorbable or slowly absorbable monofilament material (Fig. 21.16).

Open Intraperitoneal Prosthetic Mesh Repair

This alternative technique has been popularized in one or two French centers [97, 98]. The initial steps of the operation are the same as for the onlay or sublay techniques with complete excision of the peritoneal sac to the medial edge of the rectus muscles. The mesh is placed intraperitoneally with 5–6-cm overlap and secured by nonabsorbable through-and-through sutures spaced 2 cm apart and 1 cm from the border of the mesh. The sutures transverse the entire width of the muscular fascial abdominal wall and also the subcutaneous layers, and each is tied through a small incision in the skin. Protagonists of this technique claim that the prosthesis acts as a substitute for the abdominal wall avoiding suture of the two opposite fascial edges of the defect with tension. The muscular aponeurotic edges are closed in the midline as much as possible to isolate the prosthesis from possible surgical skin contamination. The authors promoting this technique have not encountered problems with enterocutaneous fistula. If this method is used, the choice of a biologic mesh will require the preservation of the hernia sac to be used as a vascularized pedicle to allow for the proper resorption of the collagen product.

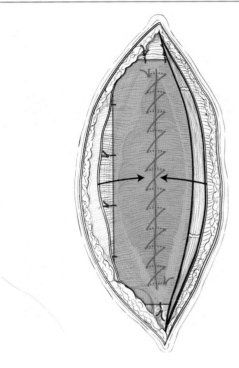

Fig. 21.15 Prosthetic mesh wide enough to cover the space behind the two rectus muscles (about 8–10 cm) and 3–4 cm longer than the midline closure is placed and secured with a few peripheral interrupted absorbable sutures

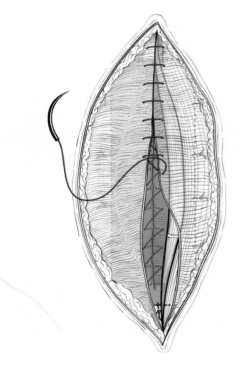

Fig. 21.16 The anterior rectus sheath is closed with a nonabsorbable or slowly absorbable continuous suture of 1 gauge suture material to achieve 4:1 suture length/wound length (<10 mm bites <10 mm intervals). Suture bites do not include muscle

Components Separation Method for Complete Closure of Abdominal Wall Defects

This major advance in abdominal wall hernia surgery was described by Ramirez in 1990 [99]. The essential element of this technique is a longitudinal incision in the external oblique aponeurosis 1 cm lateral to the rectus muscles in order to allow the muscle to move into the midline up to a distance of 10 cm on each side. Ramirez initially performed dissections on cadavers and subsequently in 11 patients to achieve his theoretical objective. An additional step in the technique is release of the posterior rectus sheath in order to obtain an extra 2–3 cm of midline movement of the rectus abdominis muscles. This technique requires significant undermining of the subcutaneous tissues into the midaxillary line to expose the aponeurosis of the external oblique. Such large skin flaps are prone to the development seroma, and it is important to perform an adequate panniculectomy (see above) to minimize this complication. Otherwise termed the sliding door technique, the prerequisite for this method is the presence of undamaged rectus muscles [100]. Not infrequently a patient with a previous stoma for transverse incision across the rectus muscle may have experienced sufficient damage, fibrosis, or postoperative infection to preclude component separation on one side of the abdomen. More recent descriptions of components separation have omitted the partition of the posterior rectus sheath but have reported high recurrence rates of over 30% [101]. The majority of these recurrences or abdominal wall defects occur through the weakened area in the external oblique aponeurosis. Therefore reinforcement of this area with a mesh prosthesis of either synthetic or biological material seems a logical extension to the component separation [80, 102]. Because of the extensive dissection of the anterior abdominal wall with this technique, wound-related complications are common with one-third of patients experiencing a minor wound dehiscence, hematoma, or infection. Additional minor procedures may also be required in 10–15% of patients [103]. The longer the delay in reconstruction, the more difficult the procedure becomes because of lateral migration of the rectus muscles, decreased compliance of the oblique muscles, suboptimal skin quality, the need for enterolysis, possible ostomy reversal, and poor pulmonary reserve. Therefore such procedures should be performed in units with significant expertise of abdominal wall reconstruction, components separation and the versatile use of prosthetic materials. Such a staged approach to the management of this problem has been confirmed in other centers with low morbidity and low technique-related mortality [104].

An important adjunct to management of these patients in the acute situation is vacuum pack-assisted temporary

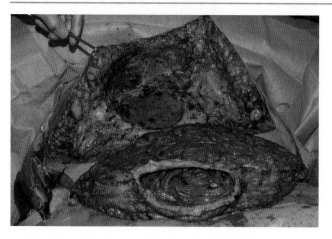

Fig. 21.17 Pseudocyst of the abdominal wall (chronic seroma)

abdominal wall closure [105]. This technique provides containment of the intra-abdominal viscera; protects them from mechanical injury, desiccation, and trauma whilst controlling egress of peritoneal fluid; and lends itself to multiple applications. When applied at the time of the formation of laparostomy, there is a higher rate of primary closure in up to 50% of patients leaving a smaller number for staged repair with its inevitable psychological impact. However, once reconstructed with complete fascial closure the mental health of these patients returns to that of the general population [106]. Over 80% of patients are then able to return to their pre-injury employment without long-term significant physical or mental health implications. It is therefore important to achieve a short time between the laparostomy and definitive abdominal wall closure.

Infected Incisional Hernia

An infected incisional hernia is a difficult problem to treat effectively. The options that are available will depend greatly if a fistula exists, prosthetic biomaterial has been used to repair the hernia, size of the fascial defect, and the amount of skin that can be used to cover the repair.

To achieve the best results previously implanted, mesh should be removed. A synthetic prosthetic should not be reintroduced into the infected area, and in this situation the use of biological mesh is recommended (see Chap. 7). Nevertheless complication rates after surgery remain high with a significant incidence of superficial wound infections, recurrence of enterocutaneous fistulas, abscess formation, and reoperation [107]. The surgeon should use all adjunctive techniques in his armamentarium including panniculectomy to avoid seroma formation, placement of suction drains, avoidance of ischemia of skin flaps, and a prolonged course of postoperative antibiotics.

Chronic Seroma (Pseudocyst of the Abdominal Wall)

Failure to adequately treat a chronic seroma will result in encapsulation of the tissue fluid by chronic granulomatous tissue and persistence of a spherical mass on the abdominal wall that is likely to be diagnosed as a recurrence of the hernia (Fig. 21.17). Pseudocysts can be treated simply by wide excision through a transverse incision and re-suture of the abdominal wall [108]. Small seromas will resolve spontaneously and only about a quarter will require aspiration on one or two occasions, and chronic seroma and pseudocyst formation is a rare event [109].

Results

Tissue repairs and suture repairs are not as successful as repairs that include the use of prosthesis. The recurrence rate is consistently improved by a factor of two or three by the use of synthetic prosthetic materials. In comparison with laparoscopic incisional hernia repair, open repair offers unique advantages, which include the ability to treat loss of domain with components separation, restoration of abdominal anatomy, and function. The simplest and most versatile technique is the onlay prefascial method [110].

Conclusions

- Specialists who have developed in interest and experience in incisional hernia repair have significantly better results than nonspecialists.
- Important predictors of recurrence are wound infection, obesity, and previous repairs.
- A choice of operative procedure is critical. Fascial closure is paramount, and mesh overlap does not need to exceed 5 cm.
- Mesh fixation should be comprehensive with a continuous peripheral suture for the onlay technique and interrupted sutures for the sublay method.
- Where there is a risk of abdominal compartment syndrome after closure of the midline fascial layer, a components separation is essential and simple.

References

1. Chan MK, Baillod RA, Tanner RA, et al. Abdominal hernias inpatients receiving continuous ambulatory peritoneal dialysis. Br Med J. 1981;283:826.
2. Engeset J, Youngson GG. Ambulatory peritoneal dialysis and hernial complications. Surg Clin North Am. 1984;64:385–92.

3. Fear RE. Laparoscopic: a valuable aid in gynecologic diagnosis. Obstet Gynecol. 1968;31:297–304.

4. Taylor GW, Jayne DG, Brown SR, Thorpe H, Brown JM, Dewberry SC, et al. Adhesions and incisional hernias following laparoscopic versus open surgery for colorectal cancer in the CLASICC trial. Br J Surg. 2010;97:70–8.

5. McDowell E. Quoted in Scharchner, A. Ephraim McDowell: Father of ovariotomy and father of abdominal surgery. Philadelphia: Lippincott; 1921.

6. Billroth T. Clinical surgery. Extracts from reports of surgical practice between the years 1860–1876. Translated from the original by C.T. Dent. London: New Sydenham Society; 1891.

7. Langenbuch. Quoted in Ponka (1980).

8. Iason AH. Hernia. Philadelphia: Blakiston; 1941.

9. Judd ES. The prevention and treatment of ventral hernia. Surg Gynecol Obstet. 1912;14:175–82.

10. Gibson CL. Operation for cure of large ventral hernia. Ann Surg. 1920;72:214–7.

11. Kirschner M. Die praktischen Ergebnisse der freien Fascien-Transplantation. Arch Klin Chir. 1910;92:889–912.

12. Gallie WE, Le Mesurier AB. The transplantation of the fibrous tissues in the repair of anatomical defects. Br J Surg. 1924;12: 289–320.

13. Rutledge RH. Theodor Billroth: a century later. Surgery. 1995;118: 36–43.

14. Leaper DJ, Pollock AV, Evans M. Abdominal wound closure: a trial of nylon, polyglycolic acid and steel sutures. Br J Surg. 1977; 64:603–6.

15. Hartley RC. Spontaneous rupture of incisional herniae. Br J Surg. 1962;49:617–8.

16. Senapati A. Spontaneous dehiscence of an incisional hernia. Br J Surg. 1982;69:313.

17. Ianora AA, Midiri M, Vinci R, Rotondo A, Angelelli G. Abdominal wall hernias: imaging with spiral CT. Eur Radiol. 2000;10:914–9.

18. Homans J. Three hundred and eighty-four laparotomies for various diseases. Boston: Nathan Sawyer; 1887.

19. Stanton E, Mac D. Post-operative ventral hernia. New York J Med. 1916;16:511–5.

20. Douglas DM, Forrester JC, Ogilvie RR. Physical characteristics of collagen in the later stages of wound healing. Br J Surg. 1969;56:219–22.

21. Akman PC. A study of 500 incisional hernias. J Int Coll Surg. 1962;37:125–42.

22. Bucknall TE, Cox PJ, Ellis H. Burst abdomen and incisional hernia: a prospective study of 1129 major laparotomies. Br Med J. 1982;284:931–3.

23. Ellis H, Gajraj H, George CD. Incisional hernias, when do they occur? Br J Surg. 1983;70:290–321.

24. Harding KG, Mudge M, Leinster SJ, Hughes LE. Late development of incisional hernia: an unrecognised problem. Br Med J. 1983;286:519–20.

25. Mudge M, Hughes LE. Incisional hernia: a ten year prospective study of incidence and attitudes. Br J Surg. 1985;72:70–1.

26. Mudge M, Harding KG, Hughes LE. Incisional hernia. Br J Surg. 1986;73:82.

27. Hodgson NCF, Malthaner RA, Ostbye T. The search for an ideal method of abdominal fascial closure: a meta-analysis. Ann Surg. 2000;231:436–42.

28. Maingot R. A further report on the 'keel' operation for large diffuse incisional hernias. Med Press. 1958;240:989–93.

29. Tagart REB. The suturing of abdominal incisions. A comparison of monofilament nylon and catgut. Br J Surg. 1967;54:952–7.

30. Ponka JL. Hernias of the abdominal wall. Philadelphia: WB Saunders; 1980.

31. Hurst JW. Measuring the benefits and costs of medical care—the contribution of health status measurement. Health Trends. 1984;16:16–9.

32. Manninen MJ, Lavonius M, Perhoniemi VJ. Results of incisional hernia repair. A retrospective study of 172 unselected hernioplasties. Eur J Surg. 1991;157:29–31.

33. Hesselink VJ, Luijendijk RW, de Wilt JHW, Heide R, Jeekel J. An evaluation of risk factors in incisional hernia recurrence. Surg Gynecol Obstet. 1993;176:228–34.

34. Rios A, Rodriguez JM, Munitz V, Alcaraz P, Perez D, Parrilla P. Factors that affect recurrence after incisional herniorrhaphy with prosthetic material. Eur J Surg. 2001;167:855–9.

35. DuBay DA, Choi W, Urbanchek MG, Wang X, Adamson B, Dennis RG, et al. Incisional herniation induces decreased abdominal wall compliance via oblique muscle atrophy and fibrosis. Ann Surg. 2007;245:140–6.

36. Mudge M, Hughes LE. Incisional hernia and post-thrombotic syndrome—an observed association. Ann R Coll Surg Engl. 1984;66:351–2.

37. Ausobsky JR, Evans M, Pollock AV. Does mass closure of midline laparotomies stand the test of time? A random controlled clinical trial. Ann R Coll Surg Engl. 1985;67:159–61.

38. Kirk RM. The incidence of burst abdomen: comparison of layered opening and closing with straight through one layered closure. Proc R Soc Med. 1973;66:1092.

39. LeBlanc KA, Booth WV, Whitaker JA, Bellanger DE. Laparoscopic incisional and ventral herniorrhaphy: our initial 100 patients. Am J Surg. 2000;180:193–7.

40. Goligher JC, Irvin TT, Johnston D, De Dombal FT, Hill GL, Horrocks JC. A controlled clinical trial of three methods of closure of laparotomy wounds. Br J Surg. 1975;62:823–7.

41. Gilbert AI. Inguinal hernia repair: biomaterials and sutureless repair. Perspect Gen Surg. 1991;2:113–9.

42. Davidson BR, Bailey JS. Incisional herniae following median sternotomy incisions—their incidence and aetiology. Br J Surg. 1986;73:995–7.

43. Knapp RW, Mullen JT. Clinical evaluation of the use of local anaesthesia for the repair of inguinal hernia. Am Surg. 1976; 42:908–10.

44. Bristol JB, Bolton RA. The results of Ramstedt's operation in a district general hospital. Br J Surg. 1981;68:590–2.

45. Kiely EM, Spitz L. Layered versus mass closure of abdominal wounds in infants and children. Br J Surg. 1985;72:739–40.

46. Luijendijk RW, Hop WCJ, van den Tol P, et al. A comparison of suture repair with mesh repair for incisional hernia. N Engl J Med. 2000;343(6):393–8.

47. Jenkins TPN. Incisional hernia repair: a mechanical approach. Br J Surg. 1980;67:335–6.

48. Israelsson LA. The surgeon as a risk factor for complications of midline incisions. Eur J Surg. 1998;164:353–9.

49. Santora TA, Roslyn JJ. Incisional hernia. Surg Clin North Am. 1993;73:557–70.

50. Rios A, Rodriguez JM, Munitz V, Alcaraz P, Perez FD, Parrilla P. Antibiotic prophylaxis in incisional hernia repair using a prosthesis. Hernia. 2001;5:148–52.

51. Bellows CF, Alder A, Helton WS. Abdominal wall reconstruction using biological tissue grafts: present status and future opportunities. Expert Rev Med Devices. 2006;3:657–75.

52. Grevious MA, Cohen M, Jean-Pierre F, Herrmann GE. The use of prosthetics in abdominal wall reconstruction. Clin Plast Surg. 2006;33:181–97.

53. Van't Riet M, Steyerberg EW, Nellensteyn J, Bonjer HJ, Jeekel J. Meta-analysis of techniques for closure of midline abdominal incisions. Br J Surg. 2002;89:1350–6.

54. Rucinski J, Magolis M, Panagopoulos G, Wise L. Closure of the abdominal midline fascia: meta-analysis delineates the optimal technique. Am Surg. 2001;67:421–6.

55. Harlaar JJ, van Ramshorst GH, Niewenhuizen J, ten Brinke JG, Hop WCJ, Kleinrensink G-J, et al. Small stitches with small suture

distances increase laparotomy closure strength. Am J Surg. 2009;198:392–5.

56. Millbourn D, Cengiz Y, Israelsson LA. Effect of stitch length on wound complications after closure of midline incisions: a randomized controlled trial. Arch Surg. 2009;144:1056–9.

57. Askar O. A new concept of the aetiology and surgical repair of para-umbilical and epigastric hernias. Ann R Coll Surg Engl. 1978;60:42–8.

58. Spencer Netto FAC, Hamilton P, Rizoli SB, Nascimento B, Brenneman FD, Tien H, et al. Traumatic abdominal wall hernia: epidemiology and clinical implications. J Trauma. 2006;61:158–61.

59. Crandall M, Popowich D, Shapiro M, West M. Post traumatic hernias: historical overview and review of the literature. Am Surg. 2009;73:845–50.

60. Dennis RW, Marshall A, Deshmukh H, Bender JS, Kulvatunyou N, Lees JS, et al. Abdominal wall injuries occurring after blunt trauma: incidence and grading. Am J Surg. 2009;197:413–7.

61. Moreno IG. Chronic eventuation and large hernias. Surgery. 1947;22:945–53.

62. Hamer DB, Duthie HL. Pneumoperitoneum in the management of abdominal incisional hernia. Br J Surg. 1972;59:372–5.

63. Forrest J. Repair of massive inguinal hernia with pneumoperitoneum and without mesh replacement. Arch Surg. 1979;114:1087–8.

64. Ravitch MM. Ventral hernia. Surg Clin North Am. 1971; 51: 1341–6.

65. Astudillo R, Merrell R, Sanchez J, Olmedo S. Ventral herniorrhaphy aided by pneumoperitoneum. Arch Surg. 1986;121: 935–6.

66. Caldironi MW, Romano M, Bozza F, Pluchinotta AM, Pelizzo MR, Toniato A, et al. Progressive pneumoperitoneum in the management of giant incisional hernias: a study of 41 patients. Br J Surg. 1990;77:306–8.

67. Van Geffen HJAA, Simmermacher RKJ. Incisional hernia repair: abdominoplasty, tissue expansion, and methods of augmentation. World J Surg. 2005;29:1080–5.

68. Mayagoitia JC, Suarez D, Arenas JC, Diazdeleon V. Preoperative progressive pneumoperitoneum in patients with abdominal-wall hernias. Hernia. 2006;10:213–7.

69. Barst HH. Pneumoperitoneum as an aid in the surgical treatment of giant hernia. Br J Surg. 1972;59:360–4.

70. Shouldice EE. The treatment of hernia. Ont Med Rev. 1953;1–14.

71. Paul A, Korenkov M, Peters S, Kohler L, Fischer S, Troidl H. Unacceptable results of the May procedure for repair of abdominal incisional hernias. Eur J Surg. 1998;164:361–7.

72. Burger JWA, Luijendijk RW, Hop WCJ, Halm JA, Verdaasdonk EGG, Jeekel J. Long-term follow-up of a randomized controlled trial of suture versus mesh repair of incisional hernia. Ann Surg. 2004;240:578–85.

73. Langer C, Schaper A, Liersch T, Kulle B, Flosman M, Fuzesi L, et al. Prognosis factors in incisional hernia surgery: 25 years of experience. Hernia. 2005;9:16–21.

74. Coda A, Bendavid R, Botto-Micca F, Bossotti M, Bona A. Structural alterations of prosthetic meshes in humans. Hernia. 2003;7:29–34.

75. Klinge U, Klosterhalfen B, Muller M, Ottinger AP, Schumpelick V. Shrinking of polypropylene mesh in vivo: an experimental study in dogs. Eur J Surg. 1998;164:965–9.

76. Garcia-Urena MA, Ruiz VV, Godoy AD, Perca JMB, Gomez LMM, Hernandez FJC, et al. Differences in polypropylene shrinkage depending on mesh positions in an experimental study. Am J Surg. 2007;193:538–42.

77. Vega-Ruiz V, Garcia-urena MA, Diaz-Godog A, Carnero FJ, Moriano AE, Garcia MV. Surveillance of shrinkage of polypropylene mesh used in repair of ventral hernias. Ciru Esp. 2006; 80:38–42.

78. Amid PK. Classification of biomaterials and their related complications in abdominal wall hernia surgery. Hernia. 1997;1:15–21.

79. Conze J, Kingsnorth AN, Flament J-B. Randomized clinical trial comparing lightweight composite mesh with polyester or polypropylene mesh for incisional hernia repair. Br J Surg. 2005;92: 1488–93.

80. Kingsnorth A. The management of incisional hernia. Ann R Coll Surg Engl. 2006;88:252–60.

81. Korenkov M, Paul A, Sauerland S. Classification and surgical treatment of incisional hernia. Results of an experts meeting. Langenbecks Arch Surg. 2001;368:65–73.

82. Israelsson LA, Smedberg S, Montgomery A, Nordin P, Spangen L. Incisional hernia repair in Sweden 2002. Hernia. 2006;10:258–61.

83. Rohrich RJ, Lowe JB, Hockney FL, Bowman JL, Hobar PC. An algorithm for abdominal wall reconstruction. Plast Reconstr Surg. 2000;105:202–16.

84. Dumanian GA, Denham W. Comparison of repair techniques for major incisional hernias. Am J Surg. 2003;185:61–5.

85. Den Hartog D, Dur AHM, Tuinebreijer WE, Kreis RW. Open surgical procedures for incisional hernias. Cochrane Database Syst Rev. 2008(3):CD006438.

86. Godara R, Pardeep G, Raj H, Singla SL. Comparative evaluation of "sublay" versus "onlay" meshplasty in ventral hernias. Indian J Gastroenterol. 2006;25:222–3.

87. Chevrel JP, Rath AM. Polyester mesh for incisional hernia repair. In: Schumpelick V, Kingsnorth AN, editors. Incisional hernia (Chap 29). New York: Springer; 2000. p. 327–33.

88. San Pio JR, Dormsgaard TE, Momgen O, Villadsen I, Larsen J. Repair of giant incisional hernias with polypropylene mesh: a retrospective study. Scand J Plast Reconstr Surg Hand Surg. 2003;37:102–6.

89. Licheri S, Erdas E, Pisano G, Garau A, Ghinami E, Pomata M. Chevrel technique for midline incisional hernia: still an effective procedure. Hernia. 2008;12:121–6.

90. Andersen LPH, Klein M, Gogenur I, Rosenberg J. Long-term recurrence and complication rates after incisional hernia repair with the open onlay technique. BMC Surg. 2009;9:6–10.

91. Downey SE, Morales C, Kelso RL, Anthone G. Review of technique for combined closed incisional hernia repair and panniculectomy status post-open bariatric surgery. Surg Obes Relat Dis. 2005;1:458–4561.

92. Kingsnorth AN, Shahid MK, Valliattu AJ, Hadden RA, Porter CS. Open onlay mesh repair for major abdominal wall hernias with selective us of components separation and fibrin sealant. World J Surg. 2008;32:26–30.

93. Rives J, Lardennois B, Pire JC, Hibon J. Les grandes eventrations: importance due "volet abdominal" et des troubles respiratories qui lui sont secondaires. Chirurgie. 1973;99:547–63.

94. Schumpelick V, Klinge U, Junge K, Stumpf M. Incisional abdominal hernia: the open mesh repair. Langenbecks Arch Surg. 2004;389:313–7.

95. Klinge U, Conze J, Krones CJ, Schumpelick V. Incisional hernia: open techniques. World J Surg. 2005;29:1066–72.

96. Kingsnorth AN, Sivarajasingham N, Wong S, Butler M. Open mesh repair of incisional hernias with significant loss of domain. Ann R Coll Surg Engl. 2004;86:363–6.

97. Hamy A, Pessaux P, Mucci-Hennekinne S, Radriamananjo S, Regenet N, Arnaud JP. Surgical treatment of large incisional hernias by an intraperitoneal Dacron mesh and an aponeurotic graft. J Am Coll Surg. 2003;196:531–4.

98. Bernard C, Polliand C, Mutelica L, Champault G. Repair of giant incisional abdominal wall hernias using open intraperitoneal mesh. Hernia. 2007;11:315–20.

99. Ramirez OM, Ruas E, Dellon AL. "Component separation" method for closure of abdominal-wall defects: an anatomic and clinical study. Plast Reconstr Surg. 1990;86:519–26.

100. Kuzbari R, Worseg AP, Tairych G, Deutinger M, Kuderna C, Metz V, et al. Sliding door technique for the repair of midline incisional hernias. Plast Reconstr Surg. 1998;101:1235–44.

101. De Vries Reilingh TS, Van Goer H, Rosman C, Bemelmans MHA, De Jong D, Van Nieuwenhoben EJ, et al. "Components separation technique" for the repair of large abdominal wall hernias. J Am Coll Surg. 2003;196:32–7.
102. Nasajpour H, LeBlanc KA, Steele MH. Complex hernia repair using component separation technique paired with intraperitoneal acellular porcine dermis and synthetic mesh overlay. Ann Plast Surg. 2011;66:280–4.
103. Shabatian H, Lee D-J, Abbas MA. Components separation: a solution to complex abdominal wall defects. Am Surg. 2008;74:912–6.
104. Jernigan TW, Fabian TC, Croce MA, Moore N, Pritchard FE, Minard G, et al. Staged management of giant abdominal wall defects: acute and long-term results. Ann Surg. 2003;238:349–57.
105. Barker DE, Kaufman HJ, Smith LA, Ciraulo DL, Richart CL, Burns RP. Vacuum pack technique of temporary abdominal closure: a 7-year experience with 112 patients. J Trauma. 2000;48:201–7.
106. Cheatham ML, Safcsak K, Llerena LE, Morrow CE, Block EFJ. Long-term physical, mental, and functional consequences of abdominal decompression. J Trauma. 2004;56:237–42.
107. Van Geffen HJAA, Simmermacher RKJ, Van Vroonhoven TJMV, Van der Werken C. Surgical treatment of large contaminated abdominal wall defects. J Am Coll Surg. 2005;201: 206–12.
108. Gaybor S-T, Tamas H, Csaba V, Tibor O. Late complication after mesh repair of incisional hernias: pseudocyst formation. Magy Seb. 2007;60:293–6.
109. Kaafarani HMA, Hur K, Hirter A, Kim LT, Thomas A, Berger DH, et al. Seroma in ventral incisional herniorrhaphy: incidence, predictors and outcome. Am J Surg. 2009;198:639–44.
110. Kingsnorth AN, Banerjea A, Bhargava A. Incisional hernia repair—laparoscopic or open surgery? Ann R Coll Surg Engl. 2009;91:631–6.

Laparoscopic Incisional and Ventral Hernia Repair

Patrice R. Carter and Karl A. LeBlanc

Introduction

Approximately 200,000 ventral hernias are repaired in the US yearly [1]. This common problem has been approached in a myriad of ways, each with various technical aspects that contribute to the long term success or failure of the repair. Laparoscopic Incisional Ventral and Hernia repair (LIVH) as first described by LeBlanc in 1993 [2], builds upon the strengths of various techniques that improve overall outcome. The significant mesh overlap in the rectro-rectus repair with transfascial fixation first described by Rives and Stoppa [3, 4] is technically similar to what is achieved in LIVH Repair.

Though some still commonly perform primary suture repair of ventral hernias, it has been shown to have a recurrence rate of 54–63% [5, 6]. When primary suture repair was compared to open mesh repair, open mesh repair was found to have a recurrence rate of 32% [6]. Though some advocate the recurrence rate to be equivalent between open mesh repair and LIVH [5, 7], multiple other studies show LIVH to be superior in the rate of hernia relapse [8, 9]. Three prospective trials comparing laparoscopic ventral hernia repair to open mesh repair show the recurrence rate for LIVH to be 2–3.3% in comparison to open mesh repair which is reported to be 1.1–10% in these studies [7, 9, 10]. LIVH has been shown to be superior to open mesh repair in postoperative wound complications, hospital length of stay, and identification of multiple defects [7–12].

The repair of incisional and ventral hernias by the laparoscopic approach should be performed by high-volume laparoscopic surgeons. The surgeon should be adept at performing the more common laparoscopic operations and also be comfortable to perform the more complex laparoscopic procedures. The assistance of another surgeon during this operation is felt to be of great benefit, if not mandatory, on most occasions. This chapter will present the concepts, technical aspects, and results of the LIVH as it is currently performed. There are variations of the technique that are presented within this chapter, as is common to every surgical procedure. This methodology is continuing to evolve and undoubtedly will be modified as newer prosthetic biomaterials and instrumentation are developed in the future. One such advancement is the laparoscopic approach to component separation. Multiple studies have shown that myofascial advancement can be achieved with minimal flap dissection and improved wound outcome [13, 14].

Preoperative Evaluation

In general, if a patient is a medically appropriate candidate for open hernioplasty, then he or she could be considered a candidate for the laparoscopic approach. Patients that have significant cardiac decompensation may experience physiological abnormalities during the procedure because of the insufflation, and resulting decrease in the venous return. Lower insufflation pressures may decrease the hemodynamic fluctuations [15].

Generally almost all hernias are candidates for the LIVH. Even the smaller hernias in obese individuals could be repaired with this technique. Recurrence rates have been shown to be higher in obese patients [16–18]. Yet the benefits of less wound complications and the ability to identify the occult defects that are missed during an open approach make LIVH a viable option for obese patients. One may opt to use the open approach in a thin patient if it is apparent that the defect is 3 cm or less [16].

A very large fascial defect that nearly encompasses the entire anterior abdominal wall may pose a difficult problem. A laparoscopic approach, however, may be feasible. The decision to attempt the laparoscopic method should be based upon the experience of the surgeon, the number of prior operative

P.R. Carter
Department of Surgery, Adventist LaGrange Hospital,
LaGrange, IL, USA

K.A. LeBlanc (✉)
Surgeons Group of Baton Rouge/Our Lady of the Lake Physician
Group, Baton Rouge, LA, USA
e-mail: Karl.LeBlanc@ololrmc.com

A.N. Kingsnorth and K.A. LeBlanc (eds.), *Management of Abdominal Hernias*,
DOI 10.1007/978-1-84882-877-3_22, © Springer Science+Business Media London 2013

procedures, mesh repairs, the type of prosthetic utilized in any previous repair(s), and the location of the potential sites. However, there are currently no "hard and fast" rules about this issue. In those patients with very large defects, a reasonable option would be to commence the operation laparoscopically and convert to an open repair if that appears to be the best alternative. More often than not, this proves to be unnecessary. A probable exception to this sequence is those individuals that exhibit a "loss of domain" of the abdominal contents. In these patients it is usually impossible to actually enter the abdomen behind the abdominal wall musculature because this musculature has been displaced laterally. In these cases, conversion to the open method would occur earlier rather than later. More commonly, however, prudence dictates that the entire procedure should be of the open type rather than even attempting the laparoscopic approach.

Absolute contraindications to the use of the laparoscopic method would be the presence of an acute surgical abdomen. A relative contraindication is intra-abdominal infection from any source. The use of a prosthetic biomaterial in the site of an overt infection may preclude the use of such a product. However, primary closure of the hernia defect with the assistance of a laparoscopic suture passer and biologic mesh, [19] may have a role in such instances though an open repair may be indicated for gross contamination. Similarly, while the presence of incarcerated bowel does not prevent the performance of the procedure, strangulation of the bowel necessitates an open hernioplasty.

Because the most common incision of the abdomen is placed in the midline, most incisional hernias occur in the midline. When a surgeon begins to perform laparoscopic incisional hernioplasty, it is recommended that he or she should repair midline defects initially to gain confidence in use of the laparoscopic technique. Once this is accomplished, the presence of a non-midline defect or multiple defects that are not adjacent to each other should not preclude the use of laparoscopy. Appropriate positioning of the patient and accurate placement of the trocars will permit an approach to the entire abdominal cavity in most cases.

Previous intra-abdominal surgery is a major consideration in the evaluation of a patient for the laparoscopic procedure. The number and type of earlier operations will influence the choice of patient position, the method of abdominal entry, trocar placement, and the position of the monitors. This preoperative assessment will allow the surgeon to plan the operative procedure and the operative suite based upon these findings. Any previous open laparotomies will, of course, be associated with more potential for adhesion formation than procedures that were performed laparoscopically. Additionally, in those patients in whom a previous incisional hernia repair included the implantation of any "unprotected" polypropylene prosthesis (see Open Ventral hernia chapter) can be expected to have dense scarring in all areas in which the material was exposed to the intra-abdominal contents. This should not deter experienced surgeons from attempting a laparoscopic approach because as many as one-third of these patients will not have any adhesions at all. It is important to note, however, that the difficulty of the procedure can be greatly magnified because of the dissection of the tenacious scarring that is encountered involving the prosthesis and the bowel and/or omentum. The risk of enterotomy is significantly increased in such instances.

Patients in whom there is an additional need for a surgical procedure such as a cholecystectomy, fundoplication of the stomach, inguinal herniorrhaphy or biopsy of an intra-abdominal or retroperitoneal structure are special subsets that deserve careful consideration. Hernia repairs in such cases are discussed later in this chapter.

Laparoscopic incisional herniaplasty should be individualized in patients with known ascites because it may be challenging to maintain a watertight closure that averts ascitic leaks. Moreover, these patients usually have a metabolic problem (e.g., chronic renal failure or hepatic disease) that can cause poor healing and predispose them to development of a hernia at the trocar sites. The use of the 5-mm. trocars, however, has made this less problematic and these patients may also be considered on occasion. Special trocars that do not cut into the abdominal muscle but dilate the tissues to enter though the wall of the abdomen should be used in these patients. The site of entry will be smaller than the actual trocar itself after it is removed thereby further minimizing the risk of leakage of ascitic fluid or subsequent herniation. Though the use of a prosthesis in patients with overt ascites is scarcely reported, some have achieved success with the LIVH in these patients with maximal optimization of ascites [20].

LIVH patients are admitted to the day-surgery unit of the hospital because they can usually be considered for discharge on the day of surgery. The number and type of comorbid conditions of the patient, the type and location of the hernia(s), the presence of incarceration and the amount of adhesiolysis required will influence the decision of timing of discharge from the hospital. Many patients now undergo laparoscopic incisional hernia repair in an ambulatory surgery center. Appropriate laboratory testing should be obtained prior to entry on the day of surgery. Patients are routinely given a preoperative dose of either a first generation cephalosporin or a fluoroquinolone. If a patient has a history of methicillin resistant staph aureus (MRSA), Vancomycin is used for preoperative prophylaxis.

Intraoperative Considerations

Patient Preparation and Positioning

LIVH repair requires the use of general anesthesia to achieve the necessary degree of relaxation and sedation. In most cases, it is not necessary to use an orogastric or nasogastric tube unless the site of entry is in the vicinity of the stomach. A urinary drainage catheter is not used if the procedure is felt to be short in length. If the operative site is close to the bladder (e.g., very low midline hernias or concomitant inguinal hernia repairs) or if the procedure will be prolonged it is then advisable to insert a urinary drainage catheter; preferably a three way catheter is used to fill the bladder for identification, if needed. Insertion of a nasogastric tube for procedures in which extensive dissection of the bowel is necessary may help to reduce the postoperative ileus that is likely to develop. It is seldom necessary to leave this tube beyond the intraoperative phase of the procedure, however.

Most patients will be placed in the supine position. Operations upon lateral defects of the abdominal wall, such as those in a subcostal or flank incision, will be facilitated by use of a semidecubitus or full decubitus position. The use of a "bean-bag" in these instances will greatly aid in the positioning of the patient. The additional use of the tilt capabilities of the operating table will assist in the manipulation of the bowel during dissection. Steep Trendelenberg or reverse Trendelenberg positions will cause the abdominal contents to move into positions that will make visualization of the contents of both the hernia and the abdomen easier. The patient's arms should be tucked in close to the body to allow sufficient room to move around the patient; this is especially important if the defect is in the lower abdomen. Occasionally this may not be feasible due to the size of the individual but, in general, it is preferred when possible. Use of a protective transparent adhesive drape is recommended.

Abdominal Entry

It is understood that the method of access into the abdomen should always be the safest approach possible. Many surgeons use the open type of Hassan entry because it is familiar to them. An open entry such as this could result in a poor seal around the trocar, which makes maintenance of insufflation pressures difficult resulting in inadequate visualization throughout the procedure. This method also requires the use of a larger trocar thereby posing a risk of herniation at that site in the future despite the best attempts at fascial closure.

In the patient with a primary ventral hernia or a single small defect, a Veress needle could be considered for insufflation before introduction of the first trocar. A "safe" area for needle insertion is usually in the right upper quadrant because it is generally free of adhesions of bowel and omentum. A site in the upper midline could also be used if it can be placed far enough away from the hernia so as not to interfere with the repair of the hernia.

Another method to gain access into the abdominal cavity uses an "optical" trocar for abdominal entry. These non-

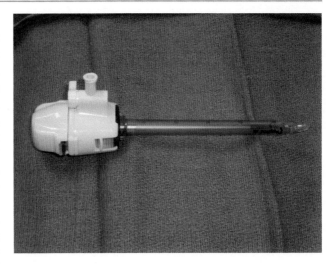

Fig. 22.1 A typical optical trocar with a clear non-cutting tip

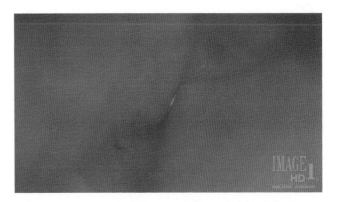

Fig. 22.2 View of subcutaneous layer through an optical trocar

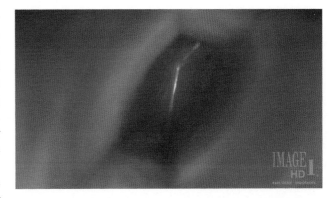

Fig. 22.3 Muscular layers seen as the optical trocar is passed into abdomen

bladed trocars are designed to provide visualization of each layer of the abdominal wall as the trocar passes through them. This is accomplished because the laparoscope is inserted into the trocar and these structures are seen as the trocar is passed. This is gaining in popularity (Figs. 22.1, 22.2, and 22.3).

In the majority of patients with an incisional hernia the view of the abdomen is, at least partially, obscured by adhesions. To enhance visualization and to free up enough space for placement of additional trocars, blunt dissection of these adhesions is necessary. The primary goal after the insertion of each of the additional trocars will be placement of the final number of necessary trocars. After the insertion of each additional trocar, the laparoscope should be placed through it to inspect the abdomen. The new view that is afforded from that vantage point will identify the optimal location of the sites of the other trocars. Additionally, the collections of these different views are important to identify any bowel that may be at risk during adhesiolysis. This is extremely important because, in some cases, neither the surgeon nor the assistant will appreciate the proximity of the bowel from only the view that is available from an individual trocar position.

When determining the best locations for the trocar positions, the selection should avoid the problem of "mirror imaging" during the manipulation of the instruments from the side in direct opposition to the viewing laparoscope. This produces an image of any manipulation that is viewed from that port that is opposite the action taken. That is, a move of the laparoscopic instrument to the left will be seen as a move to the right and vice versa. Placement of the camera in the midline of the abdomen will avoid this problem (Figs. 22.4 and 22.5). An alternative is the insertion of an additional trocar on the ipsilateral side of the location of the camera. With practice many surgeons can overcome this technical problem without the use of additional trocars. Most of this difficulty can be eliminated if the assistant surgeon can use the instruments from his or her side of the patient. One should not hesitate to insert additional trocars when this problem cannot be corrected easily to ensure the safety of the operation.

Instruments

The choice of laparoscope (0, 30, or 45°) used for incisional hernia repair depends upon the familiarity of the operating team with the instruments, the planned position of the trocars, and the habitus of the patient. While the 0° laparoscope is the primary choice of one of the authors (KAL), the majority of surgeons utilize the 30° laparoscope because it will allow good visualization of the undersurface of the abdominal wall. Additionally, one may view to the left and right of the operative field without changing the location of the optics. This is particularly beneficial in thin patients with good muscle tone. The 45° laparoscope is seldom necessary for this operation. If the optics of the camera and system are optimal, the 5-mm laparoscopes will perform as well as do the 10-mm ones. A benefit of the smaller scopes is that they

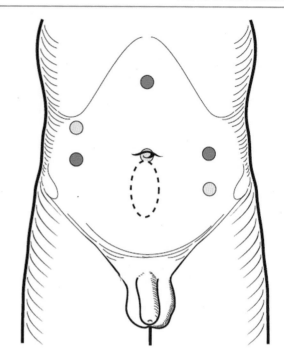

Fig. 22.4 Typical trocar positions for a lower midline hernia. The dark circles represent the location of the initial trocars. The upper midline trocar will accommodate the laparoscope. The other circles represent the location of additional trocars if these are needed to complete the procedure

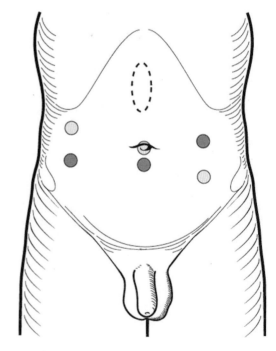

Fig. 22.5 Typical trocar positions for an upper midline hernia. The representations of the trocar sites mimic that of Fig. 22.4

utilize smaller trocars, which diminishes postoperative pain and minimizes the risk of herniation at the site of the trocar. The newer flexible tip laparoscopes are not necessary for these procedures and make their use difficult due to the distance that they must be placed to allow for the flexion of the device.

The most significant and potentially fatal complication of laparoscopic incisional herniorrhaphy is an injury to the bowel. This will occur during the dissection of the adhesions that are frequently encountered. The method of dissection is critically important in order to minimize the risk of injury to the intestine. If the adhesions encountered are few and rather filmy, one may use the scissors with the additional application of electrocautery. This should only be done if there is absolute certainty that there is no bowel adjacent to the area that will be affected by the lateral extension of the electrocautery burn. The transection of the falciform ligament is an example of this situation. In most patients dissection of omentum and/or bowel from the abdominal wall will be required. Multiple devices that limit the lateral spread of heat are available. These ultrasonic dissection devices include the Harmonic® scalpel (Ethicon Endosurgery®, Inc, Cincinnati, Ohio); the EnSeal® (Ethicon Endosurgery®, Inc, Cincinnati, Ohio) or the Ultrashears® (Covidien, Dublin, Ireland). Though these devices may be used for adhesiolysis, this should not allow the surgeon to become complacent in the use of an energy source within the abdominal cavity. The use of any type of an energy source can result in an injury to the intestine if used improperly. It is recommended that if the intestine is densely adherent to the abdominal wall or to polypropylene biomaterial from a prior failed repair, the use of scissors without cautery should be preferred. It is sometimes felt that the open procedure has less risk of intestinal injury compared to the laparoscopic approach because of the dissection of the intestine. A recent meta-analysis does not show this to be true [21]. The risk of bowel injury is generally 1.78% and cannot be absolutely avoided. One needs to ensure that the dissection proceeds in as safe a manner as surgically feasible.

Not uncommonly, the hernia contents are known to be incarcerated preoperatively and cannot be reduced with dissection and traction. In such cases, the fascial defect must be enlarged to allow reduction of the involved organs. Electrocautery scissors are used if the fascia is thick. Sometimes the ultrasonic dissector will be sufficient to cut the tissue but this is infrequent. Generally, a two or three centimeter incision into the fascia will suffice. The size of this incision is not that important because the resulting defect size will be covered by the prosthesis.

Prosthetic Biomaterials

There are currently many different products that are available for the repair of incisional hernias. The unprotected polypropylene and polyester biomaterials are prone to adhesion formation and pose a significant risk of fistulization.

Most surgeons will choose a biomaterial that has been manufactured with some method to shield the intestine from coming into direct contact with the polypropylene or polyester material. There are expanded polytetrafluoroethylene products or composites of these materials available as well. These products are described in detail in Chapter Seven.

Adhesiolysis and Identification of the Fascial Defect(s)

Before insertion of the prosthesis, the entire fascial defect(s) must be uncovered (Fig. 22.6). This usually requires removal of all the adhesions (Fig. 22.7) within the abdomen especially those attached to the anterior wall. It is best to dissect all of the adhesions that may potentially interfere with the appropriate positioning of the prosthetic material. It is also important to ensure that the parietal surface of any prosthetic material is in direct contact with the fascia and not with adipose tissue or omentum. Any fatty tissue that is interposed between the abdominal fascia and the prosthesis will inhibit the appropriate in-growth of tissue and subsequent incorporation of the biomaterial. A technical problem can develop if all of the adhesions are not adequately removed in the area of the final location of the prosthesis. If it becomes apparent that the adhesions are inhibiting the final attachment of the patch then the procedure must be temporarily delayed to allow for the additional adhesiolysis. This process can be particularly difficult once the patch is partly attached to the abdominal wall, hampering visualization and further dissection. With this in mind, it should be noted that it is particularly important to dissect either the falciform ligament or lower abdominal preperitoneal fat to expose the fascia adequately.

Dissection of the hernia sac is difficult and can result in bleeding while not producing any appreciable benefits for the patient. Therefore, it is not necessary to remove it. Some surgeons apply electrocautery or argon beam to the site of the peritoneal lining of the hernia sac in an effort to obliterate it and thereby reduce seroma formation. It is not known whether this has the desired effect. Closure of the fascial defect is not routinely performed, though some promote routine fascial closure during LIVH [19]. There is a growing opinion that this should be done when feasible, although this will be limited by the size of the defect. The security of the hernioplasty depends upon an adequate overlap of the fascial defect by the prosthesis and adequate patch fixation.

It is essential that the measurement of the hernia defect is accurate. This size of the defect will determine the size of the prosthetic. If this measurement is performed with the abdomen fully insufflated the resulting size determination will be artifactually larger than the proper measurement. The size of the defect must be measured with the insufflation pressure

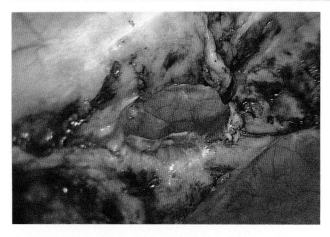

Fig. 22.6 Laparoscopic view of fully dissected incisional hernia (note the preperitoneal fat has been removed to expose the fascia)

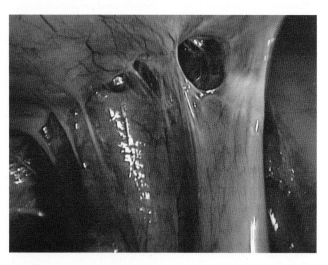

Fig. 22.7 Typical adhesions of the small intestine that require dissection from the abdominal wall

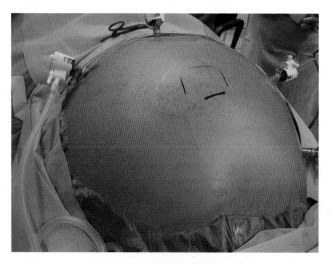

Fig. 23.8 Skin marks placed to identify the edges of the fascial defect

reduced from the working amount of 14–16 mm Hg to near zero. Reducing the pressure prevents the inflation artifact that occurs because this measurement is done on the external surface of the abdominal wall rather than on the interior surface. After desufflation, the defect is outlined on the skin over the abdomen with a skin-marking pencil (Fig. 22.8). If the choice of prosthetic size is made based on the measurement in the insufflated position, it is likely that the prosthesis will be much larger than is required. Use of that material can be exceedingly difficult because some of the trocar sites can be covered with the biomaterial. One must then trim the patch as it lies within the abdomen, which is cumbersome. The entire circumference of the defect should be identified to ascertain its maximum dimensions. To ensure adequate coverage with the prosthesis, a minimum of 6 cm is added to the maximum measurements in all directions. In other words, if the defect were 7×12 cm, the minimum patch size would be 13×18 cm. Current thought, however, is that a 5 cm overlap is ideal.

The choice of the prosthesis will be made based on the available sizes that are manufactured. In many cases, this will provide coverage in excess of 5 cm requirements. This is felt to be advantageous. If the patient is morbidly obese, it is preferred that a larger overlap disperse the intra-abdominal pressure over a larger surface area to diminish the risk of recurrence. We also believe that it is preferable to cover the entire length of the original incision even though only a portion may have an actual hernia defect. This will avoid the future occurrence of a hernia either above or below the actual repair of the original hernia. Several different techniques may be used before patch insertion to ensure that the prosthesis will be oriented properly and cover the defect adequately. A common approach is to tie ePTFE sutures (CV-0) at either side of the midpoint of the long axis of the patch and mark both sides of the midpoint of its short axis with a marking pencil prior to its insertion into the abdominal cavity [22]. It is important to mark both sides of the midpoints of the prosthesis (Figs. 22.9 and 22.10). This can be done with a marking pencil if this is possible to do so; if the biomaterial does not allow this, then one may mark these points with sutures. Once the prosthetic is inserted, the surgeon will need to visualize both surfaces of the biomaterial to assure the correct axial orientation along the abdominal wall. Some surgeons mark the short axis by placement of a contrastingly colored nonabsorbable suture, such as Prolene® or Ethibond®. Others place four or more sutures at the corners or periphery of the patches prior to insertion. The more sutures that are placed into the prosthesis prior to insertion, the more likely that there will be a tangle of suture material that can be cumbersome to separate and pull through the abdominal wall. The use of sutures in this repair continues to be discussed. Some surgeons do not believe that transfascial sutures are necessary [23] but others feel that this is absolutely indicated

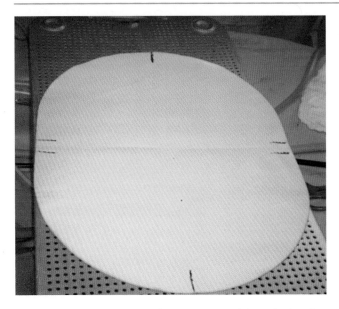

Fig. 22.9 Marks place to identify the midpoints of the parietal surface of DualMesh Plus

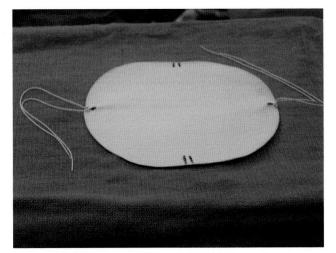

Fig. 22.10 Initial two ePTFE sutures placed at the midpoints of the long axis of the prosthesis

[22, 24, 25]. Data on prostheses and the final decision on the use of sutures will continue to evolve. Recent data does provide some guidance [26]. It seems that if the overlap is 5 cm or greater then transfascial sutures can be omitted. However, many surgeons, the authors included, believe that the benefit of the sutures out ways the risk of the few patients that may develop pain postoperatively.

The patch with any attached sutures is rolled or folded for introduction into the abdomen. The method of folding the patch is simplest if the material is folded into sequential halves after the prior fold [22]. As shown in Figs. 22.10, 22.11, 22.12, 22.13, and 22.14, the sutures are placed into the first fold and the subsequent folds result in a smaller size of the biomaterial. Early in the learning curve, it is suggested

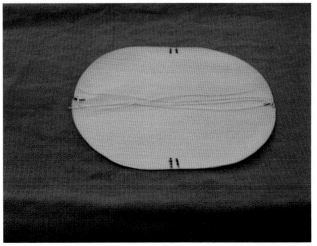

Fig. 22.11 These initial sutures are placed on the parietal surface prior to folding the mesh

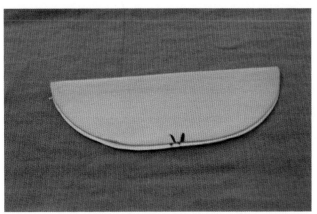

Fig. 22.12 The first fold of the prosthesis encloses these sutures (note that the edges of the mesh are offset from each other to make it easier to grasp them intraperitoneally after introduction)

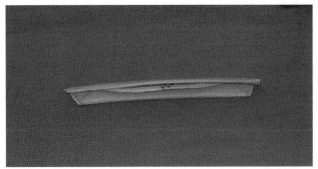

Fig. 22.13 The second fold of the mesh is shown

that 10- or 12-mm ports be utilized to insert the patches. As experience is acquired, one will find that the use of only 5-mm trocars will suffice. Some of the prostheses that are available today, such as the polypropylene- or polyester-based biomaterials, require the use of the larger trocars for

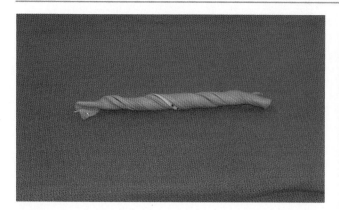

Fig. 22.14 After the folding, the product will be tightly rolled to ease introduction

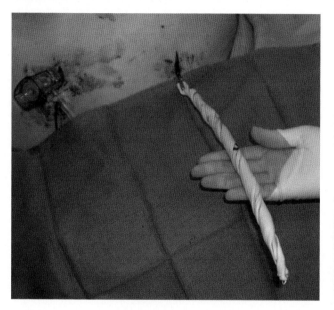

Fig. 22.15 A grasper is put through a trocar, which is then removed. The instrument will grasp the mesh and then pull it into the abdominal cavity

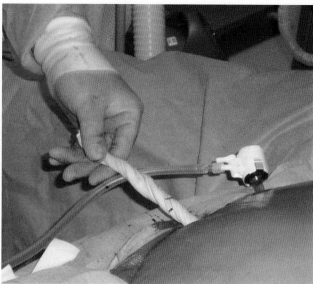

Fig. 22.16 External view of the mesh as it is pulled into the abdomen

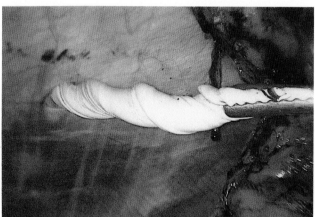

Fig. 22.17 Laparoscopic view of the mesh as it is pulled into the abdomen

their insertion into the abdominal cavity. With those products that can be compressed adequately, such as DualMesh® Plus (which is 50% air by volume), one can pull them into the abdomen with the use of the 5 mm ports. In these instances, the skin incision at the site of patch introduction should be made larger than that which is necessary for placement of the trocar itself (typically 7–8 mm). Generally, particularly for the larger patches, a grasping instrument is passed through a trocar on the opposite side of the abdomen, which is then passed outward through a trocar on the other side. The trocar through which the instrument is exited is then removed (Fig. 22.15). The tightly rolled and/or twisted biomaterial will be grasped by the instrument and pulled into the abdominal cavity (Figs. 22.16 and 22.17). The assistant surgeon can assist this maneuver by maintaining the "twist" of the patch as it is introduced. The pliability of the abdominal wall mus-

culature will accommodate the insertion of even the largest of the ePTFE patches available (24×36 cm). This maneuver can, of course, be duplicated with the larger trocars. If the larger trocars are used, however, the smaller patches can frequently be inserted directly through the trocar rather than by the above method.

Placement of the Prosthesis

Once the insertion of the prosthetic is done, the patch must be returned to its original flattened shape. The biomaterial is placed onto the viscera whereupon the surgeon and the assistant will then assist each other in the manipulation of the biomaterial to completely flatten it as much as is feasible. This will facilitate the fixation of the material to the abdominal wall. If this is not possible it may be easier to unroll the prosthesis after one or both of the initial sutures have been passed through the abdominal wall. It is preferable, however, to do this only if the above method fails because the maneuverability of the prosthesis will be impaired once the fixation is initiated.

If one has chosen to use only two initially placed sutures, these are now pulled through the entire abdominal wall with use of a sharp suture-passing instrument inserted through a small skin incision (Fig. 22.18). There are several different devices that are available for this purpose. These two sutures are placed along the long axis of the defect taking care to center the prosthesis over the defect. If necessary, the laparoscope can be placed into another port to confirm that it is centered with the necessary 5 cm minimum overlap and drawn tautly. One should remember that if a 3 cm overlap is elected, then transfascial sutures are essential. If these two facts cannot be confirmed then one or both of these sutures must be repositioned. Once the optimal position is achieved, the sutures are tied. Even in large patients, the knots can usually be pulled down to the level of the fascia. It is important to make sure that these and all the subsequent sutures are tied sufficiently tight to pull them to the fascia without any laxity. It is sometimes necessary to enlarge the skin incision slightly to allow the surgeon enough room to properly tie the suture down to the fascial level. An additional method of confirmation will be simply to examine each suture laparoscopically once tied or at the completion of the entire procedure. If the suture is loose then it must be cut and replaced.

The next step will be to confirm that the correct orientation along the short axis of the patch is correct. The surgeon and the assistant will grasp the previously marked midpoints on either side of the biomaterial. The material is then positioned over the desired final location. Either the assistant or the surgeon then uses a fixation device to attach the midpoint of one side placing only one or two tacks at that time. The tacking instrument is then given to the other surgeon and the unattached midpoint is likewise secured with one or two tacks. Inspection of the position of the biomaterial is again performed usually by moving the laparoscope to one of the other trocars to visualize the position of the biomaterial from different angles before the insertion of the additional tacks and sutures that will permanently secure the patch. After this inspection, the tacks are deployed along the periphery of the prosthesis by inserting them 2–4 mm from the edge of the patch, 1–1.5 cm apart (Fig. 22.19) [22]. Multiple tackers are available for use now: these include the titanium tacker, ProTack™ (Covidien, Norwalk, CT) and absorbable tackers such as SorbaFix™ (Bard Davol, Warwick, RI) and AbsorbaTack™ (Covidien, Norwalk,CT). The absorbable tackers are gaining in popularity and last up to 1 year.

Several authors have identified the need to place transfascial sutures to ensure adequate fixation of the biomaterial

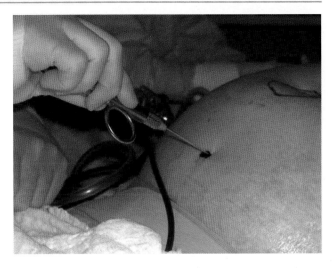

Fig. 22.18 Suture-passing instrument has been introduced to grasp one of the initial two sutures

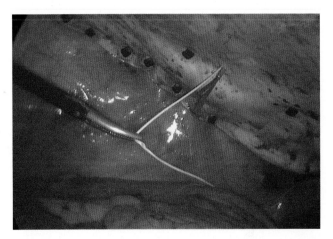

Fig. 22.19 The laparoscopic instrument has grasped an additional suture from the suture passing instrument

[22, 24, 27, 28]. It is generally believed that the insertion of the tacks is merely an initial step and serves mainly to approximate the prosthesis to the abdominal wall to ensure adequate tissue in-growth. In one study the rate of hernia recurrence without the use of these transfascial sutures resulted in a recurrence of 13% while there were no recurrences seen in those patients that had the use of sutures [27]. A recent meta-analysis showed that the degree of overlap can influence the need for transfascial sutures. Generally, in some hernioplasties with a 5 cm overlap, transfascial sutures may not be needed [26]. Tacking is followed by placement of nonabsorbable sutures (e.g., ePTFE) of size 0. These sutures will be placed through all musculofascial layers of the abdominal wall and tied above the fascia in a manner similar to the tying of the initial two sutures. During the insertion of the sutures, one should avoid clamping of any portion of the suture material that will remain within the patient. If this occurs, the suture will be permanently weakened and may fracture at that site which can lead to failure of the suture and a recurrence of the hernia.

Using the view of the laparoscope, the planned sites of suture placement are marked at intervals of 5 cm apart. A mark is made with the skin-marking pen at these points whereupon a No.11-scalpel blade is used to make a 1–2 mm skin incision at each of these points. Then at each site a suture is passed through the skin incision with one of the many fascial closure or suture-passing devices that are available (Fig. 22.20). The suture passer pierces the patch at the appropriate place. The assistant (from the opposite side of the abdomen) retrieves the suture with a grasping instrument and the suture is released (Fig. 22.21). The device is now withdrawn into the subcutaneous tissue and reinserted through the patch approximately 1 cm from the previous puncture site. The previously inserted suture is retrieved from the assistant and withdrawn from the abdomen onto the skin (Fig. 22.22). The two tails of the suture are grasped with a hemostat and the suture is cut with sufficient length to allow for the tying of the suture. These maneuvers are repeated then along the entire edge of the patch (Fig. 22.23). Once the sutures are tied the patch should lay flat and obliterate the fascial defect. A final examination of the prosthetic is performed to insure that all sutures are tight and that all edges of the patch are secured (Fig. 22.24). Any laxity of the sutures will require that these be replaced with others that provide sufficient fixation without looseness.

When the sutures are tied down, a dimple of the skin may develop at the site of the incision where the suture has been passed. This is caused by the fixation of the subcutaneous tissue that may have been grasped by the knots of the suture. This dimple can be removed by placing a fine pointed hemostat into the incision to lift the skin away from the suture (Fig. 22.25). It is important to inspect the abdominal wall with the abdomen fully insufflated after the completion of the suture fixation so that any dimples are removed. If this is not done, the cosmetic result will be unacceptable to the patient.

Rather than placing the additional sutures as described above, in some centers, an additional row of fasteners are placed near the fascial edges. The result is two concentric rows of tacks that secure the prosthesis. This "double-crown" technique is popular in some centers [23]. Current follow-up data appears to be favorable but longer-term data will be necessary to verify its effectiveness.

After the removal of the trocars and closure of the skin incisions, an abdominal binder is frequently used and left in place for at least 72 h. It is preferred, however, if the use of this binder could continue for 4–6 weeks. It is believed that the use of this binder aids in the prevention of a postoperative seroma at the site of the hernia. It assists in the management

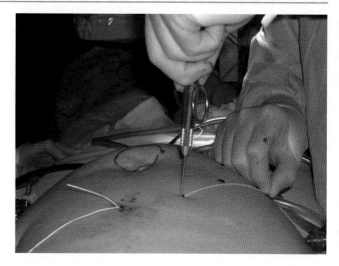

Fig. 22.20 External view of the suture passer retrieving a suture from the abdomen

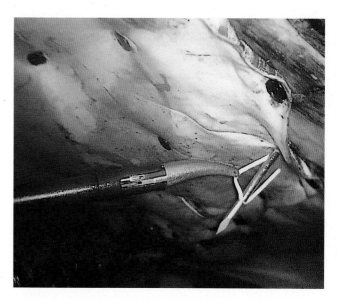

Fig. 22.21 Another view of the "hand-off" of a suture

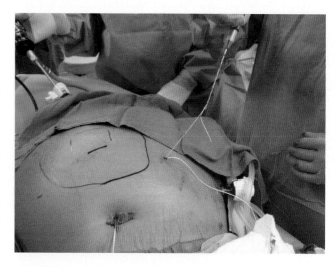

Fig. 22.22 Another view of suture retrieval

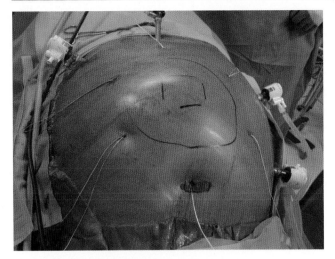

Fig. 22.23 Completed passage of the transfascial sutures

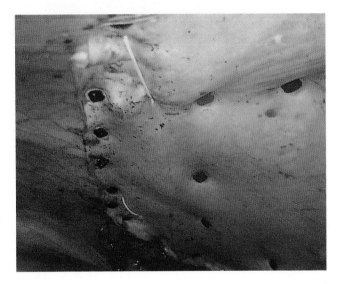

Fig. 22.24 Laparoscopic view of the completed fixation of the prosthesis with sutures and fasteners

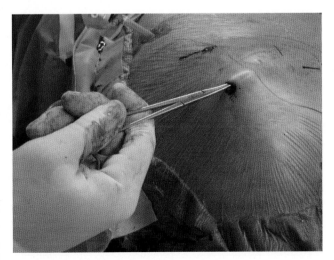

Fig. 22.25 Use of a hemostat to release the subcutaneous tissue from the suture to remove skin puckering

of postoperative pain and does not appear to affect the respiratory effort of the patient.

Immediate Postoperative Considerations

Approximately 50% of these patients can be discharged on the same day of surgery. Generally this will be the patient that has a single defect, a hernia dimension of less than 25 cm [2], few adhesions, and no incarcerated contents of the hernia. The average length of stay is 1–2 days [7, 8, 12]. Patients can consume liquids the day of surgery and resume taking any regular medications immediately. Oral and parenteral sedatives are given as needed. Postoperatively, many patients will experience some degree of abdominal distension, which is usually proportional to the extent of adhesiolysis and the extent of bowel involvement. However, most patients can resume a regular diet the day after the operation. Occasionally, some patients will experience prolongation of the ileus. This should be managed by the usual methods; which would include a nasogastric tube when necessary.

Pain may be used as the guide to determine when patients can resume their normal activities. They are allowed to shower the next day. Patients may return to their daily activities, including work, as soon as they can do so without marked pain. The majority of patients are able to drive within a week and resume job-related activities in 7–14 days. Most surgeons do not restrict the activities of these patients but allow the level of pain to dictate the increase in the level of activity.

After removal of the binder, many patients will note a firm bulge at the hernia site. The bulge may represent a seroma in the first few weeks, but subsequently this area represents the cicatricial event that occurs in the majority of these patients. Seroma formation is a common occurrence after LIVH. However, it is rarely, if ever, necessary to aspirate these fluid collections, as they will generally resolve without intervention. Aspiration will also expose the patient to a risk of the introduction of infection into the seroma.

Late Postoperative Considerations

In most patients with the cicatricial "bulge" and/or seroma at the hernia site, resolution will be noted within 2 months, depending on the size of the hernia and its contents. Occasionally the skin of the abdominal wall that overlaid the hernia will become erythematous within 4–6 days postoperatively, usually in association with a distinct surface firmness but with little tenderness and without the presence of fever, chills, or leukocytosis (Fig. 22.26). This situation, which is seen in approximately 5–7% of patients, can persist for a few weeks and can be most unsettling. This is believed to be the

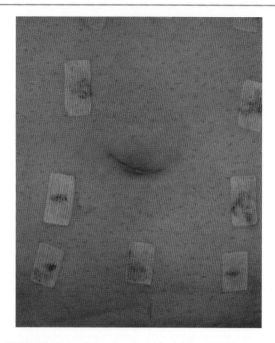

Fig. 22.26 Postoperative appearance of erythema that is not abnormal and noninfected

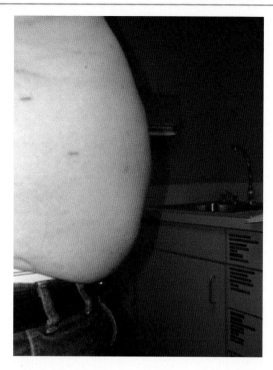

Fig. 22.28 Postoperative appearance of the same patient in Fig. 22.27 three months after LIVH

this can be treated effectively with nonsteroidal anti-inflammatory drugs or direct injections of xylocaine or other local anesthetic [30]. If this problem persists despite these maneuvers, the surgeon might consider performing a laparo-scopic examination to inspect the patch, tacks, and sutures. This is rarely necessary but occasionally transection of the offending suture will be necessary to effect a permanent relief of these symptoms.

Hernioplasty of Infrequent Defects

The majority of incisional and ventral hernias will occur in the midline of the abdomen. One will encounter other hernias that offer a particular challenge whether repaired by the open or the laparoscopic technique. One such hernia is that which lies very high in the midline, perhaps at the exit site of a mediasti-nal drainage tube used for open-heart surgery. Repair of this defect may require that the prosthetic patch be placed near or onto the diaphragm. It may be impossible to achieve an ade-quate amount of counter pressure necessary for the tacking device to provide adequate penetration of the tacks. For a defect in the pericardial area, it is advisable to use only sutures to secure the patch in order to avoid penetration of tacks into the myocardium or development of pericarditis requiring removal of the tacks. There have been anecdotal reports and unreported events of cardiac penetration and tamponade with the use of fasteners other than sutures this high in the abdomi-nal cavity. In this situation, nonabsorbable sutures should be

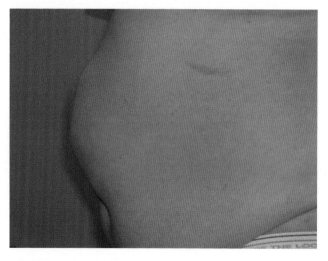

Fig. 22.27 Preoperative appearance of a large incisional hernia fol-lowing a trauma laparotomy

result of resorption of fatty tissue or the hernia sac that was left in place during the initial operation. This appears to be particularly common after the repair of hernias that had min-imal soft tissue between the skin and peritoneal sac and/or a significant amount of incarcerated tissue. No treatment is necessary unless there is a strong suspicion of infection.

Usually within 2–3 months, the abdominal wall will have completed its postoperative changes. (Figs. 22.27 and 22.28) Infrequently, an apparent seroma can still be felt. Ultrasonography or CT scan could evaluate this finding if there is a concern regarding the possibility of a recurrence of the hernia.

In less than 2% of patients, prolonged pain (>3 months) at the site of the transfascial sutures will occur [29]. Usually

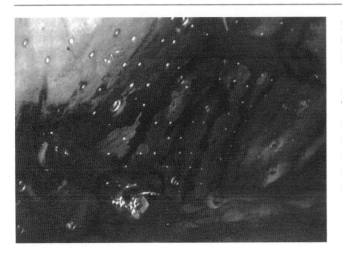

Fig. 22.29 Trocars placed through a prosthesis to place fasteners on the medial aspect of this repair

placed. Additionally an oversized patch is recommended to provide a greater overlap (8 cm or greater) than usually required due to this fixation problem.

Hernias that extend to the symphysis pubis or are associated with an inguinal hernia can also present a challenge. To repair these defects, it will be necessary to attach the lower part of the patch to Cooper's ligament. To accomplish this it will be necessary to dissect the preperitoneal space similar to the laparoscopic transabdominal preperitoneal inguinal hernia repair. This must be done to provide for strong fixation of the patch to the muscle wall of the lower abdomen and the periosteum of the pubis because transfascial sutures cannot be placed in this location. Additionally, interposing preperitoneal fat and peritoneum that remains between the patch and muscle will compromise subsequent tissue attachment. After the patch is secured, the preperitoneal flap can be secured in its usual position to the maximum extent possible.

Incisional "hernias" that occur after nephrectomy or an anterior approach to the spine are usually not true hernias as they generally do not exhibit a well-defined fascial defect. The repair of these deformities is not currently established in the literature. Surgeons that do attempt to repair these deformities must pay particular attention to the positioning of the patient. Patients with such defects should be placed in a lateral decubitus position on a "bean bag." Defects along the upper flanks that involve denervated musculature rather than a true fascial lesion require a very large patch that is secured tightly with more than the usual number of sutures to achieve an acceptable cosmetic result. The laxity of the muscles will frequently require that sutures be placed above the rib margin to secure the prosthetic biomaterial. Additionally, one may need to place sutures onto the diaphragm to ensure fixation. It is may be necessary to place additional trocars through the biomaterial itself (Fig. 22.29) to allow for the accurate placement of all the methods of fixation. In the few

patients that have undergone this repair by one of the authors (KAL), the results are encouraging but longer-term follow-up is necessary.

Hybrid procedures may be necessary for complex hernias such as the above or for patients with significant adhesions. The hybrid procedure combines open and laparoscopic techniques to achieve adequate overlap of the defect and safe adhesiolysis. Often for denervation hernias that occur after lumbar surgery, the initial muscle mobilization can be performed through the originial lumbar incision. The prosthestic of choice is placed in the abdomen after mobilization of viscera and lysis of adhesions. Transfascial or tacking sutures, such as to the diaphragm, can be placed during the open portion of the procedure. Trocars are then placed under direct vision. After the mesh is secured appropriately, the muscle layers can be plicated and the skin closed. The abdomen is then insufflated and laparoscopic suturing and tacking can be performed for adequate overlap and adherence to the abdominal wall (Figs. 22.30 and 22.31). This type of procedure has been reported in a small series of patients with 1 year follow up and no evidence of recurrence [31].

Many patients who present for laparoscopic incisional hernia repair may also require surgical treatment of a concomitant illness. This most commonly will include cholelithiasis, inguinal hernia, gastroesophageal reflux disease, or a need for biopsy of an intra-abdominal or retroperitoneal structure [27, 32]. Most commonly the primary procedure is not the incisional hernia repair and, as such, will be performed initially. If the primary operation can be completed without contamination, the hernia repair could then be performed. If contamination does occur, a prosthetic hernia repair may or may not be done. This will be dictated by the amount of contamination and the risk of infection. An open repair without the insertion of a prosthetic material could be considered but should be individualized to the patient's risk factors, prior operations and/or prior hernia repairs. Preoperative discussions with the patient should have examined this possibility. In those individuals in whom the hernia repair can be attempted subsequent to the primary procedure, placement of additional trocars may be necessary. The surgeon could plan on the future trocars at the initiation of the primary procedure but should not compromise the first procedure by the inappropriate positioning at that point. Any additional necessary trocars should be placed in the locations most appropriate for the hernioplasty once the decision is made to proceed with the second procedure. One should not avoid using more trocars when deemed necessary to carry out the second operation in a safe and effective manner.

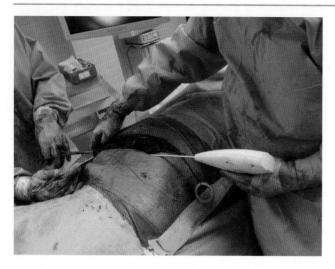

Fig. 22.30 Use of laparoscopic fixation device during the open portion of the hybrid procedure

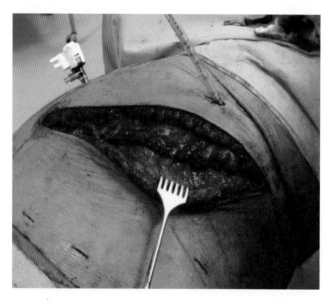

Fig. 22.31 Completed open portion of hybrid procedure with laparoscopic trocars in place

Results

In the past decade, there has been a significant amount of literature comparing LIVH to open mesh repair. This new decade alone has yielded four prospective trials, three retrospective trials and multiple meta-analysis and review papers (Table 22.1). Yet the literature fails to provide a standardization of technique in open mesh repairs. The Rives-Stoppa repair has a known recurrence rate ranging from 0 to 14% [1]; however, Burger described a recurrence rate of 32% in open mesh repairs [6]. The majority of laparoscopic repairs described in comparative trials [7, 9, 10, 12, 33–35] do adhere to the basic tenets of LIVH which include: 3 cm or greater mesh overlap and both transfascial sutures and tacks

for mesh fixation as promoted by LeBlanc and colleagues [36]. This discordant approach to open mesh repair has challenged a true comparison to LIVH in terms of overall recurrence rates.

Pring and colleagues attempted to standardize their technique by using ePTFE as an underlay with transfascial sutures in both open and laparoscopic repairs. Their results yielded a recurrence rate of 4.2% for open mesh repairs and 3.3% for laparoscopic repairs; this recurrence rate was not statistically different [7]. A meta-analysis performed by Forbes et al reviewed eight randomized controlled trials [11]. A similar study was done by Sajid et al on five randomized controlled trials and Sains and colleagues reviewed five comparative trials [37, 38]; all of these meta-analysis report no statistical difference in the recurrence rate between LIVH and open mesh repair. One of the largest meta-analysis was performed by Pierce and colleagues at Washington University. They reviewed 45 studies, of which 14 were paired studies and reported a recurrence rate of 3.1–4.3% for LIVH and 12.1% for open mesh repair [8].

In a review of recent literature, the cumulative average of operating room time for LIVH was 87 and 91.5 min for open mesh repair, which supports a number of comparative studies that report no statistical difference in OR time [9, 34, 37, 39]. However, other studies do show a statistical difference; LIVH has been shown in one meta-analysis to take 12 min longer than open mesh repair on average [35, 38]. This discrepancy is most likely secondary to the lack of standardization of open mesh repair and the learning curve for LIVH represented in earlier studies.

LIVH has been shown to have favorable results in shorter postoperative lengths of stay and overall decrease in wound infections and mesh removal [8, 11, 12, 37, 39, 40]. (Table 22.2) Pierce and colleagues found wound infections to be 4.6–8 fold higher in open mesh repairs when compared with LIVH [8]. A review of the National Surgical Quality Improvement Program (NSQIP) database, total complications were twice as high in open mesh repair in comparison to LIVH [39]. A common sequalae of LIVH is seroma formation. This complication is often underreported because it is routinely of no clinical significance. Very few studies document persistent seroma formation that required intervention.

LIVH is often accompanied with significant adhesiolysis. A dreaded consequence of extensive adhesiolyis is injury to the intestine. Injury may be a result of direct laceration secondary to sharp or blunt dissection, but heightened vigilance is required for injuries caused by traction and remote serosal injuries that may go unrecognized. In a review of the literature by LeBlanc et al, the enterotomy rate for LIVH was 1.78% out of 3925 LIVH. According to this review, approximately 18% of the time, an enterotomy is unrecognized which is associated with an increased mortality rate of 7.7%

Table 22.1 Comparison of recurrence rates, post-Op stay, OR time

	Study type	Year of publication	Recurrence rates		Post-op stay (days)		OR time (min)		Follow-up	
			Open	Lap	Open	Lap	Open	Lap	Open	Lap
Ballem [33]	Retrospective	2008	28%	29%	–	–	–	–	7.5 years[a]	7.5 years
Bencini [34]	Retrospective	2003	6%	0%	8[b]	5[b]	112	108	18 month[b]	17 month[b]
Bencini [35]	Retrospective	2009	11%	14%	2[a]	3[a]	35	70	60 month[a]	56 month[a]
Olmi [10]	Prospective	2007	1.1%	2.3%	9.9[b]	2.7[b]	151	61	24 month[a]	24 month[a]
Pring [7]	Prospective	2008	4.2%	3.3%	1[a]	1[a]	43	44	27.5 month[a]	27.5 month[a]
Lomanto [9]	Prospective	2006	10%	2%	4.7[b]	2.7[b]	93	91	20.8[b]	20.8[b]
McGreevy [12]	Prospective	2003	–	–	1.5[b]	1.1[b]	102	132	30 days[c]	30 days[c]
Forbes [11]	Meta-analysis	2009	3.6%	3.4%	–	–	–	–	6–40.8 month	6–40.8 month
Pierce [8]	Meta-analysis	2007	12.1%	3.1–4.3%	4.3[b]	2.4[b]	104.5	103	20.2[d]	25.5[d]

[a]Median
[b]Mean
[c]Completed length of follow-up
[d]Unspecified

Table 22.2 Postoperative complications

Complications	Ballem [33] Open	Ballem [33] Lap	Bencini [34] 2003 Open	Bencini [34] 2003 Lap	Bencini [35] 2009 Open	Bencini [35] 2009 Lap	Olmi [10] Open	Olmi [10] Lap	Pringe [7] Open	Pringe [7] Lap	Lomanto [9] Open	Lomanto [9] Lap	McGreevy [12] Open	McGreevy [12] Lap	Forbes [11] Open	Forbes [11] Lap	Pierce [8] Open	Pierce [8] Lap
Enterotomy	–	–	2%	5%	0%	4%	–	–	–	–	–	–	0%	1.5%[a]	0.9%	2.6%	1.2%	2.9%
Fecal obstruction	–	–	–	–	–	–	1.1%	1.1%	–	–	–	–	–	–	–	–	–	–
Ileus	–	–	10%	2%	–	–	–	–	–	–	10%	2%	4.2%	0%	–	–	–	–
Mesh Infxn/removal	–	–	–	–	–	–	–	–	–	–	–	–	–	–	3.5%	0.7%	3.2%	0.9%
Neuralgia	–	–	–	–	–	–	0%	4.7%	0%	–	–	–	–	–	–	–	–	–
Pulmonary embolism	–	–	–	–	–	–	1.1%	0%	0%	6.6%[b]	–	–	–	–	–	–	–	–
Seroma	9%	16%	10%	14%	3%	11%	1.1%	7%	33%	17%	6%	10%	4.2%	3%	15.5%	11.7%	12%	12.1%
Urinary retention	–	–	–	–	–	–	–	–	0%	6.6%	–	–	–	–	–	–	–	–
Wound Infxn	9%	7.5%	12%	0%	8%	0%	8.2%	1.1%	16.7%	3.3%	6%	4%	8.4%	0%	10.1%	1.5%	10.4%	1.3%

[a]Unrecognized
[b]Pre-existing procoagulant disorder

[21]. Should an enterotomy occur and is recognized, the injury should be repaired, of course. The next decision is whether or not to proceed with the repair of the hernia itself. The use of a prosthesis is to be avoided in conventional teaching but there is a growing opinion that the use of lower weight meshes might be considered in this situation as these seem to be less prone to infection. A primary repair of the hernia will be associated with a high risk of recurrence. Therefore, many experts recommend that the primary repair be avoided and the patient be returned to the operating room in several days [41]. With the introduction of biologic products for the repair of the hernias in contaminated fields, perhaps these could be used in this situation. This has not been reported but it has been done in some cases.

The overall cost of LIVH has been shown to be equivalent with open mesh repair. A single institution prospectively collected data on 884 incisional hernias. There was no statistical difference in overall hospital cost for LIVH when compared to open mesh repair. LIVH was shown to have shorter length of stay, though operating time and cost of supplies were higher in LIVH. LIVH costs $6,725 compared with $7,445 for open mesh repair in total hospital costs and postoperative encounters [42].

Obesity and LIVH

Obesity has been shown to be a major factor in hernia recurrence. In a study of 160 patients, obesity was compared to other risk factors for hernia recurrence such as smoking, diabetes, steroid use, and pulmonary disease. Obesity was the strongest predictor for hernia recurrence. Patients with a body mass index (BMI) of 38 were 4.2 times more likely to have a recurrent hernia in comparison to a patient with a BMI of 23 [18]. Congruent results were identified in a multi-institutional study of five academic centers. This retrospective review found the recurrence rate to be significantly higher in morbidly obese patients with an odds ratio of 4.3 [17].

Though some report a higher recurrence rate in obese patients, LIVH is safe and effective in this population of patients. LIVH has been shown to have less risk of wound complications, greater identification of multiple occult defects and wider mesh overlap. In a review of 168 patients at a single institution, perioperative complications after LIVH were not found to be statistically different from non-obese patients. Recurrence rates were related to defect size and size of mesh rather than obesity [43]. Ventral hernia repair is even promoted during laparoscopic bariatric surgery when concurrently identified. In patients who did not have their ventral hernia repaired during laparoscopic gastric bypass, there was an increased risk of intestinal incarceration during patient follow up [44].

Conclusion

LIVH has a proven track record as an effective, safe, and durable option for ventral hernia repairs. There is general consensus that LIVH has comparable recurrence rates to open mesh repair, if not less risk of recurrence as seen in some prospective trials. Wound complications and mesh infections occur infrequently. Hospital stay is shortened and increasingly, LIVH is becoming the first and only attempt at a disease that is commonly identified in 10–20% of postlaparotomy patients [1, 5, 19, 45].

References

1. Jin J, Rosen M. Laparoscopic versus open ventral hernia repair. Surg Clin North Am. 2008;88:1083–100.
2. LeBlanc K, Booth W. Laparoscopic Repair of Incisional Abdominal Hernias using expanded polytetrafluoroethylene: preliminary findings. Surg Laparosc Endosc. 1993;3(1):39–41.
3. Stoppa R, Louis D, Verhaeghe P, et al. Current surgical treatment of post-operative eventrations. Int Surg. 1987;72(1):42–4.
4. Bauer J, Harris M, Gorfine S, et al. Rives-Stoppa procedure for repair of large incisional hernias: experience with 57 patients. Hernia. 2002;6:120–3.
5. den Hartog D, Dur A, Tuinebreijer W et al. (2008) Open surgical procedure for incisional hernias. The Cochrane Collaboration.
6. Burger J, Luijendijk R, Hop W, et al. Long-term follow-up of a randomized controlled trial of suture versus mesh repair of incisional hernia. Ann Surg. 2004;240(4):578–85.
7. Pring C, Tran V, O'Rourke N, et al. Laparoscopic versus open ventral hernia repair: a randomized controlled trial. ANZ J Surg. 2008;78:903–6.
8. Pierce R, Spitler J, Frisella M, et al. Pooled data analysis of laparoscopic vs. open ventral hernia repair: 14 years of patient data accrual. Surg Endosc. 2007;21:378–86.
9. Lomanto D, Iyer S, Shabbir A, et al. Laparoscopic versus open ventral hernia mesh repair: a prospective study. Surg Endosc. 2006;20:1030–5.
10. Olmi S, Scaini A, Cesana G, et al. Laparoscopic versus open incisional hernia repair; an open randomized controlled trial. Surg Endosc. 2007;21:555–9.
11. Forbes S, Eskicioglu C, McLeod R, et al. Meta-analysis of randomized controlled trials comparing open and laparoscopic ventral and incisional hernia repair with mesh. Br J Surg. 2009;96:851–8.
12. McGreevy J, Goodney P, Birkmeyer C, et al. A prospective study comparing the complication rates between laparoscopic and open ventral hernia repairs. Surg Endosc. 2003;17:1778–80.
13. Rosen M, Williams C, Jin J, et al. Laparoscopic versus open-component separation: a comparative analysis in a porcine model. Am J Surg. 2007;194:383–9.
14. Bachman S, Ramaswamy A, Ramshaw B. Early results of midline hernia repair using a minimally invasive component separation technique. Am Surg. 2009;75(7):572–7.
15. O'Malley C, Cunningham A. Physiologic changes during laparoscopy. Anesthesiol Clin North America. 2001;19(1):1–19.
16. Hesselink VJ, Luijendijk RW, de Wilt JH, et al. An evaluation of risk factors in incisional hernia recurrence. Surg Gynecol Obstet. 1993;176(3):228–34.
17. Tsereteli Z, Pryor B, Heniford B, et al. Laparoscopic ventral hernia repair (LIVH) in morbidly obese patients. Hernia. 2008;12:233–8.

18. Sauerland S, Korenkov M, Kleinen T, et al. Obesity is a risk factor for recurrence after incisional hernia repair. Hernia. 2004;8:42–6.

19. Franklin M, Gonzalez J, Glass J, et al. Laparoscopic ventral and incisional hernia repair: an 11 year experience. Hernia. 2004;8:23–7.

20. Sarit C, Eliezer A, Mizrahi S. Minimally Invasive Repair of recurrent strangulated umbilical hernia in cirrhotic patient with refractory ascites. Liver Transpl. 2003;9:621–2.

21. LeBlanc K, Elieson M, III Corder J. Enterotomy and mortality rates of laparoscopic incisional and ventral hernia repair: a review of the literature. JSLS. 2007;11:408–14.

22. LeBlanc K. Current considerations in laparoscopic incisional and ventral herniorrhaphy. JSLS. 2004;4:131–9.

23. Carbajo M, Martin del Olmo J, Blanco J, et al. Laparoscopic treatment of ventral abdominal wall hernias: preliminary results in 100 Patients. JSLS. 2000;4:141–5.

24. Ramshaw BJ, Escartia P, Schwab J, et al. Comparison of laparoscopic and open ventral herniorrhaphy. Am Surg. 1999;65:827–32.

25. Park A, Birch DW, Lovrics P. Laparoscopic and open incisional hernia repair: a comparison study. Surgery. 1998;124:816–22.

26. LeBlanc K. Laparoscopic incisional hernia repair: are Transfascial sutures necessary? A review of the literature. Surg Endosc. 2007;21:508–13.

27. LeBlanc K, Booth W, Whitaker J, et al. Laparoscopic incisional and ventral herniorrhaphy in 100 patients. Am J Surg. 2000;180(3):193–7.

28. DeMaria EJ, Moss JM, Sugerman HJ. Laparoscopic intraperitoneal polytetrafluoroethylene (PTFE) prosthesic patch repair of ventral hernia. Prospective comparison to open prefascial polypropylene mesh repair. Surg Endosc. 2000;14(4):326–9.

29. Heniford B, Park A, Ramshaw B, et al. Laparoscopic repair of ventral hernias. Nine years' experience with 850 consecutive hernias. Ann Surg. 2003;238:391–400.

30. Carbonell A, Harold K, Mahmutovic A, et al. Local injection for the treatment of suture site pain after laparoscopic ventral hernia repair. Am Surg. 2003;69:688–92.

31. Griniatsos J, Eugenia Y, Anastasios T, et al. A hybrid technique for recurrent incisional hernia repair. Surg Laparosc Endosc Percutan Tech. 2009;19:177–80.

32. Heniford B, Park A, Ramshaw B, et al. Laparoscopic ventral and incisional hernia repair in 407 patients. J Am Coll Surg. 2000;190:645–50.

33. Ballem N, Parikh R, Berber E. Laparoscopic versus open ventral hernia repairs: 5 year recurrence rates. Surg Endosc. 2008;22:1935–40.

34. Bencini L, Sanchez L, Boffi B, et al. Incisional hernia repair. Surg Endosc. 2003;17:1546–51.

35. Bencini L, Sanchez L, Boffi B, et al. Comparison of laparoscopic and open repair for primary ventral hernias. Surg Laparosc Endosc Percutan Tech. 2009;19:341–4.

36. LeBlanc K, Whitaker J, Bellanger D, et al. Laparoscopic incisional and ventral hernioplasty: lessons learned from 200 patients. Hernia. 2003;7:118–24.

37. Sajid M, Bokhari S, Mallick A, et al. Laparoscopic versus open repair of incisional/ventral hernia: a meta-analysis. Am J Surg. 2009;197:64–72.

38. Sains P, Tilney H, Purkayastha S, et al. Outcomes following laparoscopic versus open repair of incisional hernia. World J Surg. 2006;30:2056–64.

39. Hwang C, Wichterman K, Alfrey E. Laparoscopic ventral hernia repair is safer than open repair: analysis of the NSQIP data. J Surg Res. 2009;156:213–6.

40. Misiakos E, Machairas A, Patapis P, et al. Laparoscopic ventral hernia repair: pros and cons compared with open hernia repair. JSLS. 2008;12:117–25.

41. LeBlanc K. The Critical Technical Aspects of Laparoscopic Repair of Ventral and Incisional Hernias. Am Surg. 2001;67(8):809–12.

42. Earle D, Seymour N, Fellinger E, et al. Laparoscopic versus open incisional hernia repair. A single institution analysis of hospital resource utilization for 884 consecutive cases. Surg Endosc. 2006;20:71–5.

43. Ching S, Sarela A, Dexter S, et al. Comparison of early outcomes for laparoscopic ventral hernia repair between nonobese and morbidly obese patient populations. Surg Endosc. 2008;22:2244–50.

44. Eid G, Mattat S, Hamad G, et al. Repair of ventral hernias in morbidly obese patients undergoing laparoscopic gastric bypass should not be deferred. Surg Endosc. 2004;18:207–10.

45. Perrone J, Soper N, Eagon C, et al. Perioperative outcomes and complications of laparoscopic ventral hernia repair. Surgery. 2005;138:708–16.

Parastomal Hernia

Leif A. Israelsson

Spontaneous ostomies occurring after incarcerated and fistulated abdominal wall hernias and after trauma have been reported since ancient times. A colostomy as a medically useful procedure was first suggested by Littre in 1710. The first successful colostomy was performed by Duret in 1793 on an infant with colonic obstruction due to an imperforate anus. Today creating an ostomy is a common surgical procedure utilized in both elective and emergent situations as well as by an open or a laparoscopic technique. This development has been greatly facilitated by the improvement of modern stoma bandages that nowadays enable an easy and reliable stoma care. Unfortunately the development of parastomal hernia is a very frequent complication and Goligher even considered some degree of herniation as almost inevitable after colostomy formation [1].

Parastomal hernia may present as problems of stoma care, difficulty with appliances or irrigation, a significant cosmetic deformity—or as straightforward complications of a hernia with intestinal obstruction or strangulation. The presence of a large protrusion itself may make repair a necessity irrespective of its other side effects (Fig. 23.1).

Parastomal hernia develops in 30–50% of patients supplied with an ostomy and one-third of these demand repairs. After suture repair or relocation of the stoma recurrence rates are unacceptably high. With open or laparoscopic mesh repairs considerably lower recurrence rates are reported. There are no randomized trials or long-term follow-up studies available reporting results with these various techniques for parastomal hernia repair.

In randomized trials a prophylactic prosthetic mesh placed in a sublay position has reduced the rate of parastomal hernia. In nonrandomized studies a prophylactic onlay, sublay, or intraperitoneal onlay mesh (IPOM) has also been associated with low herniation rates.

Definition of Parastomal Hernia

Pearl defined parastomal hernia as an incisional hernia related to an abdominal wall stoma [2]. Before 2004 the definition used at follow-up examination was actually given in only one report and then parastomal hernia was defined as a palpable cough impulse at the ostomy site [3]. Beginning in 2004 and thereafter many authors have reported the definition used and have then regarded any protrusion in the vicinity of the stoma as a herniation [4–11]. With a parastomal hernia detected according to this definition, patients have been demonstrated to have a poorer quality of life than matched controls, so the definition appears clinically relevant [11].

A CT scan has in some studies been added to the clinical examination at follow-up and the radiological definition then used was of any intra-abdominal content protruding along the ostomy [4, 7, 8]. However, the correlation between herniation found at clinical examination and at CT scan has in these reports not been very strong. Thus, herniation found at clinical examination may not be present at a CT scan and vice versa.

Without providing the definitions used it has in several reports been differentiated between parastomal hernia and stoma prolapse [12–18]. In a Cochrane report parastomal hernia was defined as a hernia beside the stoma, and stoma prolapse as an eversion of the stoma through the abdominal wall [19]. It is not clear how to differentiate between herniation and prolapse at clinical examination or with a prolapse present how to exclude a concomitant parastomal hernia. Many authors may have regarded both entities as a parastomal hernia at follow-up examination. This does not seem unreasonable since both entities, however they are defined, certainly represent undesired complications after stoma formation.

The anatomy of the herniation is variable. Parastomal hernia has by Kingsnorth been classified into four subtypes [20] (Fig. 23.2):

1. An interstitial type with a hernia sac within the muscle/ aponeurotic layers of the abdomen
2. A subcutaneous type with a subcutaneous hernia sac

L.A. Israelsson (✉)
Department of Surgery, Sundsvall Hospital, Sundsvall, Sweden
e-mail: leif.israelsson@lvn.se

A.N. Kingsnorth and K.A. LeBlanc (eds.), *Management of Abdominal Hernias*,
DOI 10.1007/978-1-84882-877-3_23, © Springer Science+Business Media London 2013

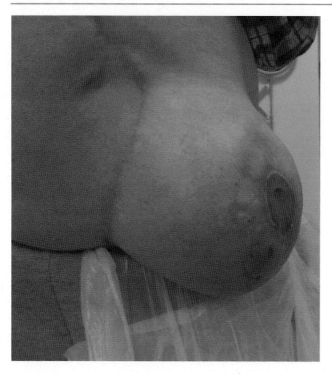

Fig. 23.1 A large parastomal hernia presenting problems of stoma care, difficulty with appliances and a significant cosmetic deformity

3. An intrastomal type in ileostomies with a hernia sac between the intestinal wall and the everted intestinal layer
4. A perstomal type or prolapse with the bowel prolapsing through a circumferential hernia sac enclosing the stoma

This classification defines the type of herniation according to the position of the hernia sac. A circumferential hernia sac within the stoma is consequently regarded as a parastomal hernia of the perstomal type or prolapse. The classification has not been used in clinical studies as it is difficult to distinguish these types of parastomal hernias by physical examination [5].

It is very difficult to compare herniation rates between different clinical reports since there has been no uniform definition of parastomal hernia. Also the rate of parastomal hernia increases with time, so herniation rates cannot be compared between reports with different time to follow-up. Follow-up examination should be no less than 12 months after the index operation, although parastomal hernias still develop after 5–10 years following ostomy formation [21].

Currently the practice is that parastomal hernia is defined as any protrusion or bulge adjacent to the stoma—detected with the patient supine with elevated legs or while coughing or straining when erect. With a CT scan added to the clinical examination parastomal hernia is defined as any intraabdominal content protruding along the ostomy.

Incidence of Parastomal Hernias

The rate of parastomal hernia is reported to occur within the very wide range of 5–81% [3, 12, 15–18, 21–28]. This broad variation is probably very much related to different definition of herniation being used as well as differences in time between the index operation and follow-up examination. Due to the lack of a uniform definition of parastomal hernia and the variable follow-up time in different reports, the true rate of parastomal hernia can only be estimated. With a more uniform approach during the last decade the rate of parastomal hernia reported after 12 months has been closer to 50%. Thus, available data indicate that 1 year after stoma formation the rate of parastomal hernia is at least 30% and probably close to 50% in general surgical practice. The rate increases during the following 5–10 years. Thus, parastomal hernia is a major clinical problem.

The rate of herniation has been suggested to be lower after an ileostomy than after a colostomy. Such a difference must be questioned, however, as it has not been perceived in a number of studies [3, 12, 29]. The proportion of parastomal hernias occurring after ileostomy using the Bricker diversion is similar to the reported rates using other ostomy techniques, since rates of 5–65% have been reported [30–36].

Loop ileostomies and loop colostomies probably produce similar rates of parastomal herniation [19, 37, 38]. Hernia rates with loop stomas cannot easily be compared with end stomas since follow-up time is often shorter with loop stomas. The shorter follow-up time is due to loop stomas often being intended as temporary and bowel continuity is then often restored. A loop stoma may also be utilized as a palliative means in patients with malignant disease and short survival time after stoma formation.

Enterostomas were previously sometimes brought out through the laparotomy wound, but this produced disastrous results in terms of infection, wound dehiscence, and herniation [1, 39–41]. An extraperitoneal construction of the stoma has been tried in order to reduce the rate of parastomal hernia [1, 27]. This was in two retrospective studies associated with a lower rate of parastomal herniation than the conventional route. These results have been challenged by others though, and the technique does not seem to have become widely used [20, 42].

To bring out the stoma through the rectus abdominis muscle has in two retrospective studies been associated with a lower rate of parastomal hernia than if brought out lateral to the muscle [25, 43]. Four other retrospective studies did not confirm these findings [3, 26, 27, 44]. There are no randomized studies available to settle this matter, but it is nevertheless probably wise to bring out enterostomas through the rectus muscle. This is obviously not associated with any disadvantages and placing the stoma as close to the midline as possible facilitates patients' stoma care.

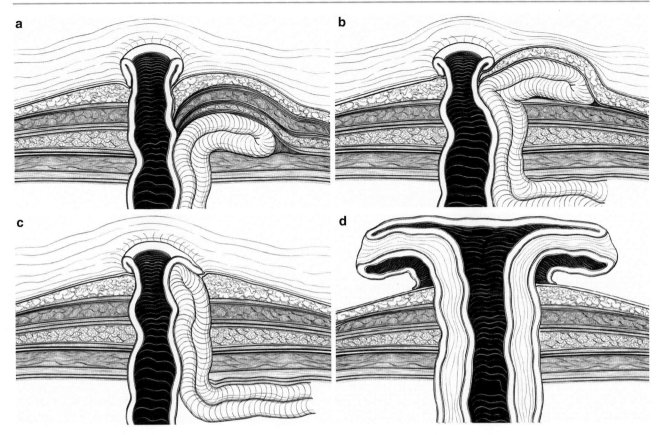

Fig. 23.2 There are four subtypes of parastomal hernia. (**a**) Interstitial. With a hernial sac lying within the muscle/aponeurotic layers of the abdominal wall. This may contain omentum, small or large intestine. In these cases the stoma is asymmetrical and is edematous and cyanotic if its vascular supply is compromised. (**b**) Subcutaneous. With herniation alongside the stoma with a subcutaneous sac containing omentum or bowel. This is the commonest form of paracolostomy hernia and not infrequently colon situated just proximal to the stoma is found in the sac. (**c**) Intrastomal. This is a problem of spout ileostomies only. A loop of intestine may herniate alongside the stoma and lie between the emergent and the everted layer of the stoma. (**d**) Perstomal or prolapse. A prolapsed stoma contains a hernial sac within itself; other viscera, especially small gut, can enter this sac and even become strangulated

Making a too large opening in the abdominal wall for the ostomy is often claimed to be the main risk factor for the development of parastomal hernia. There is actually no clinical data to support this assumption, but it nevertheless appears wise to make the opening just large enough to allow the bowel to pass through. Surgeons probably do not intentionally create a disproportionately large opening in the abdominal wall. A large opening and hence a possibly higher proportion of herniation may be more related to a bulky bowel necessitating a large opening. Fixating the mesentery or suturing the bowel to the aponeurosis has been attempted as means to lower herniation rates. Such measures can be disregarded as they have not had any effect on the rate of parastomal hernia developing [12, 27, 28, 45].

Other risk factors for parastomal hernia formation which should be taken into consideration include wound infection, old age, obesity, corticosteroid use, chronic respiratory disorders, and malnutrition [1, 20, 44, 46, 47].

Prevention of Parastomal Hernias

The most promising results in the attempt to prevent the development of parastomal hernia have been with a prophylactic prosthetic mesh placed at stoma formation. There are two randomized controlled trials available that together have randomized 108 patients to either a conventional enterostomy through the rectus abdominis muscle or to the same procedure with the addition of a mesh placed in a sublay position [8, 23]. Taken together, they report a parastomal hernia rate after 12 months of 10% with a prophylactic mesh and 45% without a mesh. One of these trials has also reported results after 5 years, and at that time the herniation rate was 13% with a prophylactic mesh and 81% without a mesh [21]. This encouraging effect on the rate of parastomal hernia with a prophylactic mesh was achieved without any increased rate of infection or any complications related to the mesh. In particular no infection of the mesh occurred.

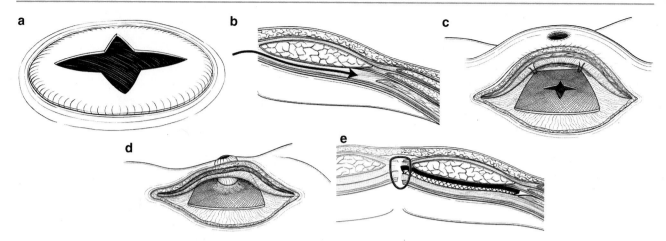

Fig. 23.3 Steps taken when placing a prophylactic mesh at stoma formation. (**a**) A circular excision of the skin is made and it is dissected through the subcutaneous tissue down to the anterior rectus aponeurosis. A cross is cut in the aponeurosis above the center of the rectus abdominis muscle. (**b**) Corresponding to the stoma site peritoneum and the posterior rectus sheath is opened along the midline for a length of more than 10 cm. Dissection is continued to the lateral border of the rectus muscle in the avascular plane dorsal to the rectus muscle. (**c**) A mesh 10 by 10 cm with a cross cut in its center is placed in the plane created. The lateral corners of the mesh are anchored to the dorsal rectus sheath with single stitches. (**d**) The bowel is brought out through the opening in the dorsal rectus sheath, the cross cut in the mesh, the split in the rectus muscle, the cross cut in the anterior rectus sheath, and the skin opening. (**e**) The medial corners of the mesh are anchored as the running suture in the anterior rectus aponeurosis incorporates also peritoneum and the mesh. Along the mesh every other stitch in the aponeurosis includes peritoneum thereby averting bowel coming into contact with the mesh

It may in view of the similarities between incisional hernias and ostomies appear rational to use a prophylactic mesh when creating a stoma. An incisional hernia is defined as intra-abdominal contents protruding through a defect in the abdominal wall. In constructing an ostomy the surgeon creates a defect in the abdominal wall for the bowel to pass through, which according to the definition produces a hernia. Therefore, the high rates of parastomal hernia encountered without a prophylactic mesh are perhaps not surprising. If ostomies are regarded as intentionally created hernias, it seems logical that parastomal herniation can be prevented in the same way as incisional hernias are repaired, i.e., with a mesh.

In the randomized trials employing a prophylactic mesh in open surgery, the abdominal cavity was accessed through the midline (Fig. 23.3). The skin at the stoma site was grasped with a clamp and a circular excision of the skin was made. After dissection through the subcutaneous tissue a cross was cut in the anterior rectus sheath.

Corresponding to the intended stoma site, peritoneum and the posterior rectus sheath were opened along the midline for a length appropriate to contain a mesh of 10 by 10 cm. Dissection was continued in the avascular plane dorsal to the rectus muscle until the lateral border of the muscle was reached.

A partly absorbable low-weight large-pore mesh was cut to 10 by 10 cm and a cross was cut in its center—just large enough to let the bowel pass through. The mesh was placed in the retromuscular plane created and the upper and lower lateral corners were anchored to the dorsal rectus sheath with single absorbable stitches.

Peritoneum and the dorsal rectus sheath were then opened by a cross incision at the intended stoma site. The stapled bowel end was first brought out through the opening in the dorsal rectus sheath and then through the opening in the mesh. The length of the bowel and the size of the opening in the mesh could then be checked and adjusted. Lastly the bowel was brought out through a split made in the center of the rectus muscle and through the openings previously made in the anterior aponeurosis and skin. The bowel was opened and sutured with a running absorbable monofilament suture with stitches placed 2–3 mm from the skin edge and with seromuscular bites in the bowel.

The medial corners of the prophylactic mesh were anchored and measures were taken to prevent the mesh unnecessarily coming into contact with abdominal contents. This was accomplished when closing the midline incision with a continuous suture technique using a slowly absorbable or nonabsorbable monofilament suture in the anterior rectus aponeurosis. Then the medial upper and lower corners of the prosthetic mesh were anchored as the running suture in the aponeurosis incorporated also the mesh and peritoneum. Along the length of the mesh every second or third stitch in the aponeurosis also included peritoneum—thereby preventing bowel from coming into contact with the mesh.

A low-weight large-pore mesh with a reduced polypropylene content and a high proportion of absorbable material in a sublay position at the primary operation has reduced the rate of parastomal hernia in two randomized trials. Experiences with a prophylactic mesh used in routine surgical practice have been reported by Jänes. In 93 consecutive

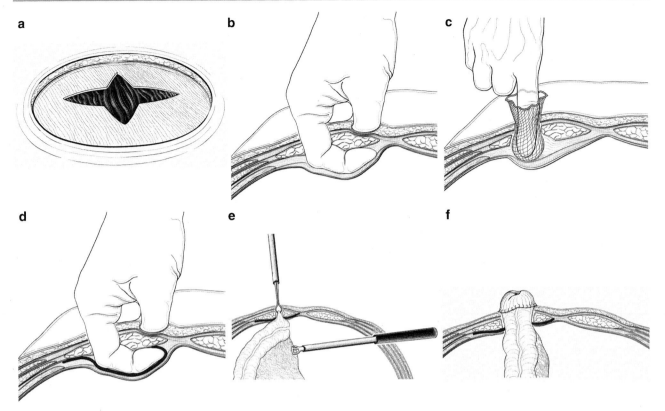

Fig. 23.4 Steps taken when placing a prophylactic mesh at laparoscopic stoma formation. (**a**) A circular excision of the skin is made and it is dissected through the subcutaneous tissue down to the anterior rectus aponeurosis. A cross is cut in the aponeurosis above the center of the rectus abdominis muscle. (**b**) The rectus muscle is split and with the index finger and a space is created bluntly in the avascular plane dorsal to the rectus muscle. (**c**) A mesh 10 by 10 cm is inserted via the skin opening. (**d**) The mesh is with the index finger spread out and positioned into the sublay position in the retromuscular space. (**e**) The sigmoid colon is held with a laparoscopic clamp close to the peritoneum at the intended stoma site. The peritoneum is then opened and as the abdomen exsufflates the colon is grabbed with a clamp inserted through the skin opening. The sigmoid colon is gently pulled through the mesh and the layers of the abdominal wall. (**f**) A running monofilament absorbable suture attached the bowel to the skin

ostomies most patients could be provided with a prophylactic mesh in a sublay position. In less than 10% of patients a mesh could not be utilized due to severe scarring of peritoneum or the abdominal wall after previous surgery. Emergency stomas in severely contaminated abdomens are probably at particularly high risk of developing a parastomal hernia. In dirty wounds with fecal peritonitis a prophylactic mesh was used in 19 patients and no infection of the mesh occurred in these patients. The rate of surgical site infection was actually lower in the group of patients provided with a mesh than in others. The higher rate of wound infection when a mesh was omitted was probably an effect of patient selection or some other bias, but it seems safe to conclude that a prophylactic low-weight large-pore mesh can be placed in severely contaminated environments.

Ostomies are sometimes formed by a laparoscopic approach. Dissection and division of the bowel is then performed laparoscopically and the bowel is brought out through an opening made in the abdominal wall with an open technique. There is no reason to assume the rate of parastomal hernia to be lower with a laparoscopic technique than with an open. Thus, there is an indication for a prophylactic mesh to be used when stomas are created with a laparoscopic technique.

The laparoscopic dissection starts by mobilizing the bowel and creating an appropriate length of the bowel before it is divided with a cutting linear stapler (Fig. 23.4). With an open technique the skin at the stoma site is grasped with a clamp and a circular excision of the skin is made. After dissection through the subcutaneous tissue a cross is cut in the anterior rectus sheath and muscle fibers are split in the center of the rectus muscle. With the index finger through this opening blunt dissection creates a space in the avascular plane dorsal to the rectus muscle. A low-weight large-pore mesh is cut to a 10 by 10 cm and is pushed through the skin opening with the index finger positioning it in the retromuscular space created. A cross is cut in the center of the mesh and peritoneum. As peritoneum is opened the abdomen will exsufflate. The bowel end that is held close to the opening with a laparoscopic clamp is then extracted through the mesh with a clamp inserted through the skin opening. This method has produced similar rates of parastomal hernia (10%) in 20 consecutive patients as with a prophylactic mesh utilized in open surgery.

There are also a number of clinical reports with the use of a prophylactic mesh in nonrandomized studies. In 1986 Bayer was the first to place a prophylactic mesh in a sublay position and reported no recurrence in 43 patients with up to 4 years of follow-up [48]. Also Marimuthu did not report any recurrence in 18 patients within 6–28 months [9]. With a prophylactic mesh placed in an onlay position Gögenur reported two parastomal hernias within 2–26 months in 24 patients [49]. A mesh was designed especially to be used as an IPOM with a flat portion and a funnel arising for the bowel to pass through. With this mesh as a prophylactic mesh in an IPOM position Berger reported no parastomal hernias or any other complications in 22 ostomies within 2–19 months [50].

Principles of Surgical Management of Parastomal Hernias

Surgical repair has been reported to be indicated in about 30% (11–70%) of patients with a parastomal hernia [5]. An accurate diagnosis and assessment of the anatomy of the hernia is essential. Therefore, the patient must be examined (a) recumbent and relaxed; (b) recumbent with the muscles tense—most easily achieved by elevating their legs; (c) in the erect position; and (d) in the erect position with the muscles tense. Investigation of the detailed anatomy with CT scanning is useful to delineate large parastomal defects in the abdominal wall and their relation to any concomitant incisional hernia. CT scanning can also detect small impalpable defects around ileostomies that present with dysfunction [51].

An accurate assessment of the anatomy of the hernia should be made. Alternative stoma sites should be considered if relocation of the stoma is needed. Care must be taken if a decision to resite a stoma is made—the help of a stoma care nurse (enterostomal therapist) is invaluable.

The patient who has had cancer surgery must be screened for recurrence before surgery is advised. Similarly, it is prudent to exclude recrudescent inflammatory bowel disease before undertaking operation in patients with ileostomies although it should be noted that the risk of para-ileostomy herniation is similar in patients with ulcerative colitis and Crohn's disease. An additional consideration that has become more commonplace is the life expectancy of the patient. An increasing number of patients of an advanced age are being seen with multiple medical problems that add to the risk of general anesthesia. If these illnesses will significantly shorten the life of the patient (e.g., less than 2–3 years) or if these

prohibit anesthesia, then one may not wish to proceed if there is no immediate need for surgical intervention.

Surgery is imperative in all cases of intestinal obstruction or strangulation related to parastomal hernia. Urgent emergency surgery is also absolutely indicated in all cases of paracolostomy hernia where perforation has occurred during irrigation.

Surgery is the treatment of choice when a parastomal hernia causes abdominal wall distortion and difficulties with fitting an appliance or irrigating a stoma. Surgery should also be considered if the stoma has become out of the patient's range of vision or if its site on a hernia bulge makes it unmanageable to elderly patients, especially those with arthritis. The disfigurement caused by a bulging parastomal hernia may warrant surgery for cosmetic reasons. In special circumstances, the repair may need to be accompanied by an abdominoplasty to permit a good fit of the appliance. In some instances local liposuction at the stoma site may reduce problems with stoma care.

Contraindications to surgery include such general problems as cardiorespiratory failure, recurrent Crohn's disease, extreme obesity, disseminated malignancy, or a short life expectancy from any disease process.

Preoperative cleansing of the colon is probably not indicated when repairing parastomal hernias. Randomized trials have shown that in colonic surgery there is nothing to be gained by subjecting patients to exhausting preoperative colonic cleansing [52]. There is no similar trial available concerning parastomal hernia repair specifically, but it seems reasonable to extrapolate findings in general bowel surgery into this field. Similarly there are no specific studies at hand concerning the use of antibiotic prophylaxis, but it is probably wise to administer prophylactic antibiotics adhering to the same principles that have been shown to be beneficial for bowel surgery in general.

Repairing Parastomal Hernias

There are several reports on attempts to repair parastomal hernias by a local procedure. The stoma is then mobilized locally, the peritoneal sac identified and its contents reduced, and the peritoneum is closed. The musculo-aponeurotic defect is closed with nonabsorbable sutures in an attempt to narrow the aperture. Results have been very poor and the method today must be regarded as obsolete. Local aponeurotic repair should not be performed since it produces an unacceptable high recurrence rate reported in the range of 50–76% [42, 47, 53–56].

Stoma relocation either with formal laparotomy or with limited transperitoneal transfer of the stoma has also been tried when treating parastomal hernias. However, relocation of the stoma into another quadrant produces a recurrence rate

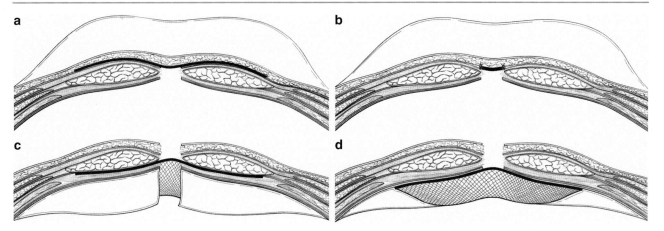

Fig. 23.5 Repairing parastomal, the mesh can be placed in an onlay, an inlay, a sublay, or an intraperitoneal onlay position. (**a**) An onlay mesh is placed anterior to the anterior rectus aponeurosis. The mesh overlap must be considerable (5–10 cm) and the mesh firmly fixated to the aponeurosis. (**b**) An inlay mesh fits the abdominal wall defect and is sutured to wound edges. This method produces inferior results.

(**c**) A sublay mesh is placed dorsal to the rectus muscle and anterior to the posterior rectus sheath. The mesh overlap must be at least 5 cm. (**d**) An intraperitoneal onlay mesh (IPOM) is placed on the peritoneum from within the abdominal cavity. The overlap must be more than 5 cm, and the mesh surface facing the abdominal cavity must not cause adhesions

at the new site that is at least as high as after the primary enterostomy and recurrence rates of 24–86% are reported [47, 53, 55, 57, 58]. If the stoma is relocated a second time, the recurrence rates are further increased [47]. Caution should be exercised when considering relocation of a stoma into a quadrant on the same side of the abdominal wall since this is associated with a higher risk of recurrence [55].

A matter of concern after relocation of an ostomy is that the defect in the abdominal wall at the parastomal hernia site may be very large. Suture repair of the defect has produced a high rate of incisional hernia at this site and Cingi reported six hernias in 23 patients on physical examination and in 11 detected with ultrasound [22]. Thus, the abdominal wall defect at a parastomal hernia site must—as with all other large abdominal wall defects—be repaired with a mesh technique.

Relocating the stoma into another quadrant is possibly a better option if a prophylactic sublay mesh is placed at the new site. This can be done in combination with a sublay mesh repair of the abdominal wall defect at the primary stoma site. This method has been reported in one nonrandomized series with no recurrence detected in 13 patients after 12 months [59].

Mesh Repair of Parastomal Hernias

There is no doubt that mesh repair has become a well-established method for repairing incisional hernias and is now evolving as the method of choice also for repairing parastomal hernias. Meshes can be placed in an onlay, an inlay, a sublay, or an intraperitoneal onlay position (IPOM) (Fig. 23.5). The mesh must be placed with considerable overlap and in all directions extend at least 5 cm beyond the edge of the abdominal wall defect. Clinical reports consistently state better results with mesh repair than with suture repair or relocation of the stoma. As of yet randomized studies comparing mesh techniques and other techniques for the repair of parastomal hernias are lacking as is also long-term follow-up.

For mesh repair of parastomal hernias all available types of meshes have been tried and results have been reported. This includes nonabsorbable, absorbable, partly absorbable, and acellular collagen matrix meshes. Polypropylene meshes and low-weight large-pore meshes can be placed in a contaminated environment without major complications [6, 60, 61]. There is a risk of inducing a major inflammatory tissue response when placing mesh in contact with bowel, and this may cause fistula formation, adhesions, and septic complications. With the IPOM technique a mesh constructed in two layers is therefore usually used. The surface facing the abdominal contents is of a nonreactive material so that adhesions are not formed. When ePTFE is used for this nonadhesive surface, there is a high risk of infection in contaminated areas and if an infection occurs the mesh must be removed.

Placement of an onlay mesh in the subcutaneous plane involves mobilization of the stoma and fixation of the prosthesis to the external oblique, after threading the stoma through a window in the prosthesis. The advantage of subcutaneous placement is that a laparotomy may not be required. The disadvantage of this and other local techniques is the risk of contamination if the stoma has to be sealed and repositioned. No matter how the stoma is sealed, there is a risk of contamination and of subsequent sepsis. If a septic complication occurs, troublesome sinuses may follow and warrant removal of the mesh. However, modern polypropylene mesh

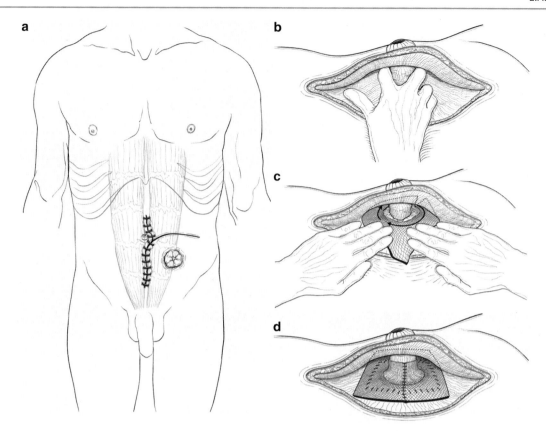

Fig. 23.6 Technique of subcutaneous parastomal hernia repair. (**a**) The old midline incision is opened, and well above the stoma the incision can be extended laterally. (**b**) The stoma is approached in the subcuta-neous layer. (**c**) The sac is reduced and the mesh introduced. (**d**) The mesh surrounds the stoma and is fixed by quilting sutures to the under-lying external aponeurosis

is tolerant of sepsis and simple local infection will usually settle with the prosthesis remaining in place.

The sublay technique places the mesh around the stoma in the plane between the posterior rectus sheath or peritoneum and the parietal muscles.

An IPOM can be placed with either an open or a laparo-scopic technique. Then the surface facing abdominal con-tents should be of a nonreactive material so that adhesions are not formed. The ePTFE mesh has previously been com-monly used although it is very prone to infection in contami-nated areas and if an infection occurs the mesh must be removed. There are today several meshes available that alleg-edly provide a nonadhesive surface towards the intestines.

The laparoscopic approach offers the surgeon the ability to visualize the entire abdominal wall so that any incisional hernias may also be repaired at the same time. This tech-nique requires that the prosthetic biomaterial be placed in the intraperitoneal position. The laparoscopic approach is described into detail in Chap. 24.

Technique of Subcutaneous Prosthetic Repair

An adherent wound drape is used to occlude the stoma and restrict contamination. A midline incision is made and extended 10 cm cranially to stoma and may also be extended laterally to enable dissection around the hernia (Fig. 23.6). The incision is deepened to the aponeurosis. The sac is found, opened, and its contents reduced. The peritoneum is closed. A sheet of polypropylene mesh is prepared with a hole in it to allow the egress of the stoma and a cut is made in the mesh so that it can be positioned. The mesh is intro-duced around the stoma and quilted down to the aponeuro-sis. The cut made in the mesh to enable it to be placed around the stoma is sutured with a nonabsorbable monofilament suture. The mesh should extend at least 5 cm outside the margins of the aponeurotic defect and is fixed by quilting sutures to the external aponeurosis. If possible, a cuff of mesh should surround the emergent stoma. Suction drains may be inserted.

Technique of Extraperitoneal Prosthetic Repair

The patient is prepared with the stoma sealed with an adherent plastic film. The original laparotomy scar is reopened. A plane of dissection is opened between the posterior sheath or peritoneum and the parietal muscles lateral to the stoma. During this dissection, the hernial contents are reduced, if possible without opening the hernia sac. This may not be possible. If the peritoneum is opened, it is closed carefully around the stoma so that the mesh can be introduced into the extraperitoneal plane (Fig. 23.7).

A sheet of polypropylene mesh is prepared, to repair the defect, with a hole in it to allow the egress of the stoma. A cut is made in the mesh so that it can be positioned. The polypropylene should fit snugly around the efferent bowel and should overlap the margins of the defect by at least 5 cm. The polypropylene is quilted into place. Suction drains may be positioned. If there is any defect in the main wound, the margin of the mesh is extended medially to overlap and repair this defect.

The Sugarbaker Technique of Open IPOM Repair

Repair in this fashion has been described by Sugarbaker and utilizes the old laparotomy incision for access to the abdominal cavity [62, 63]. Berger has developed a modified version of this method in laparoscopic repair of parastomal hernias [64, 65]. The ostomy is covered by a plastic adhesive drape to seal this site and minimize the potential for contamination. The abdomen is entered and the contents of the hernia are dissected free from the edges of the aponeurotic defect. Care must be taken to preserve the vascular supply to the bowel during this dissection. It is not necessary to dissect or remove the peritoneal sac of the hernia itself. An accurate measurement of the defect will allow the appropriate sizing of the biomaterial. A minimum of a 5-cm overlap is probably mandatory (Fig. 23.8).

The prosthesis can be fixed to the abdominal wall in a variety of methods. It is usually helpful if the colon is sutured to the lateral abdominal wall by either permanent or absorbable sutures. The mesh should be positioned to provide the necessary amount of overlap so that the intestine is "lateralized" in relation to the exit of the stoma. The biomaterial will be more easily fixed at this point by the use of tacks. The use of additional sutures provides the most assurance that the biomaterial will achieve permanent fixation. These can be placed intraperitoneal to avoid the possibility of contamination of the operative field by the contents of the ostomy.

The results reported by the above open technique in the limited number of seven patients were favorable [63]. There were no recurrences or complications after 4–7 years of follow-up. The importance of this technique today is its impact on the development of recent laparoscopic techniques.

Technique of Stoma Relocation

The new stoma site must be precise and careful. One in the lower abdomen overlying the contralateral rectus muscle and away from old incisions and skin creases is preferred. Commonly the location will be at the precise contralateral abdominal location. Preoperative consultation with the enterostomal nurse is essential to the identification of the ideal location and the site will be marked at that time.

A problem, which should be foreseen, is distortion of the abdominal wall by surgery after the operation has begun. The laxity of the musculature caused by anesthetic paralysis and the positioning of the patient on the operating table can result in a significant change in the habitus of the patient. Additionally the operative manipulation of the skin and muscle can result in lateral undermining of the tissues, which can eventuate in a poorly constructed stoma.

The ostomy is covered by a plastic adhesive drape to seal this site and minimize the potential for contamination. Approaching the operation via a midline laparotomy incision greatly facilitates the operation. The stoma is straightened out from the abdominal cavity; an everted ileostomy is uneverted, and then closed. The easiest way of closing the bowel is using one of the linear stapling devices available. This will avoid any contamination and generally results in a closed ostomy that is easy to manipulate. Theoretically, the exposed end of the staple row can be a source of infectivity and one can cover the end of the staple line with gauze if desired. The short cut off bowel end distal to the staple line is left until the operation is completed, wounds have been closed and draped, and is then easily excised through the stoma opening. This part of the bowel is most often expendable as scarring and distortion makes it useless for a new ostomy. The circular skin defect after the stoma can be narrowed with a subcuticular absorbable monofilament purse-string suture. Although this leaves a skin defect with a diameter of up to 2 cm, late cosmetic results are very good as activated dermatomyofibrils within days will contract and markedly lessen the size of the defect. As the skin opening allows the wound to drain wound infection will be rare.

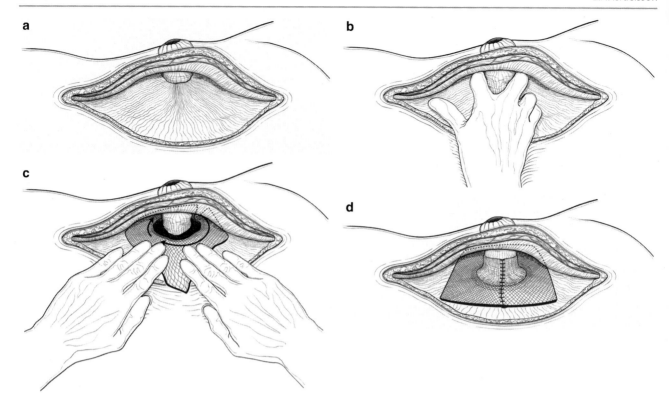

Fig. 23.7 Technique of extraperitoneal prosthetic repair. (**a**) Reopening the laparotomy incision. (**b**) Developing the extraperitoneal plane to the stoma. (**c**) Preparing the mesh to make the repair.

(**d**) Placing the polypropylene in place to the muscle layer and superficial to the peritoneum—in the extraperitoneal plane again like "ham in a sandwich"

To construct the new stoma, it is necessary to be sure of the following:

1. A very adequate length of intestine—ileum for ileostomy, colon for colostomy—must be mobilized so that the new stoma can easily be constructed with no degree of tension.
2. There is no need to close "lateral spaces" around a stoma. The stoma should be placed close to the middle of the rectus sheath; the "spaces" on either side of it are then vast and are left entirely open. Postoperative strangulation of intestine in such a large defect is unlikely.
3. A prophylactic mesh is placed in a sublay position according to the principles for a prophylactic mesh previously described. Without a prophylactic mesh recurrence rates are uncomfortably high.

A defect in the abdominal wall with a diameter of more than 2 cm usually cannot be closed by simply suturing it without a high proportion of incisional hernias developing. As the defect after a parastomal hernia is always larger than 2 cm, a mesh repair is warranted. This is the rational for combining a prophylactic mesh at the new stoma site with a large sublay mesh covering the midline incision—where a concomitant incisional hernia may be present—and the original stoma site. Provided that the midline incision can be closed and the abdominal wall defect at the primary site is not too large, one large low-weight, large-pore mesh can be used for covering all these locations. If the defects are so large that the aponeurotic edges must be sutured to the mesh, a stronger mesh should be used for the defects in the midline and at the parastomal hernia site (Fig. 23.9).

The midline is closed with a running monofilament non-absorbable or slowly absorbable suture. This suture must be with a suture length to wound length ratio of more than 4. To minimize the risk of wound infection and incisional hernia, the high suture length to wound length ratio should be achieved with many small tissue bites placed 5–8 mm from the wound edge [66]. The skin is closed with a subcuticular suture of a monofilament absorbable suture.

Postoperatively appropriate stoma care should be instituted. The general principles for fast-track abdominal surgery should be utilized with swift resumption of meals and activity together with adequate nonmorphine-based analgesics [67]. If despite these measures being taken some degree of postoperative adynamic ileus appears, it may be followed by hyperactivity of the stoma, which may necessitate intravenous fluid replacement after the operation.

Conclusions

Creating an ostomy is a common surgical procedure utilized in both elective and emergent situations. This development has been greatly facilitated by the improvement of

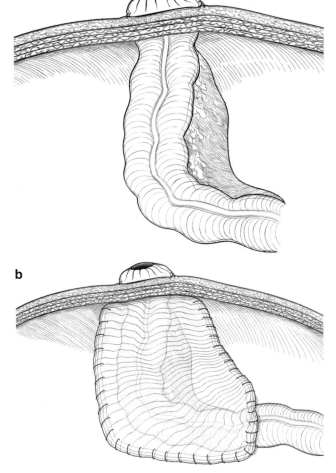

a

b

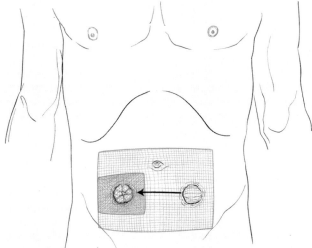

Fig. 23.9 A parastomal hernia is relocated from the left lower quadrant to the right quadrant. A low-weight large-pore mesh 10 by 10 cm is placed as a prophylactic mesh at the new stoma site. A stronger mesh covers any defect in the midline and the defect at the parastomal hernia site

Fig. 23.8 The Sugarbaker technique of open IPOM repair. (**a**) Position of the lateralized colon onto the sidewall of the abdomen prior to the placement of the biomaterial. This must usually be sutured into place to maintain this position. (**b**) Completed repair of the parastomal hernia. Note that the biomaterial covers the hernia defect as well as the lateralized intestine

modern stoma bandages that now enable an easy and reliable stoma care.

Parastomal hernia develops in 30–50% of patients supplied with an ostomy and one-third of these demand repairs.

In randomized trials a prophylactic prosthetic mesh placed in a sublay position has reduced the rate of parastomal hernia. Also in nonrandomized studies a prophylactic onlay, sublay, or IPOM has been associated with low herniation rates.

After suture repair or relocation of the stoma recurrence rates are unacceptably high. With open or laparoscopic mesh repairs considerably lower recurrence rates are reported. There are no randomized trials or long-term follow-up available presenting results with these various techniques for parastomal hernia repair.

References

1. Goligher JC. Surgery of the anus, colon and rectum. London: Baillière Tindall; 1984. p. 703–4.
2. Pearl RK. Parastomal hernias. World J Surg. 1989;13:569–72.
3. Williams JG, Etherington R, Hayward MW, Hughes LE. Paraileostomy hernia: a clinical and radiological study. Br J Surg. 1990;77:1355–7.
4. Moreno-Matias J, Serra-Aracil X, Darnell-Martin A, Bombardo-Junca J, Mora-Lopez L, Alcantara-Moral M, et al. The prevalence of parastomal hernia after formation of an end colostomy. A new clinico-radiological classification. Colorectal Dis. 2009;11:173–7.
5. Israelsson LA. Parastomal hernias. Surg Clin North Am. 2008;88:113–25.
6. Janes A, Cengiz Y, Israelsson LA. Randomized clinical trial of the use of a prosthetic mesh to prevent parastomal hernia. Br J Surg. 2004;91:280–2.
7. Cingi A, Cakir T, Sever A, Aktan AO. Enterostomy site hernias: a clinical and computerized tomographic evaluation. Dis Colon Rectum. 2006;49:1559–63.
8. Serra-Aracil X, Bombardo-Junca J, Moreno-Matias J, Darnell A, Mora-Lopez L, Alcantara-Moral M, et al. Randomized, controlled, prospective trial of the use of a mesh to prevent parastomal hernia. Ann Surg. 2009;249:583–7.
9. Marimuthu K, Vijayasekar C, Ghosh D, Mathew G. Prevention of parastomal hernia using preperitoneal mesh: a prospective observational study. Colorectal Dis. 2006;8:672–5.
10. Helgstrand F, Gogenur I, Rosenberg J. Prevention of parastomal hernia by the placement of a mesh at the primary operation. Hernia. 2008;12:577–82.
11. Kald A, Juul KN, Hjortsvang H, Sjodahl RI. Quality of life is impaired in patients with peristomal bulging of a sigmoid colostomy. Scand J Gastroenterol. 2008;43:627–33.
12. Makela JT, Turko PH, Laitenen ST. Analysis of late stomal complications following ostomy surgery. Ann Chir Gynaecol. 1997;86:305–10.
13. Hasegawa H, Yoshioka K, Keighley MR. Randomized trial of fecal diversion for sphincter repair. Dis Colon Rectum. 2000;43:961–4; discussion 4–5.

14. Steele SR, Lee P, Martin MJ, Mullenix PS, Sullivan ES. Is parastomal hernia repair with polypropylene mesh safe? Am J Surg. 2003;185:436–40.

15. Arumugam PJ, Bevan L, Macdonald L, Watkins AJ, Morgan AR, Beynon J, et al. A prospective audit of stomas—analysis of risk factors and complications and their management. Colorectal Dis. 2003;5:49–52.

16. Kronborg O, Kramhohft J, Backer O, Sprechler M. Late complications following operations for cancer of the rectum and anus. Dis Colon Rectum. 1974;17:750–3.

17. Burns FJ. Complications of colostomy. Dis Colon Rectum. 1970; 13:448–50.

18. Abrams BL, Alsikafi FH, Waterman NG. Colostomy: a new look at morbidity and mortality. Am Surg. 1979;45:462–4.

19. Guenaga KF, Lustosa SA, Saad SS, Saconato H, Matos D. Ileostomy or colostomy for temporary decompression of colorectal anastomosis. Cochrane Database Syst Rev. 2007:CD004647.

20. Devlin HB, Kingsnorth AN. Parastomal hernia. In: Devlin HB, Kingsnoth A, editors. Management of abdominal hernias. 2nd ed. London: Butterworths; 1998. p. 257–66.

21. Janes A, Cengiz Y, Israelsson LA. Preventing parastomal hernia with a prosthetic mesh: a 5-year follow-up of a randomized study. World J Surg. 2009;33:118–21.

22. Cingi A, Solmaz A, Attaallah W, Aslan A, Aktan AO. Enterostomy closure site hernias: a clinical and ultrasonographic evaluation. Hernia. 2008;12:401–5.

23. Janes A, Cengiz Y, Israelsson LA. Preventing parastomal hernia with a prosthetic mesh. Arch Surg. 2004;139:1356–8.

24. Burgess P, Matthew VV, Devlin HB. A review of terminal colostomy complications following abdominoperineal resection for carcinoma. Br J Surg. 1984;71:1004.

25. Eldrup J, Wied U, Bishoff N, Moller-Pedersen V. Parakolostomihernier. Incidens og relation till stomiens placering. Ugeskr Laeger. 1982;144:3742–3.

26. Ortiz H, Sara MJ, Armendariz P, de Miguel M, Marti J, Chocarro C. Does the frequency of paracolostomy hernias depend on the position of the colostomy in the abdominal wall? Int J Colorectal Dis. 1994;9:65–7.

27. Londono-Schimmer EE, Leong AP, Phillips RK. Life table analysis of stomal complications following colostomy. Dis Colon Rectum. 1994;37:916–20.

28. Leong AP, Londono-Schimmer EE, Phillips RK. Life-table analysis of stomal complications following ileostomy. Br J Surg. 1994;81:727–9.

29. Cheung MT. Complications of an abdominal stoma: an analysis of 322 stomas. Aust N Z J Surg. 1995;65:808–11.

30. Singh G, Wilkinson JM, Thomas DG. Supravesical diversion for incontinence: a long-term follow-up. Br J Urol. 1997;79:348–53.

31. Ho KM, Fawcett DP. Parastomal hernia repair using the lateral approach. BJU Int. 2004;94:598–602.

32. Marshall FF, Leadbetter WF, Dretler SP. Ileal conduit parastomal hernias. J Urol. 1975;114:40–2.

33. Bloom DA, Grossman HB, Konnak JW. Stomal construction and reconstruction. Urol Clin North Am. 1986;13:275–83.

34. Fontaine E, Barthelemy Y, Houlgatte A, Chartier E, Beurton D. Twenty-year experience with jejunal conduits. Urology. 1997;50:207–13.

35. Farnham SB, Cookson MS. Surgical complications of urinary diversion. World J Urol. 2004;22:157–67.

36. Wood DN, Allen SE, Hussain M, Greenwell TJ, Shah PJ. Stomal complications of ileal conduits are significantly higher when formed in women with intractable urinary incontinence. J Urol. 2004;172:2300–3.

37. Edwards DP, Leppington-Clarke A, Sexton R, Heald RJ, Moran BJ. Stoma-related complications are more frequent after transverse colostomy than loop ileostomy: a prospective randomized clinical trial. Br J Surg. 2001;88:360–3.

38. Tilney HS, Sains PS, Lovegrove RE, Reese GE, Heriot AG, Tekkis PP. Comparison of outcomes following ileostomy versus colostomy for defunctioning colorectal anastomoses. World J Surg. 2007;31:1142–51.

39. Hulten L, Kewenter J, Kock NG. [Complications of ileostomy and colostomy and their treatment]. Chirurg. 1976;47:16–21.

40. Pearl RK, Prasad ML, Orsay CP, Abcarian H, Tan AB. A survey of technical considerations in the construction of intestinal stomas. Ann Surg. 1988;51:462–5.

41. Todd IP. Intestinal stomas. London: Heinemann Medical Books; 1978.

42. Martin L, Foster G. Parastomal hernia. Ann R Coll Surg Engl. 1996;78:81–4.

43. Sjodahl R, Anderberg B, Bolin T. Parastomal hernia in relation to site of the abdominal stoma. Br J Surg. 1988;75:339–41.

44. Marks CG, Ritchie JK. The complications of synchronous combined excision for adenocarcinoma of the rectum at St Mark's Hospital. Br J Surg. 1975;62:901–5.

45. Carne PW, Robertson GM, Frizelle FA. Parastomal hernia. Br J Surg. 2003;90:784–93.

46. Leslie D. The parastomal hernia. Surg Clin North Am. 1984;64: 407–15.

47. Rubin MS, Schoetz DJ Jr, Matthews JB. Parastomal hernia. Is stoma relocation superior to fascial repair? Arch Surg. 1994;129:413–8; discussion 8–9.

48. Bayer I, Kyzer S, Chaimoff C. A new approach to primary strengthening of colostomy with Marlex mesh to prevent paracolostomy hernia. Surg Gynecol Obstet. 1986;163:579–80.

49. Gogenur I, Mortensen J, Harvald T, Rosenberg J, Fischer A. Prevention of parastomal hernia by placement of a polypropylene mesh at the primary operation. Dis Colon Rectum. 2006;49: 1131–5.

50. Berger D. Prevention of parastomal hernias by prophylactic use of a specially designed intraperitoneal onlay mesh (Dynamesh IPST). Hernia. 2008;12:243–6.

51. Toms AP, Dixon AK, Murphy JM, Jamieson NV. Illustrated review of new imaging techniques in the diagnosis of abdominal wall hernias. Br J Surg. 1999;86:1243–9.

52. Jung B, Pahlman L, Nystrom PO, Nilsson E. Multicentre randomized clinical trial of mechanical bowel preparation in elective colonic resection. Br J Surg. 2007;94:689–95.

53. Rieger N, Moore J, Hewett P, Lee S, Stephens J. Parastomal hernia repair. Colorectal Dis. 2004;6:203–5.

54. Cheung MT, Chia NH, Chiu WY. Surgical treatment of parastomal hernia complicating sigmoid colostomies. Dis Colon Rectum. 2001;44:266–70.

55. Allen-Mersh TG, Thomson JP. Surgical treatment of colostomy complications. Br J Surg. 1988;75:416–8.

56. Horgan K, Hughes LE. Para-ileostomy hernia: failure of a local repair technique. Br J Surg. 1986;73:439–40.

57. Baig MK, Larach JA, Chang S, Long C, Weiss EG, Nogueras JJ, et al. Outcome of parastomal hernia repair with and without midline laparotomy. Tech Coloproctol. 2006;10:282–6.

58. Pearl RK, Sone JH. Management of peristomal hernia: techniques of repair. In: Fitzgibbons RJ, Greenburg AG, editors. Nyhus and condon's hernia. 5th ed. Philadelphia: Lippincott Williams & Wilkins; 2002. p. 415–22.

59. Israelsson LA. Preventing and treating parastomal hernia. World J Surg. 2005;29:1086–9.

60. Vijayasekar C, Marimuthu K, Jadhav V, Mathew G. Parastomal hernia: is prevention better than cure? Use of preperitoneal polypropylene mesh at the time of stoma formation. Tech Coloproctol. 2008;12:309–13.

61. Kelly ME, Behrman SW. The safety and efficacy of prosthetic hernia repair in clean-contaminated and contaminated wounds. Am Surg 2002;68:524–8; discussion 8–9.

62. Sugarbaker PH. Prosthetic mesh repair of large hernias at the site of colonic stomas. Surg Gynecol Obstet. 1980;150:576–8.

63. Sugarbaker PH. Peritoneal approach to prosthetic mesh repair of paraostomy hernias. Ann Surg. 1985;201:344–6.

64. Berger D, Bientzle M. Laparoscopic repair of parastomal hernias: a single surgeon's experience in 66 patients. Dis Colon Rectum. 2007;50:1668–73.

65. Berger D. Parastomal hernia—persistent frustration? Hernia. 2009;13:34.

66. Millbourn D, Cengiz Y, Israelsson LA. Effect of stitch length on wound complications after closure of midline incisions: a randomized controlled trial. Arch Surg. 2009;144:1056–9.

67. Kehlet H. Fast-track colorectal surgery. Lancet. 2008;371: 791–3.

The Laparoscopic Repair of Parastomal Hernias

Dieter Berger

Introduction

The parastomal hernia is a very common complication after the creation of any ostomy [1]. Although it is generally believed that most patients with parastomal hernias do not suffer from symptoms, the contrary could be clearly shown in a recent publication [2]. In fact, more than 80% of the patients with a clinically detectable hernia have problems that interfere with their daily activities because of the hernia. Today the repair should include the use of non-resorbable meshes. Nevertheless the results of clinical studies are discouraging because of recurrence rates between 10 and 50% and a substantial frequency of wound complications [3]. However most studies only contain a limited number of patients and therefore do not allow definite conclusions.

The laparoscopic approach is gaining increasing popularity not only for the repair of incisional but also for parastomal hernias. One main advantage of the laparoscopic over the conventional approach is the reduced rate of wound complication which has been clearly demonstrated [4]. Laparoscopically the mesh is placed intraperitoneally according to Sugarbaker [5], in a keyhole fashion or using the so-called sandwich technique.

Keyhole Technique

In 2007 a group from the Netherlands published a major series using this technique [6]. An ePTFE mesh was incised, placed around the stomal loop, and closed again by sutures forming a short funnel. The results were promising; however, the observation period was only 6 weeks. An updated publication from the same group with a median observation time of 30 months revealed a recurrence rate of 37% [7]. Another study found

recurrences in 8 out of 11 patients [8]. Similarly LeBlanc et al. abandoned this approach because of a fear of the potential high failure rate, although few were seen [9]. Safadi concluded from his own results using a variety of laparoscopic techniques that laparoscopy provides only theoretical advantages [10]. McLemore et al. found two recurrences after mesh explantation in 19 patients [11]. Summarizing the results, it can be concluded that the only major series that did not provide promising results used the keyhole technique, which is also supported by smaller studies. Furthermore other studies comprising a small number of patients and incomplete or ill-defined follow-up may reveal better results.

Sugarbaker Technique

In 1985 Sugarbaker described the long-term results of seven patients treated with a mesh placed intraperitoneally, covering the stoma site, with the fascial defect, and the stomal loop [5]. Lateralizing the stomal loop between the abdominal wall and the mesh for at least 5 cm is crucial. No recurrences or any other complications have been detected. The laparoscopic adaption of that technique seems to be easy and consequently some series have been published. The recurrence rates range between 0 and 33% [8, 9, 11, 12]. However, the studies usually contain less than 20 patients. Our own experience with 41 patients treated laparoscopically according to Sugarbaker between November 1999 and April 2004 which have been consequently followed by clinical examinations was published in 2007 [13]. Despite wide parietalization and use of big meshes, the recurrence rate amounted to 20% after a median follow-up of 24 months. The common problem of the patients with a recurrence was a primarily lateral defect. The recurrence occurred laterally as well.

So in summary the laparoscopic approach according to Sugarbaker may be effective if the fascial defect is located medially but should be omitted in case of lateral defects. The studies demonstrating acceptable results mainly contain small numbers of patients and the quality of the follow-up is inconsistent or not

D. Berger (✉)
Department of General Surgery, Stadtklinik,
Balgerstrasse 50, Baden-Baden 76532, Germany
e-mail: d.berger@klinikum-mittelbaden.de

A.N. Kingsnorth and K.A. LeBlanc (eds.), *Management of Abdominal Hernias*,
DOI 10.1007/978-1-84882-877-3_24, © Springer Science+Business Media London 2013

well documented. As for the keyhole technique there is only one study with a reasonable number of patients demonstrating the weak points of the Sugarbaker technique to our knowledge.

Sandwich Technique

When we have realized that the recurrence after the Sugarbaker technique starts laterally, we decided to reinforce the complete lateral part of the abdominal wall as an added procedure. So a combination of the keyhole technique with the Sugarbaker approach was developed. Basically the keyhole mesh should reinforce the lateral part, and a larger onlay mesh will also cover the midline.

The technique follows well-known principles of the laparoscopic repair of incisional hernias. Usually the pneumoperitoneum is created using an open approach subcostally in the right anterior axillary line. Three additional trocars at the level of the umbilicus and in the right lower and left upper quadrant will be needed in cases with an ostomy in the left lower quadrant. If there is an enterostomy in the right lower quadrant, we would start in the left anterior axillary line. We always use a 30° laparoscope. The details of our technique are given in the figures. Primarily a complete adhesiolysis of the abdominal wall is performed not to miss any incisional defects. Figure 24.1 demonstrates the parastomal defect. Figure 24.2 shows the opened space of Retzius. We prepare the prevesical space in all cases in order to allow a major overlap of the lower midline incision, which is utilized in almost all cases during the primary procedure. As shown in our publications most patients not only have parastomal but also incisional hernias [13, 14]. The ligamentum teres hepatis (Fig. 24.3) must be dissected to provide firm fixation of the upper edge of the mesh. A 15×15 cm mesh is incised in a keyhole fashion and placed around the stomal loop as shown in Figs. 24.4 and 24.5. The central hole has a diameter of 1–1.5 cm. The incision is closed by two transfascial sutures and tacks which allow the adjustment of the central hole to the diameter of the stomal loop which may differ due to the amount of fatty tissue of the mesocolon. Figures 24.6 and 24.7 demonstrate the placement of the mesh according to Sugarbaker before and after fixation with tacks. The stomal loop is well parietalized between the two meshes, and the incision in the lower and upper abdominal wall is covered due to the extensive dissection of the prevesical space and the ligamentum teres hepatis.

The sandwich technique requires meshes that will be incorporated even after overlapping each other. So microporous products containing expanded polytetrafluoroethylene (ePTFE) should not be used. To our knowledge, no experimental data exists that examines the postoperative course when covered meshes are placed with an overlap.

The availability of an open mesh structure without any coverage allowing overlap and incorporation as well as prevention

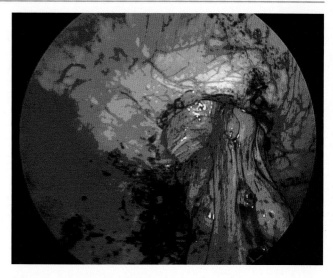

Fig. 24.1 Fascial defect of the parastomal hernia

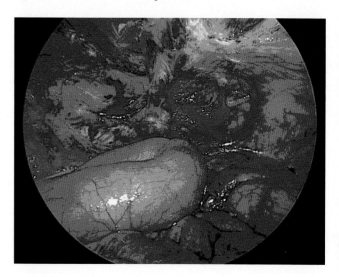

Fig. 24.2 Opened prevesical space showing the symphysis and the pubic bones

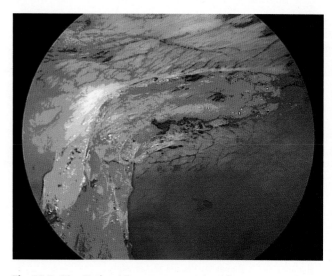

Fig. 24.3 The dissected ligamentum teres hepatis

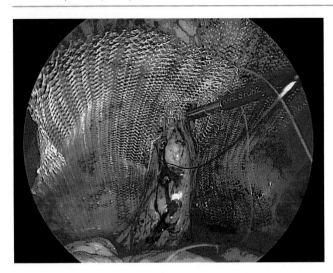

Fig. 24.4 The keyhole mesh is placed around the stomal loop showing the two transfascial sutures

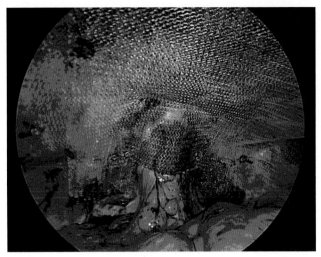

Fig. 24.7 Final intraperitoneal view of the sandwich technique

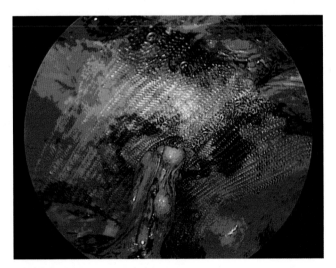

Fig. 24.5 Finally closed keyhole mesh

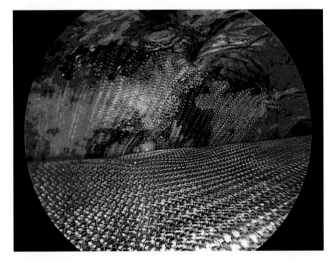

Fig. 24.6 Sugarbaker mesh widely covering the stoma place and the midline

of intra-abdominal adhesions (Dynamesh®) was the inevitable prerequisite of our technique. After a median observation time of 12 months the first 25 patients did not have any recurrences [13]. The second publication summarizing 47 patients after a median follow-up of 20 months described 1 recurrence [14]. Two patients developed an early stenosis of the stomal loop at the fascial level. These patients had predominantly subcutaneous prolapse which is usually located laterally, resulting in a sharp kink at the fascial level and the keyhole mesh. A local revision and shortening of the subcutaneous stomal loop solved the problem. It must be pointed out that the laparoscopic treatment of a subcutaneous prolapse is very difficult if not impossible.

One abscess of the hernia sac occurred which healed after VAC therapy. A deep wound infection after local revision because of a stomal stenosis again healed despite involved meshes! The total morbidity is extensively shown in the original publication and seems to be higher than in cases with incisional hernias. But the complication rate seems to be acceptable with respect to the complexity of parastomal hernia repair.

According to our own data not yet published comprising 60 patients after the sandwich technique, which were treated up to June 2009, the complication rate has remained low and no further recurrence has been observed. The median observation time approaches 30 months. In two patients we had to convert to an open procedure and another patient developed stomal stenosis. The stenosis was also treated in the manner described above.

Discussion

The parastomal hernia represents a common complication after stoma formation. Despite the fact that most patients with a clinically detectable hernia also suffer from symptoms only a small number of patients will be treated surgically. This may be explained by the high rate of recurrences and further complications even in recent studies. However these as well as former publications mainly suffer from low patient numbers and unclear or not defined observation techniques and periods. The same fact passes for almost all studies dealing with the laparoscopic approach. Nevertheless the worst results in terms of a high recurrence rate will be achieved by the keyhole technique. The Sugarbaker technique may be better but recurrence rates up to 20% are clearly too high. Our experience proved the lateral part of the abdominal wall as the weak point of the Sugarbaker technique.

Our experience also showed that 62 out of 66 patients with a parastomal hernia also have an incisional hernia [13]. The stabilization of the lateral abdominal wall and the wide coverage of the midline are best provided by the combination of the keyhole and the Sugarbaker technique, the so-called sandwich technique. The recurrence rate is low with an acceptable morbidity which can be concluded from the own cohort studies with a sufficient number of patients and adequate follow-up performed clinically [13, 14].

The prerequisite of the sandwich technique is the availability of a mesh allowing incorporation despite overlapping each other. Microporous products cannot be used; meshes of pure polypropylene or polyester should not have contact with the bowel because of adhesions and fistula [15]. Our experience with a structure made by polyvinylidene fluoride since 2004 has shown no mesh-related complications in more than 600 patients with primary and secondary ventral and parastomal hernias (unpublished data). The subcutaneous prolapse remains a problem which cannot be addressed laparoscopically and causes some asymmetry of the abdominal wall even after ideal reduction and stabilization of the parastomal hernia.

Very recently a meta-analysis allowed an insight in the real future: the prophylaxis of parastomal hernia using a mesh at the time of stoma formation [16]. Today it is absolutely clear that prophylactic meshes can be effectively used in onlay, sublay, or intraperitoneal positions and dramatically reduce the frequency of parastomal hernias. Until and if this idea will be acceptable to place that kind of prophylaxis, the laparoscopic sandwich technique should be considered as an effective treatment option of the inevitable hernia that develops.

Conclusion

After the formation of an ostomy hernias will be diagnosed in up to 70% of the patients. Cases with a clinically obvious hernia usually suffer from impairing symptoms. The surgical therapy is mainly based on mesh augmentation of the abdominal wall. Laparoscopically the meshes can be used according to Sugarbaker, in a keyhole fashion, or combining both approaches (sandwich technique). The best results by far can be achieved by the sandwich technique. According to our own results, the recurrence rate amounts to 3% with an acceptable complication rate. The literature clearly shows that the keyhole approach will be followed by a high recurrence rate. The same fact passes for the Sugarbaker technique at least in our own published experience. The laparoscopically performed sandwich technique is a surgically challenging but very effective procedure with results which cannot be achieved with any other approach.

References

1. Cingi A, Cakir T, Sever A, Aktan AO. Enterostomy site hernias: a clinical and computerized tomographic evaluation. Dis Colon Rectum. 2006;49:1559–63.
2. Moreno-Matias J, Serra-Aracil X, Darnell-Martin A, Bombardo-Junca J, Mora-Lopez L, Alcantara-Moral M, et al. The prevalence of parastomal hernia after formation of an end colostomy. A new clinico-radiological classification. Colorectal Dis. 2009;11:173–7.
3. Israelsson LA. Parastomal hernias. Surg Clin North Am. 2008;88:113–25.
4. Pierce RA, Spitler JA, Frisella MM, Matthews BD, Brunt LM. Pooled data analysis of laparoscopic vs. open ventral hernia repair: 14 years of patient data accrual. Surg Endosc. 2007;21:378–86.
5. Sugarbaker PH. Peritoneal approach to prosthetic mesh repair of paraostomy hernias. Ann Surg. 1985;201:344–6.
6. Hansson BM, Bleichrodt RP, de Hingh IH. Laparoscopic parastomal hernia repair using a keyhole technique results in a high recurrence rate. Surg Endosc. 2009;23:1456–9.
7. Hansson BM, de Hingh IH, Bleichrodt RP. Laparoscopic parastomal hernia repair is feasible and safe: early results of a prospective clinical study including 55 consecutive patients. Surg Endosc. 2007;21:989–93.
8. Muysoms EE, Hauters PJ, Van Nieuwenhove Y, Huten N, Claeys DA. Laparoscopic repair of parastomal hernias: a multi-centre retrospective review and shift in technique. Acta Chir Belg. 2008;108:400–4.
9. LeBlanc KA, Bellanger DE, Whitaker JM, Hausmann MG. Laparoscopic parastomal hernia repair. Hernia. 2005;9:140–4.
10. Safadi B. Laparoscopic repair of parastomal hernias: early results. Surg Endosc. 2004;18:676–80.
11. McLemore EC, Harold KL, Efron JE, Laxa BU, Young-Fadok TM, Heppell JP. Parastomal hernia: short-term outcome after laparoscopic and conventional repairs. Surg Innov. 2007;14:199–204.
12. Pastor DM, Pauli EM, Koltun WA, Haluck RS, Shope TR, Poritz LS. Parastomal hernia repair: a single center experience. JSLS. 2009;13:170–5.
13. Berger D, Bientzle M. Laparoscopic repair of parastomal hernias: A single surgeon's experience in 66 patients. Dis Colon Rectum. 2007;50:1668–73.
14. Berger D, Bientzle M. Polyvinylidene fluoride: a suitable mesh material for laparoscopic incisional and parastomal hernia repair! A prospective, observational study with 344 patients. Hernia. 2009;13:167–72.
15. Leber GE, Garb JL, Alexander AI, Reed WP. Long-term complications associated with prosthetic repair of incisional hernias. Arch Surg. 1998;133:378–82.
16. Tam KW, Wei PL, Kuo LJ, Wu CH. Systematic review of the use of a mesh to prevent parastomal hernia. World J Surg. 2010;34:2723–9.

Complications of Laparoscopic Incisional and Ventral Hernia Repair

V.B. Tsirline, I. Belyansky, and B. Todd Heniford

Introduction

Ventral hernia repairs are among the most common operations performed by general surgeons throughout the world. In the United States, ~105,000 ventral abdominal hernias are repaired each year. Incisional hernias, most commonly resulting from a laparotomy, occur after 3–20% of operations [1–3]. Factors predisposing patients to the formation of an initial ventral hernia include obesity, advanced age, diabetes, steroid use, pulmonary disease, and infectious wound complications. Surgical approaches to ventral hernia repair have been a subject of much research and debate for many years. Existing evidence strongly supports performing tension-free hernia repairs using prosthetic devices in most patients and all hernia sizes [4]. Recurrence rates below 20% are the norm with the currently popular Rives/Stoppa/Wantz method of the prosthetic repair of a ventral hernia. The key principles of this operation are the use of a large prosthesis as an underlay, wide fascial overlap, and tension-free repair [5, 6]. The Achilles heel of this approach is the possibility of mesh infection and the frequent wound complications, ranging from 12 to 20% [2]. The minimally invasive approach takes advantage of the wide exposure and accessibility for prosthetic placement while eliminating the large incision, extensive subcutaneous dissection and tissue flaps, the need for drains, and ultimately lowering the incidence of wound complications [7]. Since the first reports of a laparoscopic ventral hernia repair more than 15 years ago, large series as well as randomized studies have been published.

This chapter focuses on the complications of ventral and incisional hernia repairs, particularly of the minimally invasive technique. As with any major surgery, the range of complications is extensive; they include cardiovascular stressors, anesthetic side effects, bleeding, deep venous thrombosis, metabolic derangements, postoperative ileus, visceral injury, infection of the superficial or deep tissues, prolonged discomfort or musculoskeletal symptoms, and even death. With the evolution of surgical methodology, material science, and healthcare economics, the primary challenges facing the surgeons have shifted from preventing hernia recurrences to avoiding infection, maximizing patient satisfaction, and expediting recovery. As the field of ventral and incisional hernia repair continues to move forward, novel solutions are likely to alter the acuity spectrum of the complications, and we discuss them in order of historical importance.

Recurrence

The ultimate success of a hernia repair is the low rate of recurrence. As stated by Sir Cecil Wakely in 1948, "A surgeon can do more for the community by operating on hernia cases and seeing that his recurrence rate is low than he can by operating on cases of malignant disease." The use of prosthetics for defects larger than 4 cm in diameter has reduced the rate of recurrence as demonstrated in multiple studies [8, 9]. In a prospective study evaluating primary tissue repair, Luijendijk and colleagues showed unacceptably high 5-year recurrence rates of 44% for defects 3–6 cm and 73% for defects 6–12 cm in diameter [10]. Hesselink and colleagues reported a 41% recurrence rate for defects greater than 4 cm and 25% recurrence with less than 4-cm sized defects repaired primarily [11]. The use of mesh has dramatically reduced these numbers. As early as the 1980s, Stoppa noted a much higher failure rate when mesh was not applied [5]. In 2000, Luijendijk et al. reported in a sentinel paper a randomized prospective multicenter trial demonstrating 3-year cumulative recurrence rates of 46% with suture repair and 23% with mesh repair,

V. B. Tsirline
Assistant Professor Department of Surgery, AA Northwestern Memorial Hospital, Northwestern University USA

I. Belyansky, MD
Surgical Specialist at Anne Arundel, Anne Arundel Medical Center Health Sciences Pavilion, Suite 600

B.T. Heniford, MD(✉)
Department of Surgery, Carolinas Laparoscopic and Advanced Surgery Program, Carolinas Medical Center, 1025 Morehead Medical Drive, Suite 300, Charlotte, NC 28204USA
e-mail: Todd.Heniford@carolinas.org

A.N. Kingsnorth and K.A. LeBlanc (eds.), *Management of Abdominal Hernias*,
DOI 10.1007/978-1-84882-877-3_25, © Springer Science+Business Media London 2013

with a 6% recurrence for defects less than 10 cm² [4]. Further refinements in technique, prosthetic reinforcement materials, fixation devices, and perhaps patient selection continued to drive down the recurrence rates. A recent report of 505 laparoscopic hernia repairs showed a 1.8% recurrence rate [12].

There is inevitable bias in the laparoscopic hernia repair literature in the era when both laparoscopic and open repairs are widely accepted. Minimally invasive surgical specialists whose training and skill are not representative of the typical general surgeon typically report the large laparoscopic series. Illustrated in a retrospective analysis of NSQIP database from 16 VA Medical Centers, 104 laparoscopic repairs had a reported recurrence rate of 21.6% over a median follow-up of 73 months (9.1% at 1 year, 18.4% at 5 years) [13]. The authors noted that only 3 of 16 sites performed more than 10 laparoscopic repairs. These were likely highly selected patients and might not represent outcomes for the broader incisional hernia repair population.

Another source of bias is that open operations often serve as a fallback strategy for laparoscopic surgeons in complicated or multiple recurrent cases, as well as being the standard of care for emergent cases. In an attempt to eliminate this bias when comparing open and laparoscopic repairs, some authors stratify their patients into open and laparoscopic arms and report a certain conversion rate for the latter while counting the complications and recurrences within each arm. However, even in the best of hands, laparoscopic completion of the operation is not always feasible due to patient comorbidities, hernia characteristics, or other intangible factors, and patients should be counseled as such. For example, in a randomized trial, Itani et al. compared laparoscopic and open hernia repairs, reporting a recurrence rate of 12.5% (8/72) in the laparoscopic arm, which included 10 conversions with 2 recurrences [14]. Therefore, laparoscopically completed repairs had a recurrence rate of only 9.7% (6/62). Carlson and colleagues analyzed over 6,000 laparoscopic ventral hernia repairs reported in the literature and found a weighted recurrence rate of 3.6% and unweighted recurrence rate of 4.3% [15]. When weighted by the inverse of the variance in each study, the mean recurrence rate was 2.7% (with a 95% confidence interval of 2.25–3.10). Recurrent hernias are usually amenable to laparoscopic repairs [16].

Risk Factors for Recurrence

With recurrence rates in the single digits, further research focus began to shift from repair methodology to the identification of risk factors that may predict recurrence or complications in a particular patient [17–19]. A large number of potential risk factors have been implicated [11, 20–23]; however, pooled analyses do not necessarily support these findings, implying significant heterogeneity in these operations. Carlson et al., in their analysis of laparoscopic hernior-

rhaphy literature, found no correlation between follow-up duration, gender, BMI, mesh type, fixation method or overlap, and the recurrence rate reported in the literature ($p = 0.12$–0.87, $N = 24$–55 studies) [15]. This lack of correlation may be due to the fact that less experienced surgeons may avoid laparoscopy on patients with these risk factors in fear of increased complications and potential for recurrence. Only randomized prospective trials can address such selection bias. The surgeon's expertise, as measured by the total case count, has been associated with improved recurrence rates [24], although the correlation is not perfect and, therefore, likely multifactorial [15]. Likewise, the defect size, mesh size, operative time, and complications all correlate with each other and together reflect the complexity of a repair, but do not appear to increase the risk of recurrence in some series [12, 25, 26]. Despite mixed evidence, most surgeons agree that significant risk factors for recurrence include wound infections (discussed separately), previous recurrence history, and a complex interplay of mechanical factors such as obesity, hernia size, fixation methods, and mesh material.

In their retrospective review of 146 cases, Bencini et al. found significantly higher recurrence in patients with prior recurrences (67 vs. 16%) and smokers (58 vs. 23%), but the latter was not an independent predictor in their model [27]. In their analysis of nine recurrences out of 505 laparoscopic repairs, Wassenaar et al. found that 8 of 9 patients had a first-time incisional hernia with no differences in age, sex, ASA score, OR time, mesh size, and hospital stay compared to the rest; 7 of 9 recurrences had no other postoperative complications. Approximately half of the recurrences had transfascial suture fixation; the others had tacks only [16].

Mesh selection, positioning, and fixation play a significant role in recurrence after laparoscopic hernia repair. The most popular and time-tested technique for intraperitoneal onlay synthetic mesh placement is transfascial suture fixation followed by tacks around the mesh perimeter [28, 29]. Variations of this technique as well as selection of mesh, sutures, and tacks are abundantly described in the literature. Berger and colleagues used sutures to position the mesh but secured solely with tacks, resulting in a 2.7% (4/147) recurrence at a mean follow-up of 15 months [30]. Several groups reported using no fixation sutures but a "double crown" (two circumferential rows) of tacks [31] resulting in 4.4% (12/270) recurrence rate at 44 months mean follow-up [32] and 3.5% (7/200) with 22.5 months follow-up [33]. Bageacu et al. reported 15% (19/121) recurrence over a mean follow-up of 49 months and attributed the high recurrence rate to inadequate mesh fixation with metallic tacks alone [18]. In fact, the pull-off strength of suture fixation of the mesh to the abdominal wall is higher compared to the tacks [34, 35].

We believe that suture fixation of the mesh in laparoscopic ventral hernia repair is helpful, especially during the early phases of mesh integration into the abdominal wall [36].

While well-placed tacks or anchors provide adequate fixation in a static abdominal wall during the operation, they have reduced holding strength compared to sutres at about 2.5 to 1 ratio. This is also consistent with the radiologic findings of much greater mesh shrinkage after tack fixation versus fixation using sutures [37, 38]. Although the greater number of tacks may divide the tension forces among fixation points, the importance of transfascial suture fixation in larger hernias is important.

The mechanics of a laparoscopic repair of ventral defects capitalizes on the intra-abdominal forces to keep the mesh against the abdominal wall—the same forces that generate the hernia in the first place. The balance of forces, large or small, keeps the mesh in place and prevents the hernia recurrence [39]. In order to maintain this equilibrium, the mesh must overlap the fascia sufficiently in all directions. The exact amount of overlap required is not known, but most experts agree that 4–5 cm is the minimum [20, 22]. This was particularly critical with the use of heavyweight polypropylene mesh, which tends to contract significantly [40], unlike the newer lightweight synthetics [37, 41]. A systematic review of literature showed that the majority (57%) of surgeons report 3.0-cm overlap and one-third (30%) employ 4–5-cm overlap.

The laparoscopic technique allows for easier placement of prosthesis with good overlap. In the open approach, attaining an overlap of three to five centimeters requires extensive soft tissue dissection with the resultant increase in wound complications such as seromas and wound infections. Recent evidence suggests that such complications may be reduced by 50% or more by the subcutaneous application of talc [42]. Larger hernia defects require more overlap, and multiple smaller "Swiss-cheese" defects theoretically need less. Multiple retrospectives studies have shown the association between Swiss-cheese defects and lower recurrence rates [43]. On the other hand, greater overlap is recommended for patients with increased risk of recurrence [20, 28]. Mesh integration into the abdominal wall plays a pivotal role in mesh fixation [44]. Biologic meshes are discussed and possess properties that make them attractive, their tendency to stretch make them less applicable to laparoscopy. [45]. Newer, heavily cross-linked xenografts were initially met with enthusiasm; however, they lack some of the tissue integration advantages of the original products. Based on the current literature and the high cost of the biomaterials ($4–31/cm^2), there is indication for their use in clean cases, although trials are underway to address this question [46].

Morbid Obesity

Obesity is a rapidly growing problem, and morbidly obese patients increasingly present for repair of ventral and incisional hernias. Body mass index >35 kg/cm^2 is a strong predictor of postoperative wound complications, and BMI >40 kg/cm^2 has been shown to increase the risk of recurrence almost fourfold [28]. The pathophysiology of this condition is complex, but increased intra-abdominal pressure, tissue laxity due to endocrine derangements, and large amounts of subcutaneous tissues contribute to the hernia repair failures [47, 48]. This higher intra-abdominal pressure creates more strain on the mesh placed for the hernia repair, which is probably responsible for the increased incidence of incisional hernia and rate of recurrence following repair. The laparoscopic approach is ideal in the obese patient due to the smaller wounds and, theoretically, decreased wound complications [49]. In order to combat the higher recurrence rate, some authors advocate placing transabdominal sutures every 4–6 cm around the mesh perimeter [43]. A wider mesh-fascial overlap is also prudent.

What You Cannot See Can Recur

Another recognized cause of recurrence following ventral hernia repair is a missed hernia. The laparoscopic approach allows the surgeon to clearly and completely define the margins of the hernia defect and to identify additional defects that may not have been clinically apparent preoperatively. Furthermore, laparoscopic visualization of the fascia from the peritoneal side permits identification of smaller defects that could be missed in an open approach [50]. Fascial defects remote from the main hernia are common; as noted by Sharma et al., 46.6% of patients had more than one defect and 16.3% had satellite defects (some containing additional hernias) located more than 3 cm away and could only be detected laparoscopically [51]. Saber et al. found that 48% of the 146 laparoscopic ventral hernia repairs had occult defects that were not detected preoperatively [52]. Laparoscopically detected occult hernias may be one of the reasons for the lower recurrence rates following laparoscopic repair. This effect is underestimated in the literature because surgeons who encounter postoperative recurrence at a location different from the site of repair are unlikely to report them as recurrences, perhaps rightfully so. A generous mesh-fascial overlap is recommended as it may incidentally cover subtle fascial weaknesses or defects in the making, which, if present at the edges of the mesh could lead to inadequate fixation and jeopardize the repair. Some laparoscopic surgeons will make a concerted effort to cover the entire length of an incision where an incisional hernia is based to prevent these types of "recurrent herniation."

Repair of occult Swiss-cheese defects is not the only cardinal advantage of laparoscopic hernioplasty. The intra-abdominal view better identifies all of the defects and allows for better prosthetic coverage. Laparoscopy is an excellent choice for recurrent hernias that have failed prior attempts at repair, in contrast to the common bias against laparoscopy in a reoperative abdomen due to the possibility of adhesions. Laparoscopic entry into the peritoneal cavity avoids dissection through the previous operative site. This technique is ideal for patients with failed preperitoneal or onlay prosthetic repairs because the dissection avoids disrupting the colonized or previously infected mesh and risking recurrent infection. However, surgeons should gauge their experience and available expertise when embarking on complex laparoscopic reconstructions of multiple previously failed repairs, because ultimately the advantages of laparoscopy for the patients should be weighed against the high risk of re-recurrence in a less than perfect repair.

Trocar site hernias are uncommon complications with a reported incidence of less than 1%. Trocar site of larger ports (10 mm and higher) are more common and require fascial closure at the initial operation, but 5-mm trocar site hernias have also been described. Trocar site hernias occur predominantly in the midline where the fascia is fused together. In contrast, laterally, the layers of the abdominal wall shift past each other closing off the port site defect; however, suture closure of the abdominal fascia is still recommended.

Pseudo-Recurrence

Bulging and pain at the site of previous ventral hernia is sometimes noted by patients after a repair. These symptoms may be produced by seromas, hematomas, retained hernia contents, a true recurrence, or bulging of the mesh into the space formerly occupied by the hernia sac. The latter is termed a pseudo-recurrence and may mimic the symptoms of a true recurrence, without the risk of incarceration or strangulation. In a way it is similar to the diastases—the weakening of the midline fascia (and lateral displacement of the rectus abdominis muscles). Wassenaar et al. reported mesh bulging in 4 of 505 patients (0.8%), which was corrected by placing a second, larger, well-stretched mesh at the site of the initial repair [12], although the necessity of surgical correction of eventrations has been challenged [53]. Generally, the occurrence of such a phenomenon is probably due to the lack of appropriate tautness of the initial repair or insufficient fixation. Both of these can be prevented with proper technique.

Conversion

Conversion of a laparoscopic procedure to open should not be considered a complication, but may be a safety measure to obtain better exposure when laparoscopy is deemed inadequate or unsafe by the surgeon. It has been said that conversion is dependent largely on the skill and comfort level of the surgeon to proceed with laparoscopic lysis of adhesions, control of hemorrhage, organ repair, or definitive exposure.

As such, conversion rates vary greatly in the literature depending on the study setting, patient selection, and procedure choice. Conversion rate data is important for research purposes and patient counseling in terms of postoperative expectations of laparoscopic versus open procedures and the relative odds of each. In their review of literature, Carlson et al. identified 180 (3.3%) conversions in 5,411 operations. The reason for conversion to an open repair was reported in 157 cases, extensive adhesions (48%) and intraoperative complications (29%) being the most common. Whether conversion to an open procedure impacts hernia repair outcomes is impossible to estimate because the predominant factor is likely to be the reason for conversion itself; cases converted from laparoscopic to open, perhaps, should be analyzed separately and not included in the open or laparoscopic category in the surgical outcomes research.

Laparoscopy

Since ventral/incisional hernias most commonly result from a previous laparotomy, the surgeon is often faced with the task of opening a reoperative abdomen. The primary objective of this step is to establish pneumoperitoneum and obtain visualization without damaging the viscera. We prefer the conservative approach of an open cutdown. The abdominal layers are incised sequentially with careful identification of the abdominal wall structures. It is prudent to enter the abdomen away from the site of the previous incision. Even when exercising proper caution, bowel injury may be unavoidable. The advantage of the cutdown technique is that the injury is may be.

On the other end of the spectrum of possible approaches to a nonvirgin abdomen is the Veress needle approach—an insertion of a small needle away from the site of the prior operation or in one of the upper quadrants. Optical trocars offer an opportunity for entry under laparoscopic visualization and have become quite popular in these operations.

Seroma

Seroma formation is not unique to the laparoscopic approach. Seromas develop above the mesh and within the retained hernia sac with the incidence of 100% when routinely confirmed with ultrasound [30]. While the majority of patients form seromas postoperatively, they resolve spontaneously without intervention after approximately 3 months after the operation. The rate of seroma formation reported in the literature typically falls within 5–25% and represents the fraction of symptomatic patients who obtain further examination or investigation. In the largest reported laparoscopic series, the seroma rate was reported at 31% prior to the use of a postoperative pressure dressing and 20.4% after its routine application. Only 5% of patients had persistent seromas beyond 3 months, and less than 0.5% had excessive symptoms or required multiple aspirations or a reoperation; the mesh was not involved. Seromas rarely result in long-term problems, but the surgeons should inform their patients preoperatively about the likelihood of a seroma and its expectant management in the absence of additional complications.

Large, persistent seromas are fortunately uncommon in laparoscopic surgery, but they can occur. Seromas are also common after open hernia repair, especially when massive subcutaneous dissections take place. The large subcutaneous seromas can place tension on the skin leading to skin necrosis and wound breakdown and are associated with higher rates of wound infection and other complications. Drains and abdominal binders are somewhat marginally effective. Recent evidence suggests that the use of subcutaneous talc may dramatically reduce seroma formation and the incidence of postoperative wound complications in open ventral hernia repairs with extensive subcutaneous dissections [54]. In contrast, after laparoscopic hernia repairs, seromas originate in the empty hernia sac [55]. There is a suggestion that cauterization of the hernia sac lining may reduce postoperative seroma rates by facilitating cavity collapse and adhesion of the surrounding tissues together to eliminate the potential space for seroma formation, but this has not be reproduced [56].

Mesh Infection

One of the major advantages of the minimally invasive approach to ventral hernia is a significant reduction in wound and mesh infectious complications [14, 57]. The open technique of ventral hernia repair has historically been associated with a high rate of cellulitis and mesh infection. In his landmark article, Dr. Stoppa reported a 12% rate of "wound sepsis" [5]. The factors leading to infection are multiple, but local factors involve extensive tissue trauma, devascularization, creation of large subcutaneous or retromuscular spaces with postoperative accumulation of stagnant fluid, prolonged intraoperative exposure to potential contaminants, tissue hypothermia, etc. Intra-abdominal placement of mesh through a trocar minimizes tissue dissection and exposure of mesh to the abdominal surface, and since the trocar is typically inserted away from the hernia site, there is less chance of a superficial wound infection extending onto the mesh [51]. Care should be taken to avoid mesh contact with the skin; this may be facilitated by the use of iodine-impregnated adhesive drapes on the abdomen [58]. Although the incidence of mesh infection after laparoscopic hernia repair is very low, the consequences can be severe.

Infections of polypropylene meshes can be managed locally with surgical drainage and excision of exposed, unincorporated segments. Meshes containing ePTFE require removal of the prosthetic material in nearly all cases [59], although there are isolated reports of successful nonoperative management [60–62]. Mesh excision is a morbid operation, which inevitably results in the recurrence of the hernia, requiring a subsequent interval operation to repair the abdominal wall defect. The risk of infection in the subsequent operation increases dramatically due to bacterial colonization of the previous infection site.

In the pooled analysis of the literature, mesh infection rates range from 0.6 to 0.8% [15, 51]. The rate may appear slightly lower in larger series, perhaps due to the small overall incidence. This percentage compares favorably with the 12–18% rate of wound complications reported with the open prosthetic repair series [63, 64]. The most compelling argument for the laparoscopic approach to incisional hernias is the minimization of soft tissue dissection and the associated reduction in the morbidity associated with local wound complications and the potential for infection of the implanted mesh.

The mechanism of prosthetic-associated wound infections is complex. The most common pathogen, Staphylococcus aureus, produces a biofilm on the surface of the foreign body to protect itself from the host defenses and systemically administered antibiotics. For this reason antibiotic prophylaxis during surgery is less effective than surgeons might hope. The orthopedic literature, however, strongly supports antimicrobial prophylaxis for implantation of prosthetic devices [65]. Other practices based mainly on surgical opinion that might decrease the risk of infection include the use of antibacterial adhesive drapes to cover the exposed skin and prevent mesh contact with residual skin flora, avoiding mesh insertion directly through the port incision, changing surgical gloves just prior to handling the mesh, and the use of an antibiotic-impregnated mesh. The details of antimicrobial mesh coating are beyond the scope of this chapter; however, evidence suggests that antimicrobial bound mesh may hold the answer to preventing wound infections from developing. Recent animal data indicate that such strategies dramatically reduce the risk of mesh infection, preserve biologic mesh integrity, and may enable successful placement of synthetic mesh in infected wounds [66].

Bowel Injury or Visceral Injury

Bowel injury is a serious complication of ventral and incisional hernia repair, which may become problematic if the injury is not recognized. Laparoscopy does not increase the risk or severity of bowel injury. The possibility of causing a visceral injury during a laparoscopic hernia repair is real. Various strategies have been suggested to minimize the risk of such complications. Sharma reported a 2.2% enterotomy rate and attributed it to utilizing sharp adhesiolysis [51], while using cautery sparingly [28].

An intraoperatively recognized enterotomy should be repaired by open or laparoscopic approach depending on the surgeon's confidence level [67]. Fluency in laparoscopic intracorporeal suturing is a requirement for a laparoscopic repair of an enterotomy. A limited laparotomy has been described where a small incision is made to control the injury, while the rest of the procedure is performed laparoscopically. When in doubt, the surgeon can convert to a laparotomy, because a missed injury may lead to peritonitis and sepsis [14] or a chronic mesh infection with or without an enterocutaneous fistula.

In contrast, prompt recognition and repair of an enterotomy without gross contamination may not prevent mesh placement, but warrants a careful risk-benefit assessment. One of the factors to consider in such cases is the mesh prosthetic material. While ePTFE may be somewhat more susceptible to infection, polypropylene-based meshes have been placed in clean-contaminated cases with a very low rate of subsequent infections [68, 69]. The development of lightweight polypropylene composite materials has promoted this trend with evidence suggesting that such meshes may withstand measurable amounts of bacterial contamination [70]. In the face of significant contamination, however, the surgeon is wise to postpone elective hernia repair. Biologic prostheses could be used, although their long-term mechanical integrity, particularly in the face of infection, is questionable. An enterotomy increases the overall rate of postoperative complications significantly as demonstrated in a large retrospective review of the VA National Surgical Quality Improvement Program (NSQIP) data [71].

Bowel Adhesions and Mesh Erosion

Adhesions form as a result of an inflammatory reaction due to tissue dissection, mechanical shear, and certain prosthetic materials. While laparoscopic surgery minimizes direct tissue handling and generally results in fewer adhesions [72], intraperitoneal mesh placement always hold potential for adhesions. Mesh material is the principal determinant of the degree of adhesions, and dozens of mesh types have been developed over the last two decades as a result of extensive research. The original polypropylene mesh revolutionized hernia repair by providing a long-term durable reinforcement vis-a-vis an inflammatory process, which stimulates fascial ingrowth. Unfortunately, it also promotes intra-abdominal adhesions. In many cases the omentum provided the natural barrier protecting the bowel [51]; however, evidence quickly accumulated of the adverse effects of polypropylene on the bowel resulting in intestinal obstructions, erosions, and fistulas [73, 74]. Polypropylene mesh was banned from the abdomen, and extraperitoneal repairs were uniformly utilized with good results. With the advent of laparoscopy, the need arose for a safe and effective intraperitoneal mesh prosthesis. Expanded polytetrafluoroethylene (ePTFE) mesh fell into favor as it produced minimal adhesions. In addition, PTFE may be more susceptible to infection than polypropylene.

The advent of lightweight polypropylene mesh provided a more balanced option of sufficient fascial integration with low intra-abdominal adhesion characteristics [75]. Many radiographic and clinical studies extensively document the presence of adhesions with intraperitoneally placed polypropylene, and many surgeons believe that it presents an unacceptable risk. However, most reports of gastrointestinal complications and mesh erosion into bowel describe cases of mass abdominal inflammation and intestinal trauma following initial implantation, compounded by the use of heavyweight polypropylene or polyester [15]. For such cases, biologic mesh products are promoted by their manufacturers, but their benefit has only been proven in contaminated cases, where infection is otherwise inevitable. For clean cases various composite meshes have been developed, including adhesive barrier-coated polymers, partially dissolving combinations of polymers, and aggregates of PTFE on one side and polypropylene on the other. There is insufficient evidence to recommend the use of one product over another; however, they all appear relatively safe and effective as does lightweight polypropylene.

There are several isolated reports of mesh erosion with the use of polyester [76, 77]; however, a composite derivative with anti-adhesive coating is felt to be safe intraperitoneally [78]. Enteric fistula after hernia repair with polypropylene mesh is a serious but, fortunately, rare complication. Individual cases have occurred between 1 and 15 years after operations involving intraperitoneal placement of prosthetic mesh [74, 79, 80]; however, the authors of large series believe their fistula complications to be the result of an occult bowel injury [15, 51].

Pain and Quality of Life

With the advancements in hernia repair techniques and materials, attention is increasingly directed to functional outcomes, quality of life measures, and aesthetics. Multiple studies over the past decade have documented improved patient satisfaction with laparoscopic compared to open repairs [31, 81, 82]. Occasionally, after laparoscopic repairs, patients experience persistent pain at the site of the transabdominal fixation sutures. This has been reported in up to 3% of cases; however, large series not using transfascial fixation have reported persistent pain in 7.4% of cases [32]. The mechanism of transfascial suture pain is poorly understood; possible explanations include intercostal nerve entrapment, local muscle ischemia, and possible mesh contraction. On the other hand, less localized pain may be due to microabrasion of the highly sensitive parietal peritoneum by a mesh that is loosely fixed.

The postoperative discomfort at the transabdominal fixation suture sites typically resolves within 6–8 weeks [31]. The first line of treatment for persistent pain is a course of nonsteroidal anti-inflammatory medications. In refractory cases injecting local anesthetic at the sites of pain carries at least a 90% success rate [83]. The needle may be blunted to provide the surgeon tactile feedback as it passes through the fascial layers. Typically reported in the literature are clinically unapparent but statistically higher pain scores with suture fixation during the first month postoperatively with no differences at 6 months and thereafter [16, 37, 82, 84, 85]. A randomized trial showed no difference in postoperative pain and quality of life scores between absorbable transfascial sutures, double crown of tacks, and nonabsorbable sutures [16].

Various measures have been used to assess satisfaction, pain, and activity after hernia repair. The most widely used assessment both for surgical and nonsurgical pain is a visual analog scale. Another more comprehensive index is the short form 36 (SF-36) questionnaire, which takes into account patient's psychological perception, emotions and attitudes, and physical capabilities. This is a widely employed scale; however, a more sensitive and specific for hernia repair outcomes is the Carolinas Comfort Scale© (CCS) popularized over the last decade [81, 86]. On a 1–5 scale, patients rate their symptoms of pain, mesh sensation, and motion limitation for common activities such as laying down, sitting, walking—a total of eight categories. Analysis of our experience showed parallel trends in all categories, with overwhelming resolution of symptoms by the 6-month follow-up.

Readmission, Reoperation, and Mortality

Thirty-day readmission may be viewed as a composite indicator of serious postoperative complications. Hospital readmissions represent an increasing financial burden to the payers, with over $15 billion in annual expenditures according to the Medicare estimates. They are also associated with considerable patient morbidity. The rates are highly dependent on the surgical procedure and the patient population. Blatnik et al. found in their experience of 221 laparoscopic ventral hernia repairs a 5% readmission rate within 30 days of surgery [87]. They identified a number of risk factors including abdominal infection, defect size, and patient comorbidities. The primary reason for readmission was wound-related complications; not surprisingly an open repair carried a much higher readmission rate of 20% (odds ratio 35:1). While Blatnik et al. identified many potential predictors, they did not report which factors were specific to the laparoscopic group. It is clear that by drastically reducing wound complications, the laparoscopic approach eliminates the majority of immediate causes of 30-day postoperative readmission. Smoking is a strong predictor and a modifiable risk factor for wound complications [88], and many surgeons postpone elective hernia repairs in active smokers.

In their review of laparoscopic ventral hernia repair literature, Carlson et al. found a 3% (162/5,163) incidence of reoperations, nearly 40% of them for recurrence. The authors caution, however, that there was no uniform definition for the cause or the time frame for reoperation. For this reason, reoperation rates of up to 25% [43] are reported in the literature; however, most studies suggest a rate of 0–3% within 30 days [89] and 8–10% long term [90, 91].

Mortality after an elective laparoscopic ventral hernia repair is uncommon, occurring in 0.2–0.7% of operations [92–94]. In the published literature we identified 16 cases of postoperative mortality: ten due to intestinal perforation, three myocardial infarctions, one pulmonary embolism, mesenteric ischemia, and end-stage liver disease. Most deaths occurred within 3 days of the operation. Over 86% of studies on laparoscopic ventral hernia repair document no operative mortality [15].

Summary

Laparoscopic ventral and incisional hernia repair is a common operation performed throughout the world. With the widespread use of mesh, recurrence rates of 2–3% are the norm, although the incidence is higher in long-term studies. Risk factors include smoking, obesity, defect size, previous recurrences, inadequate fixation, and mesh infection. The repair should involve a 3–5-cm mesh-fascial overlap, the use of transfascial fixation sutures, and meticulous sterile technique. Fortunately, wound infections are much fewer after laparoscopic than open hernia repairs, but mesh infections are still a major source of ongoing morbidity. Traditionally, these required excision; however, there is increasing evidence of mesh salvage with antibiotic therapy, particularly with the newer, lightweight polypropylene mesh. Bowel injury is the most serious complication, and surgeons should be conscious of the possibility. Cases of mesh erosion into bowel have also been reported, but significant advances in biomaterials have virtually eliminated this risk. Early mesh-related discomfort and pain are seen in up to 20% of patients, in part due to frequent seroma formation, but these issues resolve by 6 months as a rule. With the refinement of bioprosthetics and surgical techniques, expedient recovery and postoperative quality of life have become the principal outcome measures for laparoscopic ventral hernia repairs.

References

1. Carlson MA, Ludwig KA, Condon RE. Ventral hernia and other complications of 1,000 midline incisions. South Med J. 1995; 88(4):450–3.
2. Mudge M, Hughes LE. Incisional hernia: a 10 year prospective study of incidence and attitudes. Br J Surg. 1985;72(1):70–1.

3. Read RC, Yoder G. Recent trends in the management of incisional herniation. Arch Surg. 1989;124(4):485–8.

4. Luijendijk RW, et al. A comparison of suture repair with mesh repair for incisional hernia. N Engl J Med. 2000;343(6):392–8.

5. Stoppa RE. The treatment of complicated groin and incisional hernias. World J Surg. 1989;13(5):545–54.

6. Rives J, et al. Treatment of large eventrations. New therapeutic indications apropos of 322 cases. Chirurgie. 1985;111(3):215–25.

7. Sains PS, et al. Outcomes following laparoscopic versus open repair of incisional hernia. World J Surg. 2006;30(11):2056–64.

8. Arroyo A, et al. Randomized clinical trial comparing suture and mesh repair of umbilical hernia in adults. Br J Surg. 2001;88(10):1321–3.

9. Korenkov M, et al. Randomized clinical trial of suture repair, polypropylene mesh or autodermal hernioplasty for incisional hernia. Br J Surg. 2002;89(1):50–6.

10. Luijendijk RW, et al. Incisional hernia recurrence following "vestover-pants" or vertical Mayo repair of primary hernias of the midline. World J Surg. 1997;21(1):62–5. discussion 66.

11. Hesselink VJ, et al. An evaluation of risk factors in incisional hernia recurrence. Surg Gynecol Obstet. 1993;176(3):228–34.

12. Wassenaar EB, et al. Recurrences after laparoscopic repair of ventral and incisional hernia: lessons learned from 505 repairs. Surg Endosc. 2009;23(4):825–32.

13. Hawn MT, et al. Long-term follow-up of technical outcomes for incisional hernia repair. J Am Coll Surg. 2010;210(5):648–55. 655–7.

14. Itani KM, et al. Comparison of laparoscopic and open repair with mesh for the treatment of ventral incisional hernia: a randomized trial. Arch Surg. 2010;145(4):322–8. discussion 328.

15. Carlson MA, et al. Minimally invasive ventral herniorrhaphy: an analysis of 6,266 published cases. Hernia. 2008;12(1):9–22.

16. Wassenaar E, et al. Mesh-fixation method and pain and quality of life after laparoscopic ventral or incisional hernia repair: a randomized trial of three fixation techniques. Surg Endosc. 2010;24(6):1296–302.

17. Koehler RH, Voeller G. Recurrences in laparoscopic incisional hernia repairs: a personal series and review of the literature. JSLS. 1999;3(4):293–304.

18. Bageacu S, et al. Laparoscopic repair of incisional hernia: a retrospective study of 159 patients. Surg Endosc. 2002;16(2):345–8.

19. Burger JW, et al. Long-term follow-up of a randomized controlled trial of suture versus mesh repair of incisional hernia. Ann Surg. 2004;240(4):578–83. discussion 583–5.

20. Anthony T, et al. Factors affecting recurrence following incisional herniorrhaphy. World J Surg. 2000;24(1):95–100. discussion 101.

21. Sauerland S, et al. Obesity is a risk factor for recurrence after incisional hernia repair. Hernia. 2004;8(1):42–6.

22. Vidovic D, et al. Factors affecting recurrence after incisional hernia repair. Hernia. 2006;10(4):322–5.

23. Llaguna OH, et al. Incidence and risk factors for the development of incisional hernia following elective laparoscopic versus open colon resections. Am J Surg. 2010;200(2):265–9.

24. Salameh JR, et al. Laparoscopic ventral hernia repair during the learning curve. Hernia. 2002;6(4):182–7.

25. Perrone JM, et al. Perioperative outcomes and complications of laparoscopic ventral hernia repair. Surgery. 2005;138(4):708–15. discussion 715–6.

26. Parker 3rd HH, et al. Laparoscopic repair of large incisional hernias. Am Surg. 2002;68(6):530–3. discussion 533–4.

27. Bencini L, et al. Predictors of recurrence after laparoscopic ventral hernia repair. Surg Laparosc Endosc Percutan Tech. 2009;19(2):128–32.

28. Heniford BT, et al. Laparoscopic repair of ventral hernias: nine years' experience with 850 consecutive hernias. Ann Surg. 2003;238(3):391–9. discussion 399–400.

29. Asencio F, et al. Open randomized clinical trial of laparoscopic versus open incisional hernia repair. Surg Endosc. 2009;23(7):1441–8.

30. Berger D, Bientzle M, Muller A. Postoperative complications after laparoscopic incisional hernia repair. Incidence and treatment. Surg Endosc. 2002;16(12):1720–3.

31. Eriksen JR, et al. Pain, quality of life and recovery after laparoscopic ventral hernia repair. Hernia. 2009;13(1):13–21.

32. Carbajo MA, et al. Laparoscopic approach to incisional hernia. Surg Endosc. 2003;17(1):118–22.

33. Baccari P, et al. Laparoscopic incisional and ventral hernia repair without sutures: a single-center experience with 200 cases. J Laparoendosc Adv Surg Tech A. 2009;19(2):175–9.

34. van't Riet M, et al. Tensile strength of mesh fixation methods in laparoscopic incisional hernia repair. Surg Endosc. 2002;16(12):1713–6.

35. Hollinsky C, et al. Tensile strength and adhesion formation of mesh fixation systems used in laparoscopic incisional hernia repair. Surg Endosc. 2010;24(6):1318–24.

36. LeBlanc KA. Laparoscopic incisional hernia repair: are transfascial sutures necessary? A review of the literature. Surg Endosc. 2007;21(4):508–13.

37. Beldi G, et al. Mesh shrinkage and pain in laparoscopic ventral hernia repair: a randomized clinical trial comparing suture versus tack mesh fixation. Surg Endosc. 2011;25(3):749–55.

38. Jonas J. The problem of mesh shrinkage in laparoscopic incisional hernia repair. Zentralbl Chir. 2009;134(3):209–13.

39. Cobb WS, Kercher KW, Heniford BT. Laparoscopic repair of incisional hernias. Surg Clin North Am. 2005;85(1):91–103. ix.

40. Schoenmaeckers EJ, et al. Computed tomographic measurements of mesh shrinkage after laparoscopic ventral incisional hernia repair with an expanded polytetrafluoroethylene mesh. Surg Endosc. 2009;23(7):1620–3.

41. Khan RN, et al. Does mesh shrinkage in any way depend upon the method of mesh fixation in laparoscopic incisional hernia repair? Surg Endosc. 2011;25(5):1690.

42. Klima DA, et al. Application of subcutaneous talc in hernia repair and wide subcutaneous dissection dramatically reduces seroma formation and post-operative wound complications. Am Surg. 2011;77(7):888–94.

43. Kurmann A, et al. Long-term follow-up of open and laparoscopic repair of large incisional hernias. World J Surg. 2011;35(2):297–301.

44. McGinty JJ, et al. A comparative study of adhesion formation and abdominal wall ingrowth after laparoscopic ventral hernia repair in a porcine model using multiple types of mesh. Surg Endosc. 2005;19(6):786–90.

45. Ko JH, et al. Soft polypropylene mesh, but not cadaveric dermis, significantly improves outcomes in midline hernia repairs using the components separation technique. Plast Reconstr Surg. 2009;124(3):836–47.

46. Bellows CF, et al. The design of an industry-sponsored randomized controlled trial to compare synthetic mesh versus biologic mesh for inguinal hernia repair. Hernia. 2011;15(3):325–32.

47. Raftopoulos I, et al. Outcome of laparoscopic ventral hernia repair in correlation with obesity, type of hernia, and hernia size. J Laparoendosc Adv Surg Tech A. 2002;12(6):425–9.

48. Birgisson G, et al. Obesity and laparoscopic repair of ventral hernias. Surg Endosc. 2001;15(12):1419–22.

49. Newcomb WL, et al. Staged hernia repair preceded by gastric bypass for the treatment of morbidly obese patients with complex ventral hernias. Hernia. 2008;12(5):465–9.

50. Park A, Birch DW, Lovrics P. Laparoscopic and open incisional hernia repair: a comparison study. Surgery. 1998;124(4):816–21. discussion 821–2.

51. Sharma A, et al. Laparoscopic ventral/incisional hernia repair: a single centre experience of 1,242 patients over a period of 13 years. Hernia. 2011;15(2):131–9.

52. Saber AA, et al. Occult ventral hernia defects: a common finding during laparoscopic ventral hernia repair. Am J Surg. 2008;195(4):471–3.

53. Bellows CF, Alder A, Helton WS. Abdominal wall reconstruction using biological tissue grafts: present status and future opportunities. Expert Rev Med Devices. 2006;3(5):657–75.

54. Brintzenhoff RA, et al. Subcutaneous talc decreases seroma rates and drain duration after open ventral hernia repair with skin and subcutaneous reconstruction. Chicago, IL: American College of Surgeons; 2010.

55. Sodergren MH, Swift I. Seroma formation and method of mesh fixation in laparoscopic ventral hernia repair–highlights of a case series. Scand J Surg. 2010;99(1):24–7.

56. Tsimoyiannis EC, et al. Laparoscopic intraperitoneal onlay mesh repair of incisional hernia. Surg Laparosc Endosc. 1998;8(5):360–2.

57. Forbes SS, et al. Meta-analysis of randomized controlled trials comparing open and laparoscopic ventral and incisional hernia repair with mesh. Br J Surg. 2009;96(8):851–8.

58. Swenson BR, et al. Antimicrobial-impregnated surgical incise drapes in the prevention of mesh infection after ventral hernia repair. Surg Infect (Larchmt). 2008;9(1):23–32.

59. Paton BL, et al. Management of infections of polytetrafluoroethylene-based mesh. Surg Infect (Larchmt). 2007;8(3):337–41.

60. Aguilar B, et al. Conservative management of mesh-site infection in hernia repair. J Laparoendosc Adv Surg Tech A. 2010;20(3):249–52.

61. Kercher KW, et al. Successful salvage of infected PTFE mesh after ventral hernia repair. Ostomy Wound Manage. 2002;48(10):40–2. 44–5.

62. Trunzo JA, et al. A novel approach for salvaging infected prosthetic mesh after ventral hernia repair. Hernia. 2009;13(5):545–9.

63. McLanahan D, et al. Retrorectus prosthetic mesh repair of midline abdominal hernia. Am J Surg. 1997;173(5):445–9.

64. Stoppa R. Long-term complications of prosthetic incisional hernioplasty. Arch Surg. 1998;133(11):1254–5.

65. van Kasteren ME, et al. Antibiotic prophylaxis and the risk of surgical site infections following total hip arthroplasty: timely administration is the most important factor. Clin Infect Dis. 2007;44(7):921–7.

66. Belyansky I, et al. Lysostaphin prevents mortality, preserves biologic mesh, and improves mesh integration in an infected abdomen. San Francisco, CA: American Hernia Society; 2011.

67. LeBlanc KA, Elieson MJ, Corder 3rd JM. Enterotomy and mortality rates of laparoscopic incisional and ventral hernia repair: a review of the literature. JSLS. 2007;11(4):408–14.

68. Carbonell AM, et al. The susceptibility of prosthetic biomaterials to infection. Surg Endosc. 2005;19(3):430–5.

69. Losanoff JE, Millis JM. Susceptibility of prosthetic biomaterials to infection. Surg Endosc. 2006;20(1):174–5.

70. Schug-Pass C, et al. A lightweight, partially absorbable mesh (Ultrapro) for endoscopic hernia repair: experimental biocompatibility results obtained with a porcine model. Surg Endosc. 2008;22(4):1100–6.

71. Gray SH, et al. Risk of complications from enterotomy or unplanned bowel resection during elective hernia repair. Arch Surg. 2008;143(6):582–6.

72. Garrard CL, et al. Adhesion formation is reduced after laparoscopic surgery. Surg Endosc. 1999;13(1):10–3.

73. DeGuzman LJ, et al. Colocutaneous fistula formation following polypropylene mesh placement for repair of a ventral hernia: diagnosis by colonoscopy. Endoscopy. 1995;27(6):459–61.

74. Seelig MH, et al. Enterocutaneous fistula after Marlex net implantation. A rare complication after incisional hernia repair. Chirurg. 1995;66(7):739–41.

75. LeBlanc KA. Incisional hernia repair: laparoscopic techniques. World J Surg. 2005;29(8):1073–9.

76. Ott V, Groebli Y, Schneider R. Late intestinal fistula formation after incisional hernia using intraperitoneal mesh. Hernia. 2005;9(1): 103–4.

77. Moussi A, et al. Gas gangrene of the abdominal wall due to late-onset enteric fistula after polyester mesh repair of an incisional hernia. Hernia. 2012;16(2):215–7.

78. Rosen MJ. Polyester-based mesh for ventral hernia repair: is it safe? Am J Surg. 2009;197(3):353–9.

79. Losanoff JE, Richman BW, Jones JW. Entero-colocutaneous fistula: a late consequence of polypropylene mesh abdominal wall repair: case report and review of the literature. Hernia. 2002;6(3):144–7.

80. Chew DK, Choi LH, Rogers AM. Enterocutaneous fistula 14 years after prosthetic mesh repair of a ventral incisional hernia: a lifelong risk? Surgery. 2000;127(3):352–3.

81. Hope WW, et al. Comparing quality-of-life outcomes in symptomatic patients undergoing laparoscopic or open ventral hernia repair. J Laparoendosc Adv Surg Tech A. 2008;18(4):567–71.

82. Snyder CW, et al. Patient satisfaction, chronic pain, and quality of life after elective incisional hernia repair: effects of recurrence and repair technique. Hernia. 2011;15(2):123–9.

83. Carbonell AM, et al. Local injection for the treatment of suture site pain after laparoscopic ventral hernia repair. Am Surg. 2003;69(8): 688–91. discussion 691–2.

84. LeBlanc KA, Whitaker JM. Management of chronic postoperative pain following incisional hernia repair with Composix mesh: a report of two cases. Hernia. 2002;6(4):194–7.

85. Nguyen SQ, et al. Postoperative pain after laparoscopic ventral hernia repair: a prospective comparison of sutures versus tacks. JSLS. 2008;12(2):113–6.

86. Heniford BT, et al. Comparison of generic versus specific quality-of-life scales for mesh hernia repairs. J Am Coll Surg. 2008;206(4): 638–44.

87. Blatnik JA, et al. Thirty-day readmission after ventral hernia repair: predictable or preventable? Surg Endosc. 2011;25(5): 1446–51.

88. Sorensen LT, Karlsmark T, Gottrup F. Abstinence from smoking reduces incisional wound infection: a randomized controlled trial. Ann Surg. 2003;238(1):1–5.

89. Heniford BT, et al. Laparoscopic ventral and incisional hernia repair in 407 patients. J Am Coll Surg. 2000;190(6):645–50.

90. Barbaros U, et al. The comparison of laparoscopic and open ventral hernia repairs: a prospective randomized study. Hernia. 2007;11(1): 51–6.

91. Olmi S, et al. Laparoscopic versus open incisional hernia repair: an open randomized controlled study. Surg Endosc. 2007;21(4): 555–9.

92. Egea DA, et al. Mortality following laparoscopic ventral hernia repair: lessons from 90 consecutive cases and bibliographical analysis. Hernia. 2004;8(3):208–12.

93. Bisgaard T, et al. Nationwide study of early outcomes after incisional hernia repair. Br J Surg. 2009;96(12):1452–7.

94. Elieson MJ, LeBlanc KA. Enterotomy and mortality rates of laparoscopic incisional and ventral hernia repair: A review of the literature. JSLS. 2007;11:408–14.

L. Michael Brunt

Groin injuries are a common occurrence in sport, especially in elite level athletes. Most of these injuries are muscular strains that resolve completely with standard conservative management measures. However, some groin injuries result in a significant loss of playing time and can be a source of persistent pain that limits performance. Over the last 15 years, a subset of athletes with chronic, unremitting groin pain known as "sports hernia" has become increasingly recognized. These injuries present challenging diagnostic and therapeutic management problems for athletic trainers and physicians because of the broad range of diagnostic possibilities, the subtle physical exam findings, and the anatomic complexity of the lower abdominal and groin region. In this chapter, the clinical presentation, diagnostic evaluation, and treatment options for athletes with a possible sports hernia will be reviewed. The differential diagnosis of athletic groin pain will also be discussed since surgeons who treat these athletes must understand the spectrum of injuries in order to make an accurate diagnosis.

Background and Epidemiology

Athletes who play certain sports, such as ice hockey, football, soccer, and baseball, are especially vulnerable to groin injury because of the rapid acceleration/deceleration movements and repetitive twisting and turning motions carried out at high speeds. The reported incidence of groin injuries has ranged from 5 to 28% in soccer players [1–3] (_ENREF_1) and 6–15% of ice hockey players [4, 5]. In one study, groin injuries accounted for 10–43% of all muscle injuries in elite Scandinavian league hockey players [6, 7]. Unlike most other sports injuries, athletic groin injuries are soft tissue in nature and do not result from direct physical contact.

Risk factors for groin injury have been examined by several groups. Emery and colleagues [8] analyzed injury reports from 6 NHL seasons from 1991 to 1992 through 1996–1997 involving 7,050 players with a subset analysis of the 1995/1996 and 1996/1997 seasons. Six hundred seventeen injuries were reported for an injury rate of 13.3–19 abdominal and groin injuries per 100 players. Not surprisingly, injuries were more common during training camp and early in the season. One-fourth of injuries were abdominal muscle strains and 56% of reinjuries occurred in same season. The median time lost was 7 practice or game sessions (range 0–180), and time loss was greater with abdominal injuries (median 10.6 sessions) than adductor injuries (median 6.6 sessions). Their group subsequently carried out a prospective study of National Hockey League (NHL) players over the 1998–1999 NHL training camp and regular season. Risk factors associated with an increase risk of injury were (1) <18 sport-specific training sessions (e.g., on ice) in the off-season (RR3.4), (2) history of previous groin or abdominal strain (RR 2.9), and (3) veteran player status (veteran > rookie) (RR 5.7) [9].

Reduced adductor strength relative to abductor strength was also found to be associated with a higher rate of groin injury in one study of NHL hockey players [10]. Tyler et al. prospectively studied hip strength and flexibility in one NHL team and found that players whose preseason adductor strength was <80% of abductor strength were 17 times more likely to sustain an adductor strain. Perhaps more importantly, they showed that an adductor strengthening program reduced the incidence of groin injury from 3.2/1,000 to 0.7/1,000 player game exposures.

Differential Diagnosis

The causes of groin pain in athletes are numerous and most commonly include muscular strains of the adductors, lower abdominals, and hip flexors. In addition to sports hernia, other conditions that can cause groin pain are osteitis pubis, stress fractures, hip and pelvis injuries, inguinal hernia,

L.M. Brunt, M.D. (✉)
Department of Surgery, Washington University School of Medicine,
660 S Euclid Ave., 8109, St. Louis, MO 63110, USA
e-mail: bruntm@wustl.edu

A.N. Kingsnorth and K.A. LeBlanc (eds.), *Management of Abdominal Hernias*,
DOI 10.1007/978-1-84882-877-3_26, © Springer Science+Business Media London 2013

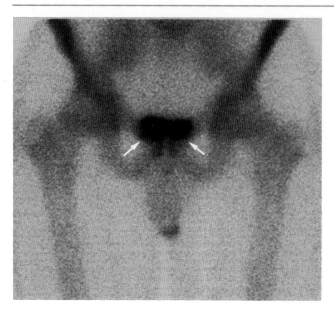

Fig. 26.1 Bone scan that shows increased uptake in both pubic rami (*arrows*) in an athlete with osteitis pubis

sports hernia, and various non-musculoskeletal-related conditions including intra-abdominal pathology. A detailed discussion of the clinical presentation and management of these various entities can be found in recent reviews on this subject [11–15] (_ENREF_9).

Stress Fractures. Stress fractures of the pelvis and hip typically are associated with extreme athletic endurance activities such as with long-distance runners and military recruits. The mechanism is thought to be due to bone breaking down faster than it can remodel. These are thought to be overuse injuries, and women at risk for osteoporosis may be especially vulnerable. Associated factors may include a change in training duration or intensity, and change in foot gear or training surface. The most common sites in the groin region are the inferior pubic ramus and femoral neck. An unrecognized stress fracture of the hip can lead to avascular necrosis; therefore, early diagnosis and treatment are essential. Plain X-rays may not reveal a fracture, and as a result, MRI is indicated in suspected cases. Pubic ramus fractures should be treated by rest and other conservative measures and usually resolve within 4–6 weeks. Femoral neck fractures may require orthopedic fixation.

Osteitis Pubis. Osteitis pubis is a condition of unknown etiology that is most likely due to overuse/repetitive trauma and abnormal biomechanics of the pubis. It is most common in runners and soccer players but also in swimmers, soccer, and hockey players. The clinical presentation consists of midline pubic symphysis pain that may be referred to adjacent areas including the adductor region. In one series, 80% had adductor pain, 30% abdominal pain, and 12% hip pain [16]. Radiographic findings in osteitis pubis may include widening of the symphysis, sclerosis along the pubic rami,

and edema on MRI. Bone scans typically show increased uptake on both sides of the pubic symphysis (Fig. 26.1). Treatment consists of a reduction in activity, pelvic stretching (especially of adductors), anti-inflammatory medications, and, for acute or refractory cases, a corticosteroid injection into the symphysis. The time frame for return to sport is unpredictable but may take several months in some cases.

Adductor Muscle Group Strains. The adductor group is the most common sports groin injury and most commonly involves the adductor longus. In one series, adductor longus injuries accounted for 62% of sports groin injuries [1]. A history of a sudden injury and even a pop in the groin is not uncommon. The mechanism involves an eccentric force on the muscle (i.e., sudden stretching when the muscle is contracted). Symptoms and findings are medial thigh or groin pain with associated pain with passive or resisted adduction movements. In acute complete tears there may be medial thigh ecchymosis and even a palpable defect. Most adductor injuries are strains and not complete tears of the tendon from its attachment to the pubis (Fig. 26.2) In chronic cases, these injuries may overlap or coexist in their clinical presentation with sports hernia and osteitis pubis. Imaging with MRI is indicated to define the extent of the injury in severe cases or those that do not resolve with conservative management. Treatment may vary according to the location and chronicity of the injury but initially should consist of rest, ice, and compression. Once symptoms subside, management should consist of progressive range of motion exercises followed by balance training/graduated strengthening, and finally sport-specific functional activities. Time to return to play may vary from a few days to several weeks depending on the severity of the injury. However, some athletes have been able to return to play from even complete adductor longus tears within 5–6 weeks of injury [17].

Iliopsoas Strain. Muscular strains of the iliopsoas present with deep groin or hip pain that is aggravated by hip flexion. The mechanism of injury is often from a hit the player sustains when the leg is extended, a common occurrence in soccer players. Symptoms consist of pain with resisted hip flexion (15°), pain with passive hip extension, and a snapping sensation in the hip. Treatment consists of nonsteroidal anti-inflammatories, rest, stretching, and strengthening exercises. A corticosteroid injection may be considered for recalcitrant cases.

Hip Injuries. Hip injuries are one of the more common causes of groin pain in athletes. These may include labral tears, femoral acetabular impingement, and femoral neck fractures. Symptoms may overlap or coexist with sports hernia type pubalgia. Labral tears present with pain in the hip or groin and mechanical symptoms such as a locking or catching sensation. Treatment is often arthroscopic debridement. Femoral acetabular impingement is a condition in which the

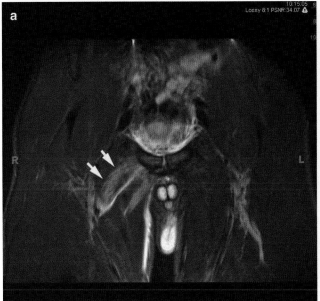
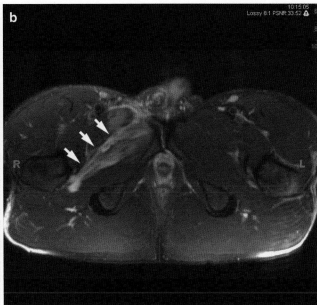

Fig. 26.2 MRI that shows extensive contusion that involves right adductor muscle group. Note the edema (bright appearance) throughout the muscle belly and feathery appearance indicating hemorrhage into the muscle planes. (**a**) STIR (short T1 inversion recovery) coronal sequences. (**b**) T2 fat-suppressed sequence

femoral head and acetabulum rub abnormally and the resultant excessive friction may lead to cartilage damage, labral tears, and early hip arthritis. Stress fractures of the femoral neck should also be considered in the differential diagnosis and may lead to avascular necrosis if unrecognized. Exclusion of hip pathology first requires examination by an experienced orthopedist. Plain hip X-rays are useful, but hip MRI is necessary to identify labral tears.

Athletic groin injuries should be managed initially with standard conservative management techniques. The vast majority of these injuries resolve and do not evolve into a sports hernia or chronic pubalgia. However, injuries that persist more than 3 months without significant improvement are associated with an increased likelihood of requiring surgical intervention. Ekstrand [18] carried out a prospective, randomized trial in soccer players with chronic groin pain of more than 3 months duration. Players were randomized into four groups—controls with no treatment, two different physical therapy groups, and a surgically treated group who underwent inguinal floor repair ± inguinal and iliohypogastric neurectomy. Only the surgically treated group showed substantial and statistically significant improvement over the 6 months of the study.

Diagnostic Evaluation

Terminology. Various terms have been used to refer to athletic injuries to the lower abdominal/inguinal region that result in a syndrome of chronic exertional pain. These include "sports hernia," athletic pubalgia [19], posterior abdominal wall deficiency [20, 21], Gilmore's groin [22, 23], and hockey groin syndrome [24]. The term sports hernia is potentially misleading because it implies the presence of a conventional hernia which is not the case. As will be discussed below, the pathophysiology is more complex than a simple hernia and, therefore, the term sports pubalgia or athletic pubalgia is preferred. Nonetheless, "sports hernia" is firmly ingrained in the athletic community and sports media and will likely continue to be used in everyday practice.

Clinical Presentation

The classic symptoms in athletes with a sports pubalgia type injury are pain that is localized to the lower abdominal and inguinal region and occurs during the extremes of exertion, such as with the initial propulsive movements of running, skating, and sudden stops, starts, or cutting movements. Ice hockey players may have pain when shooting the puck and soccer athletes with kicking the soccer ball. The onset is often insidious without a specific precipitating event and there may be associated adductor symptoms. One or both sides of the groin may be involved.

A challenge in evaluating and managing groin pain in athletes is that the clinical presentation may vary substantially and may not be limited to distal rectus and inguinal floor pathology. Meyers [25] has described 17 different clinical syndromes that involve non-hip soft tissue structures that can be primary causes of athletic groin pain. These most commonly include variations of injuries to the rectus abdominus, adductor muscle groups, or a combination thereof. Less common variants include severe osteitis variant, baseball pitcher/hockey goalie syndrome in which there is a tear of the adductor and adductor muscle belly, iliospoas variant, and rectus femoris variant. Because of the potential coexistence of more than one site of injury and overlap of symptoms with hip and other pathology, it is important that such athletes undergo careful examination by a sports orthopedist prior to referral to a hernia surgeon to exclude a source of pain from the hip and other sources. In addition, an appropriate trial of conservative management and physical therapy should first be undertaken with rare exception.

Evaluation of the athlete with a chronic groin injury should include a detailed history regarding the injury. Questions that should be asked include precise location of pain, duration, onset, involvement of thigh or hip, activities that worsen the pain, presence with sneezing or coughing, and whether pain occurs only with activity or also with rest. The level of sport activity and intensity of participation should also be determined, as many groin injuries, especially in non-collegiate or professional athletes, are related to overuse. Patients should also be queried regarding what conservative management steps such as icing, anti-inflammatory medications, and physical therapy that have been undertaken before evaluation.

Physical exam findings are a critical component of the assessment and must include evaluation of the inguinal floor, pubis, rectus abdominus, adductors and hip flexors, and hip and should include muscle-specific resistance maneuvers to identify areas of pain and tenderness. In the classic sports hernia pubalgia syndrome, the most consistent findings are tenderness in the medial portion of the inguinal canal or along the lower rectus abdominus muscle. Other findings that may be present include a dilated external inguinal ring, a palpable gap or defect over the external oblique aponeurosis and inguinal floor, and pain with a resisted sit-up or resisted trunk rotation (Fig. 26.3). Pain with resisted adduction and adductor tightness may be present, especially if there is an adductor component to the injury which is frequently the case. A true inguinal hernia is rarely present and there is typically no clinically evident hernia bulge. In our series of athletes in whom this diagnosis was made, the most common exam findings preoperatively were a weak inguinal floor (90.7%), tenderness over the medial inguinal floor/lower lateral rectus (80.2%), pain with a resisted sit-up (63.8%) or trunk rotation (73.3%), and pain with resisted adduction (56.7%) [26].

Imaging

Imaging tests are important to exclude other pathology and to help substantiate the diagnosis. Plain X-rays are usually normal but should be done if hip pathology or stress fracture

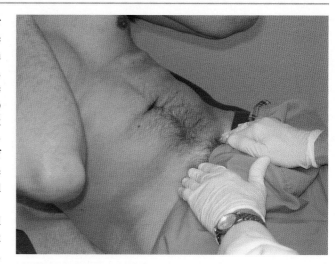

Fig. 26.3 Exam for athletic pubalgia with palpation of both inguinal floors during a sit-up

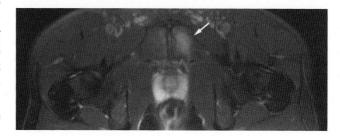

Fig. 26.4 T2 fat-suppressed MRI sequence that shows marrow edema *(arrow)* in the pubis in an athlete with sports pubalgia

is suspected. Pelvic MRI has been the most useful modality in our experience because of the details of the bony pelvis and associated muscular tears and strains it provides. In the athletes with a sports hernia seen at our center, the most common MRI findings have been edema or stress reaction and secondary cleft sign in the adjacent pubis (Fig. 26.4). Tears of the distal rectus or rectus/adductor complex may also be seen in some cases (Fig. 26.5). Adductor pathology may include tears and/or edema indicating underlying chronic tendinopathy (Fig. 26.6). Zoga and colleagues [27] recently reported results of MR imaging in 141 patients in whom athletic pubalgia was diagnosed clinically. The most common findings were rectus abdominus tendon injury, combined rectus and adductor injury, symphysis marrow edema, and a secondary cleft. The secondary cleft sign refers to an abnormal extension of the central symphyseal cleft at the anterior-inferior margin of the body of the pubis. It is thought to results from a microtear at the origin of the adductor longus and gracilis tendons [28].

Improved MRI imaging techniques have resulted in positive findings in a higher percentage of patients in recent years. Zoga [27] reported that MRI had a sensitivity of 68% and specificity of 100% for rectus abdominus tendon injury and 86% and 89% sensitivity and specificity, respectively,

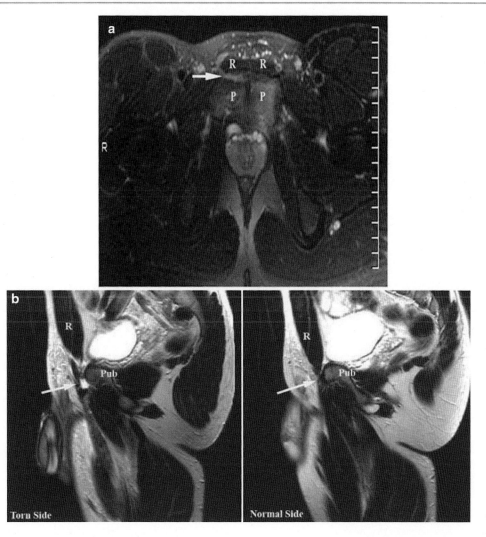

Fig. 26.5 (**a**) T2 fat-suppressed MRI of right distal rectus tear (*arrow* pointing to bright fluid in cleft where rectus is torn); *R* rectus, *P* pubis. (**b**) Sagittal fat-suppressed sequence that shows distal rectus tear with disconti- nuity (*left hand panel*) and normal contralateral side (*right hand panel*) The *arrow* on the *left panel* points to the tear (appears bright on this sequence) and to the normal rectus insertion on the *right panel*. *R* rectus, *Pub* pubis

for adductor tendon injury. MRI techniques for sports pubal- gia should center the imaging volume on the pelvis which is facilitated by use of a phase array pelvic surface coil [28]. Both fat-suppressed T1-weighted and fat-suppressed fluid- sensitive imaging sequences should be included. Imaging should be carried out in three orthogonal planes (coronal, axial, and sagittal); additionally, axial/oblique sequences may be useful for better delineating adductor tendon origins [28].

Although not often employed in North America, some groups have utilized ultrasound in the evaluation of athletic groin pain [29, 30]. Ultrasound has the advantage of real time dynamic assessment of the inguinal floor and abdomi- nal wall and can be used in conjunction with patient Valsalva maneuvers. The disadvantages are that it is operator depen- dent and, therefore, requires an experienced examiner and does not readily visualize the other bony and muscular struc-

tures around the pubis and pelvis. Muschawek and Berger [30] preferentially utilize ultrasound as the primary imaging modality in athletes with groin pain. A high-frequency trans- ducer (5–13 MHz) is used, and the motion of the inguinal canal and floor are observed with the patient supine during a stress maneuver (Valsalva). Positive findings consist of a convex anterior bulge of the posterior inguinal floor during Valsalva.

Pathophysiology

Several mechanisms have been proposed to account for the pain symptoms in athletic pubalgia syndromes. As discussed above, Meyers has proposed the concept of the "pubic joint" in which the pubis acts as the central fulcrum for the powerful abdominal and thigh muscles [31, 32].

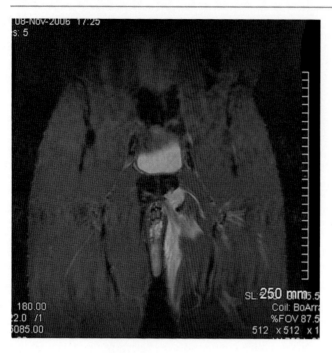

Fig. 26.6 MRI of high-grade left adductor tendon avulsion

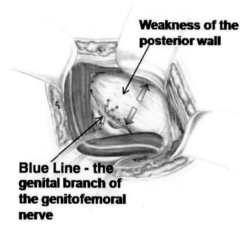

Weakness of the posterior wall

Blue Line - the genital branch of the genitofemoral nerve

Fig. 26.7 Schematic illustration of localized bulge in posterior inguinal floor with compression of the genital branch of the genitofemoral nerve (from Muschawek and Berger [35]; with permission)

Normally these muscles are symmetrically distributed. In athletes, especially those performing at high levels, tremendous torque is generated across the pelvis. If an imbalance in these forces is present, for example, from relative weakness of one or more muscle groups, then further weakening may develop leading to increased stress across the pubis and chronic pubalgia pain. The pain may result due to weakening of the rectus muscle at the pubic insertion site, which in turn results in unopposed action of the adductor longus [31] and increased pressure within the adductor compartment. Cadaver dissections have also shown that the anterior edge of the inferior pubis has fine, teethlike projections that contact the adductor muscles

and tendons, which may contribute to adductor compartment pain. The approach to repair as described below, therefore, is tailored to address these biomechanical considerations.

A second potential mechanism for athletic pubalgia involves weakening in the posterior floor of the inguinal canal. The weak posterior floor can result from an imbalance in forces between the relatively stronger hip musculature and the weaker lower abdominals [33, 34]. The weak posterior inguinal floor can lead to widening of the groin canal which in turn allows the rectus muscle to retract medially and superiorly [35]. The increased tension at the pubic bone that results causes pain at the symphysis or one or both sides of the pubis. Muschawek has theorized that compression or entrapment of the genital branch of the genitofemoral nerve by a discrete, localized bulge in the posterior wall of the inguinal canal during Valsalva maneuver is involved in the pain pathway in some athletes (Fig. 26.7). This concept has led to selective resection of the genital nerve in some athletes in her series.

Finally, the Montreal group [24, 36] has postulated that tears in the aponeurosis of the external oblique coupled with entrapment of branches of the ilioinguinal or iliohypogastric nerves are the central phathophysiologic mechanisms for athletic pubalgia pain (_ENREF_30). The external oblique tears may be central, medial, or lateral and single or multiple. These tears arise from increased intra-abdominal pressure during Valsalva that occur during sudden changes in movement or intense abdominal contraction such as that occurs in pushing against an opponent. A bulky internal oblique has also been a common operative finding and may limit space in the inguinal canal, thereby applying outward pressure on the external oblique that may ultimately lead to a tear. Tension on one or more of nerves as they exit the external oblique may sometimes be observed at operation (Fig. 26.8).

A number of findings have been described at operation that reflect the above mechanisms. These include an attenuated external oblique aponeurosis, disruption or weakness of the posterior inguinal floor, a thin or torn rectus insertion (7), and, importantly, absence of an inguinal hernia. Other findings that have been reported include a torn or hypertrophied internal oblique [24], entrapment of the ilioinguinal or iliohypogastric nerves within a torn external oblique aponeurosis with a normal posterior inguinal floor [11, 24], and compression of the genital nerve by localized bulging of the posterior inguinal floor. The most common operative findings in our athletes have been an attenuated external oblique aponeurosis (96.7%) (Fig. 26.9), weakened or disrupted inguinal floor (100%) (Fig. 26.10), torn or damaged internal oblique (63.9%), and lower rectus abnormality in 80.3% (lax insertion, muscular tears) [26]. There was only one indirect hernia identified (1.6%). Clinically insignificant cord lipomas were removed in 18%.

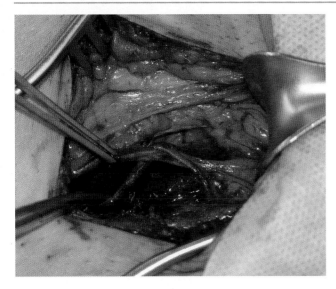

Fig. 26.8 Ilioinguinal nerve exiting through a tear in the external oblique aponeurosis medial to the external ring. Note the acute angle the nerve takes as it exits the aponeurosis, which may be a source of tension on the nerve and resultant pain

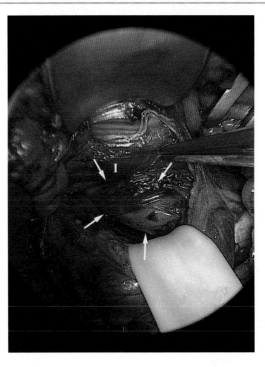

Fig. 26.10 Operative photograph showing a deficient posterior inguinal floor indicated by the *arrows*. The instrument is pointing to the internal oblique labeled I. A Penrose drain encircles the cord structures which are retracted laterally

Surgical Treatment

Surgical treatment for sports pubalgia should be reserved for patients and athletes who have the appropriate history and physical exam findings, have confirmatory evidence and/or exclusion of other significant confounding pathology with imaging (MRI or ultrasound), and who have failed a trial of conservative management. In general, surgery should be considered only after 8 weeks or more of rest, physical therapy, and other local treatment measures. For recreational athletes, the period of rest and therapy is especially important since they do not often have access to experienced athletic trainers and other resources that are available in the collegiate and professional athletic setting. In our series, the average time from onset of symptoms and injury to surgical treatment has averaged 9.7 months.

Consensus is lacking regarding the preferred surgical technique for repairing sports pubalgia injuries, which in part reflects disagreement about the pathomechanics of the injury. In general, three broad categories of repair have been employed: open primary tissue repairs, open tension-free mesh repairs, and laparoscopic mesh repair as described in detail below. Despite differences in approaches, the common goal of each of these operations is to provide support and stability of the inguinal floor and distal rectus across the pubis.

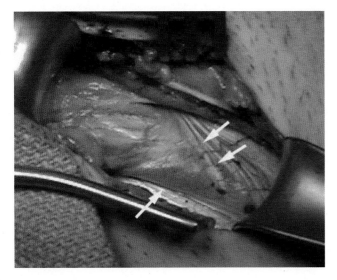

Fig. 26.9 Operative photograph showing marked attenuation in the external oblique aponeurosis

Regardless of the precise pathophysiologic mechanism of groin pain, it would appear that the central variable common to these injuries is stress across the lower abdominal wall that leads to weakening in the posterior inguinal floor or distal rectus tears or both. Whether nerve entrapment is a significant component or not is an unresolved issue, as some groups have reported successful outcomes of surgical repair without nerve resection. Factors that may contribute to the increasing incidence of these injuries include increased weight and strength training, year-round training without significant time off, single-sport focus at a young age, and lack of balance in strength and flexibility between the abdomen/core and lower body.

Surgical Approaches

Primary Pelvic Floor Repair

Two principal primary repair techniques have been described—primary pelvic floor repair by Meyers [19] and a minimal repair technique [30] by Muschaewek. Neither of these techniques employs mesh.

Meyers Technique. The precise technical details of the Meyers approach have not been shown, but consist of suture plication or reattachment of the inferolateral border of the rectus abdominus fascia to the pubis and inguinal ligament [19]. This repair is somewhat analogous to a Bassini hernia repair but with differences in the way the sutures are oriented. The goal of the operation is instead to reattach or reinforce the anterior abdominal attachments to the pubis and adjacent ligaments. In order to accomplish this, the distal rectus abdominus muscle fascia is attached directly to the pubis and the inguinal ligament, using a near vertical line of sutures and by staying as close to the pubis and as anterior possible, maximizing anterior pelvic support. A second row of sutures is placed posteriorly onto the rectus fascia to add stability to the anterior row of sutures which is the primary line of support (W Meyers, personal communication).

The pelvic floor repair operation has been coupled with an adductor release in selected athletes. In the adductor component of the procedure, the anterior epimysial fibers of the adductor longus are incised 2–3 cm from their insertion into the pubis while leaving the adductor muscle intact. Conceptually, he describes a relative compartment syndrome that may exist on one or more of the adductor muscles and that the "release" allows escape of edema due to the entrapment. It is important to recognize that this is not a complete release of the adductor tendon attachment to the pubis but rather a relative loosening of the adductor compartment. It should also be noted that release of one or more adductor muscles is sometimes carried out as an isolated procedure without accompanying pelvic floor repair.

In 2003, Muschawek developed a "minimal repair" technique for athletes with chronic sports groin injuries [30]. The goal of this operation is to stabilize the posterior inguinal floor using a nearly tension-free suture method. The operation is performed under local anesthesia with sedation and the technique is somewhat analogous to the Shouldice hernia repair but differs in that only the localized area of defect is opened and repaired and not the entire inguinal floor. In selected cases, the genital nerve is resected because of resultant pressure on the nerve from the posterior floor bulging and resultant nerve fibrosis that can result. A continuous suture is placed using a lip of iliopubic tract sutured first to itself and then over to inguinal ligament. A 2nd row of suture is then placed to lateralize the rectus abdominus fascia which

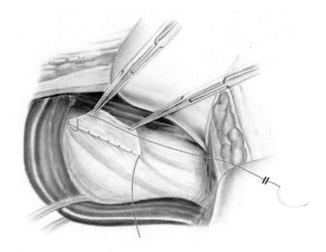

Fig. 26.11 Schematic illustration of the Muschawek minimal repair technique. Two double rows of continuous suture are placed to repair the defect (from Muschawek and Berger [35]; with permission)

she postulates has been retracted medially and cranially by the posterior floor weakness (Fig. 26.11). These lines of suture serve to counteract the tension at the pubic bone by displacement of the rectus. Lastly, a muscular collar is placed at the deep internal ring using the lateral internal oblique in order to protect the cord structures. Conceptually, mesh is avoided in order to preserve the slide bearing function and elasticity in the inguinal floor.

Open Tension-Free Mesh Repair

Since primary tissue repairs of true inguinal hernia have been replaced by tension-free mesh approaches because of fewer recurrences and earlier return to activity associated with the latter, it is logical that a tension-free mesh approach could accomplish the goals described above of providing stability and support of the posterior inguinal floor and pubic joint. As a result, several groups have preferentially used mesh to repair sports pubalgia injuries. The techniques used have employed lightweight polypropylene mesh or polytetrafluoroethylene (PTFE) meshes and have either been placed posteriorly and sutured to transversalis aponeurosis/rectus sheath and inguinal ligament similar to the Lichtenstein repair or more anteriorly to support the external oblique aponeurosis.

The approach used by this author is typically carried out under local anesthesia with sedation. The external oblique aponeurosis, which is often thin and attenuated, is opened along the plane of its fibers just as for standard inguinal hernia repair. A careful search is made for the ilioinguinal nerve, which is resected if it is entrapped by a slit in the external oblique or if it's course is such that it is vulnerable to adhesion

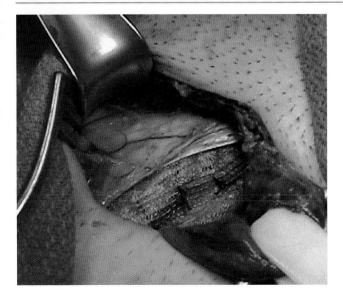

Fig. 26.12 Open tension-free mesh repair of sports pubalgia that shows mesh reinforcement of the posterior inguinal floor and distal rectus

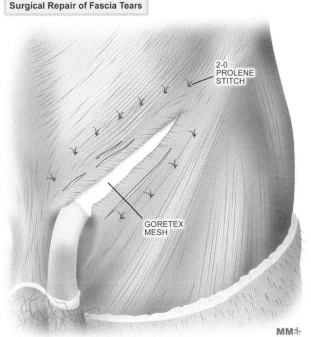

Fig. 26.13 Schematic illustration of PTFE mesh repair using the Montreal technique. The surgical repair encompasses the tears on the external oblique fascia (from Brown et al. [36]; with permission)

to the mesh or would otherwise interfere with the repair. A search is made for an indirect sac and any cord lipoma is resected. Damaged or attenuated internal oblique fibers are debrided and the floor is then reconstructed suturing the mesh medially to the transversis aponeurosis and medially to the inguinal ligament (Fig. 26.12). Although the internal ring is intact in these cases, the mesh is split like for a Lichtenstein repair and the two limbs are sutured together to the inguinal ligament so that the conformity of mesh to the posterior floor is maintained. Additionally, one or two interrupted sutures are placed to anchor the mesh and distal rectus in order to further stabilize the rectus and pubis anteriorly. The intact fibers of the external oblique are then sutured together with a heavy absorbable suture (2-0 polyglactic acid) to eliminate the area of attenuation.

The Montreal group utilizes PTFE mesh in their repair and prefers to place the mesh more anteriorly to support the external oblique layer [24, 36]. The repair is carried out under general anesthesia and the slit in the external oblique is opened generously. The patch is sutured in place to the external oblique beyond the margins of the tears using interrupted 2-0 polyprolene sutures (Fig. 26.13). The ilioinguinal and/or iliohypogastric nerves are also routinely resected.

Laparoscopic (Posterior) Mesh Repair

Laparoscopic repair is a 3rd potential option in athletes with groin pain that is preferred by some groups. However, its role in the repair of athletic pubalgia injuries is unclear. The total extraperitoneal (TEP) approach is generally used in this setting although transabdominal exploration may be indicated

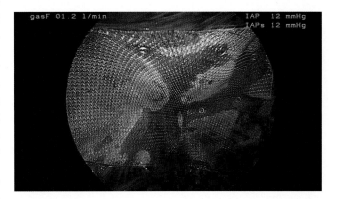

Fig. 26.14 Laparoscopic extraperitoneal mesh positioned to repair the posterior inguinal floor defect

in some athletes to exclude intra-abdominal sources of pain (e.g., inflammatory bowel disease) or gynecologic pathology in women. The technique is similar to that for standard TEP inguinal hernia repair (Fig. 26.14)

Outcomes of Surgical Treatment. A summary of reported outcomes of surgical treatment depicted by category of repair is given in Table 26.1. Reported results have in the vast majority of cases indicated a return to sport in 90% or more of cases. However, follow-up has been variable or in many cases not reported. The interval to return to sport has ranged from 4 weeks to 3–4 months. In our series of over 100 cases of repair, most athletes have returned to their sports within 8

Table 26.1 Reported results of surgical treatment of sports hernia

	Center	N	Length of follow-up	Interval to return to play	Return to sport (%)
Open primary repairs					
Polglase [41]	Australia	64	8 months	–	63
Gilmore [22]	UK	300	–	–	97
Steele [21]	Australia	47	–	4 months	77
Meyers [25]	Philadelphia	5,218	24 months	up to 3 months	95.3
Muschawek [30]	Munich	129	–	4 weeks	
Open mesh repairs					
Joesting [42]	Minnesota	45	12 months	–	90
Brown [36]	Montreal	98	–	–	97
Brunt [26]	St. Louis	57	13.6 months	8 weeks	92
Laparoscopic repairs					
Paajanen [37]	Helsinki	41	50 months	1 month	95
Van Veen [38]	Rotterdam	55	24 weeks	3 months	91
Ziprin [39]	London	17	–	42 days	94
Evans [43]	UK	287	3 months–4 years	4 weeks	90

weeks of injury, with returns as early as 5–6 weeks in some cases of in-season repair. Because many of these athletes are operated on at the conclusion of their season, the time pressures for return to play are lessened and they often extend their rehab over a period of 8–12 weeks.

Primary Repair. Meyers has reported observations from operations in 5,218 athletes out of 8,490 individuals (61.4%) evaluated for possible sports hernia pubalgia [25]. In the operated individuals, there were 26 different procedures and 121 combinations of procedures performed. The precise details of the procedures performed were not provided but appeared to primarily involve either pelvic floor repair with various combinations of release procedures. The most common sports involved were football, soccer and hockey, which accounted for 70% of cases. Complications were hematomas that required reoperation in 0.3%, wound infection in 0.4%, dysesthesia in 0.3%, and penile thrombosis in 0.1%. Recurrent problems occurred in 16 patients and reoperation after prior standard inguinal hernia repair (open of laparoscopic) at outside institutions was done in 241 patients. Further details regarding the type of symptomatic failure in these outside procedures was not reported.

Muschawek reported outcomes of a prospective cohort study of 129 patients treated from 2008 to 2009 [30]. At 4 weeks post repair, 96.1% of athletes had resumed training and full return to pre-injury sports activity had occurred in 75.8%. No recurrences were reported over the course of follow-up.

Tension-Free Mesh Repairs, Brown and colleagues [36] reported outcomes in 98 elite hockey players using the PTFE mesh approach. Overall, 97 of 98 athletes were able to return to play. Three recurrences occurred between 4 and 6 years after the original repair. All had remedial re-repair and were able to return to play.

At the Washington University Medical Center, repairs have been performed in 132 athletes. The most common sports have been hockey, football, and soccer. Level of play was professional or collegiate in 63%, high school in 7%, and recreational in 29%. Repairs were unilateral in 87% cases and bilateral in 13%. Subsequent contralateral repair was carried out in six athletes (4.5%) at a mean interval of 14.1 months later. Over 90% of repairs were done under local anesthesia as an outpatient procedure. Symptomatic outcomes were assessed at a mean interval of 13.6 months after surgical repair with successful return to athletic competition in 91% of athletes. Only one individual has required abdominal re-repair due to recurrent lower abdominal symptoms. However, five other athletes have required subsequent adductor procedures for ongoing or recurrent adductor symptoms that limited athletic performance. As a result, an adductor release procedure as described by Meyers has been added to inguinal floor repair in selected athletes with predominately adductor symptoms and pathology.

Laparoscopic Repair

In soccer players with sports hernias, successful outcomes of laparoscopic mesh repairs have been reported by some groups [37–39]. In one study of 55 athletes with chronic groin pain, incipient hernias were diagnosed in 36 cases (65%) including 9 that were bilateral, and true inguinal hernias were seen in 20 athletes (36%) [38]. Laparoscopic repair was carried out in all cases, and 5 athletes also had an adductor tenotomy performed. At 6–8 weeks, 48 of the patients (88%) had returned to normal sports activities without pain. Five patients had residual groin pain at 12 weeks that ultimately resolved with rest and physical therapy [38]. Of note is that the high incidence of true inguinal hernias in this series differs from that reported in multiple series of open repairs. Whether this observation is due to different selection criteria for surgery or an artifice of the laparoscopic viewpoint is unclear.

Table 26.2 Postoperative rehabilitation protocol

Phase	Time	Therapy	Sets	Reps	Resistance	Notes
1	0–1 weeks	Walking	1	5–60 min	3–6 mph	When patient is able to walk 20 min. continuous, begin light hamstring, quad, gastroc low back, and groin stretching
2	2–4 weeks	Active hip ROM (leg swings), treadmill incline walking, wall sits w/Swiss ball, quad stabilization, hamstring/gastroc/low back strengthen, begin bike workouts at 2 weeks	1	8 reps per exercise	As tolerated	At start of 3–4 weeks begin scar mobilization of surgical site—ART of surrounding muscle groups—at 4 weeks ART of affected psoas muscle. Avoid excessive trunk extension
3	3–4 weeks	Hip flexor stretching w/progression to resistance, light jogging, initiate exercises for transversalis and obliques, controlled rotation exercises, bridging progression, core stabilization exercises	1	8 reps per exercise	As tolerated	Continue scar mobilization
4	4–5 weeks	Increase to speed and interval training on bike or treadmill, lunges, light sport-specific activities, single-leg slideboard/theraband, lower abdominal exercises, continue core stabilization exercises	1	8 reps per exercise	As tolerated	Continue scar mobilization
5	6–8 weeks	Speed/function/volume and intensity to maximum, end stage quadruped/stabilization exercises, muscle length restored/adductor strength bilateral, drills and scrimmage w/team, MD approval and discharge				Confidence is established with timed drills/bilateral muscle strength, positive finding presurgery now negative, continues emphasis placed on maintaining muscle lengthening and symmetrical abdominal strength through adherence to stabilization program

One small prospective randomized trial has been carried out that compared laparoscopic to open repair, primarily in rugby players [40]. Open repair consisted of Bassini repair in 3 athletes and Lichtenstein type repairs in 11. Training was resumed at 4 weeks in 9 of 14 patients repaired conventionally and 13 of 14 repaired laparoscopically. Recurrent pain developed after one laparoscopic and one open repair each. Despite the apparent earlier resumption of full physical activity after laparoscopic repair, it should be noted that the role of laparoscopic repair in this setting remains controversial. Indeed, a potentially higher failure rate and need for operative reintervention in some of these athletes has been observed anecdotally by some groups [32].

Rehabilitation

Postoperative rehabilitation plays an important role in return to athletics after repair regardless of the surgical approach. Our group has described a stepwise series of activities and exercises (Table 26.2) to assist athletes and athletic trainers in guiding return to elite level athletic competition with applicability to a variety of sports [26]. A focus both on core abdominal strengthening and stabilization as well as lower body strength, flexibility, and balance with special attention to any associated adductor conditions is, we believe, essential to a successful outcome. The value of the rehab protocol was assessed by survey of ten therapists and athletic trainers who treated 21 athletes after surgery and the usefulness of the protocol in guiding therapy was rated highly (mean score 4.5 ± 0.7). Although originally developed with a focus on ice hockey, the protocol was felt to be appropriate for a variety of sports and was not overly sport specific (mean score 4.3 ± 0.7). The timetable for rehab activities and return to sport was rated 2.9 ± 0.9 (scale 1, too slow; 3, just right; 5, too fast).

The rehab protocol we have utilized was developed because of the absence of any such published guidelines when we initially began treating athletes with this problem. The protocol was structured as a series of stages for progression to full activity and a time frame for this progression and was developed to be generic enough for use in a variety of sports but also with some ice hockey-specific activities that reflected the primary population of athletes being treated. This protocol is given to the athlete early postoperatively to provide to their individual athletic trainer or physical therapist.

Other groups [24, 38] have outlined a schedule for return to sport following surgical repair but with less details than provided in our protocol. Muschawek [35] has utilized an accelerated path for return to sport in athletes undergoing the minimal repair technique. Patients are allowed to lift up to 20 kg for the first 14 days after surgery. Biking and running may be resumed as soon as the athlete is pain free and activity can be increased after the first 8 days as tolerated. This approach resulted in return to sport activity in 83% of athletes. These findings make the case for a more rapid and flexible timeline for increased activity in this population of patients that is based on symptoms and comfort level rather than a rigid time-based sequence, especially for athletes who have surgery in season, in order to minimize the number of training sessions and games missed.

Summary

In summary, groin injuries are a significant problem in athletes. A multidisciplinary team approach to evaluation and management involving the athletic trainer, orthopedist, physical therapist, and general surgeon is key to accurate diagnosis, treatment, and selection of patients for surgical intervention. Surgeons who evaluate athletes for "athletic hernia" must develop an understanding of the clinical presentation and diagnostic evaluation of related groin injuries. Surgical repair, coupled with a structured rehabilitation program that focuses on balancing strength and flexibility in the lower abdominal and thigh muscles, should allow return to competitive play within several weeks in appropriately selected athletes.

References

1. Renstrom P, Peterson L. Groin injuries in athletes. Br J Sports Med. 1980;14:30–6.
2. Ekstrand J, Hilding J. The incidence and differential diagnosis of acute groin injuries in male soccer players. Scand J Med Sci Sports. 1999;9:98–103.
3. Smodlaka VN. Groin pain in soccer players. Phys Sportsmed. 1980;8:57–61.
4. Pettersson R, Lorenzton R. Ice hockey injuries: a 4 year prosepctive study of a Swedish elite ice hockey team. Br J Sports Med. 1993;27:251–4.
5. Stuart MJ, Smith A. Injuries in Junior A ice hockey: a 3 year prospective study. Am J Sports Med. 1995;23:458–61.
6. Lorentzen R, Wedren H, Pietila T. Incidences, nature, and causes of ice hockey injuries: a three year prospective study of a Swedish elite ice hockey team. Am J Sports Med. 1988;16:392–6.
7. Molsa J, Airaksinen O, Nasman O, et al. Ice hockey injuries in Finland: a prospective epidemiologic study. Clin J Sport Med. 1997;9:151–6.
8. Emery CA, Meeuwisse WH, Powell J. Groin and abdominal injuries in the National Hockey League. Clin J Sport Med. 1999;9:151–6.
9. Emery CA, Meeuwisse WH. Risk factors for groin injuries in hockey. Med Sci Sports Exerc. 2001;33:1423–33.
10. Tyler TF, Nicholas SJ, Campbell RJ, McHugh MP. The association of hip strength and flexibility with the incidence of adductor muscle strains in professional ice hockey players. Am J Sports Med. 2001;29:124–8.
11. Lacroix VJ. A complete approach to groin pain. Phys Sportsmed. 2000;28:66–86.
12. Anderson K, Strickland AM, Warren R. Hip and groin injuries in athletes. Am J Sports Med. 2001;29:521–33.
13. Swan KGJ, Wolcott M. The athletic hernia. Clin Orthop Relat Res. 2006;455:78–87.
14. Nam A, Brody F. Management and therapy for sports hernia. J Am Coll Surg. 2008;206:154–64.
15. Caudill P, Nyland J, Smith C, Yerasimides J, Lach J. Sports hernias: a systematic literature review. Br J Sports Med. 2008;42(12):954–64.
16. Fricker PA, Taunton JE, Ammann W. Osteitis pubis in athletes: infection, inflammation, or injury. Sports Med. 1991;12:266–79.
17. Schlegel TF, Bushnell BD, Godfrey J, Boublik M. Success of non-operative management of adductor longus tendon ruptures in National Football League athletes. Am J Sports Med. 2009;37:1394–9.
18. Ekstrand J, Ringbog S. Surgery versus conservative treatment in soccer players with chronic groin pain: a prospective, randomized study in soccer players. Eur J Sports Traumatol Relat Res. 2001;23:141–5.
19. Meyers W, Foley D, Garrett W, Lohnes J, Mandelbaum B. Management of severe lower abdominal or inguinal pain in high-performance athletes. Am J Sports Med. 2000;28:2–8.
20. Hemingway AE, Herrington L, Blower AL. Changes in muscle strength and pain in response to surgical repair of posterior abdominal wall disruption followed by rehabilitation. Br J Sports Med. 2003;37:54–8.
21. Steele P, Annear P, Grove JR. Surgery for posterior inguinal wall deficiency in athletes. J Sci Med Sport. 2004;7:415–21.
22. Gilmore OJA. Gilmore's groin: ten years experience of groin disruption—a previously unsolved problem in sportsmen. Sports Med Soft Tissue Trauma. 1991;3:12–4.
23. Gilmore OJA. Gilmore's groin. Sports Med Soft Tissue Trauma. 1992;3:3.
24. Irshad K, Feldman L, Lavoie C, Lacroix V, Mulder D, Brown R. Operative management of "hockey groin syndrome": 12 years experience in National Hockey League players. Surgery. 2001;130:759–66.
25. Meyers WC, McKechnie A, Philippon MJ, Horner MA, Zoga AC, Devon ON. Experience with "sports hernia" spanning two decades. Ann Surg. 2008;248:656–65.
26. Brunt LM, Quasebarth MA, Bradshaw J, Barile R. Outcomes of a standardized approach to surgical repair and postoperative rehabilitation of athletic hernia. AOSSM Annual Meeting 2007: Calgary.
27. Zoga AC, Kavanagh EC, Meyers WC, et al. MRI findings in athletic pubalgia and the "sports hernia". Radiology. 2008;247:797–807.
28. Omar IM, Zoga A, Kavanagh EC, et al. Athletic pubalgia and "sports hernia": optimal MR imaging technique and findings. Radiographics. 2008;28:1415–38.
29. Orchard JW, Read JW, Neophyton J, Garlick D. Groin pain associated with ultrasound finding of inguinal canal posterior wall deficiency in Australian Rules footballers. Br J Sports Med. 1998;32:134–9.
30. Muschawek U, Berger L. Minimal repair technique of sportsmen's groin: an innovative open-suture repair to treat chronic groin pain. Hernia. 2010;14:27–33.
31. Meyers WC, Greenleaf R, Saad A. Anatomic basis for evaluation of abdominal and groin pain in athletes. Oper Tech Sports Med. 2005;13:55–61.
32. Meyers WC, Yoo E, Devon ON, et al. Understanding "sports hernia" (athletic pubalgia): The anatomic and pathophysiologic basis for abdominal and groin pain in athletes. Oper Tech Sports Med. 2007;15:165–77.

33. Biedert RM, Warnke K, Meyer S. Symphysis syndrome in athletes: surgical treatment for chronic lower abdominal, groin, and adductor pain in athletes. Clin J Sport Med. 2003;13:278–84.

34. Farber AJ, Wilckens JH. Sports hernia: diagnosis and therapeutic approach. J Am Acad Orthop Surg. 2007;15:507–14.

35. Muschawek U, Berger LM. Sportsmen's groin—diagnostic approach and treatment with the minimal repair technique. Sports Health. 2010;2:216–21.

36. Brown R, Mascia A, Kinnear DG, Lacroix VJ, Feldman L, Mulder DS. An 18 year review of sports groin injuries in the elite hockey player: clinical presentation, new diagnostic imaging, treatment, and results. Clin J Sport Med. 2008;2008:221–6.

37. Paajanen H, Syvahuoko I, Airo I. Totally extreparitoneal endoscopic (TEP) treatment of sportsman's hernia. Surg Laparosc Endosc Percutan Tech. 2004;14:215–8.

38. van Veen RN, de Baat P, Heijboer MP, et al. Successful endoscopic treatment of chronic groin pain in athletes. Surg Endosc. 2007;21:189–93.

39. Ziprin P, Prabhudesai SG, Abrahams S, Chadwick SJ. Transabdominal preperitoneal laparoscopic approach for the treatment of sportsman's hernia. J Laparoendosc Adv Surg Tech A. 2008;18:669–72.

40. Ingoldby C. Laparoscopic and conventional repair of groin disruption in sportsmen. Br J Surg. 1997;84:213–5.

41. Polglase AL, Frydman GM, Farmer KC. Inguinal surgery for debilitating chronic groin pain in athletes. Med J Aust. 1991;155:674–7.

42. Joesting DR. Diagnosis and treatment of sportsman's hernia. Curr Sports Med Rep. 2002;1:121–4.

43. Evans DS. Laparoscopic transabdominal pre-peritoneal (TAPP) repair for groin hernia: one surgeon's experience of a developing technique. Ann R Coll Surg Engl. 2002;84:393–8.

Index

Printed by Printforce, the Netherlands